Paul Glaser

PRINCIPLES OF RADIOGRAPHIC IMAGING

AN ART AND A SCIENCE

3RD EDITION

Richard R. Carlton, M.S., R.T.(R)(CV), FAERS
Assistant Professor of Radiologic Sciences
Arkansas State University
State University, AR

Arlene M. Adler, M.Ed., R.T.(R), FAERS
Professor and Director, Radiologic Sciences Programs
Indiana University Northwest
Gary, Indiana

Contributors
Barry Burns, Joseph R. Bittengle, Donna C. Davis, Eugene D. Frank,
Mary Ann Hovis, Bernadette M. Kaufman, Barbara J. Smith

DELMAR

™

THOMSON LEARNING

Africa • Australia • Canada • Denmark • Japan • Mexico • New Zealand • Philippines
Puerto Rico • Singapore • Spain • United Kingdom • United States

NOTICE TO THE READER

Delmar Staff

Health Care Publishing Director: William Brottmiller
Executive Editor: Cathy L. Esperti
Acquisitions Editor: Candice Janco
Developmental Editor: Marjorie A. Bruce
Editorial Assistant: Brian R. Haines
Executive Marketing Manager: Dawn Gerrain

Channel Manager: Tara Carter
Marketing Coordinator: Penelope Cartwright
Executive Production Manager: Karen Leet
Project Editor: Patricia Gillivan
Production Editor: Richard D. Killar
Technology Project Manager: Laurie Davis

COPYRIGHT © 2001
Delmar is a division of Thomson Learning. The Thomson Learning logo is a registered trademark used herein under license.

Printed in the United States of America
6 7 8 9 10 XXX 05 04 03

For more information, contact Delmar, 3 Columbia Circle, PO Box 15015, Albany, NY 12212-0515; or find us on the World Wide Web at http://www.delmar.com

Asia:
Thomson Learning
60 Albert Street, #15-01
Albert Complex
Singapore 189969
Tel: 65 336 6411
Fax: 65 336 7411

Japan:
Thomson Learning
Palaceside Building 5F
I - I - I Hitotsubashi, Chiyoda-ku
Tokyo 100 0003 Japan
Tel: 813 5218 6544
Fax: 813 5218 6551

Australia/New Zealand:
Nelson/Thomson Learning
102 Dodds Street
South Melbourne, Victoria 3205
Australia
Tel: 61 39685 4111
Fax: 61 39 685 4199

UK/Europe/Middle East
Thomson Learning
Berkshire House
168-173 High Holborn
London
WC IV 7AA United Kingdom
Tel: 44 171497 1422
Fax: 44 171497 1426

Thomas Nelson & Sons LTD
Nelson House
Mayfield Road
Walton-on-Thames
KT 12 5PL United Kingdom
Tel: 44 1932 2522111
Fax: 44 1932 246574

Latin America:
Thomson Learning
Seneca, 53
Colonia Polanco
11560 Mexico D.F. Mexico
Tel: 525-281-2906
Fax: 525-281-2656

Canada:
Nelson/Thomson Learning
1120 Birchmount Road
Scarborough, Ontario
Canada MlK 5G4
Tel: 416-752-9100
Fax: 416-752-8102

Spain:
Thomson Learning
Calle Magallanes, 25
28015-Madrid
España
Tel: 34 91446 33 50
Fax: 34 91445 62 18

International Headquarters:
Thomson Learning
International Division
290 Harbor Drive, 2nd Floor
Stamford, CT 06902-7477
Tel: 203-969-8700
Fax: 203-969-8751

Library of Congress Cataloging-in-Publication Data

Carlton, Richard R.
    Principles of radiographic imaging: an art and a science/
Richard R. Carlton, Arlene M. Adler. --3rd ed.
      p. cm.
    Includes bibliographical references and index.
    ISBN 0–7668–1300–2
    1. Radiography, Medical. I. Adler, Arlene Mckenna. II. Title.
RC78 . C34 2000
616.07'572--dc21
                                    00–043193

DEDICATION

CONTRIBUTORS

Joseph R. Bittengle, M.Ed., R.T.(R)
Chairman and Assistant Professor
Department of Radiologic Technology
College of Health Related Professions
University of Arkansas for Medical Sciences
Little Rock, Arkansas

Barry Burns, M.S., R.T.(R), DABR
School of Medicine
Division of Radiologic Science
University of North Carolina
Chapel Hill, North Carolina

Donna C. Davis, M.Ed., R.T.(R)(CV)
Instructor
Department of Radiologic Technology
University of Arkansas for Medical Sciences
Little Rock, Arkansas

Mary Ann Hovis
Associate Professor
Engineering Technologies
Lima Technical College
Lima, Ohio

Bernadette M. Kaufman, R.T.(R)(MR)
ISMRM SMRT Education Committee
Milwaukee, Wisconsin

Eugene D. Frank, M.A., R.T.(R), FASRT
Assistant Professor of Radiology
Mayo Clinic/Foundation
Rochester, Minnesota

Barbara J. Smith, B.S,. R.T.(R)(QM)
Portland Community College
Radiological Sciences
Portland, Oregon

THE FOUNDERS OF RADIOGRAPHY

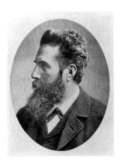

WILHELM CONRAD RÖNTGEN (1845 – 1923)

Wilhelm Conrad Röntgen became the first radiographer when he discovered x-rays on November 8, 1895, in his laboratory at the University of Würzburg in Germany. His original paper *On a New Kind of Rays* is printed in Appendix A. For his discovery he received the first Nobel prize in physics in 1901 and was decorated by Prussia, Bavaria, Great Britain, Austria, Mexico, Germany, France, the Netherlands, Sweden, Italy, Turkey, and the United States.

(Portrait courtesy of the Historical Collections of the Library, College of Physicians of Philadelphia.)

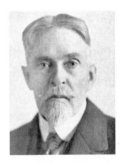

EDDY CLIFFORD JERMAN (1865 – 1936)

Ed. C. Jerman is known as "The Father of Radiography" in the United States because he was the first teacher of radiography. He began teaching x-ray techniques in 1897, he founded the American Association of Radiological Technicians (now known as the American Society of Radiologic Technologists), and personally examined the first 1,000 members of the American Registry of X-Ray Technicians. He brought order to the principles of radiographic exposure technique by naming the qualities of the radiographic image: density, contrast, detail and distortion. In 1928 he published *Modern X-Ray Technic*, the first book on radiographic principles.

(Portrait courtesy of the American Society of Radiologic Technologists.)

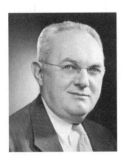

ARTHUR WOLFRAM FUCHS (1895 – 1962)

Arthur W. Fuchs is known as the inventor of the fixed kilovoltage technique of radiography. His father, Wolfram Fuchs, established the first x-ray laboratory in Chicago in 1896 but became one of the early martyrs to radiation, dying from excessive exposure. Arthur performed radiography for the United States Army in both World Wars I and II. During World War II he wrote the U.S. Army training manual, *Principles of Radiographic Exposure*, in which he outlined his success with the optimal fixed kVp technique system. In 1955 he first published his book, *Principles of Radiographic Exposure and Processing*.

(Portrait courtesy of the family of Arthur Fuchs.)

Contents

List of Tables

Foreword

"State-of-the-art" is the best term I can think of to describe this textbook. It is an excellent book written by radiographers for radiographers. This book truly reflects what radiographers should be learning in their educational process. Ms. Adler and Mr. Carlton have done a superb job of not only explaining what occurs in radiography but also how it occurs and why it occurs. The art of radiography has come a long way in 100 years and this book was written to educate radiographers for the 21st century.

When I reviewed the table of contents for this book, I immediately became intrigued by the titles of the units into which this book is divided. Upon reviewing these units I found that they live up to the promise of the table of contents. The authors have used a new approach in teaching information that is needed by radiographers.

Throughout the book the student is encouraged to use critical thinking skills in solving problems presented by their professional practice. The student is encouraged to make independent decisions and the authors have shown ways to support the decision-making process. Not only is the radiographer given "the rules" in this book, but in many cases the authors also discuss the exceptions to the rules. The authors have emphasized the responsibility of a radiographer as that of creating and analyzing the quality of an image, while the responsibility of the radiologist is to make a diagnosis from the image. Each of these professionals working together comprises the profession of radiology.

The method that has been used to write the book is educationally sound. Each of the 45 chapters has an outline, objectives, a summary, a set of review questions, and a very detailed bibliography for further reference material. Additionally, a large number of illustrations have been used in the book to further explain the content.

Ms. Adler and Mr. Carlton are to be commended for the depth of the subject matter they have incorporated into this textbook and for the clear, concise manner in which it is presented. *Principles of Radiographic Imaging* is an insightful contribution to the profession of radiologic technology and fortunate is the student who has this book from which to learn.

Marilyn Holland, B.S., R.T. (R)
Director of Radiologic Technology Education
The University of Iowa Hospitals and Clinics
Iowa City, Iowa

Preface

Introduction

As radiography educators, we designed this textbook with students and educators in mind: each chapter contains an outline, objectives, a summary, review questions, and a detailed bibliography. Although the order of the chapters is based on our experiences in teaching our students, most chapters stand alone and can be used in the order which is most appropriate within a given program.

We have made a special effort to represent our belief that professional development should be a prime objective of any radiography curriculum. This is best achieved through the demonstration of technical competence. This book is designed to assist students in developing this cornerstone of professionalism. Through technical competence and a professional demeanor students will be ready to assume their role as experts in the radiographic imaging process. In addition, we believe that true professionals take immense pride in their work to the extent that it becomes an art as well as a science.

References used extensively to assure both educator and students that we address all content expected for successful professional practice include the American Registry of Radiographic Technologists' *Content Specifications for the Examination in Radiography*, the *Curriculum Guide for Radiography Programs* by the American Society of Radiologic Technologists, and the *Curriculum Guide for Radiography* prepared by the Council on Education, Radiography, of the Canadian Association of Medical Radiation Technologists.

Content

A special attempt was made to provide an introduction to physics and the imaging modalities, as well as exploring the details of the principles of radiographic exposure techniques. The overall design of the book separates the 45 chapters into six units: Creating the Beam, Protecting Patients and Personnel, Creating the Image, Analyzing the Image, Comparing Exposure Systems, and Special Imaging Systems. This design helps organize the content for students by following a logical progression from introductory physics through the production and control of the beam to advanced modality systems.

New to This Edition

The rapid changes in technology present a challenge to textbook authors who are committed to providing current information for learners. The authors and contributors to the third edition carefully reviewed all content to identify areas requiring updating or new topics. As a result, numerous changes were made. The more significant changes are as follows:

- New Chapter 43 on digital radiography, including descriptions of current image receptor and detector systems, limitations of each currently available digital radiography system, process of acquiring the digital radiography histogram and applying the display algorithm to the collected data, image quality issues, image acquisitions elements, DICOM-3 standard, and digital radiography artifacts

- Discussion of the latest research on subnuclear structures (M theory, including string theory)

- Content on high voltage shock hazard

- Nuclear Regulatory Commission revised radiation protection standards (revised 10CFR20 regulations)

- New data and recommendations on embryo/fetus exposure (NCRP Reports 116 and 128 and Commentary 9)

- Daylight, laser, and dry film imaging systems

- "Darkroom disease" issues (including OSHA, ANSI, and ASHRAE ventilation recommendations)

- Vascular, mammography, and MRI instrumentation chapters were updated by quality experts to reflect current technology

Elements of the Third Edition

In addition to the updated and new content, this new edition continues to feature the following learning aids and critical content:

- Physical concepts are clearly explained and illustrated with many high-quality figures

- Effects of changing parameters on image quality are carefully described and illustrated with numerous images

- Criteria for image analysis are presented to help learners develop analytical skills

- High-quality radiographs are included throughout the text

- Radiation protection concepts and procedures are emphasized for both patients and radiographic personnel

- Chapter end summaries provide a quick reference to critical concepts and developments in the science of radiography

- Numerous troubleshooting tips are included to ensure quality radiographs

- Extensive references and recommended readings provide a historical perspective and provide learners a means to expand their understanding of concepts and systems

- Epigraphs and historical photos help trace the evolution of radiography to the present

- Unique emphasis on the art versus the science of radiography illustrates the broad applications of the technology

Statement of Content Accuracy

Although we assume full responsibility for any errors, including those which may be construed as arising from quoting other works out of context, we have made every effort to ensure the accuracy of the information. However, appropriate information sources should be consulted, especially for new or unfamiliar procedures. It is the responsibility of every practitioner to evaluate the appropriateness of a particular procedure in the context of actual clinical situations. Therefore, neither the authors nor the publisher take responsibility or accept any liability for the actions of persons applying the information contained herein in an unprofessional manner. This information is designed to supplement and enhance the instructional methodologies of educators in JRCERT [Joint Review Committee on Education in Radiologic Technologies (USA)] and CAMRT (Canada) approved radiography programs and should not be applied, especially to human subjects, without this background. In committing this book to print we fully realize that it is never finished, merely suspended for the time being.

Finally, as a reader your perceptions are important to is. We encourage you to communicate with us regarding facets of the book you appreciate or would like to see changed. We especially appreciate constructive comments and notice of errors. Our intention is to present the principles of radiography in an interesting format that provides a base from which true professionalism can develop. Any commentary readers care to make towards this end will be valued and welcomed.

—Richard R. Carlton
   Arkansas State University
   Radiologic Sciences, Box 910
   104 Caraway Road
   State University, AR 72467
   1-870-761-1870, fax 870-972-2004
   rcarlton@crow.astate.edu

—Arlene M. Adler
   Indiana University Northwest
   3400 Broadway
   Gary, Indiana 46408
   1-219-980-6540, fax 1-219-980-6649
   aadler@iunhaw1.iun.indiana.edu

Acknowledgments

Third Edition

Marge Bruce has been the person most responsible for our getting this edition of the book out. We know we've been difficult at times (most especially Rick), and we cannot adequately express our appreciation for her personal drive to get us into print once again. Our families remain our primary sources of inspiration. Rick's extended family now includes another grandson, Michael. The students, faculty, and staff at Arkansas State University played a major role in the third edition. Special thanks is due Dean Susan Hanrahan, Ray Winters, Jeannean Rollins, Lyn Hubbard, Tracey White, and Deanna Harris for unremitting support and constant enthusiasm for what we are trying to accomplish in the radiologic sciences.

We thank the faculty and students who have found our work valuable in the process of radiography education and practice since the first edition was published. The success of this book and the invitation to produce a new edition are a direct result of the acceptance of our work by the radiography profession, which we gratefully acknowledge.

Our families once again deserve our thanks for their understanding. Don Adler and Lynn Carlton have both given countless hours that were rightfully theirs, for which we extend a peace offering of love. Arlene's family has grown by two, and appreciation goes to her daughters Meri and Katie (who now come first) as well as to Edyta for all her help. Rick's extended family now includes grandson Nathan, who gets his time, book or not.

We again gratefully acknowledge the role played in our success by Delmar in the person of David Gordon, Marion Waldman, Marjorie Bruce, Sarah Holle, Melissa Conan, and Mary Ellen Black, all of whom have become friends. Special appreciation is due to our art and design coordinator, Richard Killar.

We cannot overemphasize the contributions made to our work by Barry Burns of the University of North Carolina, who routinely went far beyond our wildest hopes in critiquing our text, producing films to illustrate his points, disproving old wives tales in his laboratory, and generously sharing his results (and venison) with us. Much more than a friend, Barry has become a backbone of the technical aspects of this book.

Eugene Frank of the Mayo Clinic/Foundation continued his persistent and knowledgeable critique of our efforts. We are grateful for Gene's unique contributions, especially his ability to never let nearly two decades of friendship come between us and a more accurate reworking of verbiage or the details of an illustration. Gene revised his chapter on mammography instrumentation, which adds immeasurably to the depth of this work.

We also appreciate the willingness of Donna Davis and Joe Bittengle of the University of Arkansas for Medical Sciences to revise their chapter that succinctly summarizes their expertise in vascular instrumentation. The depth of their knowledge in this specialty is an important contribution to this work.

Once again, we have been assisted in our work by a wide spectrum of colleagues in the radiologic sciences and related fields. In addition to those who assisted us during the first edition, we wish to add Irven Rule of the Siemens Training and Development Center in Cary, North Carolina; Alfred Hufnagl of the Northern Alberta Institute of Technology, Canada; Penelope Roberts of the Department of Medical Physics and Medical Engineering at Southampton University Hospitals, UK; Kathheryn Root of Holyoke Community College, Massachusetts; Dr. Appel and Kevin Sisak at DuPont; Garry Harris at Agfa; and Gregory Wheeler of Wheeler and Associates, San Francisco, California.

Our ability to devote the countless hours necessary to make this book what it has become is in great part due to the support we have received from our bosses, Robert Moon at Indiana University Northwest and Sam Bassitt at Lima Technical College. Our faculties have also made significant contributions through their consistent willingness to comment on the countless details we have explored with them over the years. Thank you Jody Ellis, Sandy Piehl, Laura Richards, Marie Ross, Debra Sobota, Andy Shappell, and Deb Scroggins. Special thanks goes to Barb Hanna and Wil Reddinger who provided us with their expertise in verifying laboratory results, producing new images, and refining our clumsy attempts to illustrate many concepts. Allen Lindmark from the Department of Chemistry at Indiana University Northwest also needs our thanks for his review of our basic explanations of chemistry concepts.

And finally, we thank those fellow educators who have taken the time to sit down with us at meetings, write letters, make phone calls, compose email, and fax their comments and suggestions to us. Although we are certain we have not remembered all of you (for which we apologize), these include John Clouse of Owensboro Community College, Kentucky; Marianne Tortorici and Mike Mixdorf at the University of Nevada, Las Vegas; Bob Misiak, Orange County Community College, New York; Jack Thomas at Lakeland Community College, Ohio; Lisa Iacovelli at Crozer-Chester Medical Center, Pennsylvania; Max Grady at Kettering College of Medical Arts, Ohio; Donna Mitchell at John Peter Smith Hospital, Texas; Anita Slechta of California State University at Northridge; Elwin Tilson of Armstrong State College, Georgia; Shay Mercer at New Mexico State University; Judy Williams of Grady Memorial Hospital, Georgia; Marilyn Sinderbrand of Northern Virginia Community College; Bill Sykes of Shawnee State University, Ohio; Bart Schraa of Daniel Denhoed University, Rotterdam, Netherlands; Frank Porter at St. Vincent Infirmary Medical Center, Arkansas; Mitchell Bieber, University of Virginia Medical Center; Donna Foster at Northern New Mexico Community College; Bill May of Iatwamba Community College, Mississippi; Lorraine Henry of Orange Coast Community College, California; And Steve Dowd of the University of Alabama at Birmingham.

Appreciation is also expressed to the colleagues who reviewed the manuscripts for this edition. Their critical reviews helped to guide us in the preparation of the final manuscript.

Paul William Bober, EdD, RT(R). Radiology Department, Labette Community College, Parsons, KS

Barry Burns, MS, RT(R), DABR. School of Medicine, Division of Radiologic Science, University of North Carolina, Chapel Hill, NC

Pamela A. Intlekofer, RT(R)(MR). MRI Program, Greenville Technical College, Greenville, SC

Linda Lingar, MEd, RT(R)(M). College of Health Related Professions, University of Arkansas for Medical Sciences, Little Rock, AR

Linda S. Pressley, MS, RT(R). Health Career Programs, Sanford-Brown College, St. Louis, MO

Andrew Shappell, BS, RT(R)(MR)(CT). Medical Imaging Technology Department, Lima Technical College, Lima, OH

Edwin P. Viglia, Jr., RT(R). Radiography Program, Kankakee Community College, Kankakee, IL

Jeffrey J. Walmsley, MEd, RT(R)(QM). Lorain County Community College, Elyria, OH

First Edition Acknowledgments

The production of this book would not have been possible without the support of our spouses, Don and Lynn. In addition, we gratefully acknowledge the role played by Delmar Publishers in the person of Dave Prout, John Lent, Marion Waldman, and Leslie Boyer; Indiana University Northwest; Lima Technical College; and St. Rita's Medical Center of Lima, Ohio. Special thanks are due Dr. LaVerne Ramaeker, Sam Bassitt, Marlene Ledbetter, and Dennis Spragg for their continued support. A major contribution to the accuracy of the information and illustrations was made by the consistent presence of Eugene Frank, of the Mayo Clinic Foundation, throughout.

We are in the professional debt of many who inspired us, taught us, and collaborated with us throughout the years. Much of what is contained in this work is a direct result of these efforts. Those to whom we are especially indebted are Tracy Ahdel, Janice Akin, Judy Baron, Karen Brinkman, John Cortez, Marion Frank, Mick Jagger, Karen Jefferies, Robin Jones, Dr. George Koptik, Judy Koptik, Jon Lilly, Dr. Marzuto, Kathy Miller, Joe Mosqueda, Traci O'Donnell, LaVerne Ramaeker, Karen Schmidl, Kay Shriver, Tracy Thegze, Jean Widger, Rob Wilcoxen, and Sue Wilson. And of course our students at Indiana University Northwest, Lima Technical College, Wilbur Wright College, Malcolm X College, and Michael Reese Hospital and Medical Center.

Like our colleagues and students, we owe much to the institutions that contributed to out professional expertise. We wish to thank Indiana University Northwest, Lima Technical College, Michael Reese Hospital and Medical Center, Lutheran General Hospital, Mercy Hospital and Medical Center (Chicago), Northwestern Memorial Hospital (Chicago), Wilbur Wright College, Illinois Central College, Carl Sandburg College, Evanston Hospital, Methodist Medical Center (Peoria), and Community Memorial Hospital (Monmouth).

We owe special thanks to many people for sharing their personal expertise and material collections. One of the highest forms of professionalism, the willingness of radiologic technologists to freely give of their time and knowledge, was demonstrated again and again by everyone from whom we requested assistance in our compilation of the multitude of photographs, drawings, radiographs, and other illustrative materials in the text and those who assisted in the numerous reviews of our writing. Among these deserving special thanks are Gene Frank and Norlin Winkler of the Mayo Clinic Foundation and Ray Rossi of the University of Colorado for their commentary and technical assistance above and beyond the normal bonds of friendship; Philip W. Ballinger of the Ohio State University; Terry West of Toronto, Secretary-General of the International Society of Radiographers and Radiological Technicians; Stewart Bushong of Baylor College of Medicine; Terry Eastman of Dallas; Joe Fodor of the University of Cincinnati Medical Center; Nina Kowalczyk of Riverside Methodist Hospital, Columbus, Ohio; Denise Moore of Sinclair Community College, Dayton, Ohio; Bruce Long of Indiana University Medical Center; Marilyn Holland of the University of Iowa Hospitals and Clinics; Charles R. Griffith of FGHB Certified Radiation Physicists; Loren Garlets of Hays State University, Kansas; Pat Sharp of Gannon University, Erie, Pennsylvania; Tim Penning of Athens Regional Medical Center, Georgia; Seymour Sterling, FASRT, of Yardley, Pennsylvania; Jerome Taubel of the Mayo Clinic Foundation, Rochester, Minnesota; Bob Kobistek in Cleveland and Martin Ratner and Steve Szeglin in Carle Place, New York, both of Victoreen, Inc./Nuclear Associates; Terry Hanby of DuPont; Robert Trinkle, formerly of DuPont; Mike Wilsey of Agfa Matrix; Robert Lockery and Walter Weigl of Siemens Corporation; Robert Busic of General Electric Medical Systems; William Conklin of Orangeburg, SC; Rene Abgrall of Thoard, France; Toshinori Komba of Komazawa University, Tokyo, Japan; Angela Pickwick of Montgomery County Community College, Maryland; Jerry Conlogue of Gulf Coast Community College, Florida; Barb Imber of St. Rita's Medical Center, Lima, Ohio; Rick Halker of Lima Memorial Hospital, Ohio; The Radiology Department of Van Wert County Hospital, Van Wert, Ohio, John Stone of Emory University Medical School, Atlanta; Tom Beery and Will Wells of Lima Technical College; Judy Shaw of Lima Technical College; Doug Raver and Chris Innskeep of Lima Technical College for video and software graphics; and Jan Krietemeyer of Lima, Ohio for bibliographic research.

UNIT I

Creating the Beam

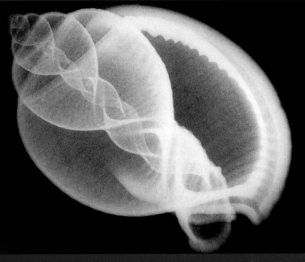

*A*n inherent quality of a professional is the possession of expertise regarding the technical aspects of a field far above that of a nonprofessional. Knowledge of the principles of radiographic image production is part of the technical expertise of the professional radiographer. Radiography programs provide students with classroom instruction, laboratory experience, and clinical practice in this subject. No other medical professional experiences as intensive or comprehensive a study of radiographic imaging. This unit is designed to provide the basics necessary for this knowledge by building a framework of information regarding the creation of the diagnostic X-ray beam.

The framework begins with an elementary review of **basic mathematics** and **radiation concepts**, including atomic theory, X-ray properties, and necessary units of measurement. Although this may be a review of previous science course work for many readers, it is important to make sure everyone is on the same wavelength before using the information in the remainder of the book. **Electricity** and **electromagnetism** are large chapters that lay the foundation for understanding how to control the beam. **X-ray equipment**, the **X-ray tube**, and **X-ray production** provide an understanding of exactly how basic physics is used to create the X-ray beam.

CHAPTER 1

Basic Mathematics

Mary Ann Hovis

*In the beginning
there were polynomials*

*differences of squares
trial and error*

*and the sum of two cubes.
X^2 minus Y^2*

*has always had
the same meaning*

John Stone, "Helping with the Math Homework."

Objectives

Upon completion of this chapter, the student should be able to:

▶ Perform functions with fractions and decimals.

▶ Determine significant digits in a number.

▶ Perform calculations in scientific notation with signed numbers and exponents.

▶ Simplify algebraic expressions.

▶ Convert units within the SI system.

*M*athematics is the language of science. Radiographers need to be able to speak this language. This math review is intended to refresh essential skills in this area.

Arithmetic

Fractions

Addition and Subtraction
To add or subtract two fractions with **like** denominators, add or subtract the numerators and keep the like denominator.

Examples:

$$\frac{3}{8} + \frac{2}{8} = \frac{5}{8}$$

$$\frac{7}{8} - \frac{4}{8} = \frac{3}{8}$$

$$\frac{a}{b} + \frac{c}{b} = \frac{a+c}{b}$$

$$\frac{a}{b} - \frac{c}{b} = \frac{a-c}{b}$$

To add or subtract two fractions with **unlike** denominators, rewrite each fraction with a like or common denominator. Then add or subtract the numerators and keep the like or common denominator.

Examples:

$$\frac{1}{4} + \frac{5}{6} = \frac{3}{12} + \frac{10}{12} = \frac{13}{12}$$

$$\frac{7}{5} - \frac{1}{3} = \frac{21}{15} - \frac{5}{15} = \frac{16}{15}$$

$$\frac{a}{b} + \frac{c}{d} = \frac{ad}{bd} + \frac{bc}{bd} = \frac{ad+bc}{bd}$$

$$\frac{a}{b} - \frac{c}{d} = \frac{ad}{bd} - \frac{bc}{bd} = \frac{ad-bc}{bd}$$

Multiplication
Multiplication can be written in several ways (Table 1–1). To multiply two fractions, multiply the numerators and multiply the denominators.

TABLE 1–1. Multiplication Notation

Throughout this review the algebraic notation for multiplication will be used.

EXAMPLE: 3×4 will be written as $3 \cdot 4$.

A $\cdot$ (dot) is used as a symbol for multiplication.

EXAMPLE: $a \times b$ will be written as $a \cdot b$ or as ab.

When two letters are used the dot is usually omitted.

EXAMPLE: $3 \times a$ will be written as $3a$ or as $3 \cdot a$.

Parentheses can also be used to represent multiplication.

EXAMPLE: 3×4 can be written as $(3)(4)$.

Examples:

$$\frac{2}{5} \times \frac{3}{7} = \frac{2 \times 3}{5 \times 7} = \frac{6}{35}$$

$$\frac{a}{b} \times \frac{c}{d} = \frac{a \times c}{b \times d}$$

Division
To divide two fractions, rewrite the division problem as a multiplication problem by multiplying the first fraction by the second fraction inverted.

Examples:

$$\frac{2}{5} \div \frac{3}{7} = \frac{2}{5} \times \frac{7}{3} = \frac{2 \times 7}{5 \times 3} = \frac{14}{15}$$

$$\frac{a}{b} \div \frac{c}{d} = \frac{a}{b} \times \frac{d}{c} = \frac{a \times d}{b \times c}$$

Decimals

Decimal number place value (columns) is determined as shown in Figure 1–1.

Addition and Subtraction
To add or subtract two decimal numbers, line up the decimal points in each number, adding or subtracting as with whole numbers. Remember to add in zeros to fill out the decimal posi-

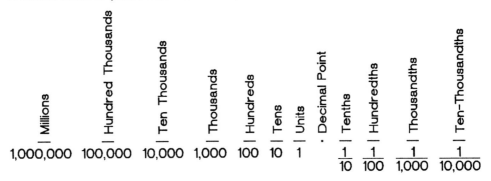

FIGURE 1 – 1. Decimal number place values.

tions if necessary. The decimal point must remain in the same position.

Examples:

Add:	Subtract:	Rewrite as:
76.81	76.1	76.10
+384.1	–2.96	–2.96
460.91		73.14

Multiplication
To multiply two decimal numbers, multiply the numbers as if they were whole numbers. Place the decimal point in the product so the number of places in the product equals the sum of the number of decimal places in each number.

Example:

Multiply:

```
    2.31        2 decimal positions
  ×  6.8        1 decimal position
   1848
   1386
  15.708        3 decimal positions
```

Division
To divide two decimal numbers, set up as if doing whole number division. Move the decimal point in the divisor to the right to make the divisor a whole number. Move the decimal point in the dividend the same number of places to the right (as was done for the divisor). Add zeros if necessary to maintain the position of the decimal. Divide the numbers as if they were whole numbers. Place the decimal point in the quotient directly above the decimal point in the dividend. Add zeros if necessary to maintain the position of the decimal.

Examples:

$$.25\overline{\smash{\big)}1250}$$

$$25.\overline{\smash{\big)}125000.}\quad\overset{5000.}{}$$

$$1.3\overline{\smash{\big)}733.2}$$

```
        564.
  13. /7332.
        65
        83
        78
        52
        52
         0
```

Convert a Fraction into a Decimal Number
To convert a fraction into a decimal, divide the denominator into the numerator.

Example: Convert 7/8 into a decimal:

```
        .875
   8 /7.000
        64
        60
        56
        40
        40
```

Convert a Percent to a Decimal
To convert a percent to a decimal move the decimal point two places to the left.

Example: Convert 78.5% to a decimal:
78.5% = .785

Convert a Decimal to a Percent
To convert a decimal to a percent move the decimal point two places to the right.

Example: Change .452 to a %
.452 = 45.2%

Computation with Values (Numbers)

Exact
Some numbers are exact values, like the counting numbers (1,2,3, . . .). For example, there are exactly four legs on a chair. Exact numbers in computations are as accurate or as precise as needed.

Significant Digits
Some values are obtained by measurement and are only as accurate as the measuring device. The last digit in the reading is usually estimated. **When dealing with these values in computations, the results will only be as accurate as the least accurate value.** This is the concept of significant digits.

To determine the number of significant digits in a value (number):

1. Count all nonzero digits.

2. Count all zeros between nonzero digits.

3. Count all zeros at the end of a decimal value.

The number of significant digits in a value is the sum of the numbers obtained in steps one, two and three.

Examples: The following are measured values from a radiation dose meter (dosimeter).
7.14 mR has three significant digits.
90.104 mR has five significant digits.
0.048 mR has two significant digits.
7300 mR has two significant digits.
6.900 mR has four significant digits.

Precision
The precision of a value refers to the decimal position of the last significant digit.

Example:
.0218 is precise to the ten-thousandths.

Rounding Off
To round a number the last digit to be retained is:

1. Left unchanged if the digit to the right of the last digit to be retained is less than 5.

2. Is increased by one if the digit to the right of the last digit to be retained is 5 or greater.

Examples
75.2581 rounded to 4 significant digits is 75.26.
6836.66 rounded to 2 significant digits is 6800.
0.0381 rounded to 2 significant digits is 0.038.
0.0299 rounded to 2 significant digits is 0.030.

Multiplication and Division of Approximate Values
When multiplying or dividing two or more approximate values, the number of significant digits in the final answer is no greater than the number of significant digits in the value with the least number of significant digits.

Example: Using the calculator, $(103.81) \bullet (1.34) =$ 139.1054. However, since 1.34 has only three significant digits, the answer should have only three significant digits. Therefore 139.1054 needs to be rounded to three significant digits, making it 139.

Addition and Subtraction of Approximate Values
When adding or subtracting two or more approximate values, the final answer should be no more precise than the **least** precise of the values.

Example: Add the following:

123.1
 89.123
103.3456
315.5686

Since the least precise number is 123.1, the answer should be rounded to 315.6.

Powers of Ten

The decimal system is based on powers of ten, as is the metric system. These are very important systems to the radiographer. When a^n is written, a is called the base and n is the exponent. Integers are defined as the numbers . . . $-3, -2, -1, 0, 1, 2, 3, \ldots$.

Positive Integer Exponents   Definition:

$$a^n = \underbrace{a \cdot a \cdot a \cdot\cdot\cdot a}_{n\,times}\ (multiply\ n\ times)$$

Examples:

$10^1 = 10$
$10^2 = 10 \cdot 10 = 100$
$10^3 = 10 \cdot 10 \cdot 10 = 1000$
$10^n = 10 \cdot 10 \cdot 10 \cdot\cdot\cdot 10 = 100\ldots0\,(n\ zeros)$

Negative Integer Exponents   Definition:

$$a^{-n} = \frac{1}{a^n}(for\ a \neq 0)$$

$$10^{-1} = \frac{1}{10} = .1$$

$$10^{-2} = \frac{1}{10^2} = .01$$

$$10^{-3} = \frac{1}{10^3} = .001$$

$$10^{-n} = \frac{1}{10^n} = .00\ldots001\,(n-1)\ zeros$$

Zero Exponents   Definition: $a^0 = 1\,(for\ a \neq 0)$

Example:
$10^0 = 1$

Scientific Notation

A number written in scientific notation is written as the product of a number between 1 (including 1) and 10 times a power of 10. In other words, $N \times 10^P$ where $1 \leq N < 10$ and p is an integer.

Examples:
7.15×10^4 is a number in scientific notation.
1.598×10^{-5} is a number in scientific notation.
7.58×10^0 is a number in scientific notation.

Converting Numbers from Ordinary to Scientific Notation   To write a number in scientific notation, the decimal point must be moved to the position following the first nonzero digit.

Examples:

$70.57 = 7.057 \times 10^1\,(p = 1)$
$.00815 = 8.15 \times 10^{-3}\,(p = -3)$
$7.58 = 7.58 \times 10^0\,(p = 0)$

In the first example, the decimal point is moved one digit to the left, making the power of ten (p), one. In the second example, the decimal point is moved three digits to the right, making the power of ten, negative three. In the third example, the decimal point is not moved and the power of ten is zero.

In general, when moving the decimal point to the left the power of ten will be the number of positions moved. When moving the decimal point to the right the power of ten will be negative the number of positions moved. When the decimal point is not moved, the power of ten will be zero.

Converting Numbers from Scientific to Ordinary Notation   To convert a number in scientific notation to ordinary notation, the decimal position is moved according to the following:

1. If the power of ten is positive move the decimal point to the right the number of positions in the exponent.

2. If the power of ten is negative move the decimal point to the left the number of positions in the exponent.

3. If the power of ten is zero the decimal remains in the same position.

In all of the above, once the decimal point has been moved, the ten and its power are dropped. Zeros are added if necessary.

Examples:

$3.7 \times 10^4 = 37,000$
$5.56 \times 10^{-5} = .0000556$
$1.34 \times 10^0 = 1.34$

Dimensional Analysis

The concept of dimensional analysis is very useful when converting from one set of units to another. The principle is based on fractions whose quotients are 1.

Example:

$$\frac{12 \text{ in}}{1 \text{ ft}} = 1 \text{ or } \frac{1 \text{ ft}}{12 \text{ in}} = 1$$

Recall that multiplying a quantity by 1 does not change the value of the quantity. In order to convert from one set of units to another, algebraic operations are performed with units in the same way they are with algebraic symbols.

Example: Convert 7.0 ft to inches.

$$7.0 \text{ ft} = 7.0 \text{ ft} \cdot \frac{12 \text{ in}}{1 \text{ ft}} = 7 \cdot 12 \text{ in} = 84 \text{ in}$$

Note that it is possible to "cancel" the feet unit, leaving the inches unit.

Convert 70.0 km/hr to m/s.

$$70.0\frac{\text{km}}{\text{hr}} =$$

$$70.0\frac{\text{km}}{\text{hr}} \cdot \frac{1000 \text{ m}}{1 \text{ km}} \cdot \frac{1 \text{ hr}}{60 \text{ min}} \cdot \frac{1 \text{ min}}{60 \text{ s}} =$$

$$70.0 \cdot 1000 \cdot \frac{1}{60} \cdot \frac{1 \text{ m}}{60 \text{ s}} = 19.4\frac{\text{m}}{\text{s}}$$

Recall that 1 km = 1000 m, 1 hr = 60 min, and 1 min = 60 s. Note that it is possible to "cancel" the km unit, the hr unit, and the min unit.

When converting cubic units or square units, extra attention needs to be given to the conversion factors. Study the following example carefully.

Example: Convert 3.8000 ft^3 (cubic feet) to cubic inches (in^3).

$$3.8000 \text{ ft}^3 = 3.8000 \text{ ft}^3 \cdot \frac{12 \text{ in}}{1 \text{ ft}} \cdot \frac{12 \text{ in}}{1 \text{ ft}} \cdot \frac{12 \text{ in}}{1 \text{ ft}}$$

$$= 6566.4 \text{ in}^3$$

or

$$3.8000 \text{ ft}^3 = 3.8000 \text{ ft}^3 \cdot \left(\frac{12 \text{ in}}{1 \text{ ft}}\right)^3 = 6566.4 \text{ in}^3$$

Example: Convert 10 roentgens per hour to roentgens per minute.

$$10.0\frac{\text{roentgens}}{\text{hour}} = 10.0\frac{\text{roentgens}}{\text{hour}} \cdot \frac{1 \text{ hour}}{60 \text{ minutes}}$$

$$= .167\frac{\text{roentgens}}{\text{minute}}$$

Algebra

Signed Numbers

Numbers are not always positive. For example, the thermometer indicates that it is very cold at $-20°$F. Negative numbers can be illustrated by using a number line (Figure 1–2). Positive numbers are assigned to the right of the zero point and negative numbers to the left of the zero point. A statement that seven is less than ten (written as $7 < 10$) indicates that 7 is to the left of 10 on the number line. A statement that minus five is greater than minus nine (written as $-5 > -9$) indicates that -5 is to the right of -9 on the number line.

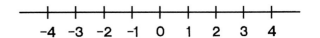

FIGURE 1–2. Number line.

Absolute Value   The absolute value of a number is the distance from 0 to that number on the number line. Since distance is a non-negative quantity, that means that the absolute value of a number is always positive or zero. The notation used for absolute value is two vertical bars (| |).

Examples:

$$|-2| = 2 \qquad |4| = 4 \qquad |0| = 0$$

Since -2 is two units from zero on the number line, the absolute value is 2. Since 4 is four units from zero on the number line, the absolute value is 4. Since 0 is zero units from zero on the number line, the absolute value is 0.

Addition   To add two positive numbers, add their absolute values and attach a positive sign to the result. The positive sign is usually omitted.

Example:

$(+7) + (+8) = +15 \qquad 7 + 8 = 15$

To add two negative numbers, add their absolute values and attach a negative sign to the result.

Example:

$(-7) + (-8) = -15 \qquad -7 + (-8) = -15$

To add two numbers with unlike signs, subtract the smaller in absolute value from the larger in absolute value and attach the sign of the larger in absolute value to the result.

Examples:

$(-10) + (3) = -7 \qquad 4 + (-9) = -5$
$(8) + (-5) = 3 \qquad -3 + (7) = 4$

Negative of a Number

The negative of a number is the opposite of the number in sign.

Examples: The negative of 7 is -7; the negative of -7 is 7.

If $b = 7$, then $-b = -7$.
If $b = -7$, then $-b = -(-7) = 7$.

Subtraction

Subtraction is rewritten as addition, as in $a - b = a + (-b)$.

Example:

$8 - 10 = 8 + (-10) = -2$
$8 - (-10) = 8 + 10 = 18$
$-8 - 10 = -8 + (-10) = -18$
$-8 - (-10) = -8 + 10 = 2$

All of the above subtraction problems are rewritten as addition and then the rules for addition of signed numbers are used.

Multiplication

To multiply two numbers, multiply their absolute values. If both numbers are positive or both numbers are negative, attach a positive sign to the result. If the numbers are opposite in sign, attach a negative sign to the result.

Examples:

$(2)(3) = 6$
$(-2)(-3) = 6$
$(2)(-3) = -6$
$(-2)(3) = -6$

Division

To divide two numbers, divide their absolute values. If both numbers are positive or both numbers are negative, attach a positive sign to the result. If the numbers are opposite in sign, attach a negative sign to the result.

Examples:

$8 \div 2 = 4$
$-8 \div -2 = 4$

$8 \div (-2) = -4$
$-8 \div 2 = -4$

Order of Operation

Order-of-operation problems may occur when parentheses are not indicated. For example, evaluate $2 + 3 \cdot 4$. Depending on whether addition or multiplication is performed first the answer might be 20 or 14. The answer actually depends on the order of operation. Rules have been established that make the correct result 14.

The difference between the unary minus sign $(-)$ and the subtraction sign $(-)$ and the difference between the unary plus sign $(+)$ and the addition sign $(+)$ must be understood before order-of-operation rules can be learned.

A subtraction sign $(-)$ is used between two numbers:

Example:
$7 - 8$ (subtraction sign)

A unary minus sign $(-)$ is used before one number.

Example:
-7 (unary minus sign)

An expression can have both a subtraction sign and a unary minus sign.

Example:
$-7 - 8$ (the first is a unary minus, the second a subtraction sign)

An addition sign (+) is used between two numbers:

Example:
8 + 10 (addition sign)

A unary plus sign (+) is used before one number.

Example:
+8

Rules for Order of Operation

1. Perform all operations inside grouping symbols (parentheses, radical symbols, fraction bar, brackets, etc.)

2. Exponentiation (raising to a power or roots)

3. Unary minus (–) or unary plus (+)

4. Multiplication and division

5. Addition and subtraction

Operations are performed from the lowest level (#1) to the largest level (#5). Operations on the same level are evaluated left to right.

Examples:

$2 + \underline{3 \cdot 4}$ (multiplication first)

$= 2 + 12$ (addition)
$= 14$

$\underline{8 \cdot 6} - \underline{12 \div 2}$ (multiplication & division first)

$= \underline{48 - 6}$ (subtraction)

$= 42$

$\dfrac{8 + 7}{2 + 3}$ (bar acts as grouping symbol)

$= \dfrac{15}{5}$ (add numerator and add denominator first)

$= 3$ (divide)

$(-2)^3$ (exponentiation first)

$= -8$

$-(2)^4$ (exponentiation first)

$= -(16)$ (unary minus sign)

$= -16$

$3(\underline{7 + 4})$ (add inside parenthesis first)

$= \underline{3 \cdot 11}$ (multiply)

$= 33$

$2(\underline{6 + 1})^2$ (add inside parenthesis first)

$= 2\underline{(7)^2}$ (exponentiation next)

$= 2 \cdot 49$ (multiply)

$= 98$

Algebraic Expressions

Algebraic expressions are letters and/or numbers that are multiplied, divided, added, subtracted or raised to a power.

Examples:

$3x^3 + 5x^2 - 7x + 8$

$\dfrac{x + 5}{y - 7}$

There are several rules for combining algebraic expressions.

Distributive Law   The statement of the distributive law is:

$a(b + c) = a \cdot b + a \cdot c$

Examples:

$7(x + y) = 7x + 7y$
$7(3 + 5) = 7 \cdot 3 + 7 \cdot 5 = 21 + 35 = 56$
$p(x + 4) = px + 4p$ (The numeral is normally written in front of the letter.)

If the addition sign were a subtraction sign, then:

$a(b - c) = a \cdot b - a \cdot c$

Examples:

$7(x - y) = 7x - 7y$

$7(3 - 5) = 7 \cdot 3 - 7 \cdot 5$
$= 21 - 35 = 21 + (-35) = -14$

$p(x - 4) = px - 4p$

Care needs to be taken when one or two negative signs are involved.

Examples:

$-7(x + y) = -7x + (-7y)$ (distributive law)
$= -7x - 7y$ (the reverse definition of subtraction)

$-7(x - y) = -7x - (-7y)$ (distributive law)
$= -7x + 7y$ (definition of subtraction)

$-7(-3 - 8) = (-7)(-3) - (-7)(8)$ (distributive law)
$= 21 - (-56)$ (multiply)
$= 21 + 56$ (definition of subtraction)
$= 77$

Addition and Subtraction of Like Terms

Like terms are terms with identical literal factors. A literal factor is a factor denoted by a letter. Like terms may be added or subtracted.

Example:

$7x + 3x = 10x$ (like terms)

Example:

$7x + 3y = 7x + 3y$ (unlike terms may not be added)

Example:

$7x - 3x = 4x$

Example:

$-7x - 3x = -7x + (-3x)$ (definition of subtraction)
$= -10x$ (combine like terms)

Example:

$-7x - (-3x) = -7x + 3x$ (definition of subtraction)
$= -4x$ (combine like terms)

Parentheses

When an algebraic expression involves parentheses, the parentheses need to be removed in order to simplify the expression.

Example:

$7(x + y) + 4(x + y)$
$= 7x + 7y + 4x + 4y$ (distributive law)
$= 11x + 11y$ (combine like terms)

Example:

$7(x + y) - 4(x + y)$
$= 7(x + y) + (-4)(x + y)$ (definition of subtraction)
$= 7x + 7y + (-4x) + (-4y)$ (distributive law)
$= 3x + 3y$ (combine like terms)

Example:

$7(x - y) - 4(x - y)$
$= 7(x - y) + (-4)(x - y)$ (definition of subtraction)
$= 7x - 7y + (-4x) - (-4y)$ (distributive law)
$= 7x + (-7y) + (-4x) + (4y)$ (definition of subtraction)
$= 3x + (-3y)$ (combine like terms)
$= 3x - 3y$ (reverse of definition of subtraction)

Example:

$x - (y - x) = x + (-1)(y - x)$
$= x + (-y) - (-x)$
$= x + (-y) + x$
$= 2x - y$

If an expression involves parentheses within parentheses, then it is simplified from the innermost parentheses out.

Example:

$7 - [6x - (x - 4)]$
$= 7 - [6x - x + 4]$ (remove innermost parentheses)
$= 7 - [5x + 4]$ (simplify within parentheses)
$= 7 - 5x - 4$ (remove parentheses [square bracket])
$= 3 - 5x$ (combine like terms)

Exponents Definition:

$$a^n = \underbrace{a \bullet a \bullet a \bullet \bullet \bullet a}_{n \text{ times}}$$

where a is the base and n is the exponent

Example:

$$3^4 = 3 \bullet 3 \bullet 3 \bullet 3 = 81$$

Laws of Exponents

Law 1: $a^m \bullet a^n = a^{m+n}$

Examples:

$$a^4 \bullet a^3 = a^{4+3} = a^7$$
$$a \bullet a^5 = a^{1+5} = a^6$$

Law 2:

$$\frac{a^m}{a^n} = \left\{ \begin{array}{l} a^{m-n} \text{ if } m \geq n \\ \dfrac{1}{a^{n-m}} \text{if } n > m \end{array} \right\} a \neq 0$$

Examples:

$$\frac{x^5}{x^2} = x^{5-2} = x^3$$

$$\frac{x^7}{x^{10}} = \frac{1}{x^{10-7}} = \frac{1}{x^3}$$

Law 3: $(ab)^m = a^m b^m$

Example:

$$(ab)^4 = a^4 b^4$$

Law 4: $\left(\dfrac{a}{b}\right)^m = \dfrac{a^m}{b^m}, b \neq 0$

Example:

$$\left(\frac{a}{b}\right)^5 = \frac{a^5}{b^5}$$

Law 5: $(a^m)^n = a^{m \bullet n}$

Example:

$$(a^4)^5 = a^{4 \bullet 5} = a^{20}$$

Definition: $a^0 = 1$ for $a \neq 0$

Examples:

$$5^0 = 1$$
$$x^0 = 1$$
$$(5x)^0 = 1$$
$$5x^0 = 5 \bullet 1 = 5$$

Definition: $a^{-n} = \dfrac{1}{a^n}$ for $a \neq 0$

Examples:

$$x^{-7} = \frac{1}{x^7}$$

$$2^{-3} = \frac{1}{2^3} = \frac{1}{8}$$

It can also be shown that:

$$\frac{1}{a^{-n}} = a^n \text{ for } a \neq 0.$$

Examples:

$$\frac{1}{5^{-2}} = 5^2 = 25$$

$$\frac{1}{x^{-5}} = x^5$$

Multiplying Numbers in Scientific Notation

When multiplying two numbers in scientific notation, the Ns are multiplied and the powers of ten are added. This is simply using the rule of exponents when the bases are the same.

Example:

$$(2.4 \times 10^3)(3.8 \times 10^{11})$$
$$= (2.4 \bullet 3.8) \times 10^{3+11}$$
$$= 9.1 \times 10^{14}$$

Dividing Numbers in Scientific Notation

When dividing two numbers in scientific notation, the Ns are divided and the exponents are subtracted. This is another example of using the rules of exponents.

Example:

$$(8.3 \times 10^4) \div (2.7 \times 10^{11})$$
$$= 8.3 \div 2.7 \times 10^{4-11}$$
$$= 3.1 \times 10^{-7}$$

Evaluating Algebraic Expressions

To evaluate an algebraic expression, replace each unknown with the given value and then perform the indicated operations.

Example:

Evaluate $2a^2 + 5b$ for $a = 3$ and $b = 4$.

$$2a^2 + 5b = 2(3)^2 + 5(4)$$
$$= 2 \cdot 9 + 20$$
$$= 18 + 20$$
$$= 38$$

Formulae are examples of equations where algebraic expressions are evaluated.

Example:

Convert 60.0° F to C.
The formula involved is C = 5/9(F − 32°).
Determine C when F = 60.0°.

$$C = 5/9(F - 32°)$$
$$C = 5/9(60.0° - 32°) \quad \text{(substitute 60.0° for F)}$$
$$C = 5/9(28°)$$
$$C = 15.6° \, C$$

Convert 20.0° C to F.
The formula to use is F = 9/5(C + 32°).
Determine F when C = 20.0°.

$$F = 9/5(20°) + 32°$$
$$F = 36° + 32°$$
$$F = 68°$$

Equations

An equation is a statement that contains an equal sign. For example, A = B is an equation. An equation can be either a true or a false statement.

Examples:

5 + 3 = 7	(false statement)
5 + 3 = 8	(true statement)

Both of these statements are equations but only one is true.

An equation that contains at least one unknown (variable) is an open equation.

Examples:

$$x + 5 = 7$$
$$3x + 5 = 7 - 2x$$

An open statement becomes either true or false when the unknown (variable) is replaced (substituted) with a numeric value.

Examples:

In $x + 5 = 7$, replace x with 3.
  3 + 5 = 7 is a false statement.
In $x + 5 = 7$, replace x with 2.
  2 + 5 = 7 is a true statement.

The solution of an equation is that numeric value which, when substituted in the equation, gives a true statement. In the example above, 2 is the solution to the equation.

There may be many solutions to an equation. For example, in the equation x + 5 = x + 5, all numeric values for x will give a true statement. **This type of equation is called an identity.**

There may be no solutions to an equation. For example, in the equation x + 5 = x + 6, there are no numbers that, when substituted in the equation, give a true statement. Therefore there are no solutions to the equation.

Equivalence Principles
The principles of equivalence are needed to solve equations. **Equivalent equations are equations that have the same solutions.**

Addition and Subtraction Principle
If the same number is added to each side or subtracted from each side of an equation, the equation remains equivalent.

Example:

x − 5 = 7	(add 5 to both sides)
x − 5 + 5 = 7 + 5	(equivalent equation to
x = 12	x − 5 = 7)

Example:

$$x + 3 = 12 \qquad \text{(subtract 3 from both sides)}$$
$$x + 3 - 3 = 12 - 3 \qquad \text{(equivalent equation to}$$
$$x = 9 \qquad\qquad x + 3 = 12)$$

Multiplication and Division Principle If the same nonzero number is multiplied or divided by each side of the equation, the equation remains equivalent.

Example:

$$\frac{x}{5} = 6 \qquad \text{(multiply each side by 5)}$$

$$5 \cdot \frac{x}{5} = 5 \cdot 6 \qquad \text{(equivalent equation)}$$

$$x = 30$$

Example:

$$3x = 12 \qquad \text{(divide each side by 3)}$$

$$\frac{3x}{3} = \frac{12}{3} \qquad \text{(equivalent equation)}$$

$$x = 4$$

To find a solution to an equation, the unknown (variable) must be isolated on one side of the equation.

Example:

Solve: $x + 7 = 12$ for x.

$$x + 7 = 12$$
$$x + 7 - 7 = 12 - 7 \quad \text{(subtract 7 from each side)}$$
$$x = 5$$

Check:

$$x + 7 = 12$$
$$5 + 7 = 12 \qquad \text{(substitute value for x)}$$
$$12 = 12 \qquad \text{(statement is true; therefore 5 is solution to equation)}$$

Example:

Solve: $\dfrac{x}{6} = 18$ for x.

$$\frac{x}{6} = 18$$

$$6 \cdot \frac{x}{6} = 6 \cdot 18 \qquad \text{(multiply both sides by 6)}$$

$$x = 108$$

Check:

$$\frac{x}{6} = 18$$

$$\frac{108}{6} = 18 \qquad \text{(substitute 108 for x)}$$

$$18 = 18 \qquad \text{(statement is true)}$$

Example:

Solve: $5a = 30$ for a.

$$5a = 30$$
$$\frac{5a}{5} = \frac{30}{5} \qquad \text{(divide both sides by 5)}$$
$$a = 6$$

Check:

$$5a = 30$$
$$5(6) = 30 \qquad \text{(substitute 6 for a)}$$
$$30 = 30 \qquad \text{(statement is true)}$$

Example:

Solve: $7x - 5 = 3x + 7$ for x.

$$7x - 5 = 3x + 7$$
$$7x - 5 + 5 = 3x + 7 + 5 \quad \text{(add 5 to both sides)}$$
$$7x = 3x + 12$$
$$7x - 3x = 3x + 12 - 3x \quad \text{(subtract 3x from both sides)}$$
$$4x = 12$$
$$\frac{4x}{4} = \frac{12}{4} \qquad \text{(divide both sides by 4)}$$
$$x = 3$$

Check:

$$7x - 5 = 3x + 7$$
$$7(3) - 5 = 3(3) + 7 \qquad \text{(substitute 3 for x)}$$
$$21 - 5 = 9 + 7$$
$$16 = 16 \qquad \text{(statement is true)}$$

To solve an equation with parentheses, the parentheses need to be eliminated using some correct procedure, usually the distributive law.

Example:

Solve: $7(x + 6) = 21$ for x.

$$7(x + 6) = 21 \qquad \text{(distributive law)}$$
$$7x + 42 = 21 \qquad \text{(subtract 42 from each side)}$$
$$7x = -21 \qquad \text{(divide each side by 7)}$$
$$x = -3$$

Check:

$$7(x + 6) = 21 \qquad \text{(substitute } -3 \text{ for x)}$$
$$7(-3 + 6) = 21$$
$$7(3) = 21$$
$$21 = 21 \qquad \text{(statement is true)}$$

Sometimes a formula needs to be rearranged. This is just like solving an equation for an unknown (variable).

Example:

Solve for t when $a = bt + c$

$$a = bt + c$$
$$a - c = bt + c - c \qquad \text{(subtract c from each side)}$$
$$a - c = bt \qquad \text{(divide by b)}$$
$$\frac{a - c}{b} = \frac{bt}{b}$$
$$\frac{a - c}{b} = t$$

Check:

$$a = bt + c$$
$$a = b \bullet \frac{a - c}{b} + c \qquad \text{(substitute } \frac{a - c}{b} \text{ for t)}$$
$$a = a - c + c$$
$$a = a \qquad \text{(statement is true)}$$

Variation

There are two types of variation that will be discussed here—direct and inverse.

Direct Variation
Direct variation means that one quantity is a multiple of a second quantity. An example of direct variation is $y = kx$ where k is the constant of proportionality. Here y is a multiple of x, making y directly proportional to x.

Another example is $y = kx^2$ where k is the constant of proportionality, making y directly proportional to the square of x. Another way to think of direct variation is that the quotient of the two quantities is always a constant. It is possible, knowing the values for the quantities, to find the constant.

Inverse Variation
Inverse variation means that when two quantities are multiplied their product is a constant.

An example of inverse variation is $y = k/x$ where k is the constant of proportionality. Here the product of x and y is a constant, namely k. This is usually read as y is inversely proportional to x.

Another example is $y = k/x^2$ where k is the constant of proportionality. Here the product of x^2 and y is a constant. This is usually read as y is inversely proportional to the square of x (or x^2).

It is also possible to combine the above. As an example, consider $y = kx/z^2$. Here y is directly proportional to x and inversely proportional to the square of z.

Units of Measurement

In order to quantify scientific phenomena, standard units of measurement have been established. These units allow scientists to describe quantities. In physics, the primary or fundamental units of measurement are **mass, length and time.** These units, although they have the same meaning and have been standardized by international organizations, are measured by the use of two widely different systems. These are the British (foot-pound-second) system, also called the United States customary system, and the metric [MKS (meter-kilogram-second) or CGS (centimeter-gram-second)] system. Although most countries utilize the metric system of measurement, attempts to switch to this system in the United States have not been very successful. In the United States, length is measured in inches and feet rather than meters and kilometers. By combining one or more of the fundamental units, scientists arrive at secondary or derived units. For example, the area of an object is derived from the fundamental unit of length. The area of a rectangle is determined by multiplying the lengths of the two sides of the object.

SI Units

In 1960, at the Eleventh General Conference of Weights and Measures, the Système Internationale d'Unites (SI) was defined and officially adopted. This system of units, used to measure various quantities, is now accepted as the metric system. In the SI system, there are seven base units (Table 1 – 2). All other units are derived from these units, although some derived units are given special names. It is important to become familiar with SI units since they have been internationally adopted.

In addition, although the United States does not use SI/metric units for the public, all scientific inquiries utilize the SI system. The seven base SI units are mass, length, time, electric current, temperature, amount of substance and luminous intensity. Radiologically important derived units are the **coulomb per kilogram** (C/kg), formerly the roentgen (R); the **gray** (Gy), formerly the rad (radiation absorbed dose); and the **sievert** (Sv), formerly the rem (radiation equivalent man). These radiologic units will be described in greater detail in Chapter 8.

Fundamental Units

Mass   Mass is the amount or quantity of matter. The standard unit of mass is the **kilogram** (kg). It is represented by a cylinder of platinum-iridium, which is kept in a vault at the International Bureau of Weights and Measures in Paris, France.

Length   The unit of length is the **meter** (m). The meter was defined in 1983 as the distance that light travels in a vacuum in 1/299,792,485 second.

Time   The unit of time is the **second** (s). The second was originally defined in terms of the rotation of the earth on its axis (the mean solar day) but, like the meter, the need for greater accuracy resulted in redefining the unit. Time is now measured by the vibrations of cesium—133 atoms. This method is sometimes called the atomic clock.

Prefixes

The metric system uses prefixes to units to denote different orders of magnitude, as shown in Table 1 – 3.

TABLE 1–2. SI Units of Measurement

BASE UNITS			
Quantity	**Unit Name**	**Symbol**	
Mass	kilogram	kg	
Length	meter	m	
Time	second	s	
Electric current	ampere	A	
Temperature	kelvin	K	
Amount of substance	mole	mol	
Luminous intensity	candela	cd	
DERIVED UNITS			
Quantity	**Unit Name**	**Symbol**	**British Units**
Absorbed dose	gray	Gy	rad
Charge	coulomb	C	esu
Electric potential	volt	v	
Dose equivalent	sievert	Sv	rem
Energy	joule	J	erg
Exposure	coulomb/kilogram	C/kg	roentgen
Frequency	hertz	Hz	cycles per second
Force	newton	N	
Magnetic flux	weber	Wb	
Magnetic flux density	tesla	T	gauss
Power	watt	W	
Radioactivity	bequerel	Bq	curie

To convert from grams to kilograms or micrograms, or to grams with any other prefix, the decimal point is moved. If the prefix moves up the table, the decimal point is moved to the left the number of exponent positions moved. If the prefix moves down the table, the decimal point is moved to the right the number of exponent positions moved. Dimensional analysis can also be used.

Examples:

23.4 g = 0.0234 kg   Move the decimal point 3 positions left.

23.4 g = 23,400 mg   Move the decimal point 3 positions right.

23.4 mg = 0.0000234 kg   Move the decimal point 6 positions left.

TABLE 1–3. SI Unit Values

Factors	Prefixes	Symbols
10^{12}	tera	T
10^9	giga	G
10^6	mega	M
10^3	kilo	k
10^2	hecto	h
10^1	deka	da
10^{-1}	deci	d
10^{-2}	centi	c
10^{-3}	milli	m
10^{-6}	micro	μ
10^{-9}	nano	n
10^{-12}	pico	p
10^{-15}	femto	f
10^{-18}	atto	a

$$23.4 \text{ kg} = 2,340,000 \text{ cg}$$

Move the decimal point 5 positions right.

Using dimensional analysis:

$$23.4 \text{ g} = 23.4 \text{ g} \frac{\text{g}}{1000 \text{ g}} = 0.0234 \text{ kg}$$

Some commonly used prefixes are shown in Table 1–4.

Conversion from one system to another is needed from time to time. For example, 1 inch = 2.54 cm is the conversion fact for changing inches to centimeters. See the section on dimensional analysis under the math review for the procedure to convert from one set of units to another.

TABLE 1–4. Commonly Used SI Prefixes

Unit	Symbol	Meaning
kilovolt	kV	10^3 volts
centimeter	cm	10^{-2} meter
milliampere	mA	10^{-3} amp
milligray	mGy	10^{-3} Gy
nanosecond	ns	10^{-9} second

Summary

A basic review of arithmetic, algebra, and units of measurement has been presented. The arithmetic review includes fractions, decimals, computation with values, powers of ten, scientific notation and dimensional analysis. The algebra review includes signed numbers, order of operation, algebraic expressions, exponents, evaluating algebraic expressions, equations, and variation. Both SI and British (U.S. customary) units of measurement are introduced.

In order to quantify science, standard units of measurement were established. The fundamental units of measurement are mass, length and time. Units of measurement were officially defined on an international level through the adoption of the SI units. The seven base SI units are mass, length, time, electric current, temperature, amount of substance and luminous intensity. Radiologically important derived units are the coulomb per kilogram (C/kg), formerly the roentgen (R); the gray (Gy), formerly the rad (radiation absorbed dose); and the sievert (Sv), formerly the rem (radiation equivalent man).

REVIEW QUESTIONS

1. $\dfrac{4}{7} + \dfrac{1}{2} =$

2. $\dfrac{2}{9} \cdot \dfrac{3}{8} =$

3. $571.1 - 182.572 =$

4. $725 \div 0.25 =$

5. Change .325 to a percent.

6. What are the significant digits of each of the following:

   a. 20.10

   b. 192

   c. 38.04

   d. 2,700

   e. 1,800.004

7. Add the following numbers, leaving the results with the correct number of significant

digits if each number is assumed to be approximate.

   a. $2.1 + 2.824$

   b. $3.2 + 4.19$

8. Change the following numbers to scientific notation:

   a. $.0081$

   b. $7,811.2$

   c. $.00024$

   d. $78,432$

9. Change the following numbers to ordinary notation:

   a. 3.614×10^2

   b. 1.876×10^{-4}

   c. 1.823×10^3

   d. 5.67×10^6

10. Convert 1,500 seconds to hours.

11. Convert 10 meters^2 to centimeters^2.

12. Simplify the following algebraic expressions:

   a. $-3(x + y) + 7(2x + 1)$

   b. $-4(x + 2y) - 8(2x - y)$

13. Simplify the following expressions, leaving the answer with only positive exponents:

   a. $a^2 \cdot b^3 \cdot a^4 \cdot b^2$

   b. $(a^4)^3 \cdot (a^2)^{-3}$

14. Evaluate the expression for $a = 5$ and $b = 3$

   $\frac{3}{8}(a^2 - b^2)$

15. Evaluate the expression for $a = 2$, $b = -4$, and $c = 6$.

   $3(a + b) - c$

16. Solve for x: $2x - 8 = 4$

17. Solve for x: $2(3x - 8) = 3(4 - x) + 6x$

18. Solve for a: $\frac{2}{3} = \frac{a}{15}$

REFERENCES AND RECOMMENDED READING

Aufmann, R. N. & Barker, V. C. (1999). *Basic college mathematics* (6th ed.). Boston: Houghton Mifflin Company.

Austin, J. C., Gill, J.C. & Isern, M. (1988). *Technical mathematics* (4th ed.). Philadelphia: Saunders College Publishing Company.

Burns, J. E. (1979). The new SI units: Problems with conversion. *The Canadian Journal of Radiography, Radiotherapy, and Nuclear Medicine. 10*(2), 60–70.

Dunworth, J. V. (1976). SI units for ionizing radiations. The use of the "Gray". *Radiography. 42*(496), 84.

Kemp, L. W. (1964). *Mathematics for radiographers* (2nd ed.). Oxford: Blackwell Scientific Publications.

The SI for the health profession. (1979). *The Canadian Journal of Medical Radiation Technology. 10*(4), 138.

Stefano, S. S. (1979). *Mathematics for technologists in radiology, nuclear medicine, and radiation therapy.* St. Louis: C. V. Mosby Company.

Washington, A. J. (1999). *Basic technical mathematics* (7th ed.). Redwood City, CA: The Benjamin/Cummings Publishing Company.

Wyckoff, H. O. (1978). The international system of units (SI). *Radiology. 128*, 833–835.

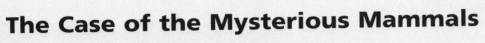

The Case of the Mysterious Mammals

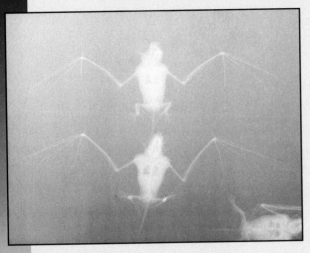

These mammals was radiographed in the deep south. What are they?

Answers to the case studies can be found in Appendix E.

CHAPTER 2

Radiation Concepts

I have discovered something interesting, but I do not know whether or not my observations are correct.

W. C. Röntgen to his friend Theodor Boveri in early December 1895.

OBJECTIVES

Upon completion of this chapter, the student should be able to:

▶ Describe the branches of science.

▶ Differentiate between matter and energy.

▶ Describe the basic structure of matter.

▶ Identify the various types of energy.

▶ Explain the basic concepts of atomic theory.

▶ Differentiate between the radiations along the electromagnetic spectrum.

▶ Describe the wave and particle theories for electromagnetic radiation.

▶ Identify the properties of x-rays.

▶ Explain the standard units of measurement.

Matter And Energy

Radiography is the recording of images created by the use of x-ray energy. It is both an art and a science. In order to perform the duties of a radiographer it is necessary to understand the art of the profession as well as the science.

Science is the use of knowledge in an organized and classified manner. The scientific method has been used by men and women to understand the world in which we live. This method systematically involves collecting facts, studying their relationships and arriving at conclusions based on analysis. Natural science is the study of the universe and its contents. It can be divided into two categories: 1) the study of nonliving matter, known as physical science, and 2) the study of living matter, known as biological science. Radiographers learn about biological science through a study of human anatomy and physiology and about physical science through a study of x-ray production and imaging processes.

Physics is a branch of physical science that studies matter and energy and their interrelationships. Matter is defined as anything that has mass and occupies space. Energy is the ability to do work.

Matter

Matter is a very general term used to describe the substance that comprises all physical objects. It has shape, form and occupies space. A principle characteristic of matter is **mass**. Mass is the quantity of matter contained in an object. It is best described by its energy equivalence although the term weight is generally used to mean the same thing. **Weight** is the force that an object exerts under the influence of gravity. An object may be weightless in a zero gravity environment, such as in space, but the mass of that object would remain unchanged.

The unit of mass is the kilogram, which equals 1,000 grams. The kilogram represents the weight of a standard piece of platinum-iridium kept at the International Bureau of Weights and Measures in Paris, France. It is equal to the mass of 1,000 cm^3 of water at 0° Celsius (C) or Centigrade.

The structure of matter has been studied throughout history. In nature, matter is most commonly found as a mixture of substances (Table 2–1). A **substance** is

TABLE 2–1. Structure of Matter

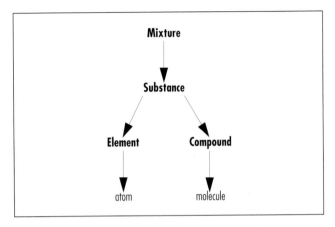

defined as a material that has a definite and constant composition. When two or more substances are combined they form a **mixture**. For example, air is a mixture of oxygen, hydrogen, nitrogen and a variety of other substances.

Substances may be either simple or complex. Simple substances are known as **elements** and complex substances are known as **compounds**. An element is a substance that cannot be broken down into any simpler substances by ordinary means. There are 92 naturally occurring elements identified on the periodic table of elements (Table 2–2). Elements include such substances as hydrogen, oxygen, carbon, calcium, copper, silver, gold, lead and barium. When two or more elements are chemically united in definite proportion, compounds are formed. Water and salt are both examples of compounds. Water is formed by the chemical union of two hydrogen atoms and one oxygen atom and is referred to as H$_2$O (Figure 2–1). Each element has an abbreviated letter or letters to identify it. These abbreviations for the elements are outlined on the periodic table. For example, in the compound salt, the element sodium (Na) is chemically combined with the element chlorine (Cl), in equal proportions, to form sodium chloride (NaCl).

When broken down and examined in its purest form, matter is actually comprised of very small invisible particles known as atoms. An **atom** is the smallest particle of an element that still possesses the chemical properties of that element. When two or more atoms are chemically united they form a **molecule**, which is the smallest particle of a compound that still possesses the characteristics

TABLE 2–2. Periodic Table of Elements

n =	1 IA	2 IIA	3 IIIB	4 IVB	5 VB	6 VIB	7 VIIB	8	9 VIIIB	10	11 IB	12 IIB	13 IIIA	14 IVA	15 VA	16 VIA	17 VIIA	18 VIIIA
K or 1	1 1.008 **H** Hydrogen																	2 4.003 **He** Helium
L or 2	3 6.941 **Li** Lithium	4 9.012 **Be** Beryllium											5 10.81 **B** Boron	6 12.01 **C** Carbon	7 14.007 **N** Nitrogen	8 15.999 **O** Oxygen	9 18.998 **F** Fluorine	10 20.179 **Ne** Neon
M or 3	11 22.990 **Na** Sodium	12 24.305 **Mg** Magnesium											13 26.981 **Al** Aluminum	14 28.086 **Si** Silicon	15 30.974 **P** Phosphorus	16 32.06 **S** Sulfur	17 35.453 **Cl** Chlorine	18 39.948 **Ar** Argon
N or 4	19 39.102 **K** Potassium	20 40.08 **Ca** Calcium	21 44.956 **Sc** Scandium	22 47.90 **Ti** Titanium	23 50.941 **V** Vanadium	24 51.996 **Cr** Chromium	25 54.938 **Mn** Manganese	26 55.847 **Fe** Iron	27 58.933 **Co** Cobalt	28 58.71 **Ni** Nickel	29 63.55 **Cu** Copper	30 65.37 **Zn** Zinc	31 69.72 **Ga** Gallium	32 72.59 **Ge** Germanium	33 74.922 **As** Arsenic	34 78.76 **Se** Selenium	35 79.904 **Br** Bromine	36 83.80 **Kr** Krypton
O or 5	37 85.47 **Rb** Rubidium	38 87.62 **Sr** Strontium	39 88.906 **Y** Yttrium	40 91.22 **Zr** Zirconium	41 92.906 **Nb** Niobium	42 95.94 **Mo** Molybdenum	43 98.91 **Tc** Technetium	44 101.07 **Ru** Ruthenium	45 102.90 **Rh** Rhodium	46 106.4 **Pd** Palladium	47 107.87 **Ag** Silver	48 112.40 **Cd** Cadmium	49 114.82 **In** Indium	50 118.69 **Sn** Tin	51 121.75 **Sb** Antimony	52 127.60 **Te** Tellurium	53 126.90 **I** Iodine	54 131.30 **Xe** Xenon
P or 6	55 132.91 **Cs** Cesium	56 137.34 **Ba** Barium	57 138.91 **La*** Lanthanum	72 178.49 **Hf** Hafnium	73 180.95 **Ta** Tantalum	74 183.85 **W** Tungsten	75 186.2 **Re** Rhenium	76 190.2 **Os** Osmium	77 192.2 **Ir** Iridium	78 195.09 **Pt** Platinum	79 196.97 **Au** Gold	80 200.59 **Hg** Mercury	81 204.37 **Tl** Thallium	82 207.2 **Pb** Lead	83 208.98 **Bi** Bismuth	84 (210) **Po** Polonium	85 (210) **At** Astatine	86 (222) **Rn** Radon
Q or 7	87 (223) **Fr** Francium	88 226.03 **Ra** Radium	89 (227) **Ac†** Actinium															

*

58 140.12* **Ce** Cerium	59 140.908 **Pr** Praseodymium	60 144.24 **Nd** Neodymium	61 (147) **Pm** Promethium	62 150.4 **Sm** Samarium	63 151.96 **Eu** Europium	64 157.25 **Gd** Gadolinium	65 158.925 **Tb** Terbium	66 162.50 **Dy** Dysprosium	67 164.930 **Ho** Holmium	68 167.26 **Er** Erbium	69 168.934 **Tm** Thulium	70 173.04 **Yb** Ytterbium	71 174.97 **Lu** Lutetium

†

90 232.04 **Th** Thorium	91 231.04 **Pa** Protactinium	92 238.03 **U** Uranium	93 237.05 **Np** Neptunium	94 (242) **Pu** Plutonium	95 (243) **Am** Americium	96 (247) **Cm** Curium	97 (247) **Bk** Berkelium	98 (251) **Cf** Californium	99 (253) **Es** Einsteinium	100 (254) **Fm** Fermium	101 (256) **Md** Mendelevium	102 (254) **No** Nobelium	103 (257) **Lr** Lawrencium

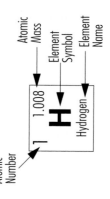

Atomic Mass — Element Symbol — Element Name — Atomic Number

1   1.008   **H**   Hydrogen

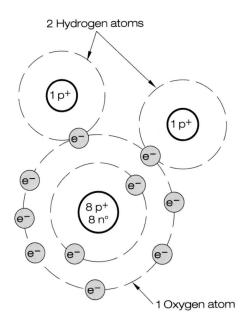

FIGURE 2–1. A water molecule is formed when two atoms of hydrogen combine with one atom of oxygen.

of the compound. For example, in the compound water, two hydrogen (H) atoms combine with one oxygen (O) atom to form one water (H_2O) molecule. With salt, one sodium (Na) atom combines with one chlorine (Cl) atom to form one sodium chloride (NaCl) molecule.

Atoms are tightly bonded to one another when a molecule is formed. These bonds cannot be broken by ordinary physical means, such as crushing. Atoms and molecules are, however, bound to one another by varying degrees of attraction. The degree of attraction between atoms or molecules will determine if the substance is a solid, a liquid or a gas. The attraction is weakest with a gas and strongest with a solid. For example, depending on the degree of molecular attraction, water can exist in its usual state as a liquid, or it can exist as a gas (steam) or a solid (ice). The state is determined by the heat or thermal energy that the substance possesses.

Energy

Energy is defined as the ability to do work. The unit of energy is the joule (J). When energy is emitted and transferred through matter it is called **radiation**. Radiation is a term applied to many forms of energy,

such as heat and light. When the burner on a stove is lit, it can be described as radiating heat. A light bulb is capable of radiating light. When any form of matter is struck by a form of radiant energy, it is described as being exposed or radiated.

There is a unique relationship between matter and energy. They are interchangeable. This relationship was described in 1905 by the German-American physicist, Albert Einstein (1879–1955), in his well-known theory of relativity. Einstein mathematically described the relationship between matter and energy in the equation:

$$E = mc^2$$

where: E = energy
m = mass
c = constant (the speed of light in a vacuum)

At the basis of Einstein's work is the Law of Conservation. This law states that the sum total of all matter and energy in the universe is a constant: matter and energy cannot be created or destroyed but can be converted from one form to another. Although recent research has demonstrated certain circumstances when Einstein's theory has been disproved, for practical purposes it is essentially true.

Atomic Theory

Matter is comprised of very small particles known as atoms. To understand how small atoms really are, it has been estimated that one teaspoon of water (about 1 cm^3) contains about three times as many atoms as the Atlantic Ocean contains teaspoons of water.

Atoms can be subdivided into three basic subatomic particles: **protons (p^+)**, **neutrons (n^0)** and **electrons (e^-)**.

Historical Overview

The composition of the atom has been a topic of scientific investigation for thousands of years. The Greeks theorized that matter has four basic components: air, water, earth and fire. They named the smallest division of these components the atom. This theory was accepted until the early 1800s, when an English schoolteacher named John Dalton (1766–1844) published his work on atomic theory. Dalton concluded that all elements could be differentiated from one another based on the characteristic of mass. He further concluded that each of the elements was composed of atoms that behaved in an identical fashion during a chemical reaction. During the mid-1800s a Russian scientist, Dmitri Mendeleev (1834–1907), developed the first periodic table of the elements. This table arranges the elements in order of ascending atomic mass and on the basis of the repetition of similar chemical properties (Table 2–2).

Investigation of the structure of matter continued and, in 1911, English physicist Ernest Rutherford (1871–1937) developed a model for the atom that contained a central, small, dense nucleus, which possessed a positive charge and was surrounded by a negative cloud of randomly placed electrons, which had a negative charge. In 1913 Niels Bohr (1885–1962), a Danish physicist, expanded on Rutherford's work and proposed a model for the atom that is considered the most representative of the structure of matter. Bohr's atom is likened to a miniature solar system where electrons orbit around a central nucleus just as the planets revolve around the sun.

Although the atom is far more complex than Bohr's simple model suggests, this model is still the most widely used in explaining the composition of matter. One key distinction between Bohr's model and an actual atom is that electrons orbit the nucleus in many planes, while the planets orbit the sun in essentially the same plane.

Bohr's simple model was difficult to apply to high atomic number elements. Both Niels Bohr and the Austrian physicist, Erwin Schrödinger, working with their associates, developed a theoretical approach to understanding atomic behavior. Both Bohr and Schrödinger were successful, but physicists primarily use Schrödinger's concept because it has been found to be more convenient. This approach is the foundation of modern physics and is known as quantum or wave mechanics.

According to the principles of quantum mechanics, orbital electrons are assigned probabilities for occupying any location within the atom. The greatest probabilities are associated with Bohr's original model.

Basic Atomic Particles

The atom is best described as having a small, dense center, known as the **nucleus**, which is surrounded by

electrons that orbit it at various levels (Figure 2–2). The nucleus contains two of the three basic particles of the atom, protons and neutrons, which are responsible for almost all of the mass of an atom. **Protons** and **neutrons** together are referred to as **nucleons**. The third basic particle, the **electron**, is located outside the nucleus and has a relatively insignificant mass, 1/1,826th that of a proton.

Electrons cannot be divided into smaller parts, but protons and neutrons are both composed of even smaller subnuclear structures called **quarks**. There are new theories that may explain them as well as find a way for quantum physics and relativity theory to work together. The overall concept is being referred to as **M theory**. It postulates that electrons and quarks may not be particles, but instead be extremely small loops of rapidly vibrating string-like matter. One idea is that matter behaves differently depending on the vibrations of the string (like a guitar string playing many different sounds depending on the position of the fingers on the frets, force applied via finger or pick, and the shape and size of the body of the guitar or the electronics in the pickup). In fact, this concept is now being called **string theory**. There are actually five different string theories and they require the

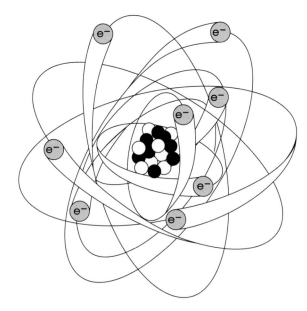

FIGURE 2–2. A three-dimensional diagram of an atom of oxygen, which contains 8 protons, 8 neutrons located within the center nucleus, and 8 electrons within orbital shells moving around the nucleus.

addition of several new dimensions in addition to the four we know (as well as the need to invent new forms of mathematics to figure out how they function). Although this begins to sound like a science fiction story, many physicists are beginning to agree that these new theories may be the next frontier for research and hold hope for better explanations about how matter behaves. It is likely that our knowledge of radiation will expand along with these theories throughout your career in the radiologic sciences.

The subatomic particles possess electrical charges. There are two types of electrical charges: positive and negative. The proton is a positively charged particle and the electron is a negatively charged particle. The neutron contains no charge and is said to be electrically neutral. When the number of positively charged protons equals the number of negatively charged electrons, the atom is neutral or stable. Because of its electrical nature, the atom is dynamic and ever moving. It is in a constant, vibrating motion because of the strong positive nuclear force field, which is surrounded by the negatively charged spinning and orbiting electrons.

Each of the elements has its own specific number of nuclear protons. This is the key characteristic that distinguishes one element from another. The number of nuclear protons in an atom is known as the **atomic number** or **Z** number. The simplest element, hydrogen, possesses only one proton and therefore has an atomic number of 1. Helium comes next on the periodic table and has two protons, giving it an atomic number of 2. Lead has an atomic number of 82, indicating that within the nucleus of an atom of lead there are 82 protons. The periodic table lists the elements in ascending order according to the element's atomic number (Table 2–2). In a neutral atom the number of protons is equal to the number of electrons. For example, in a stable, neutral atom of hydrogen there is one proton and one electron. In a stable atom of lead there are 82 protons and 82 electrons.

Although not a common occurrence in nature, when an atom of a given element loses or gains a proton that atom becomes a different element. For example, if an atom of carbon with atomic number 6 gains a proton, the atom then becomes an atom of nitrogen with atomic number 7. Atoms of one element do change to atoms of another element during the natural process of radioac-

tive decay. Radium, with an atomic number of 88, decays over a very long period of time to form the element radon, which has atomic number 86. Radon is a naturally occurring gas that is also radioactive. Recent studies have found increased radon levels in homes around the country. Radon testing kits are now commercially available to measure radon levels in the home.

Changes in the number of protons change the identity of the element completely, but this is not the case with changes in the number of neutrons or electrons. If an atom gains or loses neutrons, the result is an atom called an **isotope**. Isotopes are atoms that have the same number of protons in the nucleus but differ in the number of neutrons. Deuterium is an isotope of hydrogen. It contains the same number of protons as hydrogen but also contains one neutron.

If an atom gains or loses an electron, it is called an **ion** and the atom is said to be ionized. **Ionization** is the process of adding or removing an electron from an atom. When an electron is removed from an atom, the atom becomes a positive ion; that is, the atom possesses an extra positive charge. When an electron is added to an atom, the atom becomes a negative ion; that is, it possesses an extra negative charge (Figure 2–3).

Atomic Mass

The mass of an atom is extremely small; however, it is important to understand the differences in the mass of each of the basic particles of an atom. Each individual particle has its own unique mass. As stated earlier, the mass of an atom is almost entirely concentrated in the nucleus. The mass of a proton is approximately 1.673×10^{-27} kilograms and the mass of a neutron is almost identical, at 1.675×10^{-27} kilograms. While these numbers seem remarkably small, they are still significantly greater than the mass of an electron, at 9.109×10^{-31} kilograms. Protons have approximately 1,836 times the mass of electrons and neutrons have approximately 1,838 times more. The mass of the particles of an atom is sometimes described in **atomic mass units (amu)**.

In order for science to be as exact as possible, scientists defined an atomic mass unit as equal to one twelfth of a carbon 12 atom. The amu of a proton is approximately 1.00728, a neutron has an amu of approximately 1.00867, and an electron has an amu of approximately 0.000548.

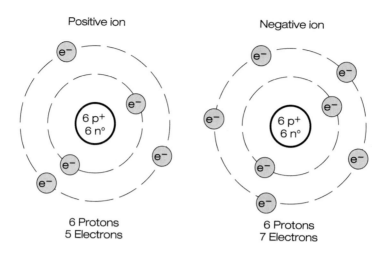

FIGURE 2–3. The ionization process. When an electron is either added to or removed from an atom, the atom is ionized. A neutral carbon atom contains 6 protons and 6 electrons; a positive ion of carbon would contain more protons than electrons and a negative ion of carbon would contain more electrons than protons.

When precision is not necessary, the mass of an atom is described by an **atomic mass number** symbolized by the letter **A**. The atomic mass number is equal to the number of protons and neutrons in the nucleus. For our purposes, each proton and neutron can be considered to have a mass number of one and an electron to have a mass number of zero (Table 2–3).

Orbital Electrons

Each of the electrons around the nucleus is in continuous motion. According to quantum mechanics, each of these electrons resides in an orbit that may be described as a "probability density." The orbital describes the region over which the electron is most likely to be at any given time.

The distance from the nucleus determines the energy level or **shell** the electron occupies. Each energy level has

TABLE 2–3. Atomic Particles

Particle	Mass Number	Mass (Kilograms)	amu	Charge
Proton	1	1.673×10^{-27}	1.00728	Positive
Neutron	1	1.675×10^{-27}	1.00867	Neutral
Electron	0	9.109×10^{-31}	0.000548	Negative

a certain **electron binding energy** (E_b). The binding energy of an electron is defined as that amount of energy needed to remove the electron from the atom. If a free electron at rest is assumed to have an energy of zero, then the total energy of an orbital electron would be zero minus the binding energy or the negative of the binding energy. The closer an electron is to the nucleus, the more tightly it is bound to its orbit or shell. The charge felt by any electron at various distances from the nucleus is termed the shielded nuclear charge.

Certain forces are responsible for maintaining the electron's position and motion in its orbit. The stability of this orbit is contributed to by two opposing forces, the centrifugal force and the attractive electrostatic force. The centrifugal force tends to cause the electron to fly out in space. The attractive electrostatic force between the positively charged nucleus and the negatively charged electron tends to cause the two to fly together. These forces are exactly equal and opposite in a stable orbital. The end result is an electron that is in motion in a specific orbit around the nucleus. The closer an electron is to the nucleus, the higher the electron binding energy is and the more difficult it is to remove the electron from the atom.

The orbital shell closest to the nucleus is called the **K-shell**; the next shell is called the L-shell, then M-, N-, O-, P-, and finally the Q-shell. These letters for the shells are actually no longer used by chemists and physicists. They identify the shells by the principle quantum number (n). The first shell (K) is designated as n=1. The second shell (L) is n=2; the third shell (M) is n=3 etc. Two additional quantum numbers, the angular momentum quantum number and the magnetic quantum number, are further used by chemists and physicists to describe more precisely the location of an electron within an atom.

In a neutral atom, the number of protons and electrons is equal. This means that each element has a different number of orbital electrons. The element hydrogen has only one proton and one electron. The electron of a hydrogen atom orbits in the K-shell. There is a maximum number of electrons that can occupy a given shell. The maximum number is determined by the formula $2n^2$, where n equals the shell or principle quantum number, starting with K as the first shell. According to this formula, the maximum number of electrons in each of the shells would be:

$$K = 2(1)^2=2$$
$$L = 2(2)^2=8$$
$$M = 2(3)^2=18$$
$$N = 2(4)^2=32$$
$$O = 2(5)^2=50$$
$$P = 2(6)^2=72$$
$$Q = 2(7)^2=98$$

Electrons may begin to appear in the next shell before a shell contains its maximum number of electrons. For example, electrons may appear in the N-shell before the M-shell has 18 electrons in it. This is because the number of electrons in the outermost shell never exceeds eight electrons. This is commonly referred to as the **octet rule**. Atoms that contain exactly eight electrons in their outermost shell are considered inert and chemically stable. The specific electron configuration will determine an element's position within the groups of the periodic table.

As the number of electrons and protons increases, so does the binding energy of a given electron. This is due to the increase in the positive charge in the nucleus. This means that the electrons in atoms of high atomic number elements are bound more tightly than the electrons in atoms of lower atomic number elements. The binding energy of electrons in the K-shell of lead is much higher than the binding energy of the K-shell electrons in hydrogen or oxygen. In addition, the binding energy of an electron decreases as the distance from the nucleus is increased (Figure 2–4). It takes more energy to remove a K-shell electron from its path than it would to remove an electron from a shell at a greater distance from the nucleus, such as the L-, M-, or N-shell. This will become important to remember when studying the effect of x-rays on atoms.

The binding energy of an electron is measured in a unit called the **electron volt (eV)**. This is the same unit used to describe x-ray energies. The electron volt is the energy one electron will have when it is accelerated by an electrical potential of one volt. Because x-ray and binding energies are great, the usual unit used to express these energies is the kilo-electron volt (keV). One keV equals 1,000 electron volts.

The atomic configuration and the approximate binding energies of certain elements are important because of their significance in radiology. These elements include hydrogen (H), carbon (C) and oxygen (O) because they are the principle elements that comprise the human body; iodine (I) and barium (Ba) because these elements are used as contrast media for a variety of radiologic examinations; tungsten (W) and molybdenum (Mo) because they are x-ray tube target materials; and lead (Pb) because it is the element used for radiation protection devices. A diagram of these elements shows that as the atomic number of an element increases, the K-shell binding energy of the element increases (Figure 2–5). This means that a K-shell electron of lead (Pb) is more tightly bound and more difficult to remove from the atom than a K-shell electron of smaller atomic number elements, such as hydrogen (H) or oxygen (O).

To remove the K-shell electron from an atom of tungsten or lead requires much more energy than would be necessary to remove a K-shell electron from an atom of hydrogen, carbon or oxygen. When an electron is removed from an atom, the atom is said to be ionized. X-rays are capable of ionizing atoms. The x-ray energy must be greater than the binding energy of the electron in order for ionization to occur (Figure 2–6).

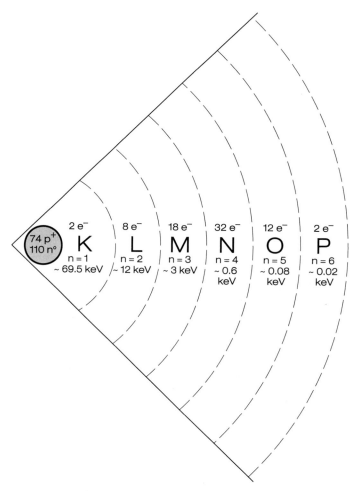

FIGURE 2–4. The closer an electron is to the nucleus, the greater will be the binding energy of the electron.

The Periodic Table

The present-day periodic table lists the 92 naturally occurring elements and an additional 11 elements that have been created in the laboratory through scientific investigation (Table 2–2). The elements are listed in ascending order based on the atomic number located in the upper left corner. The atomic mass of the element is identified in the upper right corner. Each of the elements is also arranged into one of seven horizontal periods and one of eight vertical groups. The periods represent elements with the same principle quantum number or number of electron shells and the groups represent ele-

ments with the same number of electrons in the outermost shell. For example, each element in the eighth group has eight electrons in its outermost shell. These elements are chemically very stable atoms.

The number of electrons in the outermost shell of an atom determines the chemical combining characteristic or **valence** of the element. An element that has only one electron in the outermost shell is described as having a valence of $+1$ and would be located in Group I on the periodic table. This element will freely give up this electron to bind with another element to form a compound. An element that has seven electrons in its outermost shell has a valence of -1 and would be located in Group VII.

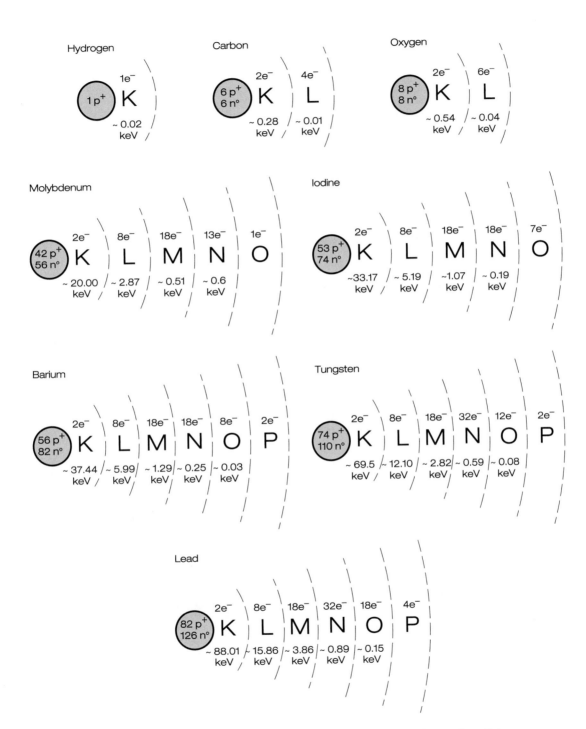

FIGURE 2–5. The atomic configurations and binding energies of elements that have significance in radiology.

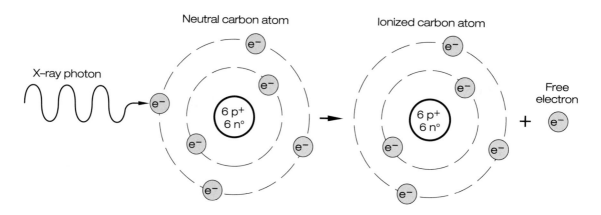

Neutral carbon atom

Ionized carbon atom

X–ray photon

6 p+
6 n°

Free electron

6 p+
6 n°

FIGURE 2–6. An x-ray photon can interact with an electron and eject it from an atom. This removal of an electron results in the ionization of the atom.

This element will freely accept an electron to form a chemical bond because atoms prefer the stable octet configuration. An example of this bond, known as an ionic bond, is the salt molecule. Sodium (Na), having a valence of +1, can easily combine with Chlorine (Cl), with a valence of −1, to form sodium chloride (NaCl), salt (Figure 2–7). The valence of an element determines the way the atoms will combine in definite proportions. Because of the element's valence number, **two** hydrogen atoms combine with **one** oxygen atom to form water. Hydrogen has a valence of +1 while oxygen has a valence of −2. Oxygen has room for two hydrogen

atoms and will share electrons, a type of bond known as a covalent bond (Figure 2–8).

Types of Energy

Energy is the ability to do work. It exists in many different forms. Regardless of form, all types of energy possess an actual or potential ability to do work. Work is the result of a force acting upon an object over a distance. It is expressed in the equation **work = force × distance**. When a force acts upon an object over a distance, ener-

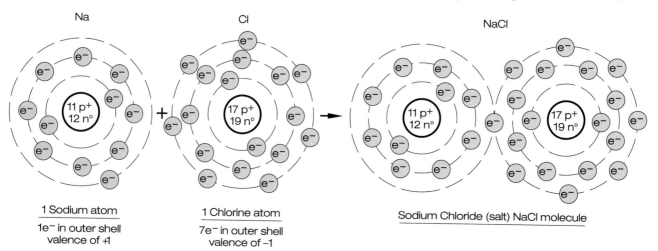

Na

Cl

NaCl

11 p+
12 n°

17 p+
19 n°

11 p+
12 n°

17 p+
19 n°

1 Sodium atom

1e⁻ in outer shell
valence of +1

1 Chlorine atom

7e⁻ in outer shell
valence of –1

Sodium Chloride (salt) NaCl molecule

FIGURE 2–7. An ionic bond is formed between sodium (Na) and chlorine (Cl) to form table salt, sodium chloride (NaCl).

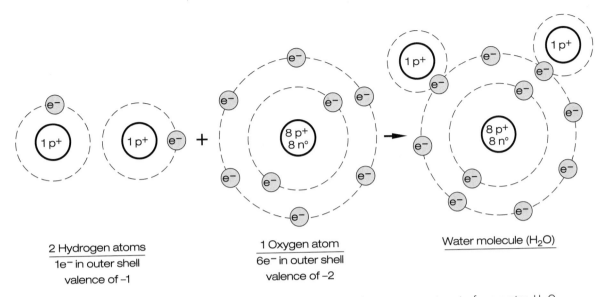

2 Hydrogen atoms
1e⁻ in outer shell
valence of –1

1 Oxygen atom
6e⁻ in outer shell
valence of –2

Water molecule (H_2O)

FIGURE 2–8. A covalent bond is formed between two hydrogen atoms and one oxygen atom to form water, H_2O.

gy is expended. For example, when a book is lifted one foot above a table, work is done and energy is expended. If the same book is lifted two feet above the table, twice as much work and energy are expended.

Mechanical
Mechanical energy is the result of the action of machines or physical movement. There are two types of mechanical energy: potential and kinetic. **Potential energy** is the energy that an object has because of its position. It is stored, by virtue of its position, in the object until it is converted to another form of energy. A car located at the top of a hill possesses more potential energy than the same car located at the bottom of a hill. If the car's brakes are released, the potential energy is then converted to kinetic energy as the car moves to the bottom of the hill (and a lower energy state). **Kinetic energy** is the energy of motion. An object in motion is able to perform work because it is moving. For example, the energy of water as it moves in a river can be used to perform work. When a dam is built across a river, the kinetic energy of the moving water can be used to produce electric energy. No electricity will be produced if the water is not moving.

Chemical
Chemical energy is the form of energy released during a chemical reaction. A battery operates

using chemical energy. The purpose of a battery is to convert chemical energy into electrical energy.

Heat
Heat, also called **thermal energy**, is the result of the motion of atoms and molecules. The faster the atoms and molecules within a substance are moving or vibrating, the greater the thermal energy of the substance. **Temperature** is a measure of thermal energy. As the temperature of a substance increases, the motion of the atoms in the substance increases. When a pan of water is placed on an electric burner, the electrical energy is converted to heat energy, which raises the temperature of the water and increases the motion of its atoms and molecules.

Electrical
Electrical energy, or **electricity**, is the result of the movement of electrons (electrical charges). Electricity is the study of resting or moving electrical charges. There are numerous appliances that operate by the use of electrical energy. When a lamp is turned on, a flow of electrons passes along a wire in a light bulb. The light bulb is a device that converts electrical energy to light, which is a form of electromagnetic energy. In a toaster, electrical energy is converted to heat, or thermal energy.

Nuclear

Nuclear energy is stored in the nucleus of each atom and holds the nuclear particles in a tight bond. A tremendous amount of energy is stored in the nucleus of an atom. In the 1940s scientists working at the University of Chicago learned how to control the release of this energy and, as a result of this knowledge, developed the atomic bomb. Today, nuclear power plants convert nuclear energy, within a very controlled environment, to electricity.

Electromagnetic

Electromagnetic energy is a form of energy that is the result of electric and magnetic disturbances in space (Figure 2–9). This type of energy travels through space as a combination of electric and magnetic fields and is produced by the acceleration of a charge. There are many very familiar forms of electromagnetic energy, including radio waves, microwaves, infrared light, visible light, and cosmic rays. X-rays are a form of man-made electromagnetic energy that is created in an x-ray tube when high-speed electrons are suddenly stopped. Physically they are identical to gamma rays, differing only in origin. Gamma rays originate from the nucleus of radioactive materials, while x-rays originate in an x-ray tube.

Electromagnetic Spectrum

Electromagnetic radiation is a natural part of the environment in which we live. Although the term may not be a common one, we are all familiar with many forms of this energy. The nature of electromagnetic radiation was discovered in scientific experiments using visible light. Visible light was shown to have both electric and magnetic properties and was therefore described as being electromagnetic. Shortly after these investigations, other forms of electromagnetic radiation, invisible to man, were studied and a theory to explain this form of energy was proposed.

Electromagnetic radiation (EM) spans a continuum of wide ranges of magnitudes of energy. This continuum is termed the **electromagnetic spectrum** (Figure 2–10). The electromagnetic spectrum details all of the various forms of EM radiation. One of the common properties of all forms of EM radiation is velocity. The velocity of EM energy is equal to the speed of light (c), which is 3

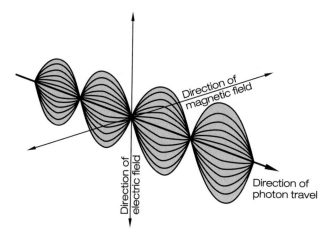

FIGURE 2–9. Overlapping sine waves, one representing an electric field and the other a magnetic field, illustrate electromagnetic radiation.

$\times\ 10^8$ meters/second (186,400 miles per second) in a vacuum.

Electromagnetic radiation with energies of approximately 10 eV and higher are capable of ionizing an atom or molecule. Ultraviolet, x-ray, and gamma radiations are all capable of ionization. When they interact with matter they can remove an electron from an orbital shell. Electromagnetic radiation is also capable of transferring energy to an atom by a process known as **excitation**. In the excitation process, electrons in an atom are moved to a higher energy state without actually being removing from the atom.

In studying EM radiation scientists found that under certain circumstances it behaved as a wave and at other times it behaved as a particle. **This dual nature is known as the wave-particle duality of radiation. To best understand x-rays, it is necessary to consider them as both waves and particles of energy.**

Wave Theory

Electromagnetic energy travels through space in the form of waves. Waves are disturbances in a medium. Ocean waves and sound waves are examples of disturbances of the mediums of water and air. When a rock is dropped into water, waves result. During speech, sound waves are created as disturbances in the air. **Electromagnetic waves are unique in that no medium is required.** They can travel in a vacuum.

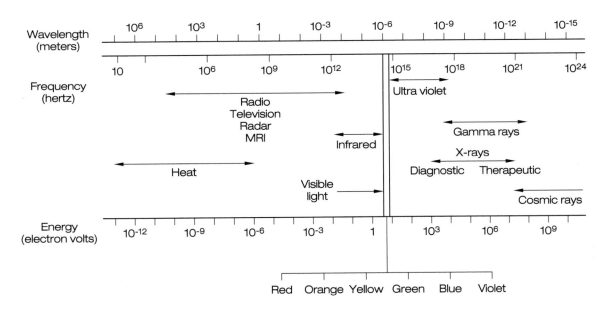

FIGURE 2–10. The electromagnetic spectrum.

All types of waves have an associated wavelength, frequency, amplitude, and period. To illustrate the wave concept, a sine wave is used because electromagnetic waves travel in the form of a sine wave (Figure 2–11). Sine waves can be mathematically described but these definitions are beyond the scope of this book. Instead, we will use the primary descriptions of electromagnetic waves: wavelength and frequency. The **wavelength** is the distance between any two successive points on a wave. Wavelength is usually measured from crest to crest or trough to trough. It is represented by the Greek letter **lambda** (λ), the character for length. Wavelengths vary from kilometers to Angstroms. The Angstrom (represented by the symbol Å) is equal to 10^{-10} meters, which is one ten-billionth of a meter. The Angstrom is of special interest because the wavelength of diagnostic x-rays is $0.1-0.5$ Å. **Amplitude** is the intensity of the wave defined by its maximal height.

The **frequency** is the number of waves that passes a particular point in a given time frame, or the number of cycles per second. It is represented by the Greek letter **nu** (ν), the initial for number. The unit of frequency is the hertz (Hz) or cycles per second (cps). **Period** is the time required to complete one cycle of the wave.

A relationship exists between the frequency, wavelength and velocity of a wave. This relationship is expressed by the formula:

velocity = frequency × wavelength,
or c = $\nu\lambda$

where: c = constant (the speed of light)
        ν = the frequency
        λ = the wavelength

This is known as the wave equation. Recall that with electromagnetic waves, velocity was a constant equal to the speed of light. Because velocity is a constant, an increase in frequency would result in an associated decrease in wavelength and vice versa. Therefore, **frequency and wavelength are inversely proportional.**

Radiation along the electromagnetic spectrum will vary according to the associated frequency and wavelength. Low frequencies and long wavelengths are at the bottom end of the spectrum with radio waves and microwaves, visible light is in the center of the spectrum, and at the top of the spectrum are gamma and x-rays, with associated high frequencies and short wavelengths.

Particle Theory

When high-frequency electromagnetic radiation interacts with matter, it behaves more like

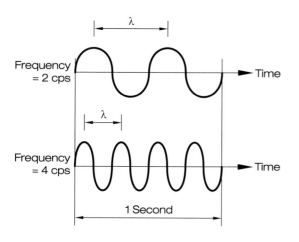

FIGURE 2-11. Two sine waves. With electromagnetic waves, if wavelength decreases, frequency will increase.

a particle than a wave. With this model, electromagnetic radiation acts like a small bundle of energy, known as a **photon** or **quantum**. The photon carries a specific amount of energy that is dependent upon frequency. **Photon energy and frequency are directly proportional.** If the frequency of an x-ray is doubled, the energy is doubled. This relationship was first described by the German physicist Max Planck (1858–1947). The relationship between photon energy and frequency is mathematically described in the formula:

$$E = h\nu$$

where: E = photon energy (eV)
 h = Planck's constant
 $(4.15 \times 10^{-15}$ eV-sec)
 ν = photon frequency (Hz)

From this formula, it is possible to calculate the frequency of an x-ray when given the x-ray photon's energy.

Example: What is the frequency of a 72 keV x-ray photon?

Answer:

$$E = h\nu$$
$$\nu = \frac{E}{h}$$

$$\nu = \frac{72\,\text{keV}}{4.15 \times 10^{-15}\ \text{eV-sec}}$$

$$\nu = \frac{7.2 \times 10^4\ \text{eV}}{4.15 \times 10^{-15}\ \text{eV-sec}}$$

$$\nu = 1.73 \times 10^{19}\ \text{Hz}$$

The Discovery of X-Rays

On November 8, 1895, the German physicist Wilhelm Conrad Röntgen discovered an unusual phenomenon while working at his laboratory at the University of Würzburg. Röntgen had been repeating various experiments with cathode rays, notably those of his colleagues Hertz, Hittorf, Crookes and Lenard. These investigators had developed equipment for exploring the effects of high tension discharges in evacuated glass tubes. By late 1895 this small group of physicists was beginning to explore the properties of cathode rays outside the tubes. Early in November of 1895 Röntgen was repeating an experiment with one of Lenard's tubes in which a thin aluminum window had been added to permit the cathode rays to exit the tube. Lenard had supplied the tube with a tightly fitting cardboard covering to protect the aluminum window from damage by the strong electrostatic field necessary to produce the cathode rays. This covering also prevented any visible light from escaping. Röntgen had successfully repeated the experiment and had observed that the invisible cathode rays caused a fluorescent effect on a small cardboard screen painted with barium platinocyanide when it was placed very close to the aluminum window.

It occurred to Röntgen that the Hittorf-Crookes tube, which had a much thicker glass wall than the Lenard tube, might also cause this fluorescent effect. In the late afternoon of November 8 he determined to test his idea. He carefully constructed a black cardboard covering similar to the one he had used on the Lenard tube. He covered the Hittorf-Crookes tube with the covering and attached electrodes to the Ruhmkorff coil to generate an electrostatic charge. Before setting up the barium platinocyanide screen to test his idea, Röntgen darkened the room to test the opacity of his cardboard cover. As he passed the Ruhmkorff coil charge through the tube, he determined that the cover was light-tight and turned to prepare the next step of the experiment. It was at this point that he noticed a faint shimmering from a bench a meter away from the tube. To be sure he tried several more discharges and saw the same shimmering effect each time. Striking a match, Röntgen discovered the shimmering had come from the location of the barium platinocyanide screen he had been intending to use next.

Röntgen spent the next few hours repeating the experiment again and again. He quickly determined that the screen would fluoresce at a distance from the tube much greater than in his previous tests. He speculated that a new kind of ray might be responsible. November 8 was a Friday, and Röntgen took advantage of the weekend to repeat his experiments and make his first notes. In the following weeks he investigated nearly all the known properties of the rays, even eating and sleeping in his laboratory.

Röntgen's discovery of x-rays was no accident and he was not working alone. With the investigations he and his colleagues in various countries were pursuing, the discovery was imminent. The idea that he just happened to notice the barium platinocyanide screen totally misrepresents his investigative powers. He had planned to use the screen in the next step of the experiment.

At one point while he was investigating the ability of various materials to stop the rays, he brought a small piece of lead into position while a discharge was occurring. Imagine Röntgen's astonishment as he saw the first radiographic image, his own flickering ghostly skeleton on the barium platinocyanide screen. He later reported it was at this point that he determined to continue his experiments in secrecy, because he feared for his professional reputation if his observations were in error.

Röntgen became the first radiographer when he produced a series of four photographs to accompany the first draft of his paper: the hand of his wife (Figure 2–12), a set of weights, a compass, and a piece of metal. Röntgen's original paper, "On a New Kind of Rays," was published 50 days later on December 28. It is translated in Appendix A. Röntgen assigned the mathematical term for an unknown, X, to the rays he discovered. In later years they were officially given his name to honor his work. Today either term, x-rays or Röntgen rays, is acceptable. Röntgen published a total of three papers on

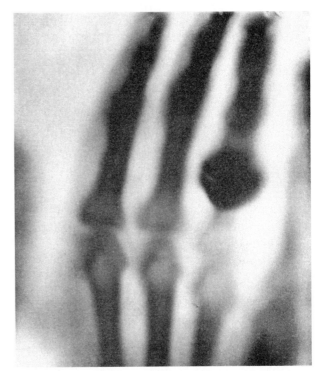

FIGURE 2-12. The first x-ray image of the human hand. The radiograph was taken by Dr. Röntgen of his wife's hand.

x-rays between 1895 and 1897. His investigative powers were so phenomenal that none of his conclusions have yet been proven false. Röntgen received many honors for his discovery, including, in 1901, the first Nobel prize for physics. He died of carcinoma of the bowel in 1923.

X-Ray Properties

When Röntgen began his study of the invisible x-rays, it was unlikely that he would be able to identify all of the properties of this new discovery. Röntgen's investigation was so thorough, however, that no scientist since has been able to add to the list of properties Röntgen identified.

Through his use of the scientific method, Röntgen found that x-rays:

1. Are highly penetrating, invisible rays which are a form of electromagnetic radiation.

2. Are electrically neutral and therefore not affected by either electric or magnetic fields.

3. Can be produced over a wide variety of energies and wavelengths (polyenergetic and heterogeneous).

4. Release very small amounts of heat upon passing through matter.

5. Travel in straight lines.

6. Travel at the speed of light, 3×10^8 meters per second in a vacuum.

7. Can ionize matter.

8. Cause fluorescence (the emission of light) of certain crystals.

9. Cannot be focused by a lens.

10. Affect photographic film.

11. Produce chemical and biological changes in matter through ionization and excitation.

12. Produce secondary and scatter radiation.

Summary

The physical universe can best be understood through physics—the study of matter and energy and their inter-relationships. Matter is the substance which comprises all physical objects. The smallest subdivision of matter is the atom, which is comprised of three basic subatomic particles: the proton, the neutron and the electron. Energy is the ability to do work. There are many forms of energy, including x-rays, which are a form of electromagnetic radiation. Matter and energy cannot be created or destroyed but are interchangeable, as described in Einstein's theory of relativity ($E = mc^2$).

The atom is best described as having a small, dense center, known as the nucleus, that is surrounded by electrons located within orbital shells. Protons and neutrons are located within the nucleus and are responsible for almost all of the mass of an atom. The electron is located outside the nucleus and has a relatively insignificant mass. Protons possess a positive charge, electrons possess a negative charge and neutrons are electrically neutral.

Each of the elements has its own specific number of nuclear protons. This is the key characteristic that distinguishes one element from another. The number of nuclear protons in an atom is known as the atomic number or Z number. The periodic table lists the elements in ascending order according to the element's atomic number.

Electromagnetic radiation behaves as both a wave and a particle. As a wave, EM radiation has an associated frequency and wavelength. As a particle, it behaves as a bundle of energy, called a photon. X-rays are a man-made form of electromagnetic radiation that is created when high-speed electrons are suddenly stopped. X-rays were discovered by Wilhelm Conrad Röntgen on November 8, 1895, in Germany. From his thorough investigation, twelve properties of x-rays were identified.

REVIEW QUESTIONS

1. What are the two major branches of natural science?

2. How do matter and energy differ?

3. Define an atom and a molecule.

4. What are the three basic subatomic particles?

5. What is ionization?

6. What is the formula used to determine the maximum number of electrons that can be contained in a given shell? How many electrons can be contained in the N-shell?

7. The periodic table of elements arranges the elements into periods and groups. How are the elements similar within each period? within each group?

8. How do radiations differ along the electromagnetic spectrum?

9. List five types of energy.

10. For electromagnetic radiation, what is the relationship between frequency and wavelength? between frequency and photon energy?

11. List five properties of x-rays.

REFERENCES AND RECOMMENDED READING

Ball, J. L. & Moore, A. D. (1986). *Essential physics for radiographers* (2nd ed.). Oxford: Blackwell Scientific Publications.

Bushberg, J. T., Seibert, J. A., Leidholdt, E. M., & Boone, J. M. (1994) *The essential physics of medical imaging.* Baltimore: Williams & Wilkins.

Bushong, S. C. (1997). *Radiologic science for technologists: Physics, biology, and protection* (6th ed.). St. Louis: C. V. Mosby.

Curry, T. S., Dowdey, J. E., Murry, R. C. (1990). *Christensen's introduction to the physics of diagnostic radiology* (4th ed.). Philadelphia: Lea and Febiger.

Eisenberg, R. L. (1992). *Radiology: An illustrated history.* St. Louis: C. V. Mosby.

Fuchs, A. W. (1960). Radiography of 1896. *Image.* 9, 4–17.

Funke, H. & Friege, H. (1980). *Das Geburtshaus Wilhelm Conrad Röntgens in Remscheid-Lennep.* Remscheid, Germany: Deutsches Röntgen-Museum.

Funke, T. (1961). William Conrad Röentgen, the German Museum, and you. *The X-Ray Technician. 32*(Nov.), 193-194.

Glasser, O. (1958). *Dr. W. C. Röentgen* (2nd ed.). Springfield, IL: Charles C. Thomas.

Graham, B. J. & Thomas, W. N. (1975). *An introduction to physics for radiologic technologists.* Philadelphia: W. B. Saunders.

Handbook of chemistry and physics (69th ed.). (1989). Boca Raton, FL: CRC Press.

Hennig, U. (1989). *Deutsches Röntgen-Museum Remscheid-Lennep.* Remscheid, Germany: Westermann.

Johns, H. E. & Cunningham, J. R. (1983). *The physics of radiology* (4th ed.). Springfield, IL: Charles C. Thomas.

Meredith, W. J. & Massey, J. B. (1977). *Fundamental physics of radiology* (3rd ed.). Chicago: Yearbook Medical Publishers.

Palmer, P. E. S. (1994). The town where Röentgen was born. *Radiology.* 193(3), 607–609.

Ridgway, A. & Thumm, W. (1973). *The physics of medical radiography.* Reading, MA: Addison-Wesley Publishing.

Röntgen, W. C. (1896). On a new kind of rays. *Nature. 53* (1369), 274–276.

Röntgen, W. C. (1869). On a new kind of rays, *Science.* 3(59), 227–231.

Selman, J. C. (1994). *The fundamentals of x-ray and radium physics* (9th ed.). Springfield, IL: Charles C. Thomas.

Sprawls, P. (1987). *Physical principles of medical imaging.* Rockville, MD: Aspen Publishers.

Streller, E. (1961). The enlarged German Röentgen Museum. *The X-Ray Technician. 32*(Nov.), 194–197.

Sutherland, C. G. (1937). Röentgen and his discovery. *The X-Ray Technician. 8,* 143–149.

Ter-Pogossian, M. M. (1967). *The physical aspects of diagnostic radiology.* New York: Hoeber Medical Division, Harper & Row.

Thumm, W. (1974). Röntgen's discovery revisited. *Canadian Journal of Radiography, Radiotherapy, and Nuclear Medicine.* 5(1), 22-28.

Tortorici, M. (1992). *Concepts in medical radiographic imaging.* Philadelphia: W. B. Saunders.

Wilks, R. J. (1981). *Principles of radiological physics.* Edinburgh: Churchill Livingstone.

CHAPTER 3

Electricity

The experience of life itself is the real test . . . for any . . . profession.

W. C. Röntgen.

OBJECTIVES

Upon completion of this chapter, the student should be able to:

- Explain the atomic nature of electricity.

- State the elementary laws of electrostatics.

- Describe the methods of electrification.

- Interpret the results of various electrostatic interactions.

- Differentiate conductors from insulators.

- Describe the basic factors of electrodynamics.

- Calculate the effect of changes in voltage, amperage and resistance according to Ohm's law.

- Calculate voltage, amperage and resistance in simple series and parallel circuits.

To control x-rays it is necessary to understand how they are produced. X-rays are produced when extremely high-energy electricity produces high-speed electrons that interact with matter. Electricity must be understood at the subatomic level for this process to become clear. The distribution and movement of electrons, along with their associated charges, make up electricity. Understanding atomic structure, including how electrons interact both in and outside of atoms, becomes the key to understanding electricity. It is the distribution and movement of atomic charges that can cause forces to interact.

Atoms contain both kinds of electrical charges, the **positive charge** of the proton, which is locked within the nucleus by very strong forces, and the **negative charge** of the electron, which is located outside the nucleus, bound by relatively weak forces. Electrons may not be associated with a nucleus at all, in which case they are called "free" electrons. In either case, **the positive charge of the proton and the negative charge of the electron are equal in strength.** Because electrons, with their negative charges, are free to move between atomic orbital shells and even between atoms, electricity concerns the distribution and movement of electrons and has little to do with the positively charged protons locked within the atomic nucleus.

Electrostatics

Electrostatics is the study of the distribution of fixed charges, or electrons that at rest. Just as all atoms are charged (neutral, positive, negative), objects become charged by their composite individual atomic charges. Some atoms include electrons in their outer shells, or beyond the outer shell but within the atom's sphere of influence, that are very easily removed. There are instances, as when walking across a heavy rug in winter, when electrons are easily transferred (literally scooped up) onto another object. It is this type of distribution and redistribution of charged electrons that makes up electrostatics.

The term **electrification** is used to describe the process of electron charges being added to or subtracted from an object. When one object has more electrons than another it also has more negative charges. Therefore it can be considered to be negatively electrified, or to

have a **negative charge**. The concept of positive electrification, a positive charge, is more complicated because protons, which carry true positive charges, are not easily distributed. Therefore a **positive charge** usually refers to something with a weaker negative charge, or fewer electrons. The so-called positively electrified, charged, object has a negative charge; it is just a weaker negative charge than the object with which it is being compared. It is less negative, and therefore termed positive, by comparison. It is important to remember that electrification is a relative term and that nearly all objects have negative charges. **When discussing electricity, the terms negative and positive refer to the relationship between two objects, not to their true atomic charges.**

In conjunction with the idea that negative and positive charges are relative to each other, another concept is required in order to establish a neutral reference point. This is done by defining the earth as **zero or ground potential**. Because the earth contains what is essentially an infinite number of charges, both positive and negative, in equal distribution, it is considered to be neutral and is the reference point for discussing charges. It has zero potential because the equally balanced charges have no potential to perform work and release energy. The symbol for ground is $\perp\!\!\!=$.

Laws of Electrostatics

Before attempting to understand how objects are electrified, it is helpful to learn five fundamental **laws of electrostatics**. These important laws have many corollaries in physics and will be used again and again throughout this book. The five laws are:

1. **Repulsion-attraction** (Figure 3–1). Like charges repel; unlike charges attract.

2. **The inverse square law** (Figure 3–2). The force between two charges is directly proportional to the product of their magnitudes and inversely proportional to the square of the distance between them. As a charged object gets further away, the influencing charge decreases because of the increased area it affects. The law is expressed as:

$$\frac{I_1}{I_2} = \frac{D_2^2}{D_1^2}$$

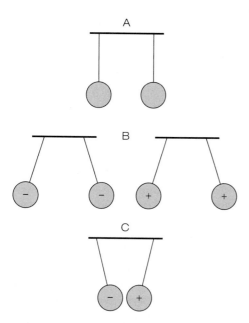

FIGURE 3–1. Repulsion-attraction law: (A) neutral charges, (B) repulsion of like charges, and (C) attraction of unlike charges.

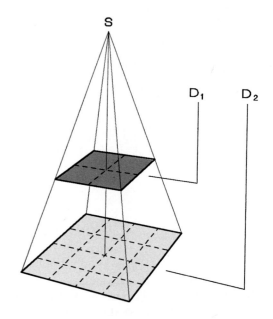

FIGURE 3–2. The inverse square law: if S is the source and D^2 is twice the distance of D^1, the area covered by the diverging field at D^2 is four times the area covered at D^1.

where:

$$I_1 = \text{old intensity}$$
$$I_2 = \text{new intensity}$$
$$D_1{}^2 = \text{old distance squared}$$
$$D_2{}^2 = \text{new distance squared}$$

Example: If an object has a charge of 4 coulombs at 4 mm, what will the charge be at 8 mm?

Answer:

$$\frac{I_1}{I_2} = \frac{D_2{}^2}{D_1{}^2}$$

$$\frac{4 \text{ coulombs}}{x} = \frac{8\text{mm}^2}{4\text{mm}^2}$$

$$\frac{4}{x} = \frac{64}{16}$$

$$64x = 64$$

$$x = 1 \text{ coulomb}$$

In this example, as the distance doubled, the charge was reduced to 25 percent of its original value. Although this inverse square formula is usually sufficient for radiographic needs, it is important to understand that the true relationship of the force between two charges is accurately expressed in Coulomb's law:

$$F = \frac{kq_1q_2}{R^2}$$

where:

$$F = \text{electrostatic force in newtons}$$
$$k = \text{constant of proportionality}$$
$$(9 \times 10^9 \text{ for coulombs and meters})$$
$$q_1 \text{ and } q_2 = \text{charges in coulombs}$$
$$R = \text{distance in square meters}$$

This formula takes into account the true definition: the force between two charges (q^1 and q^2) is directly proportional to the product of their magnitudes ($q^1 \times q^2$), and inversely proportional to the square of the distance between them ($(q^1 \times q^2)/R^2$). Ironically, although the French physicist Coulomb (1736–1806) received the credit for development of this law, the original inquiry was initiated by the American scientist Benjamin Franklin (1706–1790).

3. **Distribution** (Figure 3–3). Charges reside on the external surfaces of conductors and equally throughout nonconductors. This law is a result of the effect of the repulsion-attraction law as electrons, all with negative charges, attempt to repel each other as much as possible. In a solid conductor this results in equal distribution on the surface, which is the point where electrons can obtain maximum distance from each other. In a nonconductor, such as a cloud, charge movement is not facilitated and equal distribution throughout the object results.

4. **Concentration** (Figure 3–4). The greatest concentration of charge will be on the surface where the curvature is sharpest. If enough electrons congregate they can induce ionization of the surrounding air and even discharge to the nearest point of lower concentration. Therefore x-ray tubes, which are subjected to extremely high charges, must not have sharp or rough edges where concentrations of elec-

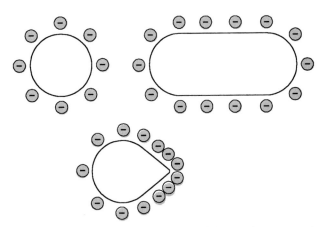

FIGURE 3–4. The law of concentration of charge: because each negative charge is repelled by all other negative charges, they tend to concentrate at points of greatest curvature.

trons could occur and discharge at the wrong moment or in an undesirable direction. Consequently, the interior components of x-ray tubes are rounded and highly polished to eliminate sharply curved surfaces.

5. **Movement.** Only negative charges move along solid conductors. Because the positive charges, the protons, are tightly bound inside the atomic nuclear field, only the electrons, which exist outside the nucleus, are easily moved along conductors.

Electrification

Objects can be electrified by three methods: **friction, contact** and **induction**.

Friction   Electrification by **friction** occurs when one object is rubbed against another and, due to differences in the number of electrons available on each, electrons travel from one to the other. Ideal conditions for electron transfer occur during cold weather when low humidity removes stabilizing electrons from the air, decreasing the resistance to electron movement between objects. An example is a common trick that delights children—rubbing a balloon against a wool sweater will permit the balloon to stick to a wall. In low humidity, electrons will transfer from the wool to the balloon, giving it a nega-

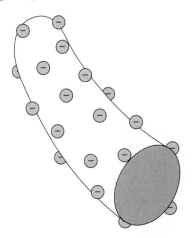

FIGURE 3–3. The law of distribution of charge: as individual electrons are repelled from one another, they distribute at the outer limits of a conductor.

tive charge which can cause it to stick to a smooth wall with a relatively positive charge. This is an example of opposites attracting one another. A common example of like charges repelling one another occurs when hair is electrified by friction during combing in low humidity conditions. The comb removes electrons from the strands of hair, often accompanied by crackling sounds, leaving each more positively charged. The strands are then repelled by those adjoining, which now also have stronger positive charges. The result is wild strands of hair standing straight out from your head. The solution to the problem is to increase the humidity, or the amount of water in the air, causing a slight condensation on all surfaces. This thin film of moisture becomes a pathway for the distribution of electrons. The use of a humidifier in a radiographic darkroom during cold weather thus helps eliminate electrostatic discharges that can cause artifacts on film.

Contact

Electrification by **contact** occurs when two objects touch, permitting electrons to move from one to the other. This process is a simple equalization of charges, with both objects having similar charges after the contact. Walking across a woolen carpet in a room with low humidity may cause shoes to scoop electrons from the carpet fibers that are then distributed over the entire body. This is an example of electrification by friction. However, when a positively charged object with fewer electrons is touched, the contact will cause electrons to move to the less negatively charged object in an attempt to equally distribute the charges. A metal doorknob or another person are examples of positively charged objects that would attract electrons from a person who had just walked across a rug. After the contact both objects would have a more equal distribution of electrons. This is caused by the individual force fields of the electrons satisfying the repulsion-attraction law over the entire surface of the conductors. In many instances actual physical contact does not occur before the electrons equalize. As soon as the oppositely charged objects are in close proximity, the electrons often jump the gap in the form of a **static discharge**. This occurs as soon as the difference in charges becomes sufficiently great and the intervening distance sufficiently small. In most cases the static discharge releases excess energy in the form of light photons. When this occurs between a piece of radiographic film and a cassette, darkroom bench or the

body of the person handling the film, the light forms an image on the film. Figure 3–5 illustrates one of the common types of static discharge that appears as a radiographic film artifact.

An electroscope is a simple device that illustrates the laws of electrostatics. It consists of a rod connected to a pair of thin, easily charged metallic leaves which are protected from air currents by a glass flask (Figure 3–6A). When a charged object (such as the metallic rod shown in Figure 3–6B) is brought into contact with the rod, the excess electrons obey the third law of electrostatics and distribute equally throughout the rod and leaves. The resultant increase in the number of electrons present on both leaves causes the two leaves to obey the first law of electrostatics and, since they possess like charges, repel each other. Consequently, it is possible to see the two leaves move further apart.

If an electroscope is subjected to an intense beam of ionizing x-ray photons, the air becomes ionized. The ionized atoms draw excess electrons from the leaves, thus

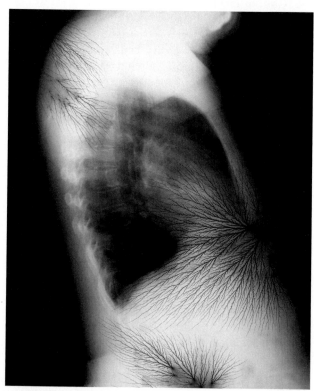

FIGURE 3–5. A typical tree-branch static discharge artifact on a radiograph.

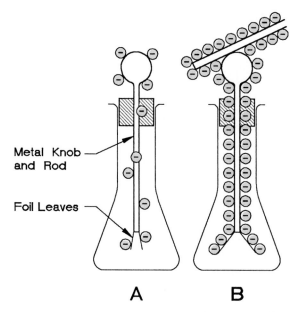

Metal Knob and Rod

Foil Leaves

A **B**

FIGURE 3–6. Charging an electroscope by contact: electrons distribute equally when they are permitted to move from one object (the rod) to another (the electroscope) by contact.

causing the charge on the leaves to be reduced. Consequently, the electroscope leaves relax and move closer together.

Induction   Electrification by **induction** is the most important method because it is the one used in the operation of electronic devices. **Induction is the process of electrical fields acting on one another without contact.** Every charged body is surrounded by a force field, much like the fields that surround individual atoms. Like atoms, force fields are a result of the composite forces of the charges residing within the object. These force fields are called **electric fields** and they can cause induction. When a strongly and a weakly charged object come close to one another, the electrical fields will begin to act on one another before contact occurs (Figure 3–7A). As can be seen in Figure 3–7B, charges will migrate to one end of an object in anticipation of contact. However, as seen in Figure 3–7C, when the stronger object is removed before contact, the charges in the weaker object will redistribute themselves as they were before the induction occurred. This temporarily induced movement of

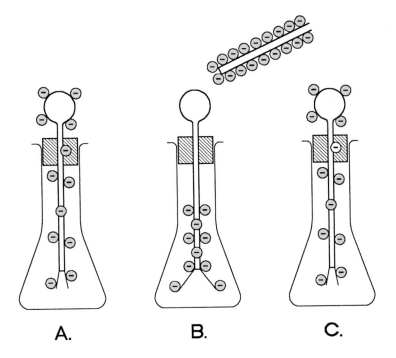

A. **B.** **C.**

FIGURE 3–7. Charging an electroscope by induction: electrons are induced to move away from the heavily charged rod (B) but return to their normal distribution when the rod is removed (A and C).

charges is useful in many electronic devices, such as motors, transformers and solenoids.

With an understanding of friction and induction electrification it becomes possible to understand one of the greatest of natural phenomena—lightning. Lightning discharges occur as the masses of atoms making up the water vapor in clouds move rapidly through the atmosphere. Under conditions where many electrons are available, such as when there are numerous storm clouds, the movement of the water vapor atoms tends to cause electrons to be picked up or lost. As an individual cloud becomes predominantly positively or negatively charged, it becomes a candidate for a huge electrostatic discharge. Clouds often pick up electrons on their upper edges and lose them on their lower edges and vice versa. In these instances the difference in charges makes the cloud a candidate for a cloud-to-cloud discharge as soon as the insulating effect of the vapor between the two surfaces has been overcome. But the most interesting part of lightning is cloud-to-ground discharges. The ground often develops a temporary opposite charge from the underside of the cloud because of the induction effect of the cloud on the ground. This causes the electrons to spread out, which in turn tends to rapidly increase the difference in charges between cloud and ground and can quickly overcome the insulating effect of the air between the cloud and the ground. The result is lightning discharges occurring much more rapidly than if induction had not taken place. Lightning discharges do not occur as a single transfer of electrons from one area to another. Instead, vast numbers of electrons may be transferred from cloud to ground, overloading the ground, which in turn transfers electrons back to the cloud, which again transfers them to the ground, over and over until the charges are somewhat equally distributed. A short lightning discharge often transfers electrons back and forth between cloud and ground many times within a microsecond.

Electrodynamics

Electrons that are moving in predominantly the same direction are often referred to as an **electric current**. A number of conditions encourage electron movement, thus permitting the flow of electric current. A **vacuum** is a space from which air has been removed. Since it has few atoms to oppose electron flow, it is especially useful in permitting electrons to reach the speed necessary to produce x-rays. Some **gasses** (such as neon) will promote the drift of electrons from a negative electrode (cathode) to a positive electrode (anode). These gasses also promote the drift of positive ions toward the negative cathode while negative ions move toward the positive anode. **Ionic solutions** can cause electrons to migrate to positive or negative poles during electrolysis, when they are subjected to an electric current.

Electrolysis becomes possible when two neutral atoms with complementary valences (i.e., -1 and $+1$) are brought together in a solution. They become ions in the solution when the positive valence atom gives up an outer-shell electron to the negative valence atom. The atom missing an electron becomes a positive ion (because a negative charge has been removed) while the one receiving the electron becomes a negative ion (because a negative charge has been added). When metallic rods are connected to a battery and immersed in the solution, the negative pole will attract the positive ions while the positive pole will attract the negative ions. This migration of electrons during the electrolytic process comprises an electrical current. **Metallic conductors**, such as copper wire, are the most common pathways provided for the movement of electrical current. The atoms of metallic conductors permit valence electrons to drift. In common household wiring the actual physical movement is about 2 mm per second (Figure 3–8). The electrical current, as a whole, is similar to a tube filled with balls, as in Figure 3–9. If the tube is full and a new ball is pushed into one end, a ball will drop instantly from the far end, although each ball moved or drifted only a short distance. Electrons move along a conductor with a similar domino effect, resulting in movement of electrons at the far end. This movement occurs extremely rapidly, nearly at the speed of light (3×10^8 meters/second).

The movement of electrons is facilitated by materials that easily permit electrons to flow. These materials are called **conductors** and **superconductors**. Examples of conductors are metals such as copper and aluminum. Conversely, electron movement is inhibited by materials that resist the flow of electrons. These nonconducting materials are called **insulators**. Examples of insulators are

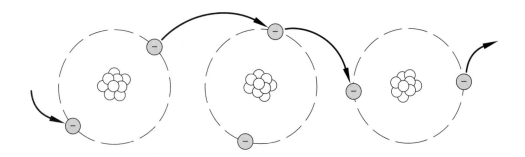

FIGURE 3–8. Electron drift along a conductor.

plastic, rubber and glass. The third classification of materials is **semiconductors**. They have the ability to conduct under certain conditions and insulate under others. The actual conditions causing these changes in conductivity are complex and are addressed later in this chapter. They result primarily from changes in the energy states of atoms, causing outer-shell electrons to move in a particular direction (Table 3–1).

An **electrical circuit** is a pathway (commonly copper wire) that permits electrons to move in a complete circle from their source, through resisting electrical devices and back to the source. As in electrostatics, an electrical circuit must have an excess charge at one end and a comparative deficiency at the other to allow electrons to flow. There are several sources of the excess electrons necessary to cause current flow. Examples include **batteries**, which convert chemical energy to electrical; **generators**, which convert mechanical energy to electrical; **solar converters**, which convert solar photons to electrical energy; and **atomic reactors**, which convert nuclear energy to electrical. Only batteries and generators are efficient devices at present. Solar converters and atomic reactors have yet to be developed to directly convert energy for widespread commercial use. Solar converters remain expensive while nuclear reactors, although efficient on a large scale, continue to meet significant public opposition. They operate by using the massive energy of the atom to produce steam, which is then used to run turbine generators.

Describing Current Flow

Electrons move from the highest concentration to the lowest. There is much confusion regarding how to describe their movement because early pioneers in electrical phenomena assumed that the moving charges were positive when actually they were negatively charged electrons. The negative pole is the source of electrons that move toward the positive receiving pole. Consequently,

TABLE 3–1. Properties of Conducting Materials

State	Material	Characteristics
Insulator	Plastic, Rubber, Glass	Large energy difference between conduction and valence bands; resists electron flow.
Semiconductor	Silicon, Germanium	Small energy difference between conduction and valence bands; conducts OR resists, depending on temperature and other conditions.
Conductor	Copper, Aluminum	Overlapping conduction and valence bands; conducts with minor resistance, varying depending on temperature and other conditions.
Superconductor	Titanium	Greatly overlapping conduction and valence bands; conducts with little or no electrical potential; most current systems require extreme cold to function although research indicates room temperature superconductors may be developed soon.

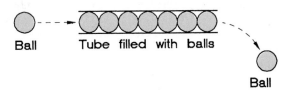

FIGURE 3–9. As when balls are pushed into a tube, each electron needs to move only a short distance for the effect of current movement to be achieved at the other end.

conventional electric current is described as going from positive to negative poles while electron flow is actually from negative to positive poles.

It is important to specify whether descriptions are of electrical current or electron flow, as they are exact opposites. It may be useful to think of negative charges moving in one direction as being equivalent to a positive charge effect in the opposite direction. The importance of these definitions will become apparent later in this text, especially when discussing the interactions of both electrical and magnetic forces.

The nature of the flow of electrons that make up an electric current can be described in many different ways. The most common factors used as descriptors are the **quantity** of electrons flowing, the **force** with which they travel, the amount of **opposition** to the current flow in the circuit and the **direction** of travel.

The **direction** of travel of the electrons is defined as either **direct current (DC)**, when all electrons move in the same direction, or **alternating current (AC)**, when electrons move first in one direction and then reverse and move in the opposite direction. Through the use of various electrical devices, which we will investigate later, it is possible to change the current from DC to AC and back, as necessary.

Current

The **quantity,** or number, of electrons flowing is sometimes referred to as the **current**. It is useful to think of the measurement of current as the number of electrons flowing past a given point per unit of time (usually per second). The French scientist André Ampère (1775–1836) did much original work in defining electricity and magnetism. Consequently, the unit of current bears his name. The **ampere** is sometimes called the **amp** for short and is represented by the symbol **A**. It consists of the movement of 6.24×10^{18} **electrons per second** past a given point; therefore the technical definition is **one coulomb of electrical charge flowing per second (1 ampere = 1 coulomb/1 second).** Earlier, the drift of electrons was given as less than 1 mm per second. The fact that one ampere flowing in a household wire causes 6,240,000,000,000,000,000 electrons to move less than 1 mm per second should help in understanding the small size of electrons. Diagnostic radiographic equipment uti-

lizes milliamperage units to regulate the number of electrons available to produce x-ray photons. The milliamperage (**mA**) is found on nearly all x-ray machines and adjustment by the radiographer operating the equipment will cause the number of electrons and the number of x-ray photons produced to vary. The adjustment of an x-ray machine to add an additional 100 mA (a common increment) causes 6.24×10^{17} more electrons per second to pass through the x-ray tube.

Example: If an x-ray machine is operating at 0.01 seconds and the amperage is 100 mA, how many electrons would move through the tube?

Answer:

$(6.24 \times 10^{17}$ electrons/second$) \times 0.01$ seconds= 6.24×10^{15} (6.24 million billion or 6,240,000,000,000,000)

The word current is used to describe the presence of electron flow as well as to describe exactly how much current is flowing. It is important to distinguish which use of the word is intended.

Potential Difference

The **force** with which the electrons travel is a function of the difference between the number of electrons in excess at one end of the circuit and the deficiency at the other end. The attempt of the unequal forces to balance is the cause of the force of electron movement. Because the difference is present while the source is connected into the circuit, **there does not have to be an actual flow of current for the difference to exist.** Therefore the simple potential for a difference is used to describe the force, or strength of movement, behind electrons.

Potential difference is the best term to describe the **force** or **strength** of electron flow. It should be remembered that potential difference continues to exist even when a switch is opened in a circuit, breaking the actual flow of electrons (current). Because potential difference is the prime force causing electrical devices to convert electrical energy to mechanical, the term **electromotive force (emf)** has also been used. Electromotive force is actually the total maximum difference of potential between the positive and negative ends of the electron source, but it is not incorrect to use the term in place of potential difference.

The unit of potential difference is the **volt**, represented by the symbol **V** (named for the Italian physicist Alessandro Volta [1745–1827]). The term voltage is also used to describe potential difference. The technical definition of a volt is **1 joule (J) of work done on one coulomb of charge (1 volt=1 joule/1 coulomb)**. A joule is the SI unit for both mechanical energy and work.

Thus, for the reasons previously stated, the force with which electrons travel can be described by the terms **potential difference, electromotive force (emf) and voltage (V).**

As the current flows along the circuit, the potential difference is reduced because the closer the electrons come to the deficient end of the circuit, the further they are from the excess end (the driving source) and the closer they are to becoming part of the deficiency themselves. With this understanding of potential difference, the concept of grounding electrical circuits for safety should become clear. When equipment is properly grounded and the radiographer, who is also grounded, comes in contact, there is no potential difference. However, when equipment is not properly grounded, the radiographer may become a better path to ground. The passage of electrons (voltage) through the radiographer may be shocking, to say the least.

High voltage is extremely dangerous because there does not have to be an actual flow of current for the potential difference to exist. This means high potential difference or voltage remains a hazard at all times (and explains why warnings must be posted in these areas). All that is required for a high difference in voltage to achieve equalization is for a conductor to present itself. If this happens to be a patient who inadvertently uses a wet hand to grasp a cracked high-voltage cable or a radiographer who touches two connection points inside a control console, the shocking result is the same.

Resistance

The amount of opposition to the current in the circuit is called the **resistance.** Research into the interrelationships of current, potential difference, and resistance was done by the German physicist Georg Ohm (1787–1854). As a result, the unit of resistance is called the **ohm**. It is represented by the symbol Ω (omega). The technical definition of an ohm is the resistance to a flow of current provided by a column of mercury 106.3 cm long with a diameter of 1 mm^2 at 0° C. A practical definition of an ohm will be provided later, based on the interaction of several characteristics of a conductor. Resistance and impedance are the terms used to describe current opposition. There are numerous factors that impede the flow of electrons, thus increasing resistance. The primary factors for electrical circuits are the **ability to conduct** electrons, the **length** of the conductor, the cross-sectional **diameter** and **temperature**.

When the expression 1/R is used, the resistance of a DC circuit is measured as **conductance** while that of an AC circuit is measured as **admittance**. The SI unit for conductance and admittance is the siemens, which is represented by the symbol S and is named after the English electrical engineer Sir William Siemens (1823–1883), brother of Werner von Siemens, founder of the German electrical and x-ray equipment corporation.

The **ability to conduct** electrons has already been discussed enough to define a **conductor** as a material that permits electrons to flow easily, and an **insulator** as one that inhibits their movement. The tendency of an atom to permit electrons nearby or within one of the orbital shells is the prime factor in determining conductivity, semiconductivity and insulation properties. The **valence energy band** (the outermost and sometimes next-to-outermost orbital shell) not only determines the chemical properties of the atom, as discussed previously, but has much to do with conductivity as well. Orbital shells lower or closer to the nucleus (and of less energy) than the valence band are normally completely full (Figure 3–10). Valence has much to do with the ability of a material to conduct electrons. Any element with one valence electron is a good conductor (i.e., copper, silver and gold). In addition, the further the valence electron is from the nucleus, the better a conductor it is. For example, gold is a better conductor than silver because its valence electron is in the sixth shell while silver's is in the fifth. Silver is a better conductor than copper because copper's valence electron is in the fourth shell. Since copper has a higher melting point and is much cheaper, it is more commonly used than silver or gold.

There is also an area beyond the valence band that is referred to as the **conduction band**. The conduction band is not an orbital shell but is within the force field

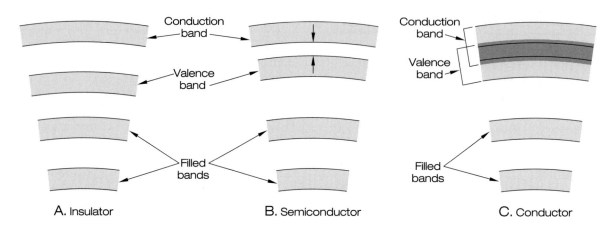

FIGURE 3–10. The arrows demonstrate the difference between the energy levels of conduction and valence bands in an (A) insulator, (B) semiconductor, and (C) conductor. Note that the conduction and valence bands overlap in a good conductor.

(area of influence) of the atom (Figure 3–10). Conductors have conduction bands that are populated by free electrons and, in solid materials, they are able to move freely from one atom's conduction band to another's, as in Figure 3–10C. This is why many of the best conductors are solids. Conversely, insulators have very poor or nonexistent conduction bands. The number of electrons in the conduction band is determined by the energy difference between the valence band and the conduction band. Although the conduction band is always at a higher energy level than the valence band, the energy required of an individual electron to place it in the conduction band will determine how many electrons can possibly exist there. In fact, the difference between the energy levels required of conduction band electrons as compared to valence band electrons is the factor that differentiates conductors from semiconductors from insulators. In Figure 3–10, the differences are shown as (C) a good conductor with overlapping valence and conduction bands, (B) a semiconductor with closely related bands, and (A) a good insulator with a wide gap between the bands. Metals often have overlapping bands with conduction bands including portions of the valence bands, thus placing large numbers of electrons into the conduction bands. Therefore metals, especially silver and copper, make the best conductors. The best insulators are materials with complex molecular structures, such as wood, plastic, glass, and rubber.

The **length** of the conductor has a directly proportional relationship to resistance. In other words, as the length of the conductor doubles, the resistance will also double. Just as a short garden hose will spray water with greater force than a long hose, so a short conductor will permit a greater force of electrons while a longer conductor offers greater resistance.

The cross-sectional **diameter** of the conductor has an inversely proportional relationship to resistance. In other words, as the cross-sectional diameter doubles, the resistance will be halved. A garden hose with a small diameter will impede water flow more than a large-diameter hose, just as a small-diameter conductor will resist electron flow more than a conductor with a large diameter.

Finally, the **temperature** of the conductor can also influence the resistance. Heat is simply a measurement of the amount of atomic and molecular energy, often seen as vibration. As temperature increases, atomic collisions provide enough energy to some electrons to permit them to jump into the atom's conduction band. In conductors, increased temperature increases free electron collisions and this in turn lessens electrical current flow. In insulators the increased number of collisions because of increased temperature causes some electrons to lose energy and fall back into the valence band, thus decreasing the energy difference between the bands and consequently decreasing the insulating ability of the material. Semiconductors become more conductive as temperature increases, for the same reason, with a resultant narrowing of the gap between their already close bands.

An approximation of these relationships is shown in Figure 3–11. A close examination of this figure illustrates that increased resistance from heat is significant. In fact, it becomes a major problem with the large heat-producing transformers used in x-ray equipment, and unique methods have been adopted to overcome its effect. In addition, extrapolation of the conductor curve to the left illustrates that if conductors can be supercooled, as they are in modern magnetic resonance imaging equipment, a significant increase in conductivity can be achieved.

In recent years, superconductivity has been achieved to reduce resistance to the point where current is apparently flowing without potential difference. Table 3–1 provides information on the conductive properties of materials important in electronics.

The total resistance is calculated as:

$$R = \frac{\rho L}{A}$$

where:

R = resistance in ohms
ρ = resistivity (a function of atomic structure and temperature) (ρ is the Greek letter rho)
L = length in meters
A = area in square meters

This total resistance formula is the true technical definition of an ohm as a unit.

Ohm's Law

Georg Ohm discovered a mathematical relationship between the factors of current, potential difference, and resistance that applies to all resistance circuits and is known as Ohm's law. The law describes the relationship between current and potential difference as **the current along a conductor is proportional to the potential difference**. It is easier to remember this relationship as a formula:

$$\frac{V}{I}$$

V = potential difference in volts
I = current in amperes

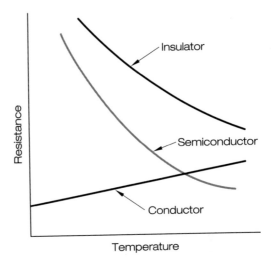

FIGURE 3–11. The effect of temperature on conductors, semiconductors, and insulators.

This expression does not include the resistance factor, which is a critical element. Therefore, Ohm's law is usually expressed as the algebraic derivation with resistance times current equal to potential difference, or:

$$V = IR$$

where:

V = potential difference in volts
I = current in amperage
R = resistance in ohms

This version solves for voltage when the current and resistance are known. Of course, Ohm's law can also be stated in its other forms to solve for unknown currents and resistances:

$$I = \frac{V}{R}$$

and

$$R = \frac{V}{I}$$

Example: What is the amperage in a circuit of 20 volts and 10 ohms?

Answer:

$$I = V/R$$
$$I = 20 \text{ volts}/10 \text{ ohms}$$
$$I = 2 \text{ amperes}$$

Example: What is the voltage in a circuit of 100 amperes and 5 ohms?

Answer:

$$V = IR$$
$$V = 100 \text{ amperes} \times 5 \text{ ohms}$$
$$V = 500 \text{ volts}$$

Example: What is the resistance in a circuit of 80 kilo-volts and 200 milliamperes?

Answer:

$$R = V/I$$
$$R = 80 \text{ kV}/200 \text{ mA}$$
$$R = 80,000 \text{ volts}/0.2 \text{ ampere}$$
$$R = 400,000 \text{ ohms}$$

A memory device used by many students is known as an Ohm's law triangle (Figure 3–12A). To determine the correct formula for one of the variables in the Ohm's law equation, V = IR, simply write the variables as shown (V over I and R), and then cover the variable to be solved with a finger. For example, Figure 3–12B is to solve for R. The correct relationship is given of V/I equals the covered R. Moving a finger around the triangle produces V/R = I and I • R = V as well.

It is useful to be able to calculate the total amount of power used in an electric circuit. **The unit of power is the watt.** Because the total amount of energy available in a circuit is determined by the current (amperage) and

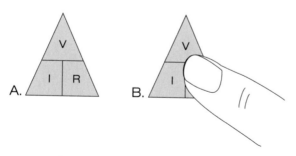

FIGURE 3–12. Ohm's law triangle.

potential difference (voltage), **the watt is defined as one ampere flowing through one volt per second.** Power is calculated with the following formula:

$$P = IV$$

where:

$$P = \text{power in watts}$$
$$I = \text{current in amperes}$$
$$V = \text{potential difference in volts}$$

Common household appliances tend to operate between 500 and 2,000 watts (most have labels indicating their wattage ratings) and all circuits in buildings have wattage safety limitations. The use of equipment whose total wattage ratings exceed the safety limit of the circuit will cause the circuit to overload and shut down because of excessive heat generation. Radiographic equipment capabilities can be measured by the power rating, usually by calculating the greatest possible energy output.

Example: What is the power rating, in kilowatts, of an x-ray generator capable of 800 milliamperes at 100 kilovolts?

Answer:

$$P = IV$$
$$P = 800 \text{ mA} \times 100 \text{ kV}$$
$$P = 0.8 \text{ A} \times 100,000 \text{ V}$$
$$P = 80,000 \text{ watts}$$
$$P = 80 \text{ kilowatts}$$

An interesting historical note for anyone who has seen car engines rated by horsepower is that one horsepower = 746 watts. We could say that an 80 kW generator is a 107 horsepower x-ray machine.

Example: If a mobile x-ray machine operates from a 110 V wall receptacle and is rated at a total resistance of 12 Ω, how much current does it draw during a one-second exposure?

Answer:

$$I = \frac{V}{R}$$
$$I = \frac{110 \text{ V}}{12 \text{ Ω}}$$
$$I = 9.2 \text{ A}$$

Example: How much power does it use per second?

Answer:

$$P = IV$$
$$P = 9.2 \text{ A} \times 110 \text{ V}$$
$$P = 1,012 \text{ W}$$

With this information it is also possible to calculate the expense of the power for a radiographic examination.

Example: If the power company charges 5¢ per kW/hour, what is the cost of the power for 10 minutes of fluoroscopy at 5 mA and 100 kV?

Answer:
The power per second is calculated as:

$$P = IV$$
$$P = 5 \text{ mA} \times 100 \text{ kV}$$
$$P = 0.005 \text{ A} \times 100,000 \text{ V}$$
$$P = 500 \text{ W}$$

The total power is calculated as:

total power = power × seconds
total power = 500 W × 10 minutes
total power = 500 W × 600 seconds
total power = 300,000 W/sec
total power = 300 kW/sec

The total cost is calculated as:

total cost = total power used × $0.05/kW/hr
total cost = 300 kW/second × $0.05/kW/hr
total cost = 5 kW/minute × $0.05/kW/hr
total cost = 0.08 kW/hr × $0.05/kW/hr
total cost = $0.004, or
total cost = 0.4¢

The heat that is produced during the operation of electrical equipment becomes of great concern as power use increases. The importance of changes in resistance to heat output can best be understood if the power formula, P = IV, is converted to what is sometimes called the **power loss formula, P=I²R**. This is calculated from:

the power formula, P = IV
substituting IR for V
(because Ohm's law states that V = IR)
resulting in P = I × IR

or $P = I^2R$ (watts per second).

This equation clarifies that power loss from current heat is proportional to the resistance, and heat power loss increases very rapidly with current increase. As illustrated in the formula, heat power loss is proportional to the square of the amperage. In other words, doubling the amperage increases power loss by a factor of 4, etc.

Series And Parallel Circuits

An electric circuit can be designed to send electrons through various resistance devices by linking them one after the other in a **series circuit** (Figure 3–13A) or by giving each component an individual branch in a **parallel circuit** (Figure 3–13B). The effect of each type of circuit on current, potential difference, and resistance is summarized in Table 3–2. The best way to understand the effects of both series and parallel circuitry is to work through a series of problems that demonstrate these differences.

Example: What is the total current in a series circuit with 3 resistances, each supplied with 10 amperes?

Answer:

$$I_t = I_1 = I_2 = I_3$$
$$I_t = 10 \text{ A} = 10 \text{ A} = 10 \text{ A}$$
$$I_t = 10 \text{ amperes}$$

TABLE 3–2. Effect of Circuit Type on Current, Potential Difference and Resistance (with an example circuit of 3 resistances)

	Series	Parallel
Current	Same in each element, each element same as total circuit, $I_t = I_1 = I_2 = I_3$	Sum of all elements equals total circuit, $I_t = I_1 + I_2 + I_3$
Voltage	Sum of all elements equals total circuit, $V_t = V_1 + V_2 + V_3$	Same in each element, each element same as total circuit, $V_t = V_1 = V_2 = V_3$
Resistance	Sum of all elements equals total circuit, $R_t = R_1 + R_2 + R_3$	Sum of reciprocal of each element is inversely proportional to the total, $\frac{1}{R_t} = \frac{1}{R_1} + \frac{1}{R_2} + \frac{1}{R_3}$

Note: A reciprocal ohm, as in 1/R, is known as a siemens (S).

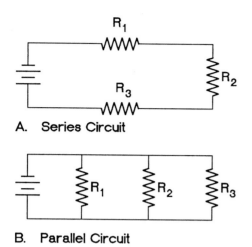

A.   Series Circuit

B.   Parallel Circuit

FIGURE 3–13. (A) Series and (B) parallel circuits.

Example: What is the total current in a parallel circuit with 3 resistances, each supplied with 10 amperes?

Answer:

$$I_t = I_1 + I_2 + I_3$$
$$I_t = 10 \text{ A} + 10 \text{ A} + 10 \text{ A}$$
$$I_t = 30 \text{ amperes}$$

Note that the series circuit supplies a current of 10 amperes while the parallel circuit supplies 30 amperes. Parallel circuits supply a greater total current than series circuits when all other factors are the same. An interesting phenomenon occurs when the effect on voltage is compared, instead of current, using resistances.

Example: What is the total voltage in a series circuit with 3 resistances, each supplied with 10 volts?

Answer:

$$V_t = V_1 + V_2 + V_3$$
$$V_t = 10 \text{ V} + 10 \text{ V} + 10 \text{ V}$$
$$V_t = 30 \text{ volts}$$

Example: What is the total voltage in a parallel circuit with 3 resistances, each supplied with 10 volts?

Answer:

$$V_t = V_1 = V_2 = V_3$$
$$V_t = 10 \text{ V} = 10 \text{ V} = 10 \text{ V}$$
$$V_t = 10 \text{ volts}$$

Note that the series circuit supplies 30 volts while the parallel circuit supplies 10 volts. Series circuits supply greater total potential difference than parallel circuits when all other factors are the same. The difference between series and parallel circuits when the same resistances are used is also notable.

Example: What is the total resistance of a series circuit with resistances of 2.5 Ω, 4.2 Ω and 6.8 Ω?

Answer:

$$R_t = R_1 + R_2 + R_3$$
$$R_t = 2.5 \ \Omega + 4.2 \ \Omega + 6.8 \ \Omega$$
$$R_t = 13.5 \ \Omega$$

Example: What is the total resistance of a parallel circuit with resistances of 2.5 Ω, 4.2 Ω and 6.8 Ω?

Answer:

$$\frac{1}{R_t} = \frac{1}{R_1} + \frac{1}{R_2} + \frac{1}{R_3}$$

$$\frac{1}{R_t} = \frac{1}{2.5\Omega} + \frac{1}{4.2\Omega} + \frac{1}{6.8\Omega}$$

$$\frac{1}{R_t} = 0.4 \text{ S} + 0.24 \text{ S} + 0.15 \text{ S}$$

$$\frac{1}{R_t} = 0.785 \text{ S}$$

$$R_t = \frac{1}{0.7 \text{ S}}$$

$$R_t = 1.274 \ \Omega$$

Note that the series circuit provides 13.5 Ω of resistance while the parallel circuit has only 1.274 Ω. Parallel circuits offer less total resistance to electrical current when all other factors are the same. In addition, parallel circuits are not broken when a single resistance is interrupted (as when a light bulb burns out). Series circuits require all resistances to be operable, otherwise there is no pathway for the current to take. The classic example of the difference is illustrated by comparing strings of Christmas lights in series versus parallel circuits. When a single series-wired light burns out, it breaks the circuit and all the lights go out. When a single parallel-wired light burns out, it breaks the circuit in its parallel branch only and the other lights continue to operate. Electrical devices use a wide variety of both types of circuits, including complicated combinations of both. It is also interesting to calculate the effect of both circuit types on amperage by figuring resistance and then applying Ohm's law.

Example: What is the total amperage in a series circuit with resistances of 2.5 Ω, 4.2 Ω and 6.8 Ω with a potential difference of 10 volts?

Answer:
The total resistance is calculated as:

$$R_t = R_1 + R_2 + R_3$$
$$R_t = 2.5\ \Omega + 4.2\ \Omega + 6.8\ \Omega$$
$$R_t = 13.5\ \Omega$$

The total amperage is calculated with Ohm's law:

$$I = \frac{V}{R}$$
$$I = \frac{10\ V}{13.5\ \Omega}$$
$$I = 0.74\ \text{amperes}$$

Example: What is the total amperage in a parallel circuit with resistances of 2.5 Ω, 4.2 Ω and 6.8 Ω and a potential difference of 10 volts?

Answer:
The total resistance is calculated as:

$$\frac{1}{R_t} = \frac{1}{R_1} + \frac{1}{R_2} + \frac{1}{R_3}$$

$$\frac{1}{R_t} = \frac{1}{2.5\ \Omega} + \frac{1}{4.2\ \Omega} + \frac{1}{6.8\ \Omega}$$

$$\frac{1}{R_t} = 0.4\ S + 0.24\ S + 0.15\ S$$

$$\frac{1}{R_t} = 0.785\ S$$

$$R_t = \frac{1}{0.7\ S}$$

$$R_t = 1.274\ \Omega$$

The total amperage is calculated with Ohm's law:

$$I = \frac{V}{R}$$

$$I = \frac{10\ V}{1.274\ \Omega}$$

$$I = 7.85\ \text{amperes}$$

Note that the series circuit operates with a current of 0.74 ampere while the parallel circuit operates with a current of 7.1 amperes. Parallel circuits operate with greater current when all other factors are the same. It is also interesting to study the effect of both circuit types on voltage by calculating resistance and then applying Ohm's law.

Example: What is the total voltage of a series circuit with resistances of 2.5 Ω, 4.2 Ω and 6.8 Ω with a current of 50 amperes?

Answer:
The total resistance is calculated as:

$$R_t = R_1 + R_2 + R_3$$
$$R_t = 2.5\ \Omega + 4.2\ \Omega + 6.8\ \Omega$$
$$R_t = 13.5\ \Omega$$

The total voltage is calculated with Ohm's law:

$$V = IR$$
$$V = 50\ A \times 13.5\ \Omega$$
$$V = 675\ \text{volts}$$

Example: What is the total voltage of a parallel circuit with resistances of 2.5 Ω, 4.2 Ω and 6.8 Ω and a current of 50 amperes?

Answer:
The total resistance is calculated as:

$$\frac{1}{R_t} = \frac{1}{R_1} + \frac{1}{R_2} + \frac{1}{R_3}$$

$$\frac{1}{R_t} = \frac{1}{2.5\ \Omega} + \frac{1}{4.2\ \Omega} + \frac{1}{6.8\ \Omega}$$

$$\frac{1}{R_t} = 0.4\ S + 0.24\ S + 0.15\ S$$

$$\frac{1}{R_t} = 0.785\ S$$

$$R_t = \frac{1}{0.7\ S}$$

$$R_t = 1.274\ \Omega$$

The total voltage is calculated with Ohm's law:

$$V = IR$$
$$V = 50\ A \times 1.274\ \Omega$$
$$V = 63.68\ \text{volts}$$

Note that the series circuit operates at 675 volts while the parallel circuit operates at 64 volts. Parallel circuits operate at lower voltage than series circuits when all other factors are the same.

Parallel circuits are used for the electrical wiring of buildings because the failure of a single device does not break the electrical supply to other devices. As can be seen from these problems, the addition of current-using devices to a series circuit causes the voltage to drop, thus reducing the potential difference to the other devices in the circuit. In a series circuit of lights, for example, the addition of more bulbs will cause all the bulbs to burn dimmer. **As more resistances are added to a parallel circuit, total resistance drops, total amperage increases and total voltage remains unchanged.** The total resistance of a parallel circuit is always less than the amount of the lowest resistor (usually about half of the lowest resistor).

A disadvantage to parallel circuits is that with the addition of resistances, the increasing amperage can short circuit the entire system. This creates the possibility of wires becoming hot enough to start a fire. To prevent this from occurring, either a **circuit breaker** or a **fuse** is placed in the line. These devices are constructed to permit the breaking of the circuit before a dangerous temperature is reached. Circuit breakers simply pop open and can be reset once the cause of the problem has been located and removed from the circuit. Fuses are constructed with a metal tab that, when dangerously heated, will melt, thus breaking the circuit. Fuses are not reusable and must be replaced.

A variable resistor called a **potentiometer** or **rheostat** permits a variable contact to slide along a series circuit of resistance coils. When resistors are connected in a series circuit Ohm's law dictates that an increase in resistance will result in a decrease in voltage and vice versa if the amperage remains unchanged. When a knob is connect-ed to the variable slide contact (as in a radio volume control), a simple twist permits voltage and amperage regulation (with a corresponding increase or decrease in speaker volume). Unfortunately, rheostats cause significant energy waste in heat, and the direct application of Ohm's law results in voltage changing when only an amperage change is desired and vice versa. For these reasons, rheostats are not practical in high-voltage situations. Their prime use is to control current but they have never been adaptable to high-voltage transformers.

Summary

The distribution and movement of electrons, along with their associated charges, make up electricity. Electrostatics is the study of the distribution of fixed charges that are at rest. When one object has more electrons than another, it also has more negative charges and is considered to have an overall negative charge. A positive charge refers to something with a weaker negative charge, or fewer electrons. The terms negative and positive refer to the relationship between two objects, not to their true atomic charges. Because the earth contains what is essentially an infinite number of charges, it is considered to be neutral, or at zero ground potential. The five laws of electrostatics are: 1) repulsion-attraction, 2) the inverse square law, 3) distribution, 4) concentration and 5) movement. Objects can be electrified by friction, contact and induction.

The movement of electrons is facilitated by materials that permit electrons to flow easily. These materials are called conductors or superconductors. Nonconducting materials are called insulators, while materials that conduct under certain conditions and insulate under others are known as semiconductors.

An electrical circuit is a pathway that permits electrons to move in a complete circle from their source, through resisting electrical devices, and back to the source. Electrons move from the highest concentration to the lowest. Conventional electric current is described as going from positive to negative poles, while electron flow is actually from negative to positive poles. It is important to specify whether descriptions are of electrical current or electron flow, as they are exact opposites.

The quantity of electrons flowing is referred to as the current and is measured in amperes. The force with which the electrons travel is referred to as the potential difference, electromotive force or voltage and is measured in volts. There does not have to be current flow for voltage to exist. The opposition to the current flow is referred to as resistance and is measured in ohms. The relationship between these factors is expressed in Ohm's law: V = IR. The resistance of metallic conductors is affected by length, diameter and temperature. When 1/R is used to express resistance in an AC circuit, it is measured in siemens.

The valence energy band of an atom has much to do with the ability of a material to conduct electrons. There is also an area beyond the valence band that is referred to as the conduction band. Conductors have conduction bands that are populated by electrons that are able to move freely from one atom's conduction band to another's. Insulators have widely separated valence and conduction bands, while semiconductors have intermediate properties.

Circuits are known by several parameters. These include the direction the electrons travel, which is defined as either direct current (DC) or alternating current (AC). It is possible to change the current from DC to AC and back, as necessary. The total amount of energy in a circuit is described as the power of the circuit and is measured in watts so that P = IV. Circuits can be described as series or parallel, depending on how the components are connected. The total resistance of a series circuit is measured in ohms, as $R_t = R_1 + R_2 + R_3$. The total resistance of a parallel circuit is measured in siemens, as

$$\frac{1}{R_t} = \frac{1}{R_1} + \frac{1}{R_2} + \frac{1}{R_3}$$

Parallel circuits operate with greater current through resistances and they supply a greater total current from the power supply than series circuits when all other factors are the same. Parallel circuits are often used because the failure of a single device does not break the electrical supply to other devices. Circuit breakers and fuses prevent damage to electrical components by permitting the breaking of an overloaded circuit before a dangerous

temperature is reached. A potentiometer or rheostat is a variable resistor.

REVIEW QUESTIONS

1. State the five elementary laws of electrostatics.
2. Describe the three methods of electrification.
3. How are conductors different from insulators?
4. Explain the difference between conventional electrical current and actual electron flow.
5. State the four basic factors that are used to describe the nature of the flow of electrons in electrodynamics.
6. What are the units used to describe potential difference, current flow and opposition to current flow?
7. State Ohm's law.
8. What is the potential difference in a circuit of 20 amperes and 10 ohms? 30 amperes and 6 ohms? 100 mA and 5 ohms?
9. What is the power rating of an x-ray generator capable of 1,000 mA at 110 kV?
10. What is the voltage in a parallel circuit of 20 amperes with resistances of 6, 10 and 15 ohms?
11. What is the amperage in a series circuit of 110 volts with resistances of 5, 10 and 20 ohms?

REFERENCES AND RECOMMENDED READING

Ball, J. & Price, T. (1989). *Chesneys' radiographic imaging.* Oxford: Blackwell Scientific Publishing.

Ball, J. L. & Moore, A. D. (1986). *Essential physics for radiographers* (2nd ed.). Oxford: Blackwell Scientific Publications.

Bushberg, J. T., Seibert, J. A., Leidholdt, E. M., Boone, J. M. (1994). *The essential physics of medical imaging.* Baltimore: Williams & Wilkins.

Bushong, S. C. (1997). *Radiologic science for technologists: Physics, biology, and protection* (6th ed.). St. Louis: C. V. Mosby.

Carroll, Q. B. (1993). *Fuchs's radiographic exposure, processing and quality control* (5th ed.). Springfield, IL: Charles C. Thomas Publishers.

DeFrance, J. J. (1969). *Electrical fundamentals.* Englewood Cliffs, NJ: Prentice-Hall.

Del Toro, V. (1993). *Principles of electrical engineering* (4th ed.). Englewood Cliffs, NJ: Prentice-Hall.

Dendy, P. P. & Heaton, B. (1987). *Physics for radiologists.* Oxford: Blackwell Scientific Publications.

Du Pont x-ray technical service product information, *Static Electricity,* Wilmington, DE: Du Pont Company, Photo Products Dept., Chestnut Run Lab, Publication E-53821.

Gates, E. D. (1987). *Introduction to electronics: A practical approach.* Albany: Delmar Publishers.

Gifford, D. (1984). *A handbook of physics for radiologists and radiographers.* New York: John Wiley & Sons.

Glasser, O., Quimby, E. H., Taylor, L. S., Weatherwax, J. L., Morgan, R. H. (1961). *Physical foundations of radiology.* (3rd ed.). New York: Paul B. Hoeber Division of Harper & Brothers.

Graham, B. J. & Thomas, W. N. (1975). *An introduction to physics for radiologic technologists.* Philadelphia: W. B. Saunders.

Hay, G. A. & Hughes, D. (1972). *First-year physics for radiographers.* London: Bailliere Tindall.

Johns, H. E. & Cunningham, J. R. (1983). *The physics of radiology* (4th ed.). Springfield, IL: Thomas.

Meredith, W. J. & Massey, J. B. (1977). *Fundamental physics of radiology* (3rd ed.). Chicago: Yearbook Medical Publishers.

Nadon, J. M., Gelmine, B. J., McLaughlin, E. D. (1989). *Industrial electricity* (4th ed.). Albany: Delmar Publishers.

Ridgway, A. & Thumm, W. (1973). *The physics of medical radiography.* Reading, MA: Addison-Wesley.

Roderick, J. F. & Sutherland, B. (1952). A study of the static electricity problems in the x-ray darkroom. *The X-Ray Technician. 23*(March).

Roller, D. & Roller, H.D. (1967). The development of the concept of electric charge: Electricity from the Greeks to Coulomb, case 8, *Harvard Case Histories in Experimental Science.* Cambridge: Harvard University Press.

Selman, J. (1994). *The fundamentals of x-ray and radium physics* (9th ed.). Springfield, IL: Thomas.

Sprawls, P. (1990). *Principles of radiography for technologists.* Rockville, MD: Aspen Publishers.

Sprawls, P. (1987). *Physical principles of medical imaging.* Rockville, MD: Aspen Publishers.

Stockley, S. M. (1986). *A manual of radiographic equipment.* Edinburgh: Churchill Livingstone.

Ter-Pogossian, M. M. (1967). *The physical aspects of diagnostic radiology.* New York: Hoeber Medical Division, Harper & Row.

Thompson, M. A., Hattaway, M. P., Hall, J. D., Dowd, S. B. (1994). *Principles of imaging science and protection.* Philadelphia: W. B. Saunders.

Thompson, T. T. (1985). *A practical approach to modern imaging equipment* (2nd ed.). Boston: Little, Brown, & Co.

Tortorici, M. (1992). *Concepts in medical radiographic imaging.* Philadelphia: W. B. Saunders.

van der Plaats, G. J. (1980). *Medical x-ray techniques in diagnostic radiology* (4th ed.). The Hague: Martinus Nijhoff Publishers.

Wilks, R. J. (1981). *Principles of radiological physics.* Edinburgh: Churchill Livingstone.

Wolbarst, A. B. (1993). *Physics of radiology.* Norwalk, CT: Appleton & Lange.

CHAPTER 4

Electromagnetism

He expressed his satisfaction and, going back to Joachim, warned him to draw in his breath and hold it until all was over. Joachim's rounded back expanded and so remained; the assistant, at the switch-board, pulled the handle. Now, for the space of two seconds, fearful powers were in play — streams of thousands, of a hundred thousand of volts.

Thomas Mann, Der Zauberberg (The Magic Mountain).

Objectives

Upon completion of this chapter, the student should be able to:

- Explain the atomic nature of magnetism.
- Classify materials according to their magnetic properties.
- State Fleming's hand rules of electromagnetics.
- Explain how a solenoid and an electromagnet function.
- Describe magnetic and electromagnetic induction.
- List the types of movement that will produce electromagnetism.
- State the factors that regulate the strength of electromagnetic induction.
- Explain self-induction.
- Illustrate the generator and motor principles.
- Explain the waveform produced by direct- and alternating-current generators and motors.
- Describe the function of a transformer.
- Calculate voltage and amperage according to the transformer law.
- Discuss various factors affecting transformer efficiency and construction.
- Explain the function of an autotransformer and a capacitor.
- Describe the function of a silicon-controlled rectifier at the atomic level.
- Describe the process of thermionic emission.
- Explain the waveforms that are produced by half-wave and full-wave rectification.

Magnetism

Magnetism is one of the fundamental forces. Materials that have the ability to attract iron are classified as having a strong magnetic force. To understand magnetism it is important to return to atomic structure for a detailed examination of the effects of particle movement around the nucleus. **When a charged particle is in motion, a magnetic force field perpendicular to the motion will be created** (Figure 4–1). In the case of the negatively charged electrons orbiting the nucleus of an atom, the closed loop of the orbit cancels all but the field that is perpendicular to the plane of the motion (Figure 4–2). This perpendicular magnetic force is called **orbital magnetic moment**.

A magnetic effect is also established by electrons spinning on their axes. The effect created by the movement of these electrons is called **spin magnetic moment**. The disruption of this axial spinning and the energy released as it reorients itself are the physical basis that permits magnetic resonance imaging (see Chapter 44).

Atoms having a significant number of electrons with their magnetic moments in the same direction, especially when the outer shells are involved, will exhibit a net magnetic field in a distinct direction (Figure 4–2A). Groups of atoms with this net magnetic field are known as **magnetic dipoles** or **magnetic domains**. This is the basis of the domain theory of magnetism. It has been theorized that 10^{15} (10,000,000,000,000,000 or 10 million billion) atoms make up a single dipole. This is not a standard number, as it has been shown that dipoles vary in size and actually grow or shrink, depending on local conditions. In nonmagnetic objects the magnetic dipoles are randomly arranged, essentially cancelling out each other. If an external force field has the time or strength to orient enough of the dipoles in the same direction and/or cause those dipoles to grow in size, the object exhibits a uniformly strong magnetic field and is referred to as a **magnet** (Figure 4–2B).

The force fields that are created when magnetic dipoles orient to create a magnet are called **lines of force, lines of flux** or the **magnetic field**. These lines of force flow not only through the magnet itself but outside the magnetic material, forming a three-dimensional field surrounding the magnet (Figure 4–2B). The stronger the magnetic field, the more lines of flux. Placing small iron filings on a surface under which a strong magnet is placed will map out the magnetic lines of flux. Figure 4–3 illustrates the lines of flux emanating from the poles of a bar and a horseshoe magnet. The ends of a magnet are defined as the north and south poles; **lines of force always flow from north to south outside a magnet and from south to north within a magnet** (Figure 4–2B). It is important to remember that **lines of force never intersect**. In some cases they are described as being parallel. However, many circumstances may cause the magnetic field to contract or expand. Under these conditions the lines of force bend closer or further from one another, no longer making them truly parallel.

The stronger the magnetic field, the greater the number of lines of flux or the greater the **flux density**. Flux density is determined both by field strength and by the area in which the lines of flux are located.

$$\text{magnetic flux} = \frac{\text{field strength}}{\text{area}}$$

There are two primary units used to measure the strength of magnetic fields. The **SI unit for magnetic flux is the Weber,** represented by the symbol Wb, (for the German physicist Wilhelm Weber [1804–1891],

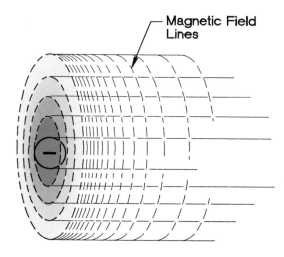

FIGURE 4–1. Magnetic field created by a charged particle in motion. The movement of a charged particle creates a magnetic field perpendicular to the motion of the particle.

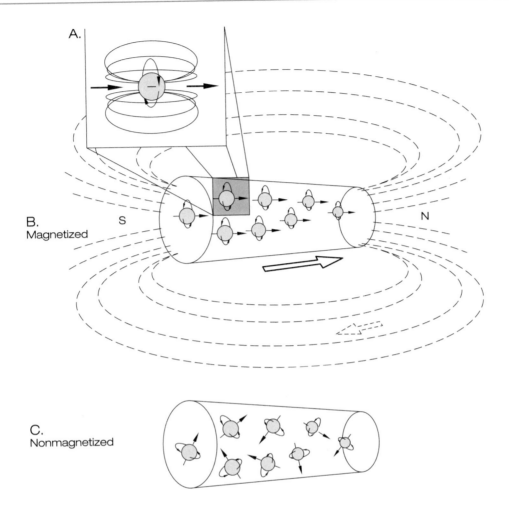

FIGURE 4–2. The concept of magnetism: (A) The spinning of an individual electron is the spin magnetic moment, and the magnetic field created by the spin is the orbital magnetic moment (heavy arrows). Groups of atoms with most of the magnetic moment force in a single direction form a magnetic dipole or domain. (B) When the magnetic dipoles or domains are in a predominant direction, a magnet is formed with an external magnetic field. (C) When the magnetic dipoles or domains are not in a predominant direction, the object is not magnetized.

who proposed the basic theory of magnetism discussed above). 1 Wb = 10^8 lines of flux. **The units for magnetic flux density are the tesla,** represented by the symbol T (for the American physicist Nikola Tesla [1857–1943]), and the gauss, represented by the symbol G (for the German mathematician Johann Gauss [1777–1855]). **1 tesla = 10,000 gauss.** 1 T = 1 Wb/m^2, or 1 Wb per square meter. The earth's magnetic field averages about 0.0001 T (1 G or 100,000 lines of flux per square meter), while an ordinary household magnet (used, for

example, to keep papers on a refrigerator) might have a strength of 0.1 T (1,000 G or 100,000,000 lines of flux per square meter). Modern magnetic resonance imaging (MRI) equipment often operates in the range of 0.3–2.0 T (3,000 to 20,000 G or 300,000,000 to 2,000,000,000 lines of flux per square meter).

Because the earth itself is a magnet, with a north and a south pole, lines of force, although relatively weak, are present everywhere. This fact is used in the design of a magnetic compass. The pointer is simply a small piece of

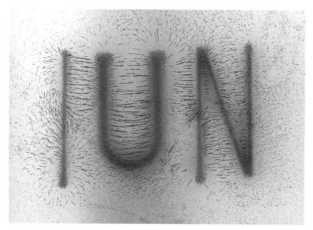

FIGURE 4–3. Strong permanent magnets placed under a surface containing loose iron filings will demonstrate magnetic lines of flux as the filings orient to the magnetic field (forming the initials of Indiana University Northwest).

permanent magnet which will align itself with the earth's magnetic lines of force and indicate direction. Because of this, a compass is a useful tool in detecting magnetic lines of force, including those induced by electrons moving in electrical circuits and devices. Worth noting is the fact that the earth's true magnetic poles are not located in Antarctica and the Arctic Ocean. Instead, the true magnetic north pole is located in Canada's far north while the true magnetic south pole is near Australia. Both poles tend to drift to new locations as geological conditions beneath the earth's crust change.

Magnets can be classified by type of production as **natural, artificial permanent** and **electromagnets. Natural magnets** are created when iron oxide (magnetite) remains in the earth's magnetic field for ages, slowly orienting the magnetic dipoles in the same direction. These natural magnets are called lodestones. They were recognized by primitive man and investigated by Greek academics. In some regions entire mountains of iron ore that have remained undisturbed for eons have magnetic properties. Natives of Thunder Bay, Ontario, delight in watching tourists follow signpost instructions to place their cars in neutral gear at the bottom of a magnetic mountain's gentle grade in hopes that the magnetic field will pull their cars up the hill.

Artificial permanent magnets are manufactured from a steel alloy called alnico, composed of aluminum, nick-

el and cobalt. While it is hot, alnico is subjected to the field of a strong commercial magnet to permit easier orientation of the magnetic dipoles. Upon cooling, the magnetic field becomes relatively permanent.

Electromagnets are temporary magnets produced by moving electric current. Because the electrons comprising the flow of current create magnetic fields in exactly the same manner as do the orbiting and spinning atomic electrons, any flow of current produces a magnetic field. When the current ceases flowing, the magnetic field collapses, making these electrical magnets temporary.

It is possible to create a fourth type of magnet by vibration. Prior to the 20th century, experienced blacksmiths were easy to spot because the tongs they used to handle heated metals had become magnetized. After many years of standing in the same position (in orientation to the earth's magnetic lines of force), heating the tongs in the forge, and then pounding the hot metal into shape on the anvil, the tongs had become well magnetized. A request to see a horseshoe hanging from a rafter would prove a smith's experience when he used the magnetized tongs to easily lift it down.

The laws governing magnetism are similar to the laws of electrostatics. However, only three are of importance for this text:

1. **Repulsion-attraction.** Like poles repel; unlike poles attract. In addition, like lines of force repel and unlike lines of force attract, when placed within each other's force fields (Figure 4–4).

2. **The inverse square law.** The force between two magnetic fields is directly proportional to the product of their magnitudes and inversely proportional to the square of the distance between them. Exactly as with electrostatics, as an object gets further away, the influencing field decreases because of the increased area it affects.

3. **Magnetic poles.** Every magnet has two poles, a north and a south, as discussed earlier. No matter how much a magnet is divided, even into individual moving electrons, both poles continue to exist.

Because the laws of electrostatics, magnetism, and gravity have so many similarities, physicists have long

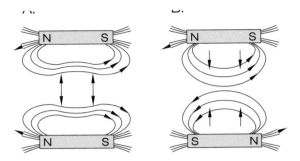

FIGURE 4–4. Repulsion-attraction of magnetic lines of force: (A) Lines of force in the same direction will repel each other. (B) Lines of force in opposite directions will attract each other.

searched for a mathematical theory to relate the three forces into a unified field theory. Albert Einstein worked unsuccessfully toward this goal until he died and the search continues to the present time, in the work of Stephen Hawking.

Magnetic Induction

When a nonmagnetized iron bar is brought within the lines of force of a strong magnet, the dipoles will temporarily align themselves with the lines of force passing through the iron bar. If the bar is removed from the field after a short time, the dipoles will return to their random orientation, thus leaving the bar unmagnetized. This process is termed magnetic induction and operates like electromagnetic induction. Instead of temporary repulsion of electrons, magnetic poles are induced through the temporary orientation of the dipoles.

The ease with which sensitive devices can be magnetized or demagnetized by stray electrical fields makes magnetic shielding desirable in many situations. Because there is no magnetic insulator, shielding is accomplished by providing a highly permeable ferromagnetic material, such as iron, through which stray magnetic fields can be directed, thus protecting sensitive devices from exposure to the stray field. This technique is used to shield some magnetic resonance imaging (MRI) units although they require radio frequency (RF) shielding as well.

Magnetic Classification of Materials

Permeability is the ease with which a material can be magnetized, while **retentivity** is the ability of a material to stay magnetized. These two factors are inversely proportional because if it is difficult to orient the dipoles (low permeability) it is also difficult to disorient them (high retentivity). The major classifications of the magnetic properties of materials according to their relative permeabilities are:

1. **Ferromagnetic** (or simply magnetic) materials such as iron, cobalt and nickel are highly permeable and greatly susceptible to induction. These materials have a majority of their dipoles lying in the same direction, thus setting up a natural magnetic field. In addition, the material must permit the atoms to be oriented, thus permitting the growth of magnetic dipoles in predominantly the same direction. Specialized alloys such as alnico, permalloy or mumetal (some alloys, strangely enough, contain no ferromagnetic elements) are designed to enhance permeability and exhibit dramatically increased magnetic field strength.

2. **Paramagnetic** materials, such as platinum and aluminum, have low permeability and weak attraction to magnetic fields. These materials have only a slight majority of dipoles in the same direction and there is little tendency for the size of the dipoles to grow.

3. **Diamagnetic** materials, such as beryllium, bismuth and lead, are actually weakly repelled by all magnetic fields, including both north and south poles. Strangely, water is slightly diamagnetic. This property is so weak that it is easily obscured by other types of magnetic induction.

4. **Nonmagnetic** materials, such as wood, glass, rubber and plastic, are not affected by magnetic fields and cannot be magnetized. Nonmagnetic materials are most often composed of atoms locked into crystalline or molecular patterns, thus forming ionic and covalent bonds and eliminating the ability of electrons to freely orient themselves to external magnetic lines of force. This classification includes most materials.

Electromagnetism

Electricity and magnetism are actually different aspects of the same force, electromagnetism. Although the study of magnetism dates to ancient times, and the study of electricity to Queen Elizabeth I's physician, William Gilbert (1540–1603), it was not until 1820, when the Danish physicist Hans Oersted (1777–1851) observed the deflection of a compass during a classroom demonstration of electrical phenomena, that the relationships between the two began to be established. Oersted's discovery, and subsequent investigations by many others, permitted the generation, control and practical use of electricity and initiated the electronic revolution that continues today.

Oersted's experiment proves that when there is no current flowing in the wire, the compass needle aligns itself with the earth's magnetic field (Figure 4–5). However, when current is flowing, the needle is deflected toward the wire and when the current stops, the needle returns to alignment with the earth's field. This led to the conclusion that **any moving charge produces a magnetic field.** As was stated earlier in the section on magnetism, this applies to even a single electron's negative charge in orbit around an atom. A slightly different arrangement of Oersted's experiment (Figure 4–6) permits the mapping of the magnetic field surrounding the flow of current.

The English scientist John Fleming (1849–1945) developed a series of easily remembered aids to help with the relationship between electricity and magnetism. They are known as **Fleming's hand rules.** There are several "hand" rules that are quite useful for remembering various electromagnetic relationships. The rules are divided into four groups: (1) **hand thumb rules along a conductor,** (2) **hand thumb rules for solenoid and electromagnet poles,** (3) **hand generator effect rules** and (4) **hand motor principle rules.** These are summarized in Table 4–1. Before learning any of the rules, it is critical to remember that **hand rules which are based on current flow (conventional current direction) and hand rules which are based on electron flow (actual direction of electron movement) will be exact opposites.** For example, the right-hand thumb rule applies to conventional current flow. This is identical to the left-hand thumb rule applied to actual electron flow.

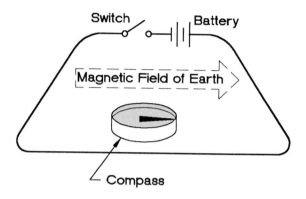

A. Without Current Flow

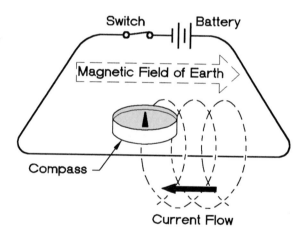

B. With Current Flow

FIGURE 4–5. Oersted's experiment: A compass placed near a wire conductor will indicate the direction of the earth's magnetic field (A) when no current is flowing in the wire. Because flowing current creates a magnetic field around the wire conductor that is stronger than the earth's field, the compass will indicate the direction of the current-induced field while the switch is closed (B).

The hand thumb rule, the first of the hand rules, applies to remembering the relationship between the direction of current along a conductor and the direction of the resulting magnetic lines of force field. **Fleming's right-hand thumb rule states that if the right hand is**

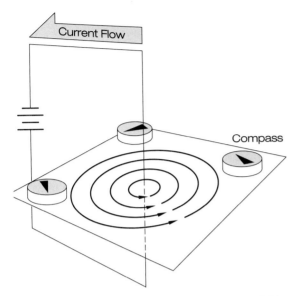

FIGURE 4–6. Relationship of induced magnetic field to direction of current flow: a variation of Oersted's experiment maps out the magnetic field induced by flowing current.

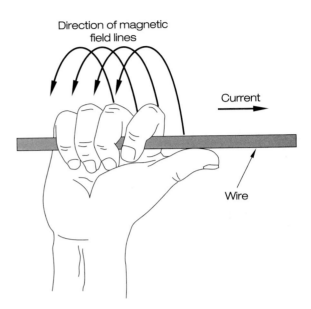

FIGURE 4–7. Fleming's right-hand thumb rule: When the right hand is positioned so the thumb points in the direction of conventional current flow, the fingers indicate the direction of the induced magnetic field. Fleming's left-hand thumb rule does the same for actual electron flow.

used to grasp a conducting wire with the thumb in the direction of the current flow, the fingers will indicate the direction of the magnetic field lines of force surrounding the conductor (Figure 4–7). (If the thumb points in the direction of actual electron flow, then a left-hand thumb rule must be used to show the direction of the magnetic field lines of force surrounding the conductor.) Table 4–1 compares this rule with the other "hand" rules.

Solenoids and Electromagnets

An interesting phenomenon occurs when conducting wire is looped (Figure 4–8A). Using the right-hand thumb rule to determine the direction of the magnetic lines of flux, it is apparent that inside the loop the magnetic fields from both sides join to double the magnetic flux density. If a series of loops are made, creating a coil (Figure 4–8B), the flux density is greatly increased. When current is flowing through this type of coil it is called a **solenoid**. The flux density can be increased further still by adding a ferromagnetic core. This configura-

tion is called an **electromagnet. The strength of solenoids and electromagnets is determined by the number of loops (or turns) of wire, the current strength and the permeability of the core.** The right-hand thumb rule can also be applied to a solenoid or an electromagnet to determine the location of the magnetic poles. **If the fingers point in the direction of the current, the thumb will point toward the north pole** (Figure 4–9). (If the fingers point in the direction of actual electron flow, then a left-hand thumb rule must be used for the thumb to point toward the north pole.) Table 4–1 compares this rule with the other "hand" rules.

Both the solenoid and the electromagnet demonstrate magnetic properties only while electric current is flowing. If the current stops flowing, the magnetic properties vanish, and if the current is adjusted up or down, the magnetic strength changes accordingly. The factors that govern the effectiveness of solenoids and electromagnets are the **diameter** of the coil, its **length** and the **current**

TABLE 4–1. Fleming's Hand Rules For Electromagnetic Relationships

	Conventional Current Flow	**Electron Flow**
Along a Conductor thumb = conventional current or electron flow fingers = magnetic field	right-hand thumb rule (see Figure 4–7)	left-hand thumb rule (left-hand version)
Solenoid and Electromagnet Poles thumb = direction of north pole fingers = conventional current or electron flow	right-hand thumb rule (see Figure 4–9)	left-hand thumb rule (left-hand version)
Generator Effect thumb = movement of conductor on armature index finger = magnetic lines of force field middle finger = current or electron flow	right-hand generator rule (see Figure 4–12)	left-hand generator rule (left-hand version)
Motor Principle thumb = movement of conductor on rotor index finger = magnetic lines of force field middle finger = current or electron flow	left-hand motor rule (see Figure 4–18)	right-hand motor rule (right-hand version)

passing along the coil. Electromagnets are used as remote control devices in circuit breakers and in the temporary locks, sometimes called detents, on radiographic equipment. In a typical circuit breaker configuration a wire from the circuit to be protected is incorporated into an electromagnet which, when the current becomes dangerously high, has been calculated to attract a movable contact which breaks the circuit.

Solenoids are often used as detent locks on the overhead crane of x-ray tubes. The detent can be activated by a switch at the x-ray tube controls. The switch activates the magnetic properties of the solenoid, which in turn attracts a metal latch or bolt. This temporarily locks the tube to the center of the x-ray table or at the proper distance from a film holder. **Electromagnetic relays** are similar to circuit breakers. They are used to protect radiographers from electrical shock by isolating control buttons on the x-ray console from the actual circuit in which high voltage is flowing.

Electromagnetic Induction

Once it became known that electrical current could generate a magnetic field, the obvious question was whether the reverse was true. The fact that it is was demonstrated by the English physicist Michael Faraday (1791–1867) the year after Oersted's discovery. The simple presence of a magnetic field is not sufficient to cause electrons to move along a wire. Faraday discovered that the magnetic lines of force and the wire must have a motion relative to each other to induce an electrical current (Figure 4–10). There are three ways to create the motion between lines of force and a conductor:

1. **Move the conductor** through a stationary, unchanging strength magnetic field.

2. **Move magnetic lines of force** through a stationary conductor with an unchanging strength magnetic field.

3. **Vary the magnetic flux** strength from a stationary magnet through a stationary conductor. As the flux strength varies, the lines of force will expand and contract, in effect causing the relative motion necessary to induce current.

The exact definitions of "magnetic flux strength" and "lines of force" are critical to understanding these differences.

There are two primary laws that govern the induction of current by magnetic fields. Faraday's law (sometimes called The First Law of Electromagnetics) states that four factors regulate the strength of induced current when magnetic lines of force and a conductor are in motion relative to one another:

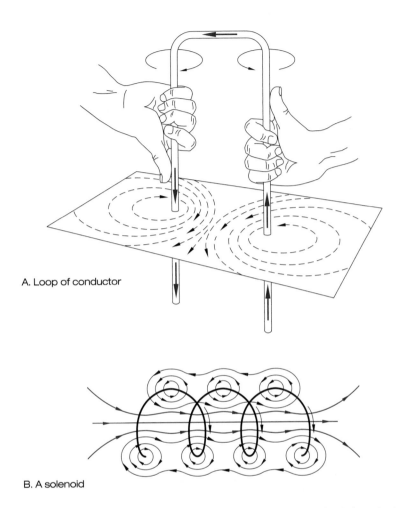

A. Loop of conductor

B. A solenoid

FIGURE 4–8. A solenoid: (A) When a conductor is looped to form a coil, the magnetic fields from both sides join to double the magnetic field strength inside the loop. (B) A solenoid is a helix coil through which current is flowing; it uses the coil loops to produce a greatly strengthened magnetic field.

1. the **strength** of the magnetic field,
2. the **speed** of the motion between lines of force and the conductor,
3. the **angle** between the magnetic lines of force and the conductor and
4. the **number of turns** in the conducting coil.

This law makes it possible to determine the direction in which the induced current will flow. This application of the law was established by the Russian scientist Heinrich Lenz (1804–1865). Lenz's law (sometimes called The Second Law of Electromagnetics) states that induced current flow sets up a magnetic field opposing the action that produced the original current, or, simply, that induced current opposes any flux change.

These two laws apply to both forms of induction: mutual induction and self-induction. **Mutual induction** occurs when two coils are placed in proximity and a varying current supplied to the first coil (as an electromagnet) induces a similar flow in the second coil (Figure 4–11). The coil supplied with current is called the **primary** coil while the coil in which the current is induced

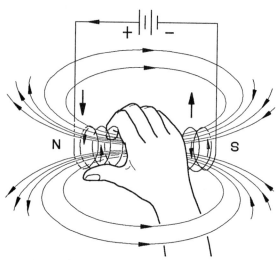

FIGURE 4–9. Fleming's right-hand thumb rule applied to determining the pole of a solenoid or electromagnet. When the fingers point in the direction of the current, the thumb will point toward the north pole.

A. Without relative motion

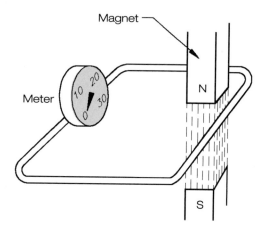

B. With relative motion

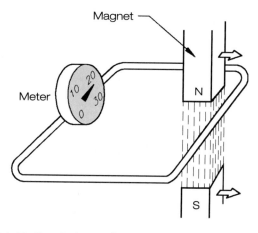

FIGURE 4–10. Faraday's experiment: a meter will not indicate current flow (A) until the magnetic lines of force from the magnet and wire have a motion relative to one another (B).

is called the **secondary** coil. The flow occurs in the secondary coil because the primary current alternates. This follows the rule that moving lines of force from a varying intensity current will induce electron flow in the wire through which it passes. In this case the secondary coil is cut by the varying (and therefore moving) lines of force from the current in the primary coil.

Self-induction is much more complicated but is more understandable when comparing a coil supplied with direct current, where there is self-induction only at the turn-on moment, with a coil supplied with alternating current, where self-induction occurs regularly. Alternating current is present when the electrons constantly change direction. A coil supplied with alternating current permits a steady flow of electrons and establishes an electromagnetic effect for half the cycle. However, at the instant the current supply reverses, the previously established electromagnetic north and south poles will induce an opposing potential difference, thus attempting to induce against the incoming supply of electrons. This tendency of an alternating current is called **inductive reactance** and is measured in ohms of resistance. Self-induction is useful when it is desirable to permit direct current to flow while at the same time hindering alternating current.

An important relationship exists between the direction of movement of a wire coil (the armature), the direction of the magnetic lines of force field and the direction in which the induced current will flow. This relationship is best remembered by the use of another "hand" rule (Figure 4–12). **Fleming's right-hand generator rule states that if the thumb points in the direction**

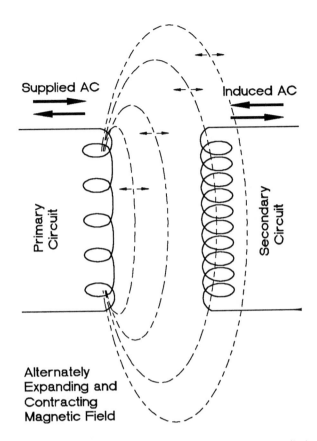

Supplied AC **Induced AC**

Primary Circuit

Secondary Circuit

Alternately
Expanding and
Contracting
Magnetic Field

FIGURE 4–11. Mutual induction: A varying current supplied to the primary coil induces a similar flow in the second coil. The constantly expanding and contracting magnetic lines of force induced in the primary coil provide the relative motion with the secondary coil necessary to induce current flow in the secondary coil.

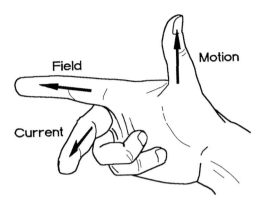

Field **Motion**

Current

FIGURE 4–12. Fleming's right-hand generator rule: When the thumb points in the direction the conductor (or armature) is moving and the index finger points in the direction of the magnetic lines of force field, the middle finger indicates the direction of conventional current flow. Fleming's left-hand generator rule does the same for actual electron flow.

the conductor (or armature) is moving and the index finger points in the direction of the magnetic lines of force field, then the middle finger will indicate the direction of the conventional current. (If the direction of actual electron flow is desired, then a left-hand generator rule must be used.) Table 4–1 compares this rule with the other "hand" rules.

Generators

A **generator,** or dynamo, is a device that converts mechanical energy to electrical energy using Faraday's discovery of moving lines of flux in relationship to a con-

ductor to induce current. This process converts the mechanical energy of the motion (any of the three ways) to electrical energy. A simple generator is composed of a conductor and magnets arranged as shown in Figure 4–13. The conductor is a coil of wire, called an **armature**, set between opposing magnetic poles so that it encounters the strongest lines of force. If the armature is rotated by a strong source of mechanical energy (such as a steam or water turbine), the generator can produce massive amounts of electrical energy. It is important to note the method that is used to convey the electrical current from the armature to the circuit. A set of **slip rings and brushes** permits the circuit to remain stationary while the armature rotates without breaking the electrical contact between them. This allows the electrons to flow without interruption. **Each slip ring connects to one end of the armature wire** (Figure 4–13.)

To understand exactly how the current is produced it is necessary to follow the production step by step (Figure 4–14). Notice that the armature coil wire is shown in cross-section at the top, three-dimensionally in the middle, and that the graph at the bottom represents the voltage produced. It is important to understand the relationship of the angle between this wire's motion and the lines of force between the stationary magnets. In Figure 4–14A the wire's motion is parallel to the lines of force.

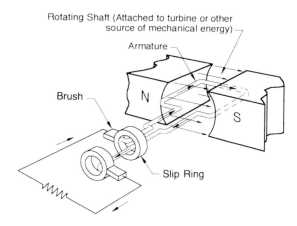

Rotating Shaft (Attached to turbine or other source of mechanical energy)

Armature

Brush

N

S

Slip Ring

FIGURE 4–13. An AC generator: Mechanical energy rotates the shaft to which the armature is attached. As the wires of the armature rotate, they cut through the magnetic lines of flux from the magnets and produce electrical current. The slip rings and brushes permit the armature to rotate while maintaining contact with the wires of the circuit.

This produces no emf, as shown on the graph. In Figure 4–14B the rotation of the armature has changed the wire's motion until it is at a 45° angle to the lines of force. Fleming's right-hand generator rule demonstrates that the conventional electrical current is moving into the page (electron flow would be out of the page). Because of the 45° angle, the magnitude of the emf, although rising, has not yet reached its peak. In Figure 4–14C, the motion of the wire is 90° to the lines of force (the maximum angle), resulting in the peak emf. As the wire begins to turn back to parallel in Figure 4–14D, the emf begins to drop back toward zero. When the wire reaches a parallel position, as in Figure 4–14E, the emf has returned to zero. As the wire begins to move into a 270° position (which is a 90° position in the opposite direction), notice that the relationship between the wire's motion and the lines of force has changed. Using Fleming's right-hand generator rule again, it is simple to see that the conventional electrical current has now reversed and is moving out of the page (while the electron flow has reversed to move into the page). **It is at this point that alternating current is produced.** This has occurred because **alternating current is produced when the wire's motion relative to the lines of force is reversed.** In Figures 4–14F, G, H, and I, the rise to peak and drop back to zero emf is repeated but in the opposite direc-

tion. This explains not only why generator-produced current must be alternating but also accounts for its pulsating nature.

The type of curve produced by an AC generator will always appear as in Figure 4–14. It is called a **sine wave** because it depends on the mathematical sine between the plane of the armature and a plane perpendicular to the lines of force. **One complete turn of the generator armature represents one cycle.** The sine wave illustrates one complete turn of the armature as the distance between two corresponding points. Note that this would be represented by the distance between *a* and *i* in Figure 4–14. **The frequency of the sine wave is determined by the number of cycles per second (cps). The unit of frequency is the Hertz, represented by the symbol Hz. 1 cps = 1 Hz.** American and Canadian generators operate at 60 Hz. Most of the rest of the world operates at 50 Hz.

Example: How many times per second do the electrons in a 60 Hz alternating current change their direction of movement?

Answer:
60 Hz x 2 directions = 120 changes per second

From Figure 4–14, it also becomes apparent that the **peak voltage is not the same as the average voltage** throughout the entire sine wave. The same is true of amperage and resistance (Ohm's law). This makes the measurement of all factors very difficult in pulsating alternating current because of the constant fluctuation of the sine wave. This is solved by using the root mean square (rms) values of the amperage and voltage. **Root mean square (rms) values of the total voltage and amperage in an alternating current are equivalent to the effect that would be produced in a direct current resistance by the same factors.** Resistance in alternating currents is calculated from a complicated series of factors, resulting in measurement of the apparent total resistance. **Apparent total resistance of an alternating current is called impedance, which is represented by the symbol Z.** This permits a revised version of Ohm's law to be applied for alternating current as:

$$I = \frac{V}{Z}$$

where:

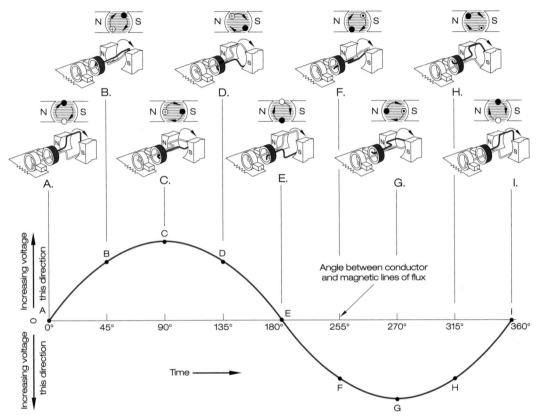

FIGURE 4–14. The production of alternating current: Armature coil wire is shown in cross section (top). Three-dimensional view of generator (middle). Graph of the voltage produced (bottom). See text for step-by-step description.

$$I = \text{rms amperage}$$
$$V = \text{rms voltage}$$
$$Z = \text{impedance}$$

When using an x-ray machine, it is worth remembering that the **kilovoltage settings represent peak kilovoltage, not average or rms values**.

A direct-current generator is made by exchanging the slip rings for a commutator ring, as shown in Figure 4–15. **A commutator is a single ring that is divided in half, with each half connected to one end of the armature wire**. The single commutator's two halves replace the pair of slip rings. Instead of each end of the armature

wire being connected to its own slip ring, each end of the armature wire is connected to half of the commutator ring. When a generator has its armature connected to a commutator, the sine wave of the output is dramatically different from that produced by a pair of slip rings. Although the armature turns exactly as in an alternating current generator, the commutator routes the current very differently. This current produces a sine wave exactly as in an alternating current generator (Figures 4–15A–C). The use of Fleming's right-hand generator rule demonstrates that the conventional electrical current is moving into the page (electron flow would be out of the page). In Figure 4–15D the wire has begun to

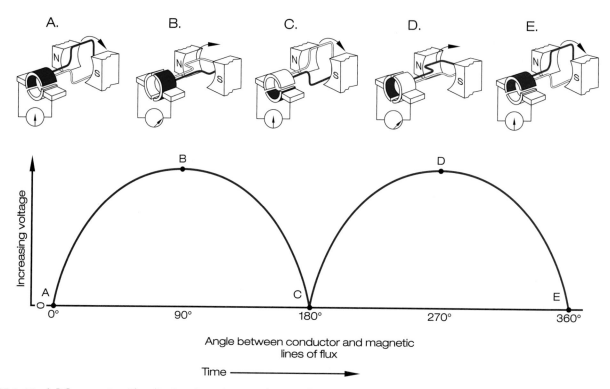

FIGURE 4–15. A DC generator: The slip rings have been exchanged for a commutator ring with each half connecting to one end of the armature wire. Although the armature turns exactly as in an AC generator, the commutator routes the current as shown on the graph. See text for step-by-step description.

move toward the second phase of the cycle. As in the alternating-current generator, the relationship between the wire's motion and the lines of force has changed. Using Fleming's right-hand generator rule again, it is simple to see that the conventional electrical current has now reversed and is moving out of the page (while the electron flow has reversed to move into the page). However, it is extremely important to note that in Figure 4–15D, the commutator ring has also changed the brush with which it was in contact. This has the same effect as switching the exiting connections on the armature wires. **Although Fleming's right-hand generator rule demonstrates the change in direction of current within the armature wire, the commutator ring has also reversed the exiting connections, thus keeping the current in the circuit flowing in the same direction. It is at this point that direct current is produced.** Note that the direct current is not as steady as would be expected with a battery source. Instead a pulsating direct current has been produced.

Multiple-coil direct-current generators are used in place of the simple single-coil generators diagrammed in Figures 4–14 and 4–15. These DC generators utilize numerous coils and a commutator divided into a corresponding number of segments, as shown in Figure 4–16A. This type of generator produces a sine wave, as shown in Figure 4–16B. The combined current generated never drops to zero and has the advantage of a much steadier flow, although the pulsations have not been completely eliminated.

Motors

A device that is supplied with electrical current to produce mechanical motion is called a motor. Motors have essentially the same parts as generators and operate

A.

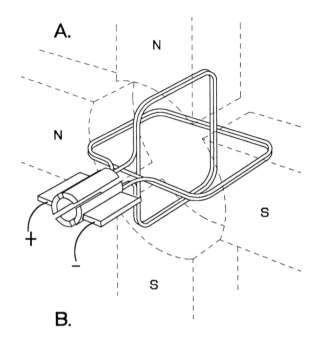

B.

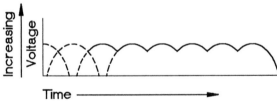

FIGURE 4–16. Multiple coil, split commutator, DC generator: More than one coil, or armature, with a split commutator (A) will produce DC current as shown in the graph (B).

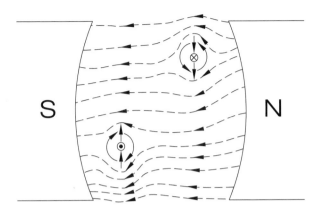

FIGURE 4–17. The motor principle: Because the conducting wires of the armature lie within the lines of force from the stationary magnets, when current begins to flow through the armature, the induced lines of force will be attracted downward for the left wire and upward for the right wire while at the same time being repelled in the other direction (upward for the left wire and downward for the right wire). The net result is that the conductor begins to move in the direction of the arrows.

on the same principles, but in reverse. In addition, some of the parts have been slightly redesigned and carry names different from those in a generator.

The motor principle is a result of the interaction of magnetic fields when an electric current is sent along a conductor that is residing in a magnetic field. As current flows through the conducting coil, a magnetic field is established, according to Fleming's right-hand thumb rule (Figure 4–17). Because the conducting coil lies within the lines of force from the stationary magnets, the induced lines of force will be attracted in one direction (downward for the left wire and upward for the right wire) while at the same time being repelled in the other

direction (upward for the left wire and downward for the right wire). The net result is that the conductor begins to move in the direction of the arrows.

Fleming's left-hand motor rule states that if the index finger points in the direction of the magnetic lines of force field and the middle finger points in the direction of the conventional current, the thumb will indicate the direction the conductor will move (Figure 4–18). (This would be a right-hand motor rule if the direction of electron flow is being considered.) Table 4–1 compares this rule with the other "hand" rules.

Different motor configurations are required depending on whether alternating or direct current is supplied. **Direct-current motors use commutator rings.** As with a DC generator, the commutator is required in order to switch the flow of current when the conducting coil begins to reach a 180° position, where the induced and stationary lines of force no longer attract or repel one another. When the current flow is switched by the commutator ring, the magnetic lines of force also reverse. Continuing this switching of current flow results in the conductor continually being simultaneously repelled and

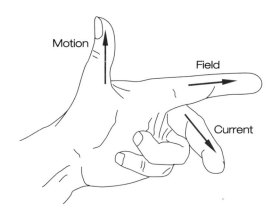

FIGURE 4–18. Fleming's left-hand motor rule: If the index finger points in the direction of the magnetic lines of force and the middle finger points in the direction of the conventional current flow, the thumb will indicate the direction the conductor will move. (This would be a right-hand motor rule if the direction of actual electron flow is being considered.)

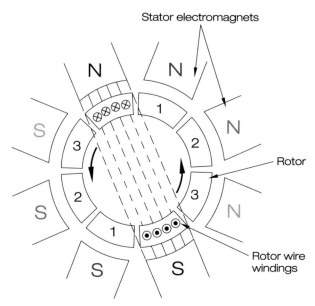

FIGURE 4–19. Alternating-current induction motor: The rotor windings obey the motor principle as they move perpendicular to the magnetic lines of flux, in the direction of the arrows. The stator electromagnets are supplied with multiphase current to activate them in sequential pairs to maintain maximum perpendicular motor principle force.

attracted in a circle, thus turning a shaft and supplying the mechanical motion as a conversion of the applied electrical energy.

These direct-current motors use many turns of wire in the conductor coil to increase the strength of the field. This requires numerous pairs of stationary magnets to force the conductor coil to cut the stationary lines of force as near to 90° (the maximum inducing angle) as often as possible (Figure 4–19).

Alternating-current motors use slip rings. Unlike direct-current motors, the incoming current switches direction, making the commutator unnecessary. There are two major types of alternating current motors.

Synchronous alternating-current motors have conducting coils that turn at the same speed as the generator armature supplying the current (or a multiple of the armature's speed). Synchronous motors are useful when a steady speed is necessary, as in a timing device. They tend to be relatively weak because insufficient motor principle force is established at the conducting coil.

Alternating-current induction motors utilize a rotor coil with the exterior magnetic field supplied by several pairs of electromagnets, thus producing a strong magnetic field, increasing the power of the motor and permitting it to run at any desired speed. Instead of sup-

plying current to the coil in the magnetic field, an induction motor uses a device called a rotor. **A rotor consists of bars of copper around an iron core** (Figure 4–19). No commutator or slip rings are required. Instead, a device called a stator is used. **A stator consists of pairs of stationary magnets (or, more commonly, electromagnets) arranged around the rotor. The stator must be supplied with multiphase current.** The stator electromagnets are energized in sequence. As the copper bars of the rotor reach a point where the motor principle forces are equalized, the multiphase current activates the next pair of electromagnets and the motor principle forces pull the rotor around to the next position. This continuing sequential energization causes the motor principle forces to continually turn the rotor. Extremely powerful induction motors are made by increasing the strength and number of pairs of electromagnets; these motors are popular for industrial and consumer uses.

Induction motors are used in rotating anode x-ray tubes where the target anode is attached to the induction motor rotor inside the glass vacuum tube. Because magnetic lines of force will pass through glass and a vacuum, the electromagnets can be positioned outside the vacuum tube, thus avoiding interference with the high voltages required to produce x-rays.

The motor principle is also used in meters: **galvanometers for direct current**, when permanent magnets are used, to indicate current and **dynamometers for alternating current**, when electromagnets are used (Figure 4–20A). To a great extent they are being replaced by digital meters that provide numerical indications of current. **When a meter is connected in series**, it measures current in amperes and is called an **ammeter** (Figure 4–20B). **When connected in parallel, it measures potential difference in volts and is called a voltmeter** (Figure 4–20C).

Controlling Electrical Current

Transformers

Alternating current, because of its changing direction, constantly establishes, collapses, re-establishes and re-collapses its surrounding magnetic field. This aspect can be used to change electricity by combining electromagnetic mutual induction with an application of Ohm's law to form a device called a **transformer**. Transformers are composed of two coils placed near one another (but without electrical connection). If current is supplied to one coil, the lines of force that are induced will pass through the other coil and induce a flow of electrons (Figure 4–11). The coil that is supplied with current is the **primary**, while the coil in which current is induced is the **secondary**.

The number of turns of wire in the primary coil is designed to be different from the number of turns of wire in the secondary. This causes the induced current to be different in the secondary coil. For example, the lines of force induced by a single primary coil loop may cut two loops of the secondary. In this case the voltage in the primary would be induced in **both** secondary loops, thus doubling the secondary voltage. When the voltage is increased from primary to secondary it is called a **step-up transformer**. When the voltage is decreased from primary to secondary it is called a step-down transformer. The **transformer law** expresses this phenomenon:

$$\frac{V_s}{V_p} = \frac{N_s}{N_p}$$

where:

V = potential difference in volts
N = number of turns of wire in the coil
p = primary coil
s = secondary coil

Example: If a transformer is supplied with 400 volts to the primary coil, has 100 turns of wire on the primary coil and 20,000 turns of wire on the secondary coil, what will the voltage be in the secondary coil?

Answer:

$$\frac{V_s}{V_p} = \frac{N_s}{N_p}$$

$$\frac{V_s}{400 \text{ V}} = \frac{20,000 \text{ turns}}{100 \text{ turns}}$$

$$100 \ V_s = 400 \ V \times 20,000 \text{ turns}$$

$$V_s = \frac{8,000,000}{100}$$

$$V_s = 80,000 \text{ volts or 80 kilovolts}$$

Example: If a transformer has 120 turns of wire on the primary coil, 80 volts in the primary coil and 20 volts in the secondary coil, how many turns of wire must there be in the secondary coil?

Answer:

$$\frac{V_s}{V_p} = \frac{N_s}{N_p}$$

$$\frac{20 \text{ V}}{80 \text{ V}} = \frac{N_s}{120 \text{ turns}}$$

$$\frac{2,400 \text{ turns}}{80} = N_s$$

$$N_s = 30 \text{ turns}$$

Transformers are used to change voltage. However, Ohm's law is in effect and the effect of the transformer on amperage, voltage and number of turns in the coils

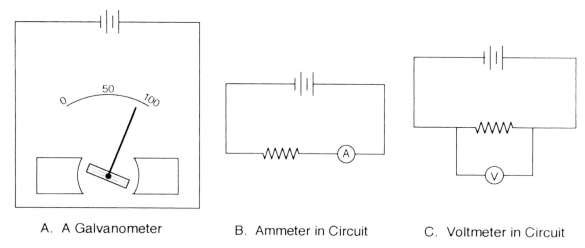

A. A Galvanometer   B. Ammeter in Circuit   C. Voltmeter in Circuit

FIGURE 4–20. (A) A simple galvanometer uses an electromagnet to attract a coil of wire to which a needle is attached. When a scale is calibrated, amperage or voltage can be measured. (B) Ammeter connection. (C) Voltmeter connection.

can be calculated by combining the transformer law with Ohm's law:

$$\frac{I_s}{I_p} = \frac{V_p}{V_s}$$

and:

$$\frac{I_s}{I_p} = \frac{N_p}{N_s}$$

It is helpful to remember that voltage and number of turns are directly proportional, while voltage and amperage are inversely proportional. Therefore, the number of turns and amperage must also be inversely proportional. It is also important to note that a step-up transformer increases voltage from primary to secondary while decreasing amperage. Conversely, a step-down transformer decreases voltage from primary to secondary while increasing amperage. Because transformers are designed to change voltages, the descriptive terms step-up and step-down refer to the voltage change, not the amperage change. You should remember that Ohm's law requires the consideration of resistance and this is indeed an important factor. However, this book will not address that aspect. **All transformers must operate on alternating current to provide the establishing and collapsing magnetic fields that induce the voltage changes in the secondary coil.**

Although transformer efficiency, the ability of a transformer to avoid power loss, is usually above 95 percent, a number of factors influence how much energy is lost. Because the high voltage transformer used in x-ray equipment must step up voltage into the kilovolt range, it uses large amounts of secondary coil windings. This massive amount of wire and the high induced voltage cause several problems that greatly affect the efficiency of the transformer.

1. **I^2R loss,** sometimes called copper loss, is caused by the inherent resistance to current flow that is found in all conductors. The power lost due to this resistance is proportional to the square of the current. It is minimized by using low-resistance wire, such as large-diameter copper, and by using high voltage and low amperage. Lost power is given off as heat. This is the reason why power transmitted long distances between cities is carried on high-voltage power lines. The high voltage permits low amperage and greatly reduced I^2R loss. Because high voltages are extremely dangerous, they are carried on high towers. Step-down transformers are used at receiving stations to lower the voltage (and increase the

amperage) to make the power safe for use in buildings.

2. **Hysteresis loss** (lagging loss) in the core occurs because energy is expended as the continually changing AC current magnetizes, demagnetizes and remagnetizes the core material. Demagnetization leaves some dipoles in the original orientation, and this residual magnetism causes the remagnetic effort to lag, thus producing more heat loss. The characteristic that requires energy to carry out this constant reorientation of the magnetic dipoles is called **coercivity.** Coercivity can be minimized by using a core material such as silicon iron.

3. **Eddy current loss** in the core is a result of currents opposing the cause which produced them, according to Lenz's law, as discussed earlier. They are produced in any conducting material subjected to changing magnetic fields. Laminating the transformer core reduces the eddy current loss by dividing the core into thin layers. This reduces the strength of the eddy currents (Figure 4–21).

These factors result in a great amount of heat build-up which can be felt by placing your hand on the exterior of the transformer cabinet in a diagnostic x-ray room. Although the transformer is highly insulated and immersed in insulating dielectric oil, there is a definite warmth to the cabinet after the machine has been in use for a few hours. The size of the x-ray transformer makes its efficiency an important factor.

There are numerous types of transformer configurations. The simple arrangement of two coils of wire in proximity to facilitate induction, that has been used so far to explain transformer function, is called an **air core** transformer. If the primary and secondary coils are filled with an iron core, the strength of the magnetic field is greatly increased, forming an **open-core** transformer. Various types of cores have been designed to enhance the lines of force and thereby increase the magnetic field strength (Figure 4–22). The field from an open core tends to diverge as it forms the external lines of force. Closing the core to form a **closed-core** transformer (by placing a top and bottom to the cores) will direct the lines of force from primary and secondary cores toward

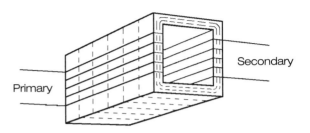

A. Closed core transformer

B. Non laminated core

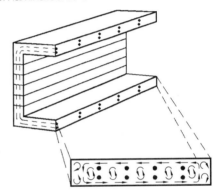

C. Eddy currents

D. Laminated core

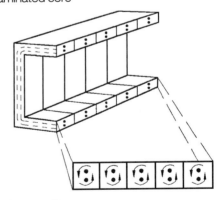

E. Eddy currents

FIGURE 4–21. (A) Closed-core transformer, (B) nonlaminated core, (C) nonlaminated core eddy currents, (D) laminated core, and (E) laminated core eddy currents.

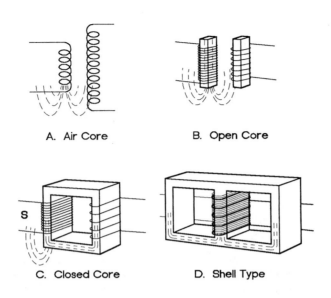

A. Air Core   B. Open Core

S

C. Closed Core   D. Shell Type

FIGURE 4–22. Various types of transformer core configurations: (A) air core, (B) open core, (C) closed core, and (D) shell type.

each other and result in a significant system net increase in field strength. The **shell type** transformer goes one step further by converging both the inside and outside lines of force through an iron core. In addition, a great efficiency is obtained by insulating the wiring and wrapping the primary and secondary coils atop one another, thus minimizing the distance between coils and maximizing the coupling effectiveness of the induction. X-ray generators use laminated core, shell type transformers, which are the most common type in use today.

Autotransformers

It is possible to construct a variable transformer, called an **autotransformer**, by connecting both primary and secondary coils in series instead of insulating them. This also permits a single coil on a central core. Connections are made along a single coil at different points for primary and secondary. The primary side has a selection of taps available to permit a variable number of turns in the primary coil (Figure 4–23). When the connections to the taps are attached to control buttons, an effective means of changing voltage is available.

Autotransformers are not suitable for use in the high-voltage transformers in x-ray machines. However, they are suitable for controlling voltage on the low-voltage side of the x-ray circuit before it has been increased by the main step-up transformer, thereby varying the voltage on the high-voltage side as well.

There are three important transformers in the x-ray circuit (Figure 4–24). The autotransformer is used to vary the incoming-line voltage to an appropriate level for the high-voltage step-up transformer. The high-voltage

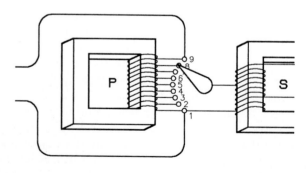

FIGURE 4–23. An autotransformer.

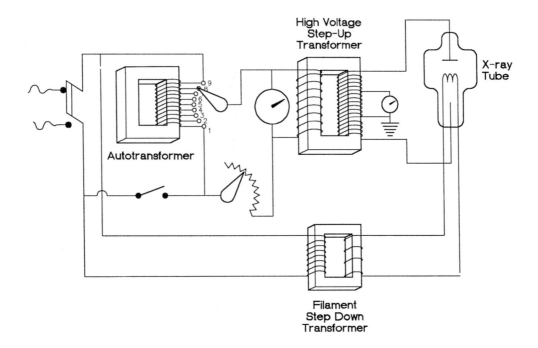

FIGURE 4–24. Three critical transformer locations in the diagnostic x-ray circuit. The autotransformer permits selection of the voltage (by controls labeled kV on the console). The high-voltage transformer steps the incoming-line voltage up to the kV range before sending it to the x-ray tube. The filament transformer steps the incoming-line voltage down to heat the x-ray tube filament.

step-up transformer is used to raise the incoming-line voltage to the kilovoltage range necessary for x-ray production. The filament step-down transformer is used to decrease the incoming-line voltage to the 5–15 volt and 3–5 ampere range used to heat the x-ray tube filament.

Capacitors

A **capacitor** is a device capable of accumulating and storing an electrical charge. A simple capacitor consists of two insulated metal plates with opposite charges (Figure 4–25). The repulsion between the charges on the two plates permits a greater number of electrons to be stored on each. The insulation between the plates is called the **dielectric** and its value is determined by the insulating ability as well as the plate size, distance between the plates, and charge. The unit of capacitance is named for Faraday but has been shortened to **farad**. It is represented by the symbol **f** and is expressed as:

$$C = \frac{q}{V}$$

where:

c = capacitance in farads
q = charge on either plate in coulombs
V = potential difference between plates in volts

Because of the immense size of the coulomb, the farad is very large, making the microfarad (μf) the more common unit.

Capacitors must be charged to be operable; this is done by applying a direct-current voltage. The capacitor will accept a charge until it equals the DC voltage. When discharged, the capacitor has the ability to deliver the stored charge in short and easily controlled intervals. This uniform direct current is especially useful in mobile x-ray units where it is convenient to have a battery charge a capacitor and then initiate a burst of high volt-

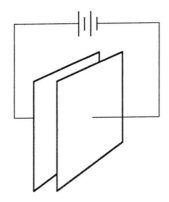

FIGURE 4–25. A simple parallel plate capacitor.

age for the x-ray exposure. Capacitors are also used to supply a more constant voltage to the x-ray tube in some stationary units.

Rectification

X-ray tubes operate best when receiving direct current. In fact, there is a danger in supplying alternating current because if a flow of electrons occurs in the wrong direction the tube may be damaged beyond repair. **Rectification is the process by which alternating current is changed to pulsating direct current**, and requires the use of one-way electrical devices called rectifiers. Although solid-state semiconductor diodes are most commonly used, it is easier to understand the operation of a vacuum-tube rectifier. Both of these devices create electrical "one-way streets" by permitting electrons to flow easily in one direction while offering a high resistance to movement in the other direction.

The operation of semiconductors was mentioned earlier, in Chapter 3, during the discussion of conductor valence bands. There are numerous types of semiconductors but they all operate in the same manner. The simplest to explain is the p-n junction semiconductor, which is composed of solid materials of two predominant categories, n-type and p-type. N-type materials have loosely bound electrons that move freely between an atom's conduction bands. P-type materials have electron traps made up of positively charged holes that tend

to attract and hold electrons instead of permitting them to move freely to another atom. Both types of materials are affected by slight amounts of impurities which are intentionally added to change the conduction properties. For example, arsenic has a valence that permits it to form covalent bonds with silicon crystals, but it makes an extra electron available for conduction, thus forming an n-type material. Conversely, gallium also has a valence permitting covalent bonding with silicon, but it leaves a need for an additional electron, thus forming an electron "hole" and a p-type material.

A rectifying semiconductor called a **diode** is made by sandwiching a p-type crystal with an n-type to form a p-n junction (Figure 4–26). When a potential difference is established with the positive charge at the p side of the junction and the negative charge at the n side, the positive holes from the p side are attracted to the junction, as are the available electrons from the n side. This permits easy movement of electrons into the p holes. **In a diode, electrons flow from the n to the p side of the p-n junction and conventional electrical current moves from the p to the n side.** When alternating current reverses and the positive charge is at the n side of the junction and the negative charge is at the p side, the positive holes from the p side are repelled from the junction, as are the available electrons from the n side. This makes movement of electrons from the n side of the junction to the p side very unlikely, as both the repulsion-attraction of the charges and the distance between p holes and electrons are working against the electron movement. The result is that no electrons move across the junction, thus creating a one-way street for electrons. The electronic symbol for a diode reflects this movement for conventional electrical current (Figure 4–26D). Remember that electron flow will be opposite the direction of the arrow.

A thyristor, or silicon-controlled rectifier (SCR), is a more complex semiconductor that has proven useful for high-speed switching of the primary high-voltage x-ray circuit. SCRs are composed of two p-type and two n-type layers, making three p-n junctions (Figure 4–27). Both n-p-n-p and p-n-p-n sequences are possible. In either case, the third section serves as a gate. This gate can change the polarity of the entire SCR by receiving a given charge. Rapid pulses of current to the gate permit it to hold or release large amounts of current. The SCR functions extremely rapidly and has replaced mechanical

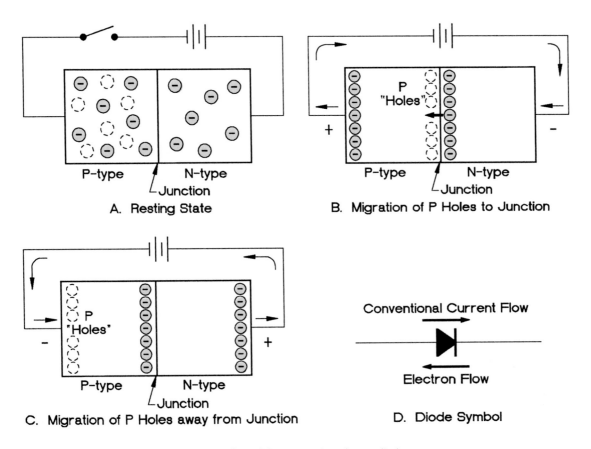

FIGURE 4–26. The functioning of a p-n junction of a solid-state semiconductor diode.

switchers and thyratrons (gas-filled predecessors to thyristors) in high kilowattage x-ray generators.

A valve tube was a vacuum tube that operated in the same manner as a diode but was constructed like an x-ray tube. Although they are no longer used in x-ray circuitry, they are a useful example in learning how a modern diode circuit functions. The difference between a valve tube and an x-ray tube is that a valve tube operated at energies below the range necessary to produce x-ray photons. The cathode and anode were arranged to permit electrons to jump without requiring the energy necessary to produce x-rays (Figure 4–28). Current could flow from cathode to anode because the jump to the massive anode was easy. However, as electrons repelled one another they spread out over the entire surface of the anode and could not develop sufficient repulsive force to

jump to the cathode. This made the tube a one-way street for electrons to move from cathode to anode.

The **cathode included a coil of small-diameter tungsten wire, called the filament, through which current was passed.** Of course the small diameter of the wire caused a greatly increased resistance to the flow of electrons. This resulted in heat increase to the extent that electron movement actually ejected individual electrons from the surface of the wire. Sometimes this phenomenon is described as a boiling of electrons from the surface. The result was the formation of an electron cloud (Figure 4–28B). This process is called **thermionic emission** because the heat (therm) has caused ionization (ionic), resulting in electrons being expelled (emission) from the surface of the wire. This effect is sometimes called a **space charge cloud.** It is important to note that the small diam-

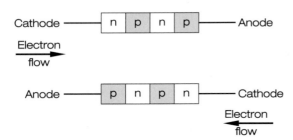

FIGURE 4–27. Silicon-controlled rectifier (SCR) n-p-n-p and p-n-p-n junctions.

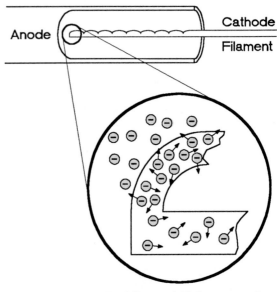

B. Filament Enlargement

FIGURE 4–28. Anode and cathode of a valve tube.

eter of the cathode's thin filament wire makes it extremely fragile. At the high kilovoltages supplied to x-ray tubes, a single electron striking the heated filament would cause it to break, thus rendering the tube useless. All modern x-ray machines use safety devices to prevent the anode side of the tube from receiving electrons, even during the opposing flow of alternating current.

The anode is a relatively large metallic surface, usually a cup, disk or flat plate, depending on the desired function of the tube. The shape of the anode varies between a valve tube and an x-ray tube and this accounts for the fact that x-ray tubes emit primarily x-ray range photons while valve tubes do not. Diagnostic x-ray tubes utilize angled disks, while dental x-ray tubes and other types of relatively low-voltage tubes use flat-plate anodes. A valve-tube anode consists of a cold metallic cup that surrounds the coiled filament (Figure 4–28).

Valve tubes permit electrons to flow from cathode to anode when a large enough potential difference exists to cause the electrons of the thermionically emitted cloud to be simultaneously repelled from the cathode and attracted to the anode. This is done by creating a **negative charge at the cathode and a positive charge at the anode** (Figure 4–29). **Remember that electron flow will always be from cathode to anode and this means conventional electrical current will always be from anode to cathode.** It is important to note that electrons cannot move from anode to cathode due to the charges and to the shapes of the anode and cathode. The anode is shaped much larger than the cathode filament and this causes the electrons to distribute themselves over the entire surface as they follow the law of repulsion in regard to one another (see Figure 4–29). With such a

large distribution surface, the electrons should not build up enough repulsion or heat to make movement from anode to cathode possible. When direct current causes the anode to remain positive at all times, there is a force of attraction working to keep the electrons on the anode. On the other hand, the cathode is relatively small and carries a negative charge at all times. The small size not only causes heating, it also restricts the flow of electrons so much that thermionic emission is enhanced. The negative charge works to encourage thermionic emission by actively repelling the electrons from the filament surface. Together these forces make the anode very attractive to electrons, while making the cathode undesirable. Consequently, as electron movement from cathode to anode is made easy, movement from anode to cathode is made extremely difficult. This creates a one-way street for electron flow, just as in a diode.

Half-Wave Rectification

In both solid-state diodes and valve tubes the forces create an electronic one-way street and effectively sup-

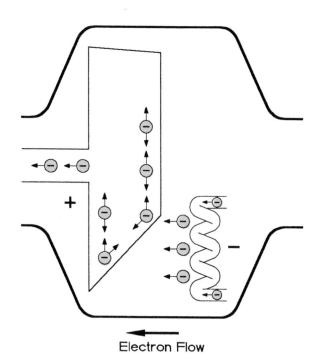

Electron Flow

FIGURE 4–29. Electron flow through an x-ray tube.

press the opposing half of the incoming current flow. A supply of alternating current to either type of rectifier will result in a pulsating direct current due to the suppression of half of the incoming wave (Figure 4–30). This type of suppression rectification is called **half-wave**

rectification because only half of the incoming alternating current is being converted to pulsating direct current. The opposing half of the flow is simply ignored and not utilized. In early radiography this type of circuit was called **self-rectification** (Figure 4–31). The danger was that overheating of the anode might cause thermionic emission. This condition could result in electrons moving to the cathode filament during the half of the alternating-current cycle when the anode was negatively charged. This of course would break the filament and destroy the x-ray tube. In even the simplest of modern x-ray equipment the x-ray tube is protected from this occurrence by the addition of a single rectifier on the anode side of the circuit (see Figure 4–30). This protects the x-ray tube anode from receiving a negative charge. In addition, if overheating should occur, the protecting rectifier would be destroyed and could be replaced, costing much less than it would to replace the x-ray tube.

Full-Wave Rectification

It is possible to convert the opposing half of the incoming electron flow so that electrons are always moving in the same direction, instead of discarding half the cycle by suppression. This is done through an ingenious arrangement of four rectifiers in a bridge circuit called a **full-wave rectification circuit** (Figure 4–32). A full understanding of the circuit requires following the electron flow completely from the secondary coil of the high-voltage step-up transformer to the x-ray tube dur-

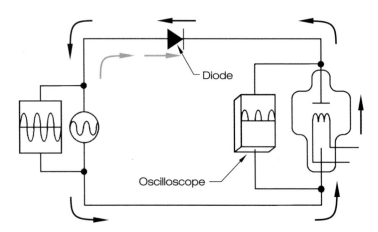

Diode

Oscilloscope

FIGURE 4–30. Half-wave rectification with one diode rectifier on the anode side of the x-ray tube circuit. Note the wave forms that would result if an oscilloscope was connected to the circuit.

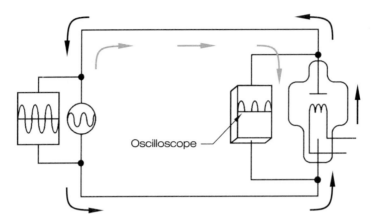

Oscilloscope

FIGURE 4–31. Half-wave rectification without a diode rectifier (self-rectification).

ing both halves of the AC cycle. Figure 4–32A illustrates the electron flow by the sequence of numbered arrows.

1. Electron flow is induced from the secondary coil of the high-voltage step-up transformer.

2. Electron flow reaches the first circuit junction and flows both ways.

3. Electron flow on this path reaches the anode of valve tube II and distributes over the large, unheated surface, attempting to build up enough charge to jump to the cathode.

4. Electron flow on this path reaches the heated cathode of valve tube I and easily jumps to the anode (thus never permitting enough charge to accumulate for the electron flow at arrow 3 to jump across valve tube II).

5. Electron flow reaches the second junction and flows both ways.

6. Electron flow on this path reaches the anode of valve tube III and distributes over the large, unheated surface, attempting to build up enough charge to jump to the cathode.

7. Electron flow on this path moves without resistance toward the x-ray tube.

8. Electron flow reaches the x-ray tube heated cathode and jumps to the anode.

9. X-rays are produced as a result of the electrons striking the anode.

10. Electron flow from the anode moves without resistance back toward the rectification circuit.

11. Electron flow reaches the third junction and flows both ways.

12. Electron flow on this path reaches the heated cathode of valve tube II but cannot jump to the anode because the anode is still loaded with the charge moving at arrow 3. Because these are like charges, they repel one another.

13. Electron flow on this path reaches the heated cathode of valve tube IV and easily jumps to the anode.

14. Electron flow reaches the fourth junction and flows both ways.

15. Electron flow on this path reaches the heated cathode of valve tube III but cannot jump to the anode because the anode is still loaded with the charge moving at arrow 6. Because these are like charges, they repel one another.

16. From this point on, electron flow on this path moves without resistance toward the secondary coil of the high-voltage step-up transformer. This completes the circuit.

Following the same logic, to trace the current path for the opposite half of the alternating current cycle in Figure 4–32 results in reorientation of the direction of

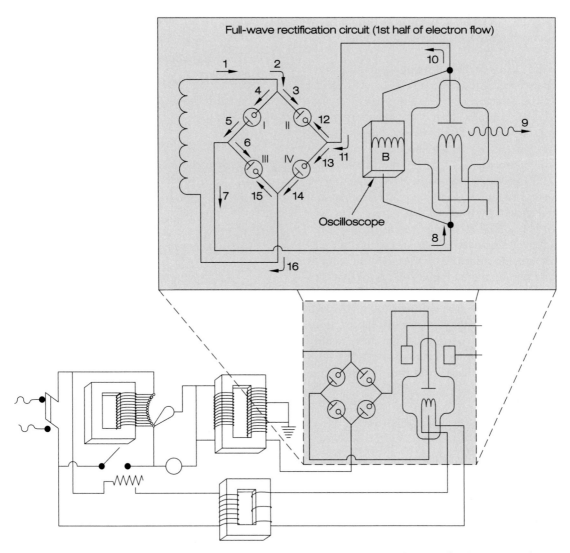

FIGURE 4–32. Full-wave rectification circuit from within a basic diagnostic x-ray circuit. (See text for description of electron flow.)

electron flow. This is full-wave rectification and it produces the sine wave shown in Figure 4–32B.

Note that **the x-ray tube will emit x-ray photons during both halves of the full-wave rectified AC cycle**. The double efficiency of full-wave rectification permits a significant increase in the power output capability of radiographic equipment. This results in an ability to use higher mA and kVp settings. Consequently, nearly all modern x-ray equipment is full-wave rectified.

Summary

A magnetic force field surrounds all charged particles when they are in motion. These force fields are magnetic lines of force. Electromagnets are temporary magnets produced by moving electric current. The laws governing magnetism are similar to the laws of electrostatics. Electromagnetic induction is an important phenomenon basic to nearly all electrical devices. It is produced by movement between magnetic lines of force and a conductor.

A generator is a device that converts mechanical energy to electrical energy. Either AC or DC current can be produced through the use of either slip rings or a commutator ring. One complete turn of the generator armature represents one cycle (1 Hz). A device that is supplied with electrical current to produce mechanical motion is called a motor. Motors have essentially the same parts as generators and operate on the same principles, but in reverse. A meter may be connected in parallel to measure current or in series to measure voltage.

A transformer is used to change voltage through the use of Ohm's law. A capacitor is a device capable of accumulating and storing electrical charge. Rectification is the process by which alternating current is changed to pulsating direct current. Silicon-controlled rectifiers are solid-state semiconductors that are used for high-speed switching of the primary high-voltage x-ray circuit. Both self-wave and half-wave rectification are infrequently used in modern x-ray equipment. Diodes replaced valve tubes as one-way circuits that permit full-wave rectification.

● REVIEW QUESTIONS

1. What is magnetism?
2. What is an electromagnet?
3. Explain the difference between electron flow and conventional current flow.
4. What is indicated by the direction of the thumb, index, and middle finger in one of Fleming's hand rules?
5. What are the three ways to induce electromagnetic current flow in a conductor?
6. Name the four factors controlling the strength of electromagnetically induced current.
7. What is the difference between a generator and a motor?
8. Describe the functions of slip rings and of a commutator ring.

9. How is an ammeter different from a voltmeter?
10. What is the function of a transformer?
11. State the transformer law.
12. What is the function of an autotransformer?
13. What is a diode?
14. What is rectification?
15. What components are necessary to produce a full-wave rectified circuit?

● REFERENCES AND RECOMMENDED READING

Ball, J. & Price, T. (1989). *Chesneys' radiographic imaging.* Oxford: Blackwell Scientific Publishing.

Ball, J. L. & Moore, A. D. (1986). *Essential physics for radiographers* (2nd ed.). Oxford: Blackwell Scientific Publications.

Boylestod, R. L. (1987). *Introductory circuit analysis* (5th ed.). Columbus: Merrill Publishing Company.

Bushberg, J. T., Seibert, J. A., Leidholdt, E. M., Boone, J. M. (1994). *The essential physics of medical imaging.* Baltimore: Williams & Wilkins.

Bushong, S. C. (1997). *Radiologic science for technologists: Physics, biology, and protection* (6th ed.). St. Louis: C. V. Mosby.

Carroll, Q. B. (1993). *Fuchs's radiographic exposure, processing and quality control* (5th ed.). Springfield, IL: Charles C. Thomas Publishers.

DeFrance, J. J. (1969). *Electrical fundamentals.* Englewood Cliffs, NJ: Prentice-Hall.

Del Toro, V. (1993). *Principles of electrical engineering* (4th ed.). Englewood Cliffs, NJ: Prentice-Hall.

Dendy, P. P. & Heaton, B. (1987). *Physics for radiologists.* Oxford: Blackwell Scientific Publications.

Du Pont x-ray technical service product information, *Static Electricity,* Wilmington, DE: Du Pont Company, Photo Products Dept., Chestnut Run Lab, Publication E-53821.

Gates, E. D. (1987). *Introduction to electronics: A practical approach.* Albany: Delmar Publishers.

Gifford, D. (1984). *A handbook of physics for radiologists and radiographers.* New York: John Wiley & Sons.

Glasser, O., Quimby, E. H., Taylor, L. S., Weatherwax, J. L., & Morgan, R. H. (1961). *Physical foundations of radiology* (3rd ed.). New York: Paul B. Hoeber Division of Harper & Brothers.

Graham, B. J. & Thomas, W. N. (1975). *An introduction to physics for radiologic technologists.* Philadelphia: W. B. Saunders.

Hay, G. A. & Hughes, D. (1972). *First-year physics for radiographers.* London: Bailliere Tindall.

Hendee, W. R. & Ritenour, R. (1993). *Medical imaging physics* (3rd ed.) St. Louis: C. V. Mosby.

Johns, H. E. & Cunningham, J. R. (1983). *The physics of radiology* (4th ed.). Springfield, IL: Thomas.

Loper, D. E., Ahr, A. F., Clendenning, L. R. (1973). *Introduction to electricity and electronics.* Albany: Delmar Publishers.

Meredith, W. J. & Massey, J. B. (1977). *Fundamental physics of radiology* (3rd ed.). Chicago: Yearbook Medical Publishers.

Nadon, J. M., Gelmine, B. J., & McLaughlin, E. D. (1989). *Industrial electricity* (4th ed.). Albany: Delmar Publishers.

Ridgway, A. & Thumm, W. (1973). *The physics of medical radiography.* Reading, MA: Addison-Wesley.

Roderick, J. F. & Sutherland, B. (1952). *A study of the static electricity problems in the x-ray darkroom.* The X-Ray Technician. *23*(March).

Roller, D. & Roller, H. D. (1967). The development of the concept of electric charge: Electricity from the Greeks to Coulomb, case 8, *Harvard Case Histories in Experimental Science.* Cambridge: Harvard University Press.

Selman, J. (1994). *The fundamentals of x-ray and radium physics* (9th ed.). Springfield, IL: Thomas.

Sprawls, P. (1990). *Principles of radiography for technologists.* Rockville, MD: Aspen Publishers.

Sprawls, P. (1987). *Physical principles of medical imaging.* Rockville, MD: Aspen Publishers.

Stockley, S. M. (1986). *A manual of radiographic equipment.* Edinburgh: Churchill Livingstone.

Ter-Pogossian, M. M. (1967). *The physical aspects of diagnostic radiology.* New York: Hoeber Medical Division, Harper & Row.

Thompson, M. A., Hattaway, M. P., Hall, J. D., Dowd, S. B. (1994). *Principles of imaging science and protection.* Philadelphia: W. B. Saunders.

Thompson, T. T. (1985). *A practical approach to modern imaging equipment* (2nd ed.). Boston: Little, Brown, & Co.

Tortorici, M. (1992). *Concepts in medical radiographic imaging.* Philadelphia: WB Saunders.

van der Plaats, G. J. (1980). *Medical x-ray techniques in diagnostic radiology* (4th ed.). The Hague: Martinus Nijhoff Publishers.

Wilks, R. J. (1981). *Principles of radiological physics.* Edinburgh: Churchill Livingstone.

Wolbarst, A. B. (1993). *Physics of radiology.* Norwalk, CT: Appleton & Lange.

CHAPTER 5

X-Ray Equipment

Suspended in icy silence
I look at myself from far off
Calmly, I feel free

Even though I'm not, now
Or ever:

The metal teeth of death bite
But spit me out
One more time:

When the technologist says breathe
I breathe.

Patricia Goedicke, "One More Time."

Objectives

Upon completion of this chapter, the student should be able to:

▶ Describe various diagnostic equipment, table, tube-support, and ancillary equipment configurations.

▶ State incoming line current characteristics.

▶ Describe the differences between single-phase and three-phase power.

▶ Explain the functions of the basic components of the main and filament x-ray circuits.

▶ Discuss the differences between single-phase, three-phase six- and twelve-pulse, and high-frequency waveforms on generator output.

▶ Describe the function of capacitor discharge and battery-operated mobile units.

▶ Explain the function of a falling load generator.

▶ Differentiate phototimers from ionization chamber automatic exposure controls.

> ▶ Describe the placement and function of a phototimer and an ionization chamber automatic exposure control.
>
> ▶ Describe potential problems that could be caused by minimum reaction times.
>
> ▶ Justify the use of backup time when using automatic exposure controls.

Types of X-Ray Equipment

*A*vast number of uses for x-rays have been found in medicine and this has led to the development of a wide variety of categories and types of equipment (Figure 5–1). Medical x-ray units can be classified as **diagnostic** or **therapeutic**. Most diagnostic units are designed for specific procedures, such as general procedures, cardiac catheterization, head procedures, fluoroscopy, etc. All of these units operate within the diagnostic x-ray range. This range is approximately $10-1,200$ milliamperes (mA), $0.001-10$ seconds, at a peak kilovoltage (kVp) of approximately 25 to 150. Therapeutic equipment operates at much higher energies, ranging from 4 to 40 million electron-volts (meV). Because of the extremely high voltages used, therapy equipment operates below 20 mA and with time settings in the range of 1 to 60 minutes.

Tables

The radiographic table is designed to support the patient in a position that will enhance radiographic examination. As any patient can attest, comfort is not the primary purpose of the table, although some institutions permit foam pads for lengthy examinations.

The tabletop must be uniformly radiolucent to easily permit x-rays to pass through. A Bakelite or similar surface is most common, although specialized applications, such as angiography, may use a carbon graphite fiber to reduce absorption of photons. Although flat tops are most common, curved tops are available. Curved (or dished) tops are usually used for fluoroscopic examinations. They are usually more comfortable for the patient and permit the body part to be placed slightly closer to the film for a more accurate image. Curved tops have

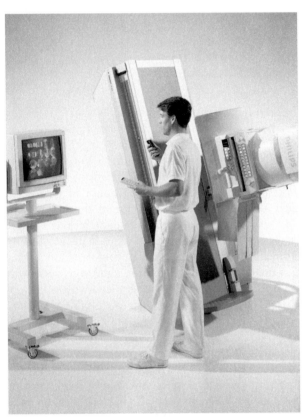

FIGURE 5–1. A typical diagnostic radiographic and fluoroscope room. *(Courtesy of Philips Medical Systems, Shelton, CT)*

two serious disadvantages. It is difficult for the radiographer to maintain a patient accurately in an oblique or lateral position on a curved top, and the top is entirely useless as a level support surface for a film cassette during tabletop radiography.

The tabletop must be **easily cleaned, hard to scratch, and without crevices where radiographic contrast media**

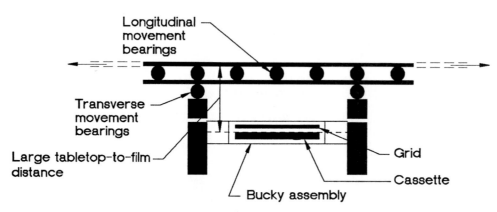

FIGURE 5–2. A diagnostic radiographic floating top table. *(Used by permission from Stockley, S. M. [1986]. A manual of radiographic equipment. Edinburgh: Churchill Livingstone.)*

can accumulate. It is sometimes necessary to remove body fluids after an examination and this must be possible to achieve in a quick and sanitary manner.

The table must **include space for a tray to hold film cassettes and a radiographic grid** (Figure 5–2). The tray is often called a "Bucky tray" in honor of Dr. Gustav Bucky (1880–1963), the inventor of the radiographic grid that is installed over the film cassette tray. The grid installation usually consists of a mechanism that will automatically move the grid during exposure. Many units include automatic exposure control sensors in the tray. Some tables use a stationary tray with a movable tabletop. Others use a tray that is movable along rails extending the length of the table with a stationary tabletop. Still others use a tray and top that are both partially movable. Some tabletops are motor driven and movable along their length. Others are floating tops which can be moved along their length and width simultaneously when an electromagnetic brake is released. The brake may be controlled by hand, knee, or foot. Floating tops save radiographers significant amounts of time and effort, especially when positioning large patients.

Tables are available in **fixed** and **tilting** models. Fixed tables do not permit tilting the patient's head or feet down. They are designed for diagnostic radiographic work only. Tilting tables are sometimes described by their tilting capability (for example, 90–15 would indicate a table capable of tilting 90° in one direction and 15° in the other). Rooms designed to perform both diagnostic radiographic and fluoroscopic (R&F) examina-

tions are equipped with tilting tables, although some rooms designed only for radiographic examinations may also use them.

The table is usually at a height that reduces physical strain on the radiographer, who must stretch and bend over and around the table as the patient, ancillary equipment, film, and x-ray tube are positioned. This is usually 30–40 inches or 75–100 cm from the floor. This is not a safe or convenient height for patients and it causes problems for ambulatory patients who are not in good physical condition. A primary concern for all radiographers must be proper assistance to these patients when they are getting onto and down from the table. Fixed tables are available in adjustable models that can be lowered while a patient is assisted onto the table and then raised to a working height.

Ancillary equipment for tilting tables includes a **footboard** for patients to stand on when the table is upright. The footboard is often used for gastrointestinal studies when the patient begins the examination in an erect position and is then brought horizontal during the procedure, or vice versa. In these instances it is critical to ascertain that the footboard is securely in place and will support the full weight of the patient. This is best done when the table is horizontal by pulling hard on the footboard. Procedures requiring tilting the patient's head down, such as myelography, may require the use of **shoulder supports** to keep patients from sliding off the table. In these instances **handgrips** give the patient an added feeling of security.

Compression bands serve two functions: they restrain patients who are unable to cooperate, and they compress abdominal tissue for a more uniform subject density. Both functions improve radiographic image quality. A compression band should never be used as the sole restraint device.

Tube Supports

The tube support system is designed to permit the x-ray tube to be manipulated to the various locations necessary to obtain examination procedure projections and to hold the tube immobile during the exposure. Tube suspension systems are available in five versions: **overhead, floor-to-ceiling, floor, mobile and C-arm**. Both flexibility and cost are reflected in this order, with overhead supports being the most flexible and costly.

The **overhead suspension system**, sometimes called ceiling suspension, includes **two sets of rails** for controlling **longitudinal** and **transverse** positioning and a **telescoping column** for controlling vertical distance (Figure 5–3A). The end of the telescoping column can be capable of **angling** up to a 300° arc toward the head or foot of the table, **rotating** up to 360° around the column, and **rolling or pitching** up to 60° transversely (side to side) (Figure 5–3B). A properly installed overhead suspension system will be perfectly counterbalanced and will not drift toward one side or corner of the room when the positioning locks are released. A well-designed system will permit the radiographer to remove the locks and "carry" the tube to any position within the room.

Each of these complex motions is locked into place by a solenoid with a control placed where it can be easily

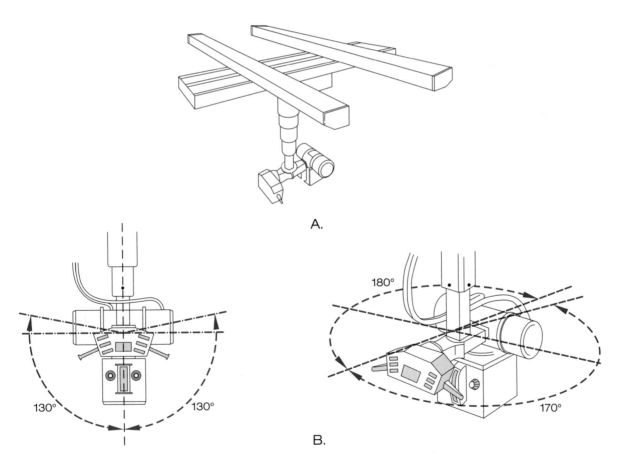

FIGURE 5–3. An overhead (or ceiling) tube suspension system.

reached by the radiographer. Also included in the control mechanisms are "detents," or centering locks, to verify common tube positions (for example, centered to the film cassette in the Bucky tray or at a routine distance from the table or upright Bucky unit). Unfortunately, each manufacturer uses a different placement and labeling for these controls. For this reason, it is helpful to practice manipulating the controls prior to using the equipment to perform radiographic procedures.

The **floor-to-ceiling suspension system** uses a pair of rails, one on the ceiling and one on the floor, for longitudinal positioning. Rooms with extremely high ceilings may use an overhead rail suspended from a wall (Figure 5–4). This system uses a telescoping arm for transverse positioning and a main column collar that slides up and down for vertical distance and pivots for additional maneuverability. The tube may also be able to angle and roll or pitch but it is not capable of rotating. One of the

disadvantages of a floor-to-ceiling tube is that rotation must be accomplished by pivoting the main column collar and then bringing the tube back into position by longitudinal and transverse adjustments.

A **floor suspension system** uses a tube-support column mounted on the floor. Stationary columns are fixed to the table while movable columns run on either one or two rails mounted on the floor (Figure 5–5). The operation of this system is similar to the operation of a floor-to-ceiling system. The system must be carefully counterbalanced to avoid tipping. This is usually accomplished by adding a counterweight to the back of the telescoping tube arm and requires that both tube system and table be installed further from the back wall than other systems. Some floor suspension systems are not designed to permit pivoting of the collar, which limits their positioning capability severely.

There are many types of **mobile** systems. The tube suspension systems for mobile units vary tremendously but most are based on the floor suspension system (Figure 5–6). Another type of system is simply a tube mounted on a mobile stand for use during special procedures, such as angiography. The basic radiography system (BRS) developed by the International Society of Radiographers and Radiological Technicians (ISRRT)

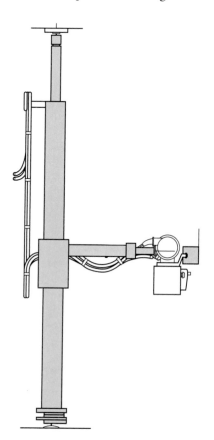

FIGURE 5–4. A floor-to-ceiling tube suspension system.

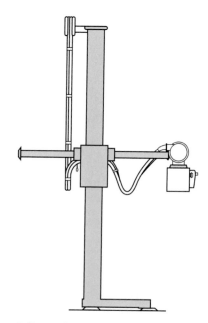

FIGURE 5–5. A floor tube suspension system.

and the World Health Organization (WHO) for use in developing regions is a very simple system designed to facilitate the provision of services to these areas. This extremely portable system can be mounted on a tripod or patient lift support.

A **C-arm tube suspension system** utilizes a C-shaped arm to support the tube and image receptor (Figure 5–7). The tube and image receptor are fixed to opposite ends of the C-arm. When the clamp or lock holding the C-arm in position is released, it permits both tube and image receptor to be rotated to a new position. C-arms (or U-arms) are used in head units, mobile fluoroscopy units and ceiling-suspended angiography and surgical units.

Head Units

A **head unit** is a specialized adaptation of the floor-to-ceiling unit and is designed to enhance radiography of the cranium and facial bones. A head unit consists of an x-ray tube and a Bucky tray unit but does not include a table (Figure 5–8). The patient can be radiographed standing, sitting in a chair, or pulled over the Bucky tray

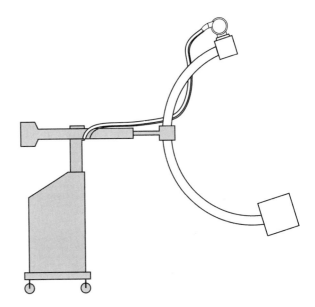

FIGURE 5–7. A C-arm tube suspension system.

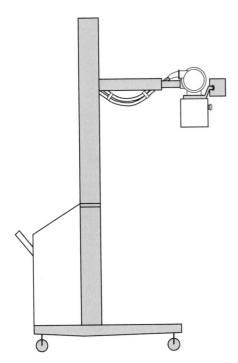

FIGURE 5–6. A mobile tube suspension system.

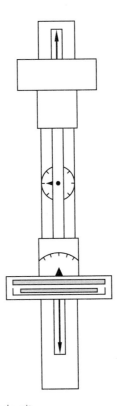

FIGURE 5–8. A head unit.

from a locked cart. The advantage of a head unit is that it can be added to a radiographic room with an existing tube and table and can usually be operated from an existing generator and console. It improves head radiography by regulating tube angles, decreasing the distance from the patient to the film and minimizing the positioning of the patient (especially advantageous for trauma patients). The unit consists of a floor-to-ceiling tube mount with a C-arm or U-arm attachment on the pivoting collar.

Upright Units

An upright film cassette holder or Bucky unit is a common and useful ancillary piece of equipment in any radiographic room (Figure 5–9). Chest radiography should routinely be done in an upright position and there are numerous other procedures that are best done upright (for example, acromio-clavicular joints, abdominal obstructive procedures, cervical spine, etc.). Upright film cassette holders may or may not include a radiographic grid. Upright Bucky units may include the same equipment as the Bucky tray located in a table (movable radiographic grid, film cassette tray and automatic exposure control sensors).

Other Specialized Diagnostic Equipment

Other types of equipment have been developed to meet specialized needs. They include chest units designed to automate chest radiography by combining an upright Bucky unit with an automatic film handling mechanism, **mammography** units for breast studies, **tomography** units with tubes that move in an arc during exposure, **head units** for cranial studies (as previously discussed), **panoramic dental and facial units** for combined tomography of facial structures, **computed tomography** units for computerized sectional images, radiation therapy **simulator** units to verify radiation therapy treatment set-ups prior to actual treatment, **urologic** units to facilitate urological and genital studies and units custom built to nearly any specifications.

Power For X-Ray Generation

A diagnostic x-ray generator is composed of numerous basic electrical devices. An x-ray circuit is established when these devices are connected in a sequence capable of accelerating electrons to the speed necessary to cause the production of x-ray photons within an x-ray tube. The incoming line power may be modified in several ways to establish these conditions.

Incoming Line Current

Electricity is usually supplied to buildings in the United States and Canada by 60 Hz alternating current with a nominal rms of 200–240 volts. These are termed nominal because, as users operate various resistances, the voltages constantly fluctuate, as illustrated by Ohm's law. This power is called the **incoming line current** (sometimes called the **mains**) and is supplied in the form of a three-phase power cycle (Figure 5–10). One of the "hot" wires is always half the incoming voltage above-ground potential while the other is always the same voltage below-ground potential. In the United States and

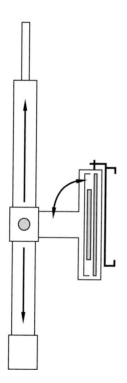

FIGURE 5–9. An upright Bucky unit.

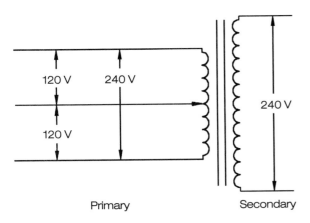

FIGURE 5–10. Three-phase, 60 Hz, 240 V incoming line current.

Canada each carries 110–120 volts. With 60 Hz alternating current, the two hot wires reverse their polarity 120 times per second. Bringing incoming line current from the neutral (or ground) wire and one of the hot wires produces a potential difference of 110–120 volts. Because the two lines are not in phase with one another, using incoming current from both hot wires produces a potential difference that is less than the sum of the two single phases. The usual result is about 210 V. Nearly all x-ray equipment operates from an incoming line of 210–220 volts.

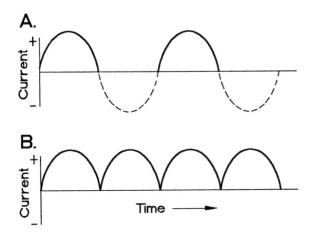

FIGURE 5–11. Single-phase power: (A) incoming line, (B) full-wave rectified.

Single-Phase Power

Single-phase power permits the potential difference to drop to zero with every change in the direction of current flow (Figure 5–11A) and is represented by the symbol 1ϕ. In a full-wave rectified circuit (direct pulsating current), this means the x-ray tube is experiencing no potential difference and is producing no x-ray photons 120 times each second on a 60 Hz line (Figure 5–11B). With the 60 Hz line, an exposure of 0.1 second with a single-phase full-wave rectified unit results in twelve intervals of no photon production (Figure 5–12). In addition, the photons produced during the low-voltage periods are of such low energy that they may not exit the tube, or they do not contribute to the radiographic image because they are absorbed before reaching the image receptor (film). The root mean square (rms) voltage of a single-phase sinusoidal wave is usually given as 70.7 percent of the peak voltage.

Example: What is the approximate rms voltage of a single-phase sine wave with a peak of 80 kVp?

Answer:

$$\text{rms voltage} = 70.7\% \text{ peak kVp}$$
$$\text{rms voltage} = 70.7\% \times 80 \text{ kVp}$$
$$\text{rms voltage} = 56.6 \text{ kVp}$$

Obviously this is not as efficient as desired. A solution is to combine several waveforms of current slightly out of step with one another to create **three-phase power**.

Three-Phase Power

Three-phase power is produced by the generator and is the common form in which power is supplied to users by power companies. Three-phase power is generated as is shown in Chapter 4 by Figure 4–16 and is represented by the symbol 3ϕ. As each wave peak begins to drop toward zero, the overall potential difference is boosted back to peak by the next phase wave. The result is that the sum of the phasing never drops to zero (Figure 5–13A). When full-wave rectification is applied, the net voltage produces a **voltage ripple**. Three-phase current produces a voltage ripple of 3 pulses per half cycle, which is 6 pulses per Hz and 360 pulses per second. (See Figure 5–17.)

Whenever any of the phases is at zero, the other two phases are of equally opposite values so that the sum of

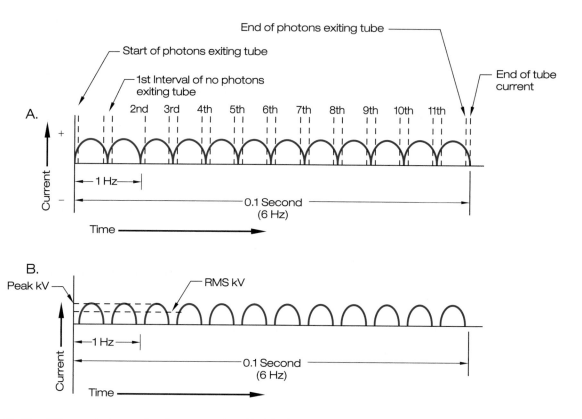

FIGURE 5–12. The difference between the photons produced inside the x-ray tube during an exposure and the photons emitted from the tube during the same exposure. (A) X-ray production during an exposure of 0.1 second with a 1φ full-wave rectified unit. (B) Emission of photons from an x-ray tube during an exposure of 0.1 second with a 1φ full-wave rectified circuit.

the three currents is always zero. This fact is used in connecting the generator windings to combine the current. A **wye or star connection** (Figure 5–14A) combines phases 1, 2 and 3 to achieve the waveform seen in Figures 5–13A&B. Although the wye or star connection is more popular because it permits a single phase to be easily tapped from the same line, a **delta connection** is also possible (Figure 5–14B).

A Basic X-Ray Circuit

The basic x-ray circuit can be divided into the **main** and **filament** circuits. **The main circuit supplies the x-ray tube with properly modified power.** Its purpose is to produce x- rays. **The filament circuit supplies the fila-**

ment of the x-ray tube with properly modified power. Its purpose is to create the appropriate thermionically emitted electron cloud at the filament. These two circuits are distinct from each other although they are interconnected (Figure 5–15).

The Main X-ray Circuit

The main x-ray circuit modifies the incoming-line power to produce x-rays by a sequence of devices, as shown in Figure 5–16. The circuit must boost the voltage to the range necessary to produce x-rays and to permit the radiographer to adjust the amperage, voltage and length of exposure, as well as incorporate appropriate circuitry to increase the efficiency of x-ray production.

The **main switch** and **circuit breakers** are usually enclosed in an electrical power box. The **exposure switch**

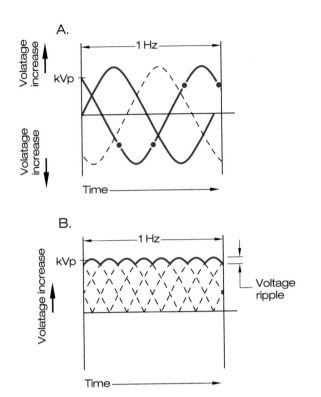

FIGURE 5–13. (A) Three-phase incoming line current. (B) Full-wave rectified three-phase current.

is simply a remote control switch that permits current to flow through the circuit. Diagnostic x-ray control exposure switches are designed to begin but not end exposures. The **timer** circuit is intended to end the exposure at an accurately measured, preset time. For this reason, whenever the exposure switch is depressed it must be held until both the audible and visible indicators (usually a buzzer and a light) have ceased. For example, if a radiographer is accustomed to making short exposures of less than 0.5 second, failure to hold the exposure switch for a 2.5 second exposure of a large abdomen would prematurely terminate the exposure.

The Exposure Switch

The exposure switch can be connected to the switch that activates the rotating anode of the x-ray tube. The anode must be turning at a sufficiently high speed to avoid melting of the target area by the high kilovoltage exposure. To avoid the possibility of error, all x-ray units that utilize rotating anodes have circuitry that prevents an exposure until the anode is turning at the correct speed. It is usually convenient to combine the anode rotor and the exposure switch in a two-step button. Therefore, most exposure switches are depressed halfway to activate the anode rotation and then depressed completely to initiate the x-ray exposure. Tube manufactur-

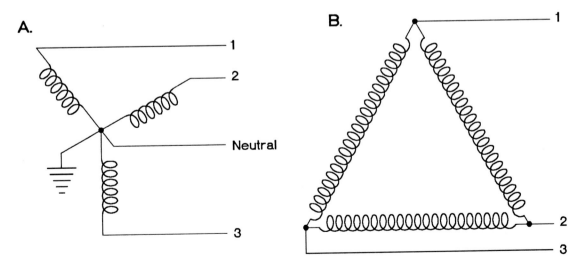

FIGURE 5–14. Three-phase connections: (A) wye or star, (B) delta. Phases 1, 2, and 3 are combined in a wye or delta configuration to achieve incoming three-phase power.

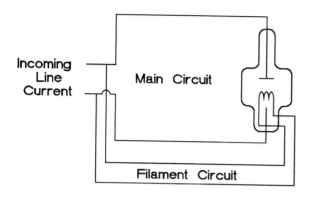

FIGURE 5–15. Main and filament circuits.

ers recommend that these buttons be depressed completely in one motion. This helps to extend the life of the x-ray tube.

The exposure switch must be attached to the control console in such a manner that it is impossible for the operator to be exposed. In addition, the equipment must be designed to prohibit the x-ray tube from being manipulated into a position where it could expose the user. On mobile equipment the switch must be on a cord with a minimum length of six feet. This is to permit the radiographer to move as far as possible from the x-ray tube during an exposure. All exposure switches must be of the "dead-man" type, in which x-ray exposure may occur only while the switch is depressed. Release of the switch must terminate the exposure. This prevents the exposure from continuing when the operator enters the radiation area.

The Timer Circuit

The timer circuit can be of several types. All are designed to regulate the length of time the x-ray tube is part of the circuit and thereby control the number of x-ray photons produced.

Synchronous Timers

Synchronous timers operate from a simple motor that is turning at the same rate as the generator. The number or percentage of rotations can be converted into time increments. Units equipped with synchronous timers are easily recognized as the time increments tend to be multiples of 1/60th (1/30, 1/20, 1/15, etc.). They require a short recycling time and

therefore cannot be used for serial exposures.

Electronic Timers

Electronic timers are the most common timers in use today. They are capable of accurate exposures as short as 0.001 second with only a 1 msec delay. Most electronic timers operate by charging a silicon-controlled rectifier (SCR) which then triggers the exposure. It is linked with a microprocessor that calculates the length of time the current will need to reach a trigger value. This level is set by the variation of the timer controls on the console unit by the radiographer.

Milliampere-Second Timers

Milliampere-second timers are used in falling load generators as well as some capacitor discharge units. They monitor the product of mA and time on the secondary side of the high-voltage step-up transformer. When the desired mAs level is reached, these timers interrupt the circuit to stop the exposure. Because the high-voltage capacitor, timer and x-ray tube are operating on the same circuit, mAs value remains constant even when there is a slight fluctuation in the capacitor charging current.

Automatic Exposure Control Timers

Automatic exposure controls or automatic exposure devices are also used, as described later in this chapter. The **autotransformer**, with its taps controlled by the kVp selectors on the control console, modifies the incoming line voltage in anticipation of the kilovoltage that will be produced by the step-up transformer. Some units divide the kVp adjustments into major and minor regions. Usually a major adjustment will change in units of 10 kVp while minor adjustments will change in units of 1 or 2 kVp.

The Filament Circuit

The filament circuit modifies the incoming line power to produce the thermionic emission from the filament wire of the x-ray tube by a sequence of devices (Figure 5–16). The incoming line must be modified to about 3–5 amperes and 6–12 volts. The filament circuit's supply is drawn directly from the main circuit's supply. Current control devices regulate the amperage supplied to the filament in the x-ray tube. This control device can be adjusted by the radiographer at the control console. It is not labeled by the actual amperage it controls. Instead it is marked in increments representative of the mA that will be available at the filament when the high-voltage supply is released at exposure. Filament circuits are usually adjustable to the equivalent of mA ratings of 50, 100, 200, 300, 400, 500, 600, 800, 1,000 and 1,200. Not all equipment will have all mA settings and some may have other unusual settings, as discussed in the section on timers. Most 1φ units do not go beyond 500 mA. Specialized tomographic equipment generators may also include 10, 15, 20, 25, 30 and 40 mA stations.

Many units include a meter at this point to provide an accurate reading of the amperage delivered. After regulation, the current is then sent to a step-down transformer that modifies it to the appropriate amperage that will reach the filament itself. A very slight shift in the quantity of electrons in the thermionic cloud around the filament can have a dramatic effect on the quantity of x-ray photons produced when the kilovoltage exposure occurs. Therefore, filament circuits also incorporate several types of current stabilization devices, including frequency compensators, voltage stabilizers and space charge compensators.

The main and filament circuits are combined to form the complete basic x-ray circuit (Figure 5–16). The radiographer adjusts the various factors from a control console which must be located in a radiation-shielded location outside the radiographic exposure room. **All of the radiographer-operated controls are located on the low-voltage side of the circuit to protect operators from high-voltage shock hazards.** The controls that are likely to be located on this console are included in Table 5–1.

Generators

Single-Phase Generators

Single-phase generators with full-wave rectification produce a voltage ripple of 2 pulses per Hz or 120 pulses per second. This produces two usable pulses per cycle

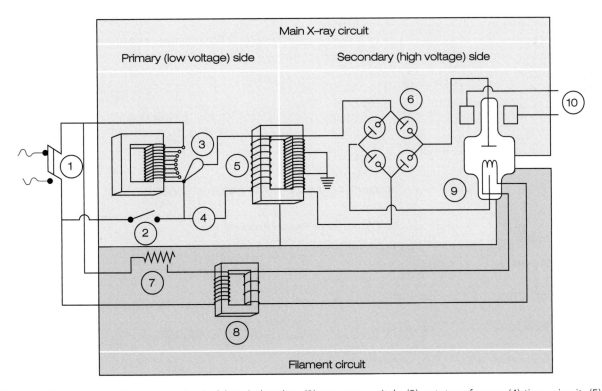

FIGURE 5–16. The complete basic x-ray circuit: (1) main breaker, (2) exposure switch, (3) autotransformer, (4) timer circuit, (5) high-voltage step-up transformer, (6) four-diode rectification circuit, (7) filament circuit variable resistance, (8) filament step-down transformer, (9) x-ray tube and (10) rotor stator.

(1ϕ 2P waveform) with a ripple of 100 percent. This means the voltage in the tube drops to 0 twice per period or cycle. These relationships are shown in Figure 5–17. Figure 5–18 illustrates the entire waveform changes.

Three-Phase Generators

When full-wave rectification is applied to 3ϕ current, it produces a voltage ripple of 6 pulses per Hz or 360 pulses per second. This produces six usable pulses per cycle, which is known as a **three-phase, six-pulse** (3ϕ 6P) waveform. Three-phase, six-pulse power produces a ripple of 13–25 percent. This means the voltage in the x-ray tube never falls below 75–87 percent of the peak kilovoltage setting on the console. These relationships are shown in Figure 5–17. Figure 5–19 illustrates the entire circuit with the waveform changes. **A full-wave rectified, three-phase, six-pulse waveform produces approximately 35 percent more average photon energy than full-wave rectified, single phase.** This will become an important point to remember when setting technical factors.

Equipment is also available with a **three-phase, twelve-pulse** waveform. This is accomplished by a complicated combination of twelve diodes with one wye and two delta windings so as to create two transformer windings that are out of step with one another. The voltage peaks from one of the wye transformers are then inserted into the line to fill in the ripples between the voltage peaks from one of the delta transformers. When full-wave rectified, this configuration produces a voltage rip-

ple of 4–10 percent, with tube voltage never dropping below 90–96 percent of the peak kilovoltage setting. These relationships are shown in Figure 5–17. Figure 5–20 illustrates the entire circuit with the waveform changes. **A full-wave rectified, three-phase, twelve-pulse waveform produces approximately 41 percent more average photon energy than full-wave rectified, single-phase.** This is also an important point to remember when setting technical factors. Voltage ripple varies as higher voltage loads are applied; the percentage figures given are approximations under average loads.

Generator power ratings are determined by the greatest load the generator is capable of sending to the x-ray tube. Power is calculated as voltage times amperage. The unit of power is the watt, so $V \times A = W$. This formula applies to a 3ϕ generator. Because 1ϕ generators have a lower average photon emission energy, the formula must be corrected by using a constant. For a 1ϕ generator the power rating formula is $V \times A \times 0.7 = W$. Since x-ray generators operate in the kilovoltage and milliamperage range, their power ratings are stated in kilowatts.

Example: What is the power rating for a 3ϕ generator capable of delivering 150 kVp at 1,000 mA to the tube?

Answer:

$$V \times A = W$$
$$150 \text{ kV} \times 1,000 \text{ mA} = W$$
$$150,000 \text{ V} \times 1.0 \text{ A} = 150,000 \text{ W}$$
$$= 150 \text{ kW}$$

TABLE 5–1. Common Diagnostic X-Ray Console Controls

Control	Factor	Electrical Device and Location in Circuit
kVp selection	kVp level	Autotransformer (between incoming line and exposure switch)
mA selection	Filament current	Variable resistor (in filament circuit between incoming line and step-down transformer)
Time selection	Length of exposure	Timer circuit (between exposure switch and step-up transformer)
Rotor switch	Speed of rotating anode	Stator (separate circuit from stator of anode motor)
Exposure switch	Moment of exposure	Switch (between autotransformer and timer circuit)

Example: What is the power rating for a 1φ generator
capable of delivering 120 kVp at 300 mA to the tube?

Answer:

$$V \times A \times 0.7 = W$$
$$120 \ kV \times 300 \ mA \times 0.7 = W$$
$$120{,}000 \ V \times 0.3 \ A \times 0.7 = 25{,}200 \ W$$
$$= 25.2 \ kW$$

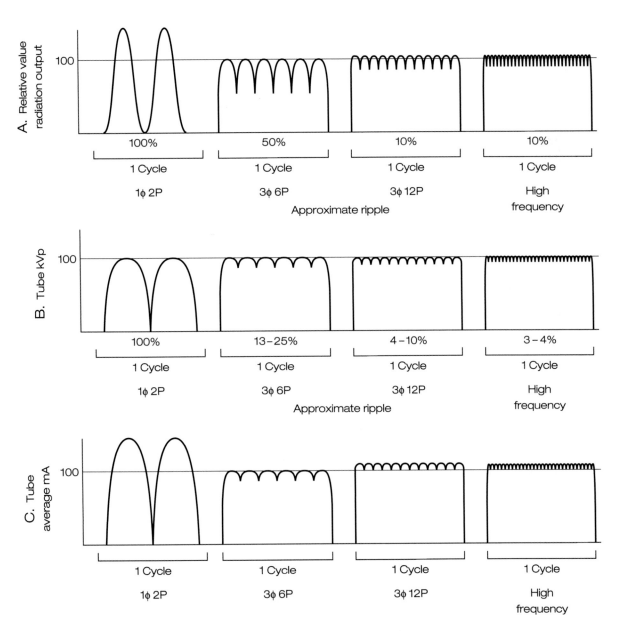

FIGURE 5–17. The relationships between (A) relative value radiation output and approximate ripple, (B) tube kVp and approximate ripple, and (C) tube average mA. Each relationship is shown for one cycle of 1φ 2P, 3φ 6P, 3φ 12P, and high-frequency generator configurations.

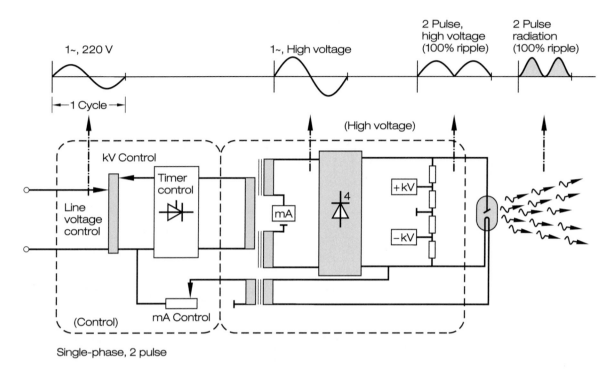

FIGURE 5–18. Single-phase, two-pulse generator.

These ratings serve as a guideline for comparing the capability of various generators. Generator power often varies as kilovoltage changes so a high-power generator at 150 kVp may not be as powerful when the kVp is lowered into the middle diagnostic range.

High Frequency

High-frequency generators use AC and DC power converters to change the incoming-line voltage frequency from 60 Hz to the 6,000 Hz range (Figure 5–21A). When a high-frequency current is supplied with full-wave rectified power, a 12–13 kHz waveform can be produced. An oscillator controls the pulses sent through the circuit, sending them at a much larger frequency (closer together), as shown in Figure 5–21B. When this wave is applied to the x-ray tube, the peak kilovoltage is achieved in about 10 percent of the time necessary for 3φ generators and with only 3–4% voltage ripple. Figure 5–17 illustrates the complex conversions used in a high-frequency generator to create the various waveforms prior to achieving the final multi-pulsed radiation beam. Full-

wave rectified high-frequency generator ripple ranges from 4–15 percent, depending on the total load, which is comparable to 3φ 12P generators. These relationships are shown in Figure 5–17. Figure 5–22 illustrates the entire circuit with the waveform changes. Because of the higher-frequency current, transformers for these units are significantly smaller.

Capacitor Discharge Mobile Units

It is also possible to operate an x-ray tube with the power generated from the discharge of a high-voltage capacitor. The capacitor operates exactly as explained in Unit II but in the kilovoltage range necessary to produce x-rays. In these units, depression of a charge button causes the rectification circuit to charge a capacitor instead of the x-ray tube. A signal indicates readiness when the capacitor fills to the appropriate level, and depression of the exposure switch triggers a discharge to the x-ray tube.

The disadvantage of a capacitor discharge unit is that the capacitor may continue to discharge after the usable exposure. Figure 5–23A shows the charging curve, the

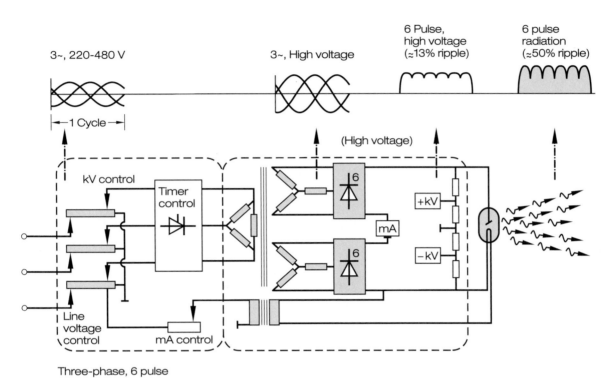

FIGURE 5–19. Three-phase, six-pulse generator.

exposure period, and the discharging curve. Exposure begins at the peak voltage and then decreases (Figure 5–23B). This is sometimes called wavetail cutoff. **Capacitor discharge units provide an rms voltage significantly lower than the peak voltage.** The ending kV is approximately 1 kV per mAs lower than the initial kVp. Therefore the rms voltage is about 0.5 kV/mAs lower than the initial kVp. Because capacitors discharge more slowly as potential difference decreases, considerable residual kV may exist after the desired exposure time. This can create a leakage of radiation, although several devices help avoid the problem. Grid-biased x-ray tubes can be used to cut the photon emission at a set time by reversing the charge polarity of a wire grid in front of the filament. Additionally, the tube collimator can be designed to automatically close its lead shutters after the desired exposure, thus stopping radiation leakage.

Capacitor discharge units are most commonly used for mobile equipment. The capacitor circuit is supplied from batteries which are charged from line current. This permits the unit to be mobile without having to be plugged into a wall outlet. Instead, the batteries can be recharged periodically when the unit is parked.

Battery-Operated Mobile Units

Mobile units are also available that operate on nickel-cadmium (NiCd) battery-supplied AC current. The batteries supply nonpulsating direct current to a rotary converter which provides current similar to 3ϕ 12P or even greater frequencies. Compared to capacitor discharge machines, these units have the obvious advantage of 3ϕ exposure consistency, higher rms voltage, and no leakage possibility. They also have all the advantages of mobility, with recharging capabilities, and for these reasons they have become extremely popular.

Falling Load Generators

Falling load generators usually are specially designed 3ϕ or high frequency generators. They take full advan-

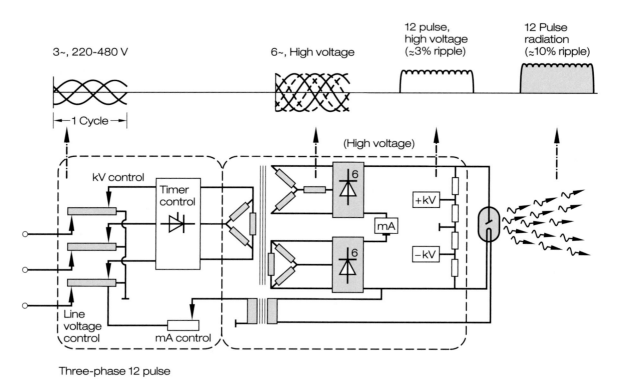

Three-phase 12 pulse

FIGURE 5–20. Three-phase, twelve-pulse generator.

tage of the current loading capability of the x-ray tube by beginning the exposure with a high amperage and then allowing it to fall during the exposure. This can be accomplished with a constant potential generator. It requires that both the mA and the kV be regulated independently.

Falling load generators are a solution to this problem as they permit greater use of the acceptable tube limits. They do so without requiring a higher-power (and more expensive) generator that would permit higher mA loading. For example, in Figure 5–24, a constant potential generator exposure of 240 mAs is compared to the same falling load exposure. A falling load generator permits the same tube to achieve 240 mAs in 0.5 second. This is accomplished by beginning the exposure at 600 mA for the first 0.1 second. At this time the 600 mA tube limit is reached and the generator is programmed to automatically reduce the mA to 500 until the tube limit is again reached (0.2 second later, or 0.3 second from exposure

start). Once again the generator reduces the mA to 400 until the limit is reached (0.2 second later, or 0.5 second from exposure start). This produces 240 total mAs.

A falling load generator utilizes the tube's loading potential to a much greater extent than the constant-potential generator. This is made evident by comparing the falling load of the 240 mAs example with a constant-potential load for the same mAs. In actual practice a margin of error is allowed for the tube loading. Most falling load generators will step down the mA at 70–80 percent of the tube loading capacity. This feature has a disadvantage in that constant-potential generators may actually make better use of tube loading capacity on very short exposures, where they may use 80–90 percent of the tube loading capacity.

Falling load generators begin exposures at the highest possible mA. This removes control of the mA from the radiographer, and there are instances when this is undesirable. For example, some examinations, such as those

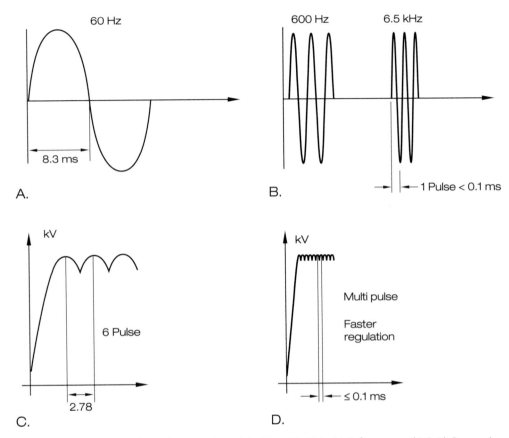

FIGURE 5–21. High-frequency waveforms: (A & B) Conversion of 1φ 2P to 3φ 6P to high frequency. (C & D) Comparison of time interval necessary to reach peak kV on 3φ 6P and high-frequency generators. *(Courtesy of Siemens AG, Medical Engineering Group)*

for the lateral thoracic vertebra (spine) and sternum, require a "breathing technique" in which low mA and long-time exposures are used to blur superimposing structures from the image. Unless falling load consoles are equipped with special controls (often as tomographic options) to permit starting exposures at low mA, these examinations cannot be performed correctly.

There are several factors that should be understood before using falling load generators. Because they function with an mA that is unknown to the operator, it is impossible for the operator to set the correct time to achieve the desired mAs. Therefore, falling load generators must be used with automatic exposure controls, or rely on an mAs timer, instead of independent mA and time controls. The kVp across the tube varies for a brief

moment as the mA is adjusted. This is an Ohm's law effect during the continuous mA reductions and results in a slightly lower average kVp. Falling load generators can shorten x-ray tube life considerably as they use higher mA settings, thus causing the filament to wear out more quickly. The advantages of falling load generators are shorter times in heavy-load situations, and simpler operation.

When comparing the various types of generators it is most important to evaluate the radiation output from the tube as this is the factor that influences both patient exposure and image quality. Figure 5–17 assists in this process by illustrating the various transformations that occur in the x-ray tube milliamperage and kilovoltage as well as the all-important relative value of radiation output.

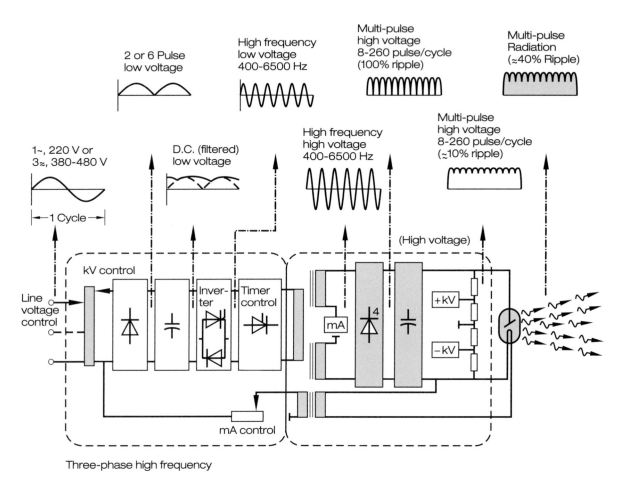

FIGURE 5–22. Three-phase, high-frequency generator.

Automatic Exposure Controls

All automatic exposure controls do exactly what their name indicates; they are programmed to terminate the radiographic exposure time. It is important to remember that automatic exposure controls do not control any factor except time. Milliampere-seconds and kVp remain under the control of the radiographer in all but falling load generators. Even falling load units leave the kVp under the radiographer's control.

There are two types of automatic exposure controls: **phototimers and ionization chamber devices. The term phototimer is often used to refer to all automatic expo-** sure controls. They are also referred to as automatic exposure devices and the acronyms AEC and AED occasionally appear in professional literature. Actually, phototimers are seldom utilized in modern radiography. Most of the devices that are called phototimers today consist of ionization chambers.

All automatic exposure controls function by measuring a preset quantity of radiation and breaking the timer circuit when a dose sufficient to produce the desired film density has been reached.

Phototimers

Old-fashioned phototimer devices used a thyratron to regulate exposure automatically. The x-ray beam would

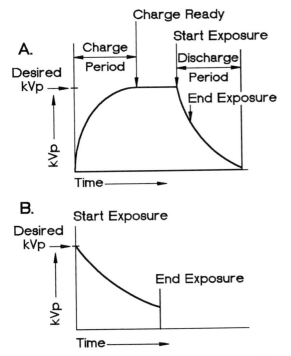

FIGURE 5–23. (A) Capacitor discharge unit waveform. (B) Wavetail cut-off.

pass through the patient, tabletop, and cassette before it struck a fluorescent screen that had the ability to absorb the x-rays and produce light photons. The light photons were then directed toward a photomultiplier tube. A photomultiplier tube had the ability to produce multiple electrons from each light photon. The electrons then established a charge on the capacitor. When the capacitor reached its preset value, it discharged, triggering a thyratron and opening the relay to terminate the exposure. Phototimers were calibrated by setting the capacitor-discharge point (usually controlled by a set screw in the electronics cabinet) at a level that produced a satisfactory density on the radiographic film in the cassette. This was done by a trial-and-error procedure with a radiographic phantom. Radiographs were exposed at various combinations of kVp, time, and mAs until a satisfactory diagnostic quality image was consistently obtained.

Ionization Chambers

Ionization chamber automatic exposure control is quite different (Figure 5–25). The x-ray beam passes through the patient and tabletop before striking the ionization chamber. Unlike with the old phototimers, the cassette and film are positioned under the ion chamber. Until the development of a thin, parallel-plate ionization chamber, it was impossible to locate the chamber in this position because it would cast an objectionable shadow artifact on the film. Because thin, parallel-plate chambers are only about 5 mm in thickness, this is not a problem (Figure 5–26). It is critical that the exact size, shape and position of the ionization chamber be known to the radiographer.

Minimum Reaction Time

All automatic exposure controls have a **minimum reaction (or response) time**, which is determined by the length of time necessary for the AEC to respond to the radiation and for the generator to terminate the exposure. This delay is caused primarily by the turn-off delay in the high-voltage circuits. Old phototimers had a minimum reaction time of 0.05 second or less. Modern ionization chambers with SCRs may have a minimum reaction time of less than 0.001 second. Automatic exposure controls are sometimes incapable of terminating exposures quickly enough, especially with extremely high-speed films and intensifying screens during high kVp chest radiography. In this instance, radiographic technology has outstripped itself and either a manual time or a slower film and screen combination must be used, although some manufacturers use an exposure-monitoring circuit to terminate low dose rate exposures quickly.

Backup Time

Nearly all automatic exposure equipped units permit (and may have electronic interlocks that require) a manual backup time to be set. There are numerous reasons why an automatic exposure control may be improperly set. For example, if one forgets to activate the AEC in a wall unit, this may leave an AEC in a table unit waiting for exposure by a tube that is directed toward the wall (and through a patient). Because the wall AEC is not receiving any radiation dose, the exposure would not cease until the tube overload protector activated. Not only is this an expensive waste of tube life, but the radiographer error causing excessive radiation dose to the patient is completely unwarranted. The fact that the

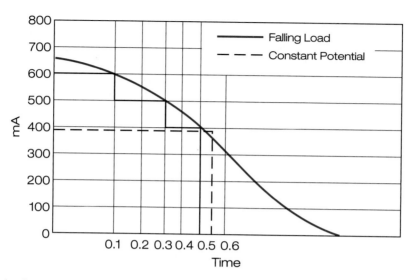

FIGURE 5–24. Falling load generator versus constant-potential tube limit curve. In the example shown, the mAs is calculated as follows:

mA	Time in sec	mAs achieved
600	0.1	60
500	0.2	100
400	0.2	80
Total	0.5	240

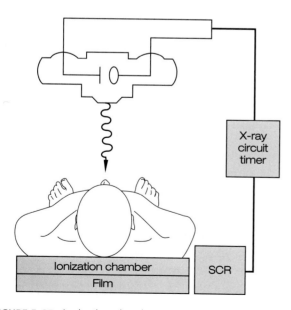

FIGURE 5–25. Ionization chamber AEC circuit.

radiograph would be overexposed, requiring it to be repeated, adding to the patient's dose again, simply makes matters worse. **Backup times cannot exceed the tube limit and should be set at 150 percent of the anticipated manual exposure mAs.** According to U.S. Public Law 90–602, generators must terminate the exposure at 600 mAs for exposures above 50 kVp and 2,000 mAs for exposures below 50 kVp (primarily during mammography).

Summary

Medical x-ray units can be classified as diagnostic or therapeutic. Diagnostic units operate within a range of 10–1,200 milliamperes (mA), 0.001–10 seconds and at a peak kilovoltage (kVp) of approximately 25 to 150.

Radiographic equipment includes a wide variety of units with different tube stand configurations, including ceiling suspension, floor-to-ceiling, floor mounted and C-arms. Nearly all x-ray equipment operates from an

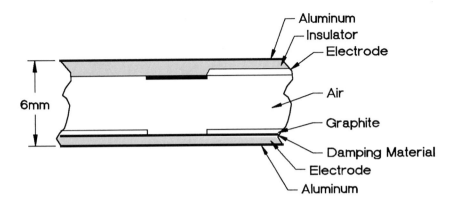

FIGURE 5–26. Parallel-plate ionization chamber AEC. *(Courtesy of Siemens Medical Systems, Inc.)*

incoming line of 210–220 volts, which is then used for single-phase or three-phase power.

The basic x-ray circuit can be divided into the main and filament circuits. The main circuit supplies the x-ray tube with properly modified power, while the filament circuit supplies the filament of the x-ray tube with properly modified power. The basic circuit includes the exposure switch, timer, high-voltage step-up transformer and rectifier circuit.

Although waveforms differ depending on incoming line and rectification, differences occur in both voltage ripple and the interval between initiation of the exposure and the peak kilovoltage.

Generator power ratings are determined by the greatest load the generator is capable of sending to the x-ray tube. Power is expressed in watts and varies by incoming line current and rectification. Falling load generators permit more effective use of the tube loading capacity but eliminate mA and time settings from consideration.

Although often called phototimers, automatic exposure controls (AECs) today are almost always ionization chambers. When using an AEC, problems may be avoided by considering the minimum reaction time and the backup time.

REVIEW QUESTIONS

1. Name three types of diagnostic radiographic tube-support systems.

2. What are the two types of incoming line current?

3. How many pulses are there per Hz for 1φ and 3φ power?

4. What device in the x-ray circuit controls kVp? mA? time? rectification?

5. What is the approximate voltage ripple for 1f 2P equipment? 3φ 6P? 3φ 12P?

6. What happens to the tube mA during an exposure using a falling load generator?

7. What is the difference between an ionization chamber and a phototimer?

8. What factor determines the minimum reaction time?

REFERENCES AND RECOMMENDED READING

Ammann, E. (1986). Update on technology of x-ray generators, Radiological Society of North America Refresher Course, Chicago, Illinois, December 1.

Ball, J. & Price, T. (1989). *Chesneys' radiographic imaging.* Oxford: Blackwell Scientific Publishing.

Baranoski, D. (1985). High frequency and speed 500. The *Canadian Journal of Radiography, Radiotherapy, and Nuclear Medicine.* 16(2), 55–59.

Barnes, G. T. & Tishler, J. M. (1981). Fluoroscopic image quality and its implications regarding equipment selection and use. *The Physical Basis of Medical Imaging.* Editors: Coulam, C. M., Erickson, J. J., Rollo, F. D., James, A. E. New York: Appleton-Century-Crofts, 93–106.

Braun, M. (1976). Considerations on the falling load principle. *Optical Engineering. 15*(4), 338–343.

Curry, T. S., Dowdey, J. E., Murry, R. C. (1990). *Christensen's introduction to the physics of diagnostic radiology* (4th ed.). Philadelphia: Lea and Febiger.

DeFrance, J. J. (1969). *Electrical fundamentals.* Englewood Cliffs, NJ: Prentice-Hall.

Evans, S. A., Harris, L., Lawinski, C. P., Hendra I. R. F. (1985). Mobile x-ray generators: A review. *Radiography. 51*(595), 89.

Gray, J. E., Winkler, N. T., Stears, J., & Frank, E. D. (1988). Radiologic exchange. *Radiologic Technology.* (August).

Gray, J. E., Winkler, N. T., Stears, J., & Frank, E. D. (1983). *Quality control in diagnostic imaging.* Baltimore: University Park Press.

Harrison, R. M. & Forster, E. (1984). Performance characteristics of x-ray tubes and generators. *Radiography. 50*(594), 245.

Joseph, E. S. & Schneble, J. E. (1975). X-ray automatic exposure timing and control circuitry. *Application of Optical Instrumentation in Medicine, IV. 70,* 166–170.

Lin, P. P. (1975). Phototimers, user's point of view. *Application of Optical Instrumentation in Medicine, IV. 70,* 196–200.

Morgan, J. A. (1968). The development and application of multi-phase x-rays in medical radiography. *Radiologic Technology. 40*(2), 57.

Morgan, R. H. (1943). The automatic control of exposure in photofluorography. *Public Health Reports. 58*(42), 1533–1541.

Nadon, J. M., Gelmine, B. J., McLaughlin, E. D. (1989). *Industrial electricity* (4th ed.). Albany: Delmar Publishers.

Ridgway, A. & Thumm, W. (1973). *The physics of medical radiography.* Reading, MA: Addison-Wesley.

Seeram, E. (1985). *X-Ray imaging equipment.* Springfield, IL: Charles C. Thomas.

Selman, J. (1994). The *fundamentals of x-ray and radium physics* (9th ed.). Springfield, IL: Thomas.

Sprawls, P. (1990). *Principles of radiography for technologists.* Rockville, MD: Aspen Publishers.

Sprawls, P. (1987). *Physical principles of medical imaging.* Rockville, MD: Aspen Publishers.

Stears, J. G., Gray, J. E., Webbles, W. E., & Frank, E. D. (1988). Radiologic exchange (automatic exposure control function). *Radiologic Technology. 59*(6), 521–522.

Sterling, S. (1988). Automatic exposure control: A primer. *Radiologic Technology. 59*(5), 421–427.

Stockley, S. M. (1986). *A manual of radiographic equipment.* Edinburgh: Churchill Livingstone.

Ter-Pogossian, M. M. (1967). *The physical aspects of diagnostic radiology.* New York: Hoeber Medical Division, Harper & Row.

Thompson, M. A., Hattaway, M. P., Hall, J. D., & Dowd, S. B. (1994). *Principles of imaging science and protection.* Philadelphia: W. B. Saunders.

Thompson, T. T. (1985). *A practical approach to modern imaging equipment* (2nd ed.). Boston: Little, Brown, & Co.

Thornburn, D. S. Physical characteristics of falling load generators. Shelton, CT: Philips Medical Systems, Inc.

Tortorici, M. (1992). *Concepts in medical radiographic imaging.* Philadelphia: W. B. Saunders.

van der Plaats, G. J. (1980). *Medical x-ray techniques in diagnostic radiology* (4th ed.). The Hague: Martinus Nijhoff Publishers.

Weigl, W. (1989). A new high-frequency controlled x-ray generator system with multi-pulse wave shape. *Journal for Radiological Engineering. 1*(1), 7–19.

Weigl, W. (1988). Design of falling load generators. Unpublished paper presented at American Association of Physicists in Medicine seminar.

Wilks, R. J. (1981). *Principles of radiological physics.* Edinburgh: Churchill Livingstone.

Wolbarst, A. B. (1993). *Physics of radiology.* Norwalk, CT: Appleton & Lange.

The Case of the Unidentified Flying Object in the Skull

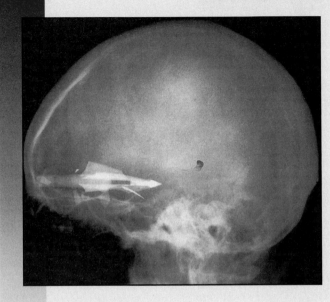

This lateral skull radiograph was obtained on a patient in the emergency room. What could this rocket-shaped object be?

Answers to the case studies can be found in Appendix E.

CHAPTER 6

The X-Ray Tube

. . . circumstances led me to the construction of experimental high vacuum tubes with a heated tungsten filament as cathode and a tungsten disc as anode . . . . The tube was then stable and controllable . . . .

W. D. Coolidge, "Experiences with the Roentgen-ray tube."

Objectives

Upon completion of this chapter, the student should be able to:

▶ Draw a complete dual-focus cathode assembly.

▶ Discuss the necessary characteristics of filament metals and construction.

▶ Describe the control of thermionic emission from the filament.

▶ Select exposure factors and techniques that will extend tube life.

▶ Explain the function and design of a grid-biased focusing cup.

▶ Draw a complete rotating anode assembly.

▶ Discuss the characteristics of anode targets.

▶ Explain the line-focus principle and its effect on anode target design.

▶ Explain the anode heel effect and its effect on primary beam intensity.

▶ Explain the production of off-focus radiation.

▶ Describe the function of a rotating anode induction motor, stator and rotor.

▶ Discuss the construction of the glass envelope and protective housing.

▶ Calculate safe exposures when provided with a tube rating chart, anode cooling curve, and housing cooling curve.

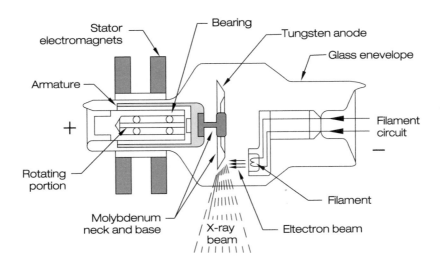

FIGURE 6–1. A rotating anode x-ray tube.

*T*he electrical production of x-rays is only possible under very special conditions including a source of electrons, an appropriate target material, a high voltage and a vacuum. The x-ray tube is the device that permits these conditions to exist, and it is within the tube that x-ray photons come into existence. The tube consists of a **cathode** and an **anode** enclosed within a **glass envelope** and then encased in a **protective housing** (Figure 6–1). X-ray tubes, whose useful life can be significantly extended by proper care and handling by professional radiographers, can cost over $10,000.

The Cathode Assembly

The cathode is the negative side of the x-ray tube. The function of the cathode is to produce a thermionic cloud, conduct the high voltage to the gap between cathode and anode and focus the electron stream as it heads for the anode. The cathode is a complex device and can be referred to as the **cathode assembly**. This assembly consists of the **filament** or filaments, **focusing cup** and associated **wiring** (Figure 6–2).

The Filament

The filament is a small coil of thin thoriated tungsten wire. The wire is about 0.1–0.2 mm thick and the coil

1–2 mm wide by 7–15 mm long. It is set in the cathode assembly within the focusing cup (Figure 6–3). Tungsten is the material of choice because of its high melting point (3,370°C) and because it is difficult to vaporize (turn into a gas). Rhenium (melting point of 3,170°C) and molybdenum (melting point of 2,620°C) are also desirable materials. The high melting point permits the filament to operate at the high temperatures required of an x-ray tube. In addition, tungsten is not easily vaporized. Vaporization produces particles that deposit on other surfaces and reduce the vacuum within the tube. The length and width of the filament have a great effect on the ability of the particular x-ray tube to image fine details.

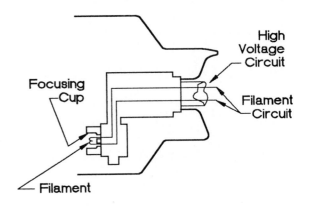

FIGURE 6–2. A cathode assembly.

Most diagnostic x-ray tubes have dual filaments called a **dual focus** arrangement (Figure 6–3). The wiring for dual filaments does not require separate ground conductors. Instead a common ground is used (Figure 6–4).

As we have discussed previously, the function of the filament is to provide sufficient resistance to the flow of electrons so that the heat produced will cause thermionic emission to occur. (A tungsten filament will not exhibit significant thermionic emission below 2,200°C.) This process causes electrons to leave the surface of the filament wire and form a thermionic cloud. When the high voltage is released at exposure the entire cloud is available to be driven toward the anode target where x-ray photons will be produced. This provides many more times the number of electrons than would be available from a cold cathode.

Not all of the electrons that are thermionically emitted from the filament are driven to the anode or return to the filament. A very small percentage of the electrons are permanently vaporized from the filament and they contribute to reducing the vacuum, thus making the tube gassy. Vaporized tungsten (from both filament and anode) is also gradually deposited on the inner surface of the glass envelope. This deposit causes old tubes to have a mirrored appearance and can eventually cause high-

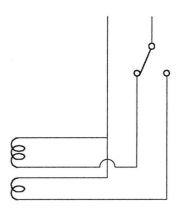

FIGURE 6–4. Dual-filament wiring.

voltage arcing when sufficient current is attracted to a deposit during an exposure. Arcing of this type immediately destroys the tube. Evaporization deposits on the glass envelope also cause increased filtration of the primary beam and this decreases tube efficiency. Tubes with a metal or ceramic envelope can be grounded to significantly reduce this problem.

Another major cause of tube failure is the breaking of the filament itself. Filaments become increasingly thin as vaporization continues. When about 10 percent of the diameter has vaporized, a filament becomes subject to breaking, exactly the way a light bulb filament will burn out. However, older tubes are much more sensitive to rough handling and a thin filament that is jarred can break prematurely.

When the x-ray machine is first turned on, a mild current is sent to the filament. The filament remains in this preheated mode until immediately prior to an exposure. When the switch labeled "rotor" is activated prior to an exposure, not only does the rotor begin to turn but a higher current is sent to the filament to bring the thermionic cloud to the proper size for the mA selected. This increase in filament heating is what causes most of the vaporization of the filament. An average diagnostic x-ray tube filament life is only about 6–9 hours (10,000–20,000 exposures) at this heating level. One of the primary causes of premature tube failure is the radiographer's habit of holding the rotor switch prior to making exposures. Every second the rotor switch is

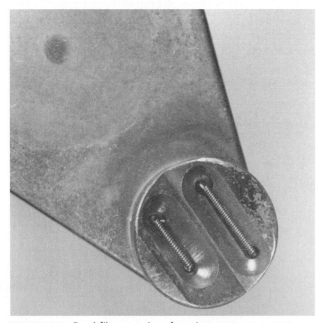

FIGURE 6–3. Dual filaments in a focusing cup.

depressed, life is removed from the filament. Routinely delayed exposures while the filament is enduring maximum current can shorten tube life by 50–60 percent (to 5,000–6,000 exposures).

Most tube manufacturers recommend that two-step exposure switches be **fully depressed in one motion**. All units have electronic interlocks that will not permit the exposure to occur until the rotor has brought the anode up to the proper speed. Holding the rotor switch (and filament heat) can be justified in cases where the patient is unable to cooperate. In these instances (such as with pediatric patients) the rotor and filament must be readied to permit an instant exposure to avoid patient breathing and motion. Single-phase generators are usually capable of initiating exposure within 10 milliseconds (0.01 second) and 3ϕ generators may be a quick 1 millisecond (0.001 second). Routine clinical examinations seldom need to be timed closer than these limitations.

Historical Notes   In the earliest days of radiography a cold cathode with an unheated filament was used. It was not until the American physicist William D. Coolidge (1873–1975) developed the Coolidge tube for the General Electric Corporation in 1915 that the hot filament became available. Prior to the development of the Coolidge tube, the radiographer kept a selection of tubes of various mA values on a rack, usually in the darkroom (Figure 6–5). When a change of mA was required, the radiographer disconnected the tube and replaced it with a different one from the rack. Coolidge's contribu-

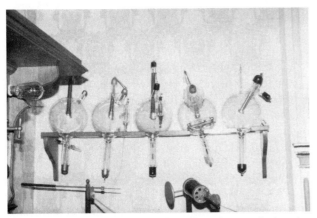

FIGURE 6–5. A selection of cold filament tubes as displayed at the Deutsches Röntgen Museum, Remscheid-Lennep, Germany. (*Photograph courtesy of Philip W. Ballinger*)

tions to radiography included not only the hot filament, but also the focusing cup, the imbedded anode target, and various anode cooling devices (including the unique water-cooled tube).

The Focusing Cup

The focusing cup is a shallow depression in the cathode assembly designed to house the filament (Figure 6–2). It is made of nickel and its purpose is to narrow the thermionic cloud as it is driven toward the anode. Because electrons all possess negative charges, their tendency is to diverge rather than to travel in straight lines. The focusing cup is provided with a low negative potential which, because of its geometry, focuses the electrons toward one another in a convergence pattern (Figure 6–6). Most x-ray tubes have the focusing cup at the same potential as the filament. It is possible to decrease the size of the focal spot by using a **biased** focusing cup. A biased focusing cup maintains the cup at a more negative voltage than the filament. This causes the exiting electron beam to be focused into a narrower stream as it heads towards the anode. In mammographic x-ray tubes focusing cup biasing is used when the small focal spot is selected.

As more and more electrons build up in the area of the filament, their negative charges begin to oppose the emission of additional electrons. This phenomenon is called the **space charge effect** and it limits x-ray tubes to maximum mA ranges of 1,000–1,200.

Saturation current is another filament phenomenon that affects the efficiency of the x-ray tube. As kVp increases, a greater percentage of the thermionically emitted electrons are driven toward the anode. This relationship is shown by a filament emission chart (Figure 6–7). The filament amperage curve flattens out when the kVp is driving the entire thermionic cloud toward the anode. The filament saturation current has been achieved when there are no further thermionic electrons to be driven toward the anode. At this point an increase in kVp will not increase the tube mA. Further mA increases must be achieved by increasing the filament amperage. Close examination of a filament emission chart demonstrates that something must be done to compensate for the tube mA increase when kVp is changed. For example, an exposure at 100 kVp will produce a significantly greater tube mA than the same expo-

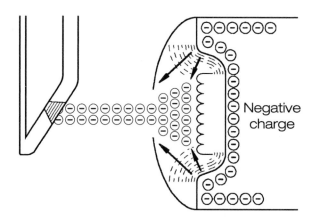

FIGURE 6–6. The geometry of the negative charge on the cathode focusing cup.

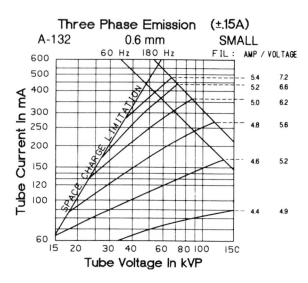

FIGURE 6–7. A filament emission chart showing saturation as a function of filament amperage, tube voltage, and tube current. *(Courtesy of Varian EIMAC)*

sure at 60 kVp. The filament amperage must be adjusted to compensate for these changes and the x-ray circuitry does this automatically whenever factors are changed by the operator.

Grid-Biased Tubes

In some applications, such as cine-film recording or capacitor discharge generators, it is desirable to quickly regulate the flow of electrons producing x-ray photons. The addition of a more negative potential difference (approximately 2,000 volts) at the focusing cup causes the cup to attract the thermionic cloud. This attraction very cleanly removes electrons from use for x-ray production when the focusing cup charge is pulsed from negative to positive in synchrony with another device (such as the shutter of a cine camera), it becomes possible to regulate, pulse and synchronize x-ray production very precisely. The third wire is the only physical difference between a normal and a grid-biased tube. In older tubes an actual grid of wires was placed between the filament and anode. These types of tubes are sometimes called **grid-pulsed**, **grid-biased** or **grid-controlled**.

The Anode Assembly

The anode is the positive side of the x-ray tube and has three functions: it serves as a target surface for the high-voltage electrons from the filament, thereby becoming the source of the x-ray photons; it conducts the high voltage from the cathode back into the x-ray generator circuitry and it serves as the primary thermal conductor. The anode target surface is where the high-speed electrons from the filament are suddenly stopped, resulting in the production of x-ray photons. The entire anode is a complex device referred to as the **anode assembly**. This assembly consists of the **anode**, **stator** and **rotor** (Figure 6–8) and serves as the path for the high-voltage flow during exposure.

The Anode

Anodes are divided into two types: **stationary and rotating** (Figure 6–9). Rotating anodes, developed in 1936, turn during the exposure, thus presenting a much larger target area. Modern rotating anodes permit bombardment of a given area of the target for only 7–50 microseconds. The faster the anode rotates, the better the heat dissipation. The use of stationary anode x-ray tubes has become limited to low-power functions, such as those of dental units. Nearly all units designed for diagnostic radiography utilize rotating anodes because of their greater efficiency.

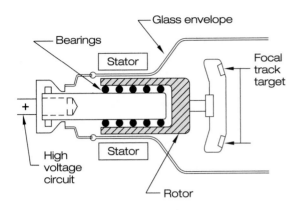

FIGURE 6–8. The anode assembly with anode, target, rotor, bearings, and stator.

1. high atomic number,

2. high melting point and

3. heat-conducting ability.

Tungsten's atomic number (74) enhances the production of diagnostic-range photons. During normal use, the focal track reaches a temperature between 1,000–2,000°C but the temperature can go higher if the tube load increases. Because of tungsten's high melting point, it can withstand normal operating temperatures. Tungsten also conducts heat very well. The rhenium provides greater elasticity when the focal track expands rapidly due to the intense heat. To assist in the dissipation of heat in heavy load situations, specialized anodes may have the anode disk backed by a thicker layer of molybdenum or graphite. Graphite-backed anodes can double heat-loading capabilities without increasing bearing wear.

Specialized x-ray tubes for mammography utilize molybdenum (atomic number 42) as the primary target material due to its ability to emit a more uniform range of lower energy photons. The lower characteristic energy photons permit a better soft tissue image. Molybdenum also has a high melting point, as discussed above. These tubes also utilize a specialized glass envelope window made of beryllium because the glass used in most x-ray tubes absorbs too much of the low-energy beam.

Normal use of a rotating anode will eventually vaporize sufficient target focal track material to roughen or pit the target area (Figure 6–11). Pitting reduces the efficiency of the tube; the term pitted or pitting is often used to describe an older tube's focal track.

The anode is composed of several different metals, each designed to contribute the maximum to the overall function of the anode. Stationary anodes are composed of rhenium-alloyed tungsten imbedded in a 45° angled end of a copper rod. Rotating anode disks range from 5–13 cm in diameter and are composed of molybdenum. The anode's function as the source of x-ray photons and as the primary thermal conducting device is enhanced by the use of rhenium-alloyed tungsten as the target focal track material (Figure 6–10). Tungsten is the metal of choice for the source of x-ray photons for three primary reasons:

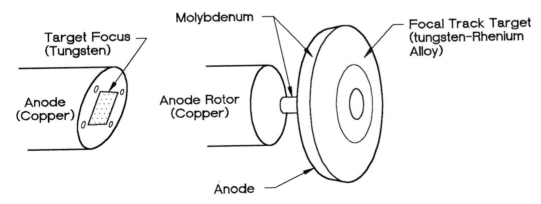

FIGURE 6–9. A stationary and a rotating anode.

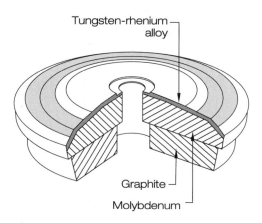

FIGURE 6–10. Rotating anode construction.

When first activating an x-ray unit, it is important to use an **anode warm-up procedure**. These procedures are specified by the tube manufacturers and are designed to bring the anode heat from room temperature to near the

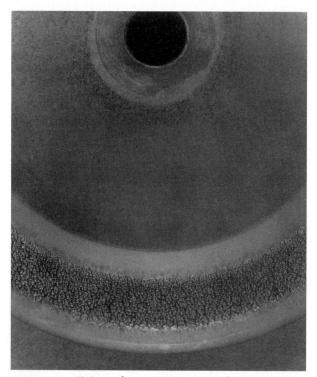

FIGURE 6–11. Pitting of a rotating anode focal track from extended use.

range of operation. The procedure also permits the heat from the hot anode to serve as a "vacuum pump" to maintain a strong vacuum inside the glass envelope. This is why x-ray tubes should be warmed up regularly, even when the unit is not being used for patients. A normal procedure might require an average kVp and mA station for a one-second exposure to be followed by two more two-second exposures. Failure to follow the warm-up procedure can cause the entire anode to crack if the molybdenum absorbs the heat too rapidly and exceeds its expansion capability. Many newer anodes are stress relieved (Figure 6–12). A stress-relieved anode dissipates heat much more efficiently and does not require an elaborate tube warm-up procedure.

The Target Area   The portion of the anode where the high-voltage electron steam will impact is called by various names: the **target**, the **focus**, the **focal point**, the **focal spot** or the **focal track** (although this last term has a more specific definition, it is the target area). This is the precise point at which the x-ray photons are created. The target is considered to be a point source of x-ray photons and it is from this point that all tube-to-object and image-receptor (film) distances are measured. Some x-ray tube housings have a line drawn on them to indicate the exact level of the target within. All measuring devices have their zero point at this level. This is why a tape measure attached to the side or bottom of a tube collimator may begin at 12 cm. It is attached 12 cm from the target but is calculated to measure target-to-image-receptor distances.

Stationary anodes have a static target area. Rotating anodes have a dynamic target area and are designed to

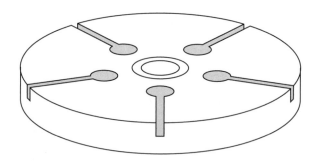

FIGURE 6–12. The back of a stress-relieved anode.

greatly increase the target area (Figure 6–9). A rotating anode can increase the target area up to 300 times, depending on the diameter of the anode disk. Rotating anodes have much greater heat loading capacities than stationary anodes. High- speed anodes have higher heating capacities than regular-speed anodes (often 50 percent greater).

When discussing a rotating anode target area, the term **focal track** is used to represent the circular path that will be impacted by the electron beam. The terms **target, focus, focal point** and **focal spot** refer to the area of the focal track that is impacted by the electron beam at one time. In addition, the term **actual focal spot** is used to describe the physical area of the focal track that is impacted. The term **effective focal spot** is used to describe the area of the focal spot that is projected out of the tube toward the object being radiographed (Figure 6–13).

Line-Focus Principle

The **line-focus principle** is used to reduce the effective area of the focal spot. This permits the best resolution of detail while permitting as large an actual area as possible (to increase thermal conductivity). **The effective focal-spot size is controlled by** the size of the actual focal spot (which is controlled by the length of the filament) and the anode target angle. As the actual focal-spot size increases, the effective focal-spot size also increases (Figure 6–13).

When the target angle is less than 45°, the effective focal spot is smaller than the actual focal spot (Figure 6–14). This is accomplished by the line-focus principle. This principle can best be understood by holding a pencil straight up and then sloping it towards oneself so that the pencil is seen end on. The perceived dimensions of the pencil change as the angle changes. In the x-ray tube, changing the angle of the target changes the effective focal spot.

The most common diagnostic radiography target angle is 12°. However, tubes are available with angles ranging from 7° to 17°. When the angle is decreased, smaller focal spots can be achieved. A disadvantage of extremely small target angles is that the geometry of the angle can limit the size of the primary beam field at short source-to-image receptor distances (Figure 6–15). To cover a 14" x 17" field at 40", a minimum of a 12° target angle is required. It has been shown that at large heat loads, target angles can decrease due to "warping" of the anode. In these instances, the anode end of the primary

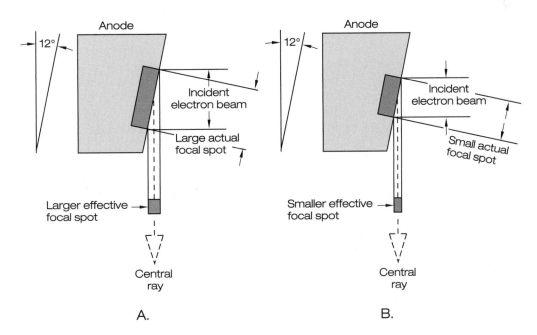

FIGURE 6–13. Effect of actual focal-spot size on effective focal-spot size.

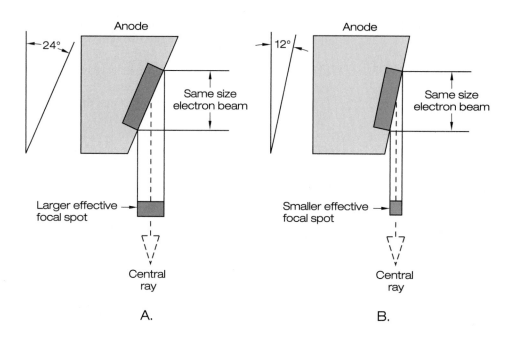

FIGURE 6–14. Use of the line-focus principle to obtain an effective focal spot smaller than the actual focal spot.

beam field can be reduced enough to cut off structures near the collimated edge. A slight angle of the tube will compensate for this effect. Target angles of less than 14° have been shown to produce some degree of cut-off as they age. Some tubes have offset filaments with two different focal tracks, which can be set at different target angles.

X-ray tube focal spots are rectangular because the line-focus principle applies only in the direction of the angle. It does not apply horizontally across the anode focal track because there is no angle in this direction. X-ray tube targets must be narrow to maintain the small effective focal-spot size in the horizontal direction, usually not over 2 mm. The line-focus principle permits the actual focal spot's vertical dimension to be as much as 6 mm to gain the maximum thermal conductivity. **The effective focal spot's vertical dimension is the one that is stated as the focal-spot size.**

The National Electrical Manufacturers Association (NEMA) establishes standards for focal spot size. These standards provide tolerance ranges for 23 focal spot sizes. For example, a 1.0 mm focal spot is within tolerance if it measures up to 1.4 mm in width and 2.0 mm in length.

It is important to remember that in some instances, focal spots may be considerably larger than their stated size. Diagnostic tubes are available with focal spots of 0.1 mm to 3.0 mm. Occasionally the term **fractional focal spot** is used to refer to a very small focal spot, one that is a fraction of a millimeter in size.

In normal usage, the term focal-spot size refers to the effective focal spot size. Most diagnostic x-ray tubes have dual focal spots to include one for fine detail studies and the other for heavy tube loads. The small focal spot will not permit the use of higher mA stations. If the x-ray unit allows the radiographer to choose the focal-spot size, an exposure cannot be made with a high mA station and the small focal spot. Automatic systems link the focal-spot size selection with the appropriate mA station. Therefore, the radiographer should realize that the focal-spot size may be mandated by the mA station. When a small focal spot is desired, it is important to use only low mA stations, even though this may require a longer exposure time.

Focal-spot size increases, or blooms, as milliamperage is increased. For example, the focal spot is slightly larger during an exposure of 80 kVp, 800 mA and 0.1 second

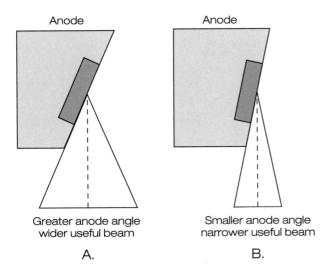

FIGURE 6–15. Anode target angle as a function of maximum primary beam field size.

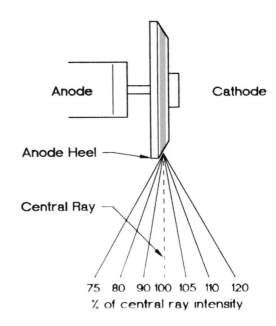

FIGURE 6–16. The anode heel effect.

than it is during an exposure of 80 kVp, 100 mA and 0.8 second. Although originally considered to be a significant factor, recent research has indicated that focal-spot blooming does not have a resounding effect on recorded detail.

Anode Heel Effect

The use of the line-focus principle causes a problem that is known as the **anode heel effect** (Figure 6–16). Because of the geometry of an angled anode target, the **radiation intensity is greater on the cathode side**. As electrons bombard the target, x-rays are produced and most are emitted at angles between 45 and 90 degrees in the direction of the electron travel. These are absorbed by the anode itself or by the tube housing. Those photons that are emitted from the surface of the target are emitted in all directions. The intensity of the radiation which is emitted will vary between the cathode end of the tube and the anode end of the tube. This is because photons that are emitted toward the anode end are more likely to be absorbed by the target material itself than those that are emitted toward the cathode end (Figure 6–17). This can cause as many as 20 percent more photons at the cathode end of the tube and 25 percent fewer photons at the anode end (Figure 6–18). A total variation of approximately 45 percent exists parallel to the anode-cathode axis. No significant variation occurs perpendicular to the anode-cathode axis.

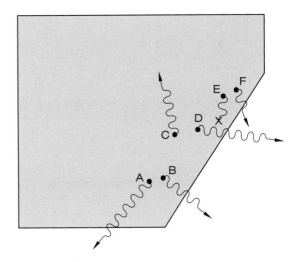

FIGURE 6–17. A–E represent photons created in the target. A exits at anode end of tube while B exits at cathode end of the tube. Notice the greater distance photon A must travel through the target material itself as compared to photon B. Most photons are absorbed as in C. C is absorbed in the anode D, which exits the anode but is absorbed in the housing, and E, which is heading toward the anode end but does not exit the anode. F exits at the cathode end because it has a shorter distance to travel through the anode.

The 45 percent variation is significant enough to cause a visible difference in film density during radiographic examinations **when large film sizes are used at short distances**. The anode heel effect is the reason why each radiographic table has a standard or natural "head" end. The tube anode is established at the head of the table to utilize the anode heel effect to best advantage. No significant variations will be seen in density from side to side.

Because the cathode end of the x-ray tube has a more intense beam, it should be positioned toward the denser (thicker) part of the body.

Example: In which direction should the cathode be placed for an anteroposterior examination of the thoracic vertebral column?

Answer: Because the inferior thoracic region is more dense, the cathode's more intense beam should be positioned inferiorly to help increase the film density in that region.

The Stator

The induction-motor electromagnets comprise the stator that turns the anode. The stator is the only part of cathode or anode assemblies that is located **outside** the vacuum of the glass envelope (Figure 6–8). The electromagnetic effect that causes the rotor to turn can function through the glass, permitting electrical isolation of the stator coils from the high voltage of the exposure. The kilovoltage range of the exposure would destroy the stator's electromagnets. The switch labeled "rotor" that must be activated prior to an exposure actually sends current to the stator, which then causes the rotor to turn the anode. If the stator fails, the rotor will cease to turn the anode, resulting in the immediate melting of a spot on the target because rotating anode targets are not designed to absorb the heat of a high-voltage exposure while stationary (Figure 6–19).

The Rotor

The rotor is located inside the stator and inside the glass envelope. It is composed of a hollow copper cylinder or cuff that is attached to the anode disk by a molybdenum shaft. The cuff is the true rotor that is affected by the electromagnetic field of the stator, causing it to turn.

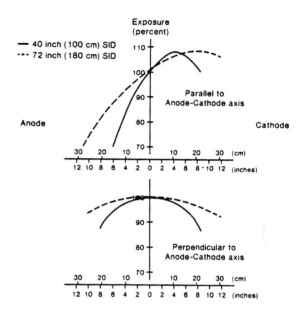

FIGURE 6–18. Variation in intensity of x-ray emissions parallel and perpendicular to anode-cathode axis. *(By permission of Mayo Foundation, [1983]. Quality control in diagnostic imaging,* Aspen Publishers, Inc., Rockville.)

Common rotating anodes revolve at 3,200–3,600 revolutions per minute (rpm). High-speed rotating anodes that operate at 10,000–12,000 rpm are also available to assist in dissipating heat.

The inside of the rotor contains silver-plated steel ball bearings around a shaft that is anchored to the glass envelope (Figure 6–8). The ball bearings use silver plating as a high-temperature lubricant between the cuff and the anode shaft. Liquids tend to produce gas at high temperatures and this would reduce the vacuum in the tube. When the rotor switch is depressed prior to an exposure, the sound that is heard from the tube is actually the sound of the ball bearings turning at high speed. A new tube rotor with fresh bearings should coast for about 60 seconds after a 3,000 rpm exposure before stopping. When the coasting time slows to less than 20 seconds, the bearings are usually near binding.

High-speed anodes have a particular problem that is caused by the tone produced by their rotating. At between 5,000 and 7,000 rpm the harmonics produced by the rotating cuff are at a frequency capable of shattering the glass envelope. Consequently, at the end of an

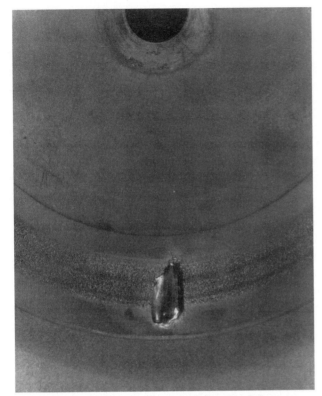

FIGURE 6–19. Anode melt due to rotor-bearing failure.

exposure, direct current is run through the stator to quickly slow the rotor safely through the dangerous harmonic range. Another problem associated with high-speed anodes is the gyroscopic effect produced by the centrifugal force of the rotation. This force is great enough that if a high-speed anode tube housing is quickly rotated from one position to another (for example, from horizontal to perpendicular), the gyroscopic effect can cause trauma to the anode disk and bearing, causing the destruction of the tube. Usually the reversal of the stator prevents this problem but constant rough handling of this sort can cause undue wear on the rotor bearings. Any rough or extremely fast movement of the housing is not healthy for an x-ray tube and should be avoided.

A common cause of tube failure is bad bearings caused by long use at high temperatures. Although the molybdenum shaft that attaches the anode disk is designed to conduct a minimal amount of heat, the ball bearings eventually become imperfectly round. This

leads to a grinding noise and wobbling of the rotor. Rotor wobble throws the focal track off center and tube efficiency drops dramatically.

Another effect of stator or rotor failure is that the electron stream overheats the target area of the anode focal track. When the temperature exceeds the melting point of tungsten, melting will occur. Superheated melted tungsten that drips onto the glass envelope will destroy the tube.

Any tube is dangerous to use when these events occur. A wobbling or melting anode disk can crack from the heat of exposure. A cracked anode can divert the electron and/or photon stream toward the glass envelope. Either instance will crack the envelope, permitting implosion of the vacuum, which can suck the insulating oil into contact with the superheated anode assembly. This can cause vaporization of the oil in a violent explosion that can blow out the rubber expansion seals of the housing, permitting hot oil to drop from the tube housing. Superheated oil is a severe hazard to the patient and the normal response should be emergency removal of the patient from under the tube. In nearly all instances, it is quicker to pull the patient from under the tube than to release the locks necessary to manipulate the tube away from the patient. In an angiographic laboratory or surgical situation, the breaking of sterile aseptic technique would be justified. A blown tube is a rare event and should never occur if proper tube loading, quality control and maintenance procedures are followed.

The Glass Envelope

The entire cathode assembly and all of the anode assembly except the stator are enclosed within a glass envelope commonly called the tube (Figure 6–20). A common glass envelope is made by sculpting several different types of heat-resistant Pyrex glass together to form a tube about 10" long, 6" in diameter at the center and 2" in diameter at the ends. The glass is joined to the metal of the cathode assembly at one end and the anode assembly at the other. The envelope is constructed around both the cathode and anode assemblies and must be sealed tight to maintain a high vacuum. At the point where the primary x-ray beam exits the glass envelope, a **window** segment is constructed. In some tubes this is

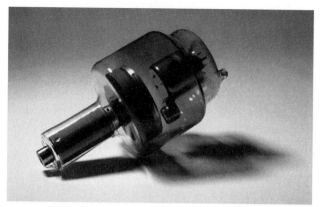

FIGURE 6–20. A complete diagnostic x-ray tube with glass envelope, cathode assembly, anode disk, and rotor. *(Courtesy of Varian Interay, North Charleston, SC)*

simply a thinner section of the envelope to allow less absorption or scatter of the photons. Some special application tubes have other types of windows. For example, a molybdenum target tube for mammography uses a special metallic beryllium window to avoid attenuating the lower-energy photons, as discussed earlier.

The Vacuum

The primary function of the glass envelope is to maintain the vacuum between the cathode and anode. After construction, the air is removed from the tube until a pressure of less than 10^{-5} mm mercury (Hg) is achieved. This is done by use of a vacuum pump through a special vent, which is then permanently sealed. **The removal of the air permits electrons to flow from cathode to anode without encountering the gas atoms of air** and greatly increases the efficiency of the tube's operation.

Historical Notes   Röntgen discovered x-rays with a Crookes or Hittorf tube which did not enclose a vacuum but instead contained known volumes of various gasses. Specialized tubes were quickly developed to meet the increasing need for x-ray production and the vacuum tube was an early improvement. The x-ray pioneers simply placed the glass envelope within a leaded glass bowl. This was convenient when tubes had to be changed manually during the era of cold cathodes. Rapidly increasing awareness of the biological effects of ionizing radiation led to the development of metallic housings for x-ray tubes.

Protective Housing

Modern x-ray tubes must be mounted inside a protective housing (Figure 6–21). **The housing controls leakage and scatter radiation, isolates the high voltages and provides a means to cool the tube.**

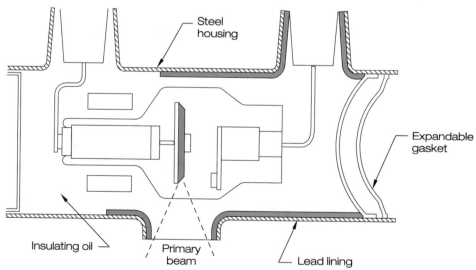

Steel housing

Expandable gasket

Insulating oil

Primary beam

Lead lining

FIGURE 6–21. A diagnostic x-ray tube housing.

Control of Leakage Radiation and Scatter Radiation

When x-ray photons are produced at the anode they are emitted isotropically (in all directions). The primary beam consists of photons emitted through the glass window. The remaining photons are unwanted and the tube housing is designed to absorb them. The protective housing is composed of cast steel and is capable of absorbing most of the unwanted photons. The housing is usually lined with lead for additional absorption only at the cathode end because of the direction of the photons being emitted from the anode. The housing is equipped with a window to permit unrestricted exit for the useful photons from the glass envelope window. Any photons that escape from the housing except at the port are **leakage radiation. Leakage radiation must not exceed 100 mR/hr at 1 meter.** The housing also serves to cushion the x-ray tube from rough handling by operators.

High-Voltage Isolation and Tube Cooling

A special dielectric oil is used to fill the space between the glass envelope and the tube housing. The dielectric property of the oil insulates the high-voltage components from the tube housing, which is handled by the radiographer. In addition, the oil absorbs much of the heat that is produced by x-ray production. One end of the tube housing is sealed with an expandable gasket to permit the oil to expand as it is heated (Figure 6–21). This gasket can be blown out by an imploded tube that has vaporized some of the insulating oil, thereby presenting a hazard to the patient. Many tube housings include a small air fan to remove heat from the housing itself. In tubes that are subjected to extremely high loads, such as computed tomography tubes, the oil may be routed through a recirculation system (heat exchanger) to further cool it. Under no circumstances should anyone be in contact with a tube housing during an exposure.

Off-Focus Radiation

An often overlooked factor that can cause serious degradation of radiographic image quality is **off-focus or extrafocal radiation. Off-focus radiation is composed of photons that were not produced at the focal spot.** It occurs when the high-voltage electrons striking the focal spot produce scattered electrons or photons. In some cases these scattered electrons or photons have sufficient energy remaining that when they strike another object in the tube (the cathode assembly, vaporized metal on the glass envelope, off-target sites on the anode, etc.) they produce photons. These photons are produced away from the focal spot and are therefore considered off-focus. The tube housing will absorb the majority of off-focus radiation but enough will be produced at a proper angle that they will exit through the tube window, housing port and collimator (Figure 6–22). These photons can cause "ghosting" of structures adjacent to the edge of the primary beam (Figure 6–23). This is not the result of scatter from the patient. Patient scatter is not capable of creating a diagnostic image of anatomical structures. Off-focus radiation may contribute as much as 25–30 percent of the total primary beam. However, all off-focus radiation is of significantly lower energy than the primary beam itself. X-ray tubes are available with a grounded metal and ceramic envelope to absorb off-focus radiation. These tubes may also use two sets of

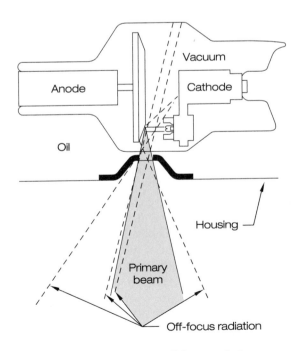

FIGURE 6–22. The production of off-focus radiation.

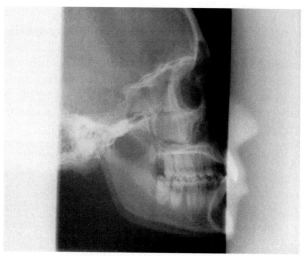

FIGURE 6–23. Off-focus radiation producing an image of the nose on a collimated sinus radiograph.

bearings to increase the heat-loading capacity. They have received limited acceptance because of their cost and the fact that they will not fit most existing tube housings. However, they can increase the total tube life by up to three times.

Rating Charts And Cooling Curves

Three types of rating charts are available to help radiographers avoid thermal damage to x-ray tubes: **radiographic tube rating charts, anode cooling charts and housing cooling charts.** Radiographic rating charts, sometimes called **tube rating charts**, are the most valuable because they provide a guide regarding the maximum technical factor combinations that can be used without overloading the tube. All radiographic tube rating charts plot milliamperage, kilovoltage and time (the three most important factors set by the radiographer). Various manufacturers plot these factors in different ways (Figure 6–24). In most instances any combination of factors at or under the curve is safe. However, the radiographer should verify this fact by establishing that lower

technical combinations lie under the curve. (If both the x and the y axes have lower values at the lower left corner of the chart, safe factors are under the curves.) **Each filament of each tube has a unique radiographic tube rating chart.** The radiographer must ascertain that the correct chart for the **tube and filament** is being used.

Example: Is an exposure of 80 kVp, 0.1 second and 200 mA within the limits of the 1φ, 0.6 mm focal-spot tube rating chart shown in Figure 6–24?

Answer: When the intersection of the 80 kVp and 0.1 second lines is located on the tube rating chart, it is below the 200 mA line. Since the lower technical combinations lie below the mA lines, this is within limits.

Example: Is an exposure of 90 kVp, 0.08 second and 600 mA within the limits of the 3φ, 1.2 mm focal-spot tube rating chart shown in Figure 6–25?

Answer: When the intersection of the 90 kVp and 0.08 second lines is located on the tube rating chart, it is above the 600 mA line. Since the higher technical combinations lie above the mA line, it is not within limits.

Anode cooling charts permit the calculation of the time necessary for the anode to cool enough for additional exposures to be made (Figure 6–26). All cooling charts

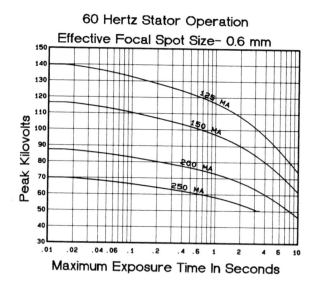

FIGURE 6–24. Example tube rating chart for 1φ full-wave rectification. (*Courtesy of Varian EIMAC*)

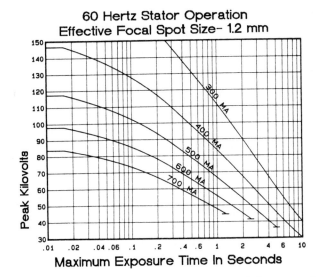

FIGURE 6–25. Example tube rating chart for 3ϕ full-wave rectification. (Courtesy of Varian EIMAC)

are calculated in terms of radiographic heat units. **A heat unit is calculated as kVp x mA x time x rectification constant.** The heat unit (HU) constants are given in Table 6–1. (Radiographic heat units are based on 1 kVp × 1 mA = 1 watt × 1 sec = 1 watt/sec × 0.71 rms voltage = 1 heat unit. Technically 1 radiographic heat unit= 0.78 joules.)

Example: How many heat units are generated by an exposure of 80 kVp, 200 mA and 0.2 second on a 1ϕ full-wave rectified unit?

Answer:

$$80 \text{ kVp} \times 200 \text{ mA} \times 0.2 \text{ sec}$$
$$\times 1.00 = 3,200 \text{ HU}$$

TABLE 6–1. Heat Unit Rectification Constants

Rectification	Constant
1ϕ 2 pulse (Full wave)	1.00
3ϕ 6 pulse	1.35
3ϕ 12 pulse	1.41
High frequency	1.45

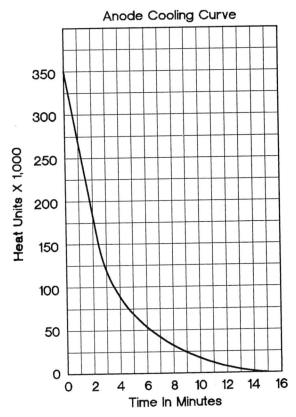

FIGURE 6–26. Example anode cooling chart.

Example: How many heat units are generated by an exposure of 70 kVp, 300 mA and 0.15 sec on a 3ϕ 6 pulse unit?

Answer:

$$70 \text{ kVp} \times 300 \text{ mA} \times 0.15 \text{ sec}$$
$$\times 1.35 = 4,253 \text{ HU}$$

Example: How many heat units are generated by two exposures of 65 kVp, 400 mA and 0.05 sec on a 3ϕ 12 pulse unit?

Answer:

$$65 \text{ kVp} \times 400 \text{ mA} \times 0.05 \text{ sec}$$
$$\times 1.41 \times 2 \text{ exposures}$$
$$= 3,666 \text{ HU}$$

To use the chart, the exposure factors must first be calculated in heat units. The length of time for the anode to cool can then be calculated by the following steps:

1. Find the total heat units applied on the vertical scale.

2. Read from the heat units over to the cooling curve and then down to read the corresponding time.

3. Calculate the time necessary for the anode to cool to any desired level and subtract the corresponding time of the initial exposure. (Or make the corresponding time of the initial exposure zero and calculate the time necessary for the anode to cool to any desired level from this point.)

For example, with the anode cooling chart in Figure 6–26, if a series of exposures produces 200,000 hu, the corresponding time is 2 minutes. The anode will cool to 150,000 HU in 2.5 minutes, so it will take 0.5 minute for the anode to cool from 200,000 HU to 150,000 hu. Similarly, the anode will cool to 100,000 HU in 1.5 minutes, to 50,000 HU in 4 minutes, and to room temperature (0) in 13 minutes.

Example: Use the anode cooling curve in Figure 6–26 to calculate the length of time necessary for the anode to cool to 50,000 HU after five exposures of 80 kVp, 500 mA and 0.5 second on a 1ϕunit.

Answer:

$$80 \text{ kVp} \times 500 \text{ mA} \times 0.5 \text{ sec} \times 1.00$$
$$\times 5 = 100,000 \text{ HU}$$
$$50,000 \text{ HU} = 6 \text{ minutes on cooling curve}$$
$$100,000 \text{ HU} = 3.5 \text{ minutes on cooling curve,}$$
$$\text{so 6 min} - 3.5 \text{ min} = 2.5 \text{ min to}$$
$$\text{cool from } 100,000 \text{ to } 50,000 \text{ HU}$$

A more practical application of an anode cooling curve is to solve a problem regarding whether a desired exposure will overload the anode. For example, again using Figure 6–26, how long would it be after a load of 250,000 HU before a series of exposures equal to 150,000 HU could be made? Since the total HU capacity of the anode is 350,000 hu, it must cool to 200,000 HU in order to take the additional 150,000 hu. The question becomes,

"How long will it take the anode to cool from 250,000 to 200,000 hu?" It will take 0.75 minute (2–1.25 min), or 45 seconds, before the new series of exposures can be made because 250,000 HU corresponds to 1.25 minutes and 200,000 HU corresponds to 2 minutes.

Example: Use the anode cooling curve in Figure 6–26 to calculate the length of time necessary for the anode to cool sufficiently from 350,000 HU to accept a series of exposures totaling 150,000 HU on a 1ϕ unit.

Answer:

350,000 HU – 150,000 HU = 200,000 HU as level to which anode must cool
350,000 HU = 0 minutes
200,000 HU = 2 minutes
It will be 2 minutes (2 – 0 min) before the series of exposures can be made.

After working through several of these problems for most tube anodes, it becomes apparent that modern x-ray tubes are designed to withstand most exposures within the diagnostic range for average patients. It is when a series of exposures must be made (as occurs routinely in angiographic procedures) that most radiographic tube rating and anode cooling charts must be consulted.

Housing cooling charts permit the calculation of the time necessary for the housing to cool enough for additional exposures to be made (Figure 6–27). As with anode cooling charts, they are calculated in terms of radiographic heat units. They are used in exactly the same manner as an anode cooling chart. In actual practice the anode will usually reach its limits long before the housing. However, there are instances, as when the forced-air fan for the housing is not functioning, when these charts can be useful.

Recommendations For Extending Tube Life

There are many things that the professional radiographer can do to extend the life of an x-ray tube. Warming up the anode according to the manufacturer's recom-

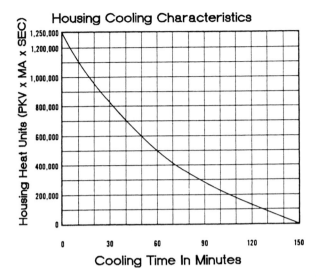

FIGURE 6–27. Example housing cooling chart. *(Courtesy of Varian EIMAC)*

mendations prevents thermal shock (cracking of a cold anode). Cracking can occur when a nonstress-relieved anode is unable to expand rapidly enough to absorb a room temperature-to-operating heat level exposure. Holding the rotor switch unnecessarily should be avoided. The rotor switch increases the filament's thermionic emission to exposure levels. Thermionic emission removes the electrons from the filament, deposits vaporized electrons on tube surfaces and decreases the tube vacuum, all of which can cause tube failure. In addition, the rotor switch causes stress to the rotor bearings, which can also decrease tube life. To avoid these problems, double-press switches should be completely depressed in one motion and dual switches should have the exposure switch depressed first, followed by the rotor switch. Lower mA stations should be used when possible because high mA increases filament thermionic emission. The lower-speed rotor should be used when possible because the high-speed rotor increases rotor bearing wear. Repeated exposures near tube loading limits should not be made as total heat units may approach anode or housing loading limits. Rotating the tube housing rapidly from one position to another should be avoided because the gyroscopic effect may crack or otherwise

damage the rotor. A tube should not be used when loud rotor bearings can be heard (unless it has been checked by a qualified service person) because a wobbling anode disk can cause tube failure. These recommendations are summarized in Table 6–2.

Summary

X-ray production requires a source of electrons, an appropriate target material, a high voltage and a vacuum. The x-ray tube is the device that permits these conditions to exist. It consists of a cathode and an anode enclosed within a glass envelope and then encased in a protective housing.

The cathode is the negative side of the x-ray tube. The function of the cathode is to produce a thermionic cloud, conduct the high voltage to the gap between cathode and anode and focus the electron stream as it heads for the anode. The cathode assembly consists of the filament or filaments, focusing cup and associated wiring. The filament is a small coil of thin, thoriated tungsten wire. The focusing cup serves to narrow the thermionic cloud as it is driven to the anode.

The anode is the positive side of the x-ray tube. Anodes are divided into two types: stationary and rotating. Anodes are made using tungsten because of its high atomic number, high melting point and good heat-conducting ability. The anode assembly consists of the anode, the stator and the rotor. The portion of the anode

TABLE 6–2. Recommendations for Extending Tube Life

1. Warm up the anode following manufacturer's recommendations.
2. Do not hold the rotor switch unnecessarily. Double-press switches should be completely depressed in one motion. Dual switches should have exposure switch depressed first, followed by rotor switch.
3. Use lower mA stations when possible.
4. Use lower-speed rotor when possible.
5. Do not make repeated exposures near tube loading limits.
6. Do not rotate the tube housing rapidly from one position to another.
7. Do not use a tube when you can hear loud rotor bearings (unless it has been checked by a qualified service person).

where the high-voltage electron stream impacts is called the target, focus, focal point, focal spot or focal track. The term actual focal spot is used to describe the physical area of the focal track that is impacted. The term effective focal spot is used to describe the area of the focal spot that is projected out of the tube toward the object being radiographed.

The line-focus principle is used to reduce the effective area of the focal spot. This permits the best resolution of detail in as large an actual area as possible. The effective focal-spot size is controlled by the filament size and the anode target angle. When the target angle is less than 45°, the effective focal spot is smaller than the actual focal spot.

The anode heel effect states that radiation intensity is greater on the cathode side than on the anode side.

An often overlooked factor that can cause serious degradation of radiographic image quality is off-focus or extrafocal radiation. Off-focus radiation is composed of photons that were not produced at the focal spot.

Three types of heating charts are available to help radiographers avoid thermal damage to x-ray tubes: radiographic tube rating charts, anode cooling charts and housing cooling charts. Radiographic rating charts, sometimes called tube rating charts, are the most valuable because they provide a guide regarding the maximum technical factor combinations that can be used without overloading the tube. There are many things a radiographer can do to extend the life of an x-ray tube.

REVIEW QUESTIONS

1. What conditions must exist for x-rays to be produced?

2. What are the basic parts of a cathode assembly?

3. What is the purpose of the focusing cup?

4. Explain the space charge effect.

5. Why is tungsten the best metal for the x-ray source?

6. Explain the line-focus principle.

7. How does the anode heel effect affect radiation intensity?

8. What is the advantage of a high-speed rotor?

9. Why is it necessary for a vacuum to exist within the glass envelope?

10. Define leakage radiation.

11. How is off-focus radiation produced?

12. What is the function of rating charts and cooling curves?

13. Define a heat unit.

14. Name five things a radiographer can do to extend the life of an x-ray tube.

REFERENCES AND RECOMMENDED READING

Ball, J. & Price, T. (1989). *Chesneys' radiographic imaging.* Oxford: Blackwell Scientific Publishing.

Brookstein, J. J. & Steck, W. (1971). Effective focal spot size. *Radiology. 98,* 31–34.

Bushberg, J. T., Seibert, J. A., Leidholdt, E. M., & Boone, J. M. (1994). *The essential physics of medical imaging.* Baltimore: Williams & Wilkins.

Carroll, Q. B. (1993). *Fuchs's radiographic exposure, processing and quality control* (5th ed.). Springfield, IL: Charles C. Thomas Publishers.

Coolidge, W. D. (1945). Experiences with the Röentgen-ray tube. *American Journal of Roentgenology. 54,* 583–589.

Coolidge, W. D. (1913). A powerful Röntgen ray tube with a pure electron discharge. *The Physical Review. 2*(6).

Cullinan, J. E. (1968). Fractional-focus x-ray tubes. *Radiologic Technology. 39*(6), 333.

Curry, T. S., Dowdey, J. E., & Murry, R. C. (1990). *Christensen's introduction to the physics of diagnostic radiology* (4th ed.). Philadelphia: Lea and Febiger.

Dendy, P. P. & Heaton, B. (1987). *Physics for radiologists.* Oxford: Blackwell Scientific Publications.

De Vos, D. C. (1990). *Basic principles of radiographic exposure.* Philadelphia: Lea & Febiger.

Dietz, K. *The x-ray tube in diagnostic applications.* Erlangen, West Germany: Siemens Aktiengesellschaft, Medical Engineering Group, publication MR A 5/1241.121.

Drew, P. G. (1989). Lowly x-ray tube may be in for some big changes, *Diagnostic imaging.* (Jan.), 50.

Eisenberg, R. L. (1992). *Radiology: An illustrated history.* St. Louis: C. V. Mosby.

Engel, T. L. (1979). Effect of kilovoltage and milliamperage on focal spot size, *Radiologic Technology. 50*(5), p 559–561.

Everson, J. D. & Gray, J. E. (1987). Focal-spot measurement: comparison of slit, pinhole, and star resolution pattern techniques. *Radiology. 165*(1), 261–264.

Fairbanks, R. & Doust, C. (1979). Methods for studying the focal spot size and resolution of diagnostic x-ray tubes. *Radiography. 45*(533), 89.

Fodor, J. (1988). Recent advances in x-ray tube design. *Radiologic Technology. 60*(1), 33.

Fuchs, A. W. (1947). The anode 'heel' effect in radiography, *The X-Ray Technician. 18*, 158–163.

Gifford, D. (1984). *A handbook of physics for radiologists and radiographers.* New York: John Wiley & Sons.

Glasser, O. (1958). *Dr. W. C. Röentgen* (2nd ed.). Springfield, IL: Charles C. Thomas.

Glasser, O. (1936). What kind of tube did Röntgen use when he discovered x-ray? *Radiology. 27,* 138–140.

Grigg, E. R. N. (1965). *The trail of the invisible light: From x-Strahlen to radio(bio)logy.* Springfield, IL: Charles C. Thomas Publisher.

Harrison, R. M & Forster, E. (1984). Performance characteristics of x-ray tubes and generators. *Radiography. 50*(594), 245.

High and normal speed rotors: Effect on focal spot size, resolution and density. (1981). *Radiologic Technology. 53*(1).

Machlett Laboratories, Inc. *"Trade-offs" A guide to the selection of diagnostic x-ray tubes.* Stamford, CT: The Raytheon Corporation publication ST-2859-1.

Matsui, H. & Katsuhiro, O. (1985). A uniform focal spot x-ray tube with improved MTF and KW rating. *Radiology.* 227.

National Electrical Manufacturers Association. (1985). Measurements of dimensions and properties of focal spots of diagnostic x-ray tubes. NEMA Standards Publication No. XR-5-1984.

Ridgway, A. & Thumm, W. (1973). *The physics of medical radiography.* Reading, MA: Addison-Wesley.

Seeram, E. (1985). *X-ray imaging equipment.* Springfield, IL: Charles C. Thomas.

Seeram, E. (1977). Recent x-ray tube innovations. *Canadian Journal of Radiography, Radiotherapy, and Nuclear Medicine. 8*(4), 192–197.

Selman, J. (1994). *The fundamentals of x-ray and radium physics* (9th ed.). Springfield, IL: Thomas.

Sprawls, P. (1990). *Principles of radiography for technologists.* Rockville, MD: Aspen Publishers.

Sprawls, P. (1987). *Physical principles of medical imaging.* Rockville, MD: Aspen Publishers.

Stears, J. G., Gray, J. E., Frank, E. D. (1979). Overcoming tube failure in a special procedures room. *Radiologic Technology. 51*(1), 89.

Stears, J. G., Gray, J. E., Frank, E. D. (1986). Half-value layer increase owing to tungsten buildup in the x-ray tube: Fact or fiction? *Radiology.* 837.

Stears, J. G., Gray, J. E., Webbles, W. E., & Frank, E. D. (1989). Radiologic exchange (resolution according to focal spot size). *Radiologic Technology. 60*(5), 429–430.

Stears, J. G., Gray, J. E., Webbles, W. E., & Frank, E. D. (1988). Radiologic Exchange (tube warm-up and leaving x-ray units on). *Radiologic Technology. 59*(4), 325–326.

Stears, J. G., Gray, J. E, Webbles, W. E., & Frank, E. D. (1987). The three limits to prevent x-ray tube damage. *Radiologic Technology. 58*(5), 423.

Stockley, S. M. (1986). *A manual of radiographic equipment.* Edinburgh: Churchill Livingstone.

Suleyman, R. & Doust, C. (1979). The management of the kilovoltage applied to an x-ray tube. *Radiography. 45*(540), 263.

Ter-Pogossian, M. M. (1967). *The physical aspects of diagnostic radiology.* New York: Hoeber Medical Division, Harper & Row.

Thomas, J. B. & Roderick, J. F. (1946). The use and abuse of x-ray tubes. *Radiologic Technology. 18*(2), 62.

Thomas, S. R. (1983). Radiation physics — Characteristics of extrafocal radiation and its potential significance in pediatric radiology. *Radiology.* (March), 793.

Thompson, M. A., Hattaway, M. P., Hall, J. D., & Dowd, S. B. (1994). *Principles of imaging science and protection.* Philadelphia: W. B. Saunders.

Thompson, T. T. (1985). *A practical approach to modern imaging equipment* (2nd ed.). Boston: Little, Brown, & Co.

Tortorici, M. (1992). *Concepts in medical radiographic imaging.* Philadelphia: W. B. Saunders.

Trigg, C. N. (1979). X-ray tube failures and prevention: A preliminary report. *Radiologic Technology. 50*(4), 430.

van der Plaats, G. J. (1980). *Medical x-ray techniques in diagnostic radiology* (4th ed.). The Hague: Martinus Nijhoff Publishers.

Wallace, R. J. Diagnostic x-ray tube failure and prevention, *Radiologic Technology,* 48: No. 5, p 565, 1977.

Wilks, R. J. (1981). *Principles of radiological physics.* Edinburgh: Churchill Livingstone.

Wolbarst, A. B. (1993). *Physics of radiology.* Norwalk, CT: Appleton & Lange.

CHAPTER 7

X-Ray Production

I did not think, I investigated.

*Professor Wilhelm Röntgen to Sir James Mackenzie-Davidson during his
only recorded interview, when asked what he thought when he discovered x-rays.*

Objectives

Upon completion of this chapter, the student should be able to:

▶ State the percentage of electron energy that is converted to x-ray photon energy in the x-ray tube.

▶ Describe a bremsstrahlung target interaction.

▶ Describe a characteristic target interaction.

▶ Identify factors affecting characteristic K-shell photon production.

▶ Explain the shape of the x-ray photon emission spectrum curve.

Conditions

X-ray photons are produced when the high-speed electrons from the cathode strike an anode target. The fact that they are man-made is the only difference between x-rays and gamma rays (which are products of nuclear radioactive decay). An understanding of how x-ray photons are created from the atoms of the target material permits the radiographer to assert full control over the production of the primary beam.

The electrons that form the thermionic cloud around the filament arrive at the anode target (2 cm distant) traveling at nearly half the speed of light. A true understanding of the force contained in a kilovoltage-level exposure can be obtained by realizing that these electrons were accelerated from zero to half the speed of light in about 2 cm. These incoming electrons are called **incident electrons** and are represented in drawings by a solid arrow. In contrast, photons are represented by a wave arrow.

When incident electrons strike the target, they convert their tremendous kinetic energy to the atoms of the target material and this interaction produces x-ray photons. The greater the mass or speed of the incident electrons, the greater the quality (energy) and quantity (number) of photons produced. This process occurs through two very different **target interactions**. All target interactions occur within 0.25 to 0.5 mm of the surface of the target. After giving up their energy to the target atoms, the electrons slow down enough to be conducted through the anode and the remainder of the high-voltage circuit. However, the incident electrons often experience 1,000 or more interactions before reaching this state.

Target Interactions

Heat Production

The target interactions that produce the x-ray photons consist of **less than one percent** of the total kinetic energy of the incident electrons. **Over 99** percent of the kinetic energy of the incident electrons is converted to heat. This is the reason why so much technical research has gone into the development of the thermal aspects of x-ray tubes. In spite of the cost and performance capabilities of modern x-ray tubes, they are tremendously inefficient because they waste over 99 percent of the energy they use. This is true only in the range of diagnostic x-rays. As the kinetic energy of the incident electrons increases, so does the efficiency of photon production. By the time the therapeutic MeV range is reached, the majority of the energy is producing photons instead of heat.

Because they have such high kinetic energy, incident electrons seldom transfer enough energy to the outer shells of target atoms to cause ionization. Instead, they transfer enough energy to excite the outer-shell electrons to the point where they will emit infrared radiation as heat. These electrons then return to their normal state — where they will be re-excited again and again, each time emitting infrared radiation as heat.

There are two types of target interactions that can produce diagnostic-range x-ray photons: **bremsstrahlung interactions and characteristic interactions**. The interaction which will occur depends on the **electron kinetic energy** and the **binding energy of the electron shells** of the atom. Tungsten and rhenium are used as target materials in an effort to provide appropriate atomic number atoms, and a maximum number of similar electron shell binding energies.

Bremsstrahlung Interactions

Bremsstrahlung interactions are named by the German word for braking or slowing. The abbreviation "brems" is also used. **Brems interactions may occur only when the incident electron interacts with the force field of the nucleus.** The incident electron must have enough energy to pass through the orbital shells and approach the nucleus of the atom. Because atomic nuclei have a positive charge and the incident electron has a negative charge, there is a mutual attraction between them. When the incident electron gets close to the nucleus, the powerful nuclear force field is much too great for the electron to penetrate. Instead, the force field causes the incident electron to slow down (or brake) and then it diverts the electron's course. As a result, the electron loses energy and changes direction. The energy that is lost during the braking (or bremsstrahlung) is emitted as an x-ray photon. **These emissions are called bremsstrahlung photons and their energy is exactly the difference between the entering and exiting kinetic energy of the electron** (Figure 7–1). The amount of kinetic energy lost by the incident electron in a brems interaction is determined by the distance the electron is from the nucleus. At larger distances very little kinetic energy is lost, resulting in low energy brems radiation. At closer distances more energy is lost, resulting in higher energy brems radiation. The incident electron can also have a direct impact with the nucleus, resulting in the loss of all of the electron's kinetic energy. Because of the relatively small size of the nucleus, the chance of a direct impact is very low.

These energies are individually unpredictable and can range from the total value of the incident electron (which could be as high as the peak kilovoltage) to such a minimal amount of energy that it is immeasurable. Statistically, it is possible to predict their energies quite

accurately by a study of the x-ray emission spectrum, as will be discussed later in this chapter. Only when the incident electron loses all of its excess kinetic energy would the electron drift away to join the current flow. A single incident electron can cause numerous brems interactions in many different atoms before losing enough energy to become included in the current flow.

Characteristic Interactions

Characteristic interactions may occur only when the incident electron interacts with an inner-shell electron (Figure 7–2). The incident electron must have enough energy to knock an inner-shell electron from orbit, thereby ionizing the atom. The incident electron will usually continue but in a slightly different direction. More important is the fact that the electron "hole" that has been created in the inner shell makes the atom unsta-

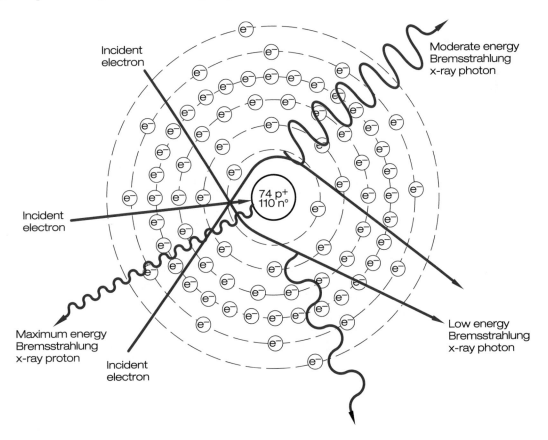

FIGURE 7–1. The bremsstrahlung interaction in a tungsten atom.

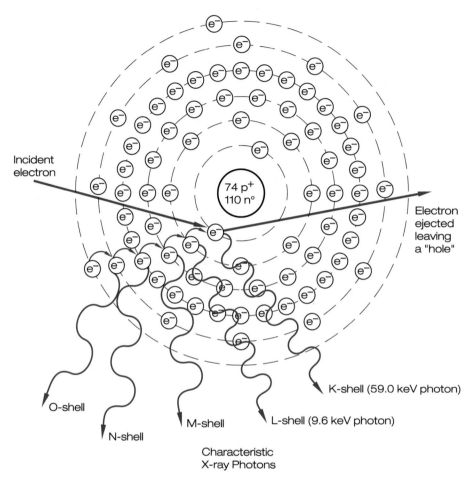

FIGURE 7–2. The characteristic interaction in a tungsten atom. Only the K-shell characteristic photon has sufficient energy to be a part of the useful beam.

ble. An electron from another shell will immediately drop into the "hole." This dropping of an electron from an outer, higher-energy state into an inner, lower-energy state results in the energy difference between the two shells being emitted as an x-ray photon. **These emissions are called characteristic photons because their energy is exactly the difference between the binding energy of the outer and inner shells between which the electron dropped.** After an outer shell electron has dropped to fill the "hole," another electron will drop to fill the "hole" it left and so on until only the outermost shell is missing an electron. This process is called a **characteristic cascade** and it can produce numerous x-ray photons for each electron that leaves the atom.

The first electron that was knocked from position in an inner orbital shell often has sufficient energy that it, too, may cause further interactions before it loses enough energy to become part of the current flow. Of course this will also contribute to the total number of photons created.

Unlike brems photons, characteristic photon energies are so predictable that the science of x-ray spectroscopy uses measurements of these photon energies to determine what types of atoms make up the sun, stars and other celestial bodies.

A tungsten atom, with its high atomic number of 74, has sufficient electron shells to produce relatively high-energy characteristic photons. Tungsten has a total of 74 electrons, with 2 electrons in the K-shell, 8 in L, 18 in M, 32 in N, 12 in O and 2 in the P-shell (Figure 2–5). The binding energies of the electrons in these shells are 69.5 keV for the K-shell electrons, 12.1 keV for L-shell electrons, 2.8 keV for M, 0.6 keV for N and 0.08 keV for the O-shell electrons. The electron that drops into the "hole" may be from any shell further away from the nucleus. Of course the further out the dropping electron's original position, the greater the energy imparted to the characteristic photon.

Characteristic photons can be created from incident electron ionization of any shell and "hole" filling from any shell. For example, K-shell ionizations can result in characteristic photons from electron drops between shells L and K, M and K, N and K, etc. Characteristic photons can also result from L-shell ionizations with electron drops between shells M and L, N and L, and so on. A wide variety of characteristic photon energy levels are thus produced (Table 7–1). The filling of a "hole" from an adjacent shell results in a lesser energy photon than non-adjacent shell transitions. For example, a K-shell vacancy filled by an L-shell electron will result in a weaker characteristic photon than the same vacancy filled by an M-shell electron. That is the result of the lower binding energy for the M-shell electrons. In addition, within each shell there are discrete energy states for individual electrons. As a result, slightly different energies can result from an L to K transition depending on the specific energy state of the electron involved in the

transition. Note that only electron drops into the K-shell will produce characteristic photons within the diagnostic x-ray range. Characteristic photons from the other shells (L, M, N, etc.) have energies that are too low to be significant in diagnostic radiology.

A single incident electron can cause a variety of interactions in many different atoms before losing enough energy to become included in the current flow (Figure 7–3). Remember, most of these interactions will result in the production of heat.

TABLE 7–1. Characteristic Photon Emissions from X-Ray Target Materials

TUNGSTEN

K-Shell Characteristics Photons		L-Shell Characteristics Photons	
L to K	59.0 keV		
M to K	67.2 keV	M to L	9.6 keV
N to K	69.1 keV	N to L	11.0 keV
Effective energy	69.5 keV	Effective energy	12.1 keV

MOLYBDENUM

K-shell Characteristics Photons	
L to K	17 keV
M to K	20 keV
Effective energy	18 keV

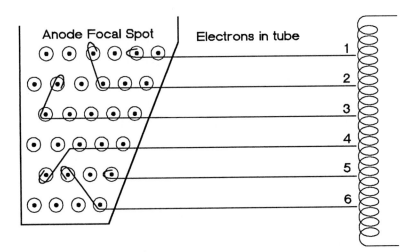

FIGURE 7–3. Sample paths of interactions for incident electrons striking the tube target.

Emission Spectrum

Within the diagnostic x-ray range most photons are produced by bremsstrahlung target interactions. Characteristic photons will not comprise any of the useful beam until the kVp is above 70 because removal of a K-shell electron from tungsten requires 69.5 keV. Between 80–100 kVp about 80–90 percent of the primary beam is produced by brems interactions and 10–20 percent by characteristic interactions.

As mentioned previously, the K-shell emissions are the only ones within the diagnostic x-ray range, although the L-shell emissions form a similar group and the M- to P-shell emissions form a third group. Both brems and characteristic emissions combine to form the complete primary beam spectrum (Figure 7–4). The L-shell characteristic emissions are included within the total spectrum, but when filtration is added to the tube these photons do not have sufficient energy and are absorbed by the filter. The K-shell emissions form a **characteristic peak** at their effective energy range of 69 keV. This char-

acteristic peak is worthy of special note as it can cause strange results for the radiographer who is operating the x-ray tube slightly above the K-shell peak and needs a slight decrease in radiation output. A slight decrease that sets the tube potential directly on the 69 keV K-shell peak would greatly increase the tube output instead of decrease it, as anticipated. Modern x-ray equipment is capable of somewhat overcoming these fluctuations by programmed switching and the use of tungsten alloys (such as molybdenum) in the target to smooth out characteristic peaking. However, characteristic peaks are a point of consideration, not only in the target material but in the construction of x-ray tabletops, grids, cassettes, intensifying screens and any other object through which the primary beam must pass. **The kilovoltage peak of the exposure is the maximum possible energy for any photon that exits the x-ray tube.**

Example: At what kVp was the exposure made that produced the graph in Figure 7–4?

Answer: As the maximum brems photons were at 80 keV, the kVp was set at that level.

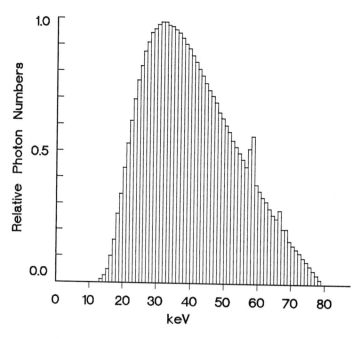

FIGURE 7–4. The x-ray emission spectrum with a tungsten target. This graph is the result of an exposure made with 2.8 mm Al/Eq filtration at constant potential, producing 17.8 mR/mAs at 30 in. (75 cm). The effective photon energy was 31 keV. *(Courtesy of Raymond P. Rossi, University of Colorado Health Science Center)*

What is interesting about Figure 7–4 is that it clearly demonstrates an often overlooked fact about radiographic exposures. **The average primary beam photon has a keV energy of only about 30–40 percent of the kVp.**

The emission spectrum for a mammographic molybdenum target is quite different from that of a tungsten target. The K-shell characteristic peak is about 18 keV and the average photon energy range is between 20–40 keV, which is perfect for soft-tissue visualization.

It is very useful to examine the effect on the primary beam emission spectrum of various factors under the control of the radiographer. When **mA, time or mAs** is changed, all of which control the quantity (number) of electrons striking the target, the result is a change in the **amplitude** of the emission graph (Figure 7–5). Note that each point on the higher curve represents exactly twice the number of photons on the lower curve. When **kVp,** which controls the quality (energy) of electrons striking the target, is changed, the result is a change in the **number of higher-energy photons as well as in the amplitude** of the emission graph (Figure 7–6). Note that there are more higher-energy photons on the higher curve, as well as an increase in the number of photons (seen in the increased amplitude). There was no increase in the total number of electrons striking the target. The increase in amplitude represents more emitted photons due to the higher energy of each incident electron striking the target.

The x-ray emission spectrum is affected by the quantity and composition of the materials through which it must pass to exit the x-ray tube and housing. This is the filtration, which is the subject of the next chapter. As the x-ray beam passes through the filtering materials, some

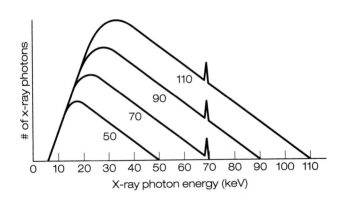

FIGURE 7–6. The effect of kVp on the x-ray emission spectrum.

of the lower-energy photons are absorbed. This **decreases** the intensity of the beam but at the same time **increases** the average photon energy. Increased filtration decreases image density, and vice versa.

The generator phasing also has an effect on the emission spectrum. As the efficiency of x-ray production increases—from 1ϕ 2 pulse to 3ϕ 6 pulse to 3ϕ 12 pulse to constant potential—the emission spectrum changes (Figure 7–7). As generator phasing efficiency increases, the x-ray beam increases in intensity and there is also an increase in the average photon energy. Decreased phasing efficiency decreases both intensity and average photon energy.

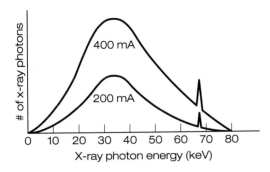

FIGURE 7–5. The effect of mA changes on the x-ray emission spectrum.

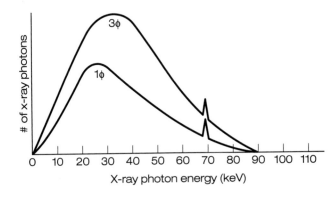

FIGURE 7–7. The effect of generator phase on the x-ray emission spectrum.

Summary

X-ray photons are produced when the high-speed electrons from the cathode strike an anode target. When incident electrons strike the target, they convert their tremendous kinetic energy to the atoms of the target material and this interaction produces x-ray photons. The greater the mass or speed of the incident electrons, the greater the quality (energy) and quantity (number) of photons produced.

The two target interactions that produce x-ray photons are bremsstrahlung (brems) and characteristic interactions. Less than one percent of the total kinetic energy of the incident electrons produces these interactions. Over 99 percent of the kinetic energy of the incident electrons is converted to heat.

Brems interactions occur when the incident electron interacts with the force field of the nucleus. This force field causes the incident electron to slow down (or brake) and then it diverts the electron's course. As a result, the electron loses energy and changes direction. The energy that is lost during the braking is emitted as a bremsstrahlung photon and the photon energy is exactly the difference between the entering and exiting kinetic energy of the electron.

Characteristic interactions occur when the incident electron interacts with an inner shell electron. The incident electron knocks out an inner shell electron and continues in a slightly different direction. An electron "hole" is created in the inner shell, making the atom unstable. An electron from another shell will immediately drop into the "hole," which results in the emission of an x-ray photon. This emission is called a characteristic photon because the energy is exactly the difference between the binding energy of the outer and inner shells between which the electron dropped.

Within the diagnostic x-ray range most photons are produced by bremsstrahlung target interactions. An x-ray emission spectrum graph illustrates the relationship between the two target interactions within the primary beam. The average primary beam photon has a keV energy of only about 30–40 percent of the kVp.

When mA, time or mAs is changed, all of which control the quantity (number) of electrons striking the tar-get, the result is a change in the amplitude of the emission spectrum graph. When kVp is changed, which controls the quality (energy) of electrons striking the target, the result is a change in the number of higher-energy photons, as well as in the amplitude of the emission spectrum graph.

REVIEW QUESTIONS

1. What is the approximate percentage of electron energy that is converted to x-ray photon energy in the x-ray tube?

2. The majority of the electron energy in the x-ray tube is converted to what form of energy?

3. Describe a bremsstrahlung target interaction.

4. Describe a characteristic target interaction.

5. What is a characteristic cascade?

6. What is the average keV of the primary beam as compared to the kilovoltage peak?

7. What effect does increasing mAs and kVp have on the total x-ray emission spectrum?

REFERENCES AND RECOMMENDED READING

Bushberg, J. T., Seibert, J. A., Leidholdt, E. M., & Boone, J. M. (1994). *The essential physics of medical imaging.* Baltimore: Williams & Wilkins.

Bushong, S. C. (1997). *Radiologic science for technologists: Physics, biology, and protection* (6th ed.). St. Louis: C.V. Mosby.

Dendy, P. P. & Heaton, B. (1987). *Physics for radiologists.* Oxford: Blackwell Scientific Publications.

Erickson, J. J. & Coulam, C. M. (1981). Production of x-rays. *The Physical Basis of Medical Imaging.* Editors: Coulam, C. M., Erickson, J. J., Rollo, F. D., & James, A. E. New York: Appleton-Century-Crofts, 37–46.

Fewell, T. R. & Shuping, R. E. (1977). Photon energy distribution of some typical diagnostic x-ray beams. *Medical Physics.* 5(3), 187–197.

Irfan, A. Y., Pugh, V. I., & Jeffery, C. D. (1985). Some practical aspects of peak kilovoltage measurements. *Radiography. 51*(599), 251–254.

Johns, H. E. & Cunningham, J. R. (1983). *The physics of radiology* (4th ed.). Springfield, IL: Thomas.

Mahoney, G. J. (1957). The nature of x-ray production. *Radiologic Technology. 29* (2), 84.

Sprawls, P. (1987). *Physical principles of medical imaging.* Rockville, MD: Aspen Publishers.

Stears, J. G., Gray, J. E., Webbles, W. E., & Frank, E. D. (1989). Radiologic exchange (kVp measurements). *Radiologic Technology. 60*(3), 233–236.

Storm, E. & Israel, H. I. (1970). Photon cross sections from 1 keV to 100 MeV. *Nuclear Data Tables*, CRC Press.

Ter-Pogossian, M. M. (1967). *The physical aspects of diagnostic radiology.* New York: Hoeber Medical Division, Harper & Row.

Thompson, M. A., Hattaway, M. P., Hall, J. D., & Dowd, S. B. (1994). *Principles of imaging science and protection.* Philadelphia: W. B. Saunders.

Tortorici, M. (1992). *Concepts in medical radiographic imaging.* Philadelphia: W. B. Saunders.

Trout, E. D. (1963). The life history of an x-ray beam. *Radiologic Technology. 35*(3), 161–170.

van der Plaats, G. J. (1980). *Medical x-ray techniques in diagnostic radiology* (4th ed.). The Hague: Martinus Nijhoff Publishers.

Wilks, R. J. (1981). *Principles of radiological physics.* Edinburgh: Churchill Livingstone.

Wilson, P. (1977). Theoretic basis of the nature and origin of x-radiation. *Canadian Journal of Radiography, Radiotherapy, and Nuclear Medicine. 8*(1), 12–27.

Wolbarst, A. B. (1993). *Physics of radiology.* Norwalk, CT: Appleton & Lange.

UNIT ▐▐

Protecting Patients and Personnel

*A*critical skill of the radiographer is the ability to protect both patients and other personnel from excessive exposure to ionizing radiation. This includes the radiographer as well. A thorough knowledge of basic radiation physics, personnel monitoring procedures, and advanced procedures for reducing exposure are expected of all radiographers.

Prior to beginning to function in a clinical setting, the radiographer must learn the **basics of radiation protection concepts and equipment.** The critical skill is the ability to apply this information to the **radiation protection procedures for patients and personnel.**

The chapters on **filtration** and the **prime factors** explain how to shape and mold the beam to minimize radiation exposure while obtaining maximum diagnostic information. **X-ray interactions** open the door to exactly what occurs to the biological systems that are being imaged as well as laying groundwork for future understanding of problems in image production.

Finally, advanced procedures for **minimizing patient dose** are provided to provide the practicing radiographer with real clinical skills that will achieve the theory presented in this unit.

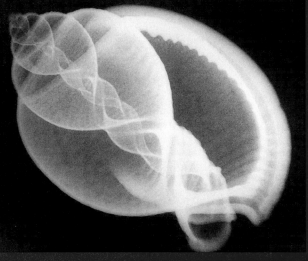

CHAPTER 8

Radiation Protection Concepts and Equipment

One aspect of the wide use of the x-rays perturbed Röntgen greatly. From laboratories in the United States, England, Germany, and France came more and more reports of a peculiar skin reaction similar to a sunburn in persons working with the rays, some of these reactions being particularly serious . . . . It distressed Röntgen to believe that these effects were due to x-rays. . .

Otto Glasser from the biography Dr. W. C. Röntgen

Objectives

Upon completion of this chapter, the student should be able to:

▶ Describe the nature of ionizing radiation.

▶ Identify the types of biological effects of ionizing radiation.

▶ Identify the principle sources of ionizing radiation.

▶ Define the quantities and units used for measurement of radiation.

▶ Describe devices used to detect and measure radiation, including field survey instruments and personnel monitoring devices.

The Basics of Radiation Protection Principles and Practice

*I*n medical applications exposure to ionizing radiation carries with it both a benefit and a risk. The benefit of information from an x-ray examination regarding the clinical management of the patient examination is weighed against the small, but nonetheless finite, risk when a physician requests the examination. The diagnostic benefit of a radiologic procedure far outweighs the risk resulting from the associated x-ray exposure. The information about the clinical condition of a patient received by the physician from a radiologic examination is an essential part of the practice of modern medicine.

It is the responsibility of the radiographer to ensure that each patient receives the minimal dose of radiation that will produce a diagnostic image consistent with the requirements of the examination. Radiographers must also ensure that all individuals are properly protected from unnecessary radiation exposure.

The Nature of Ionizing Radiation

Ionizing radiation is capable of creating positively and negatively charged particles when it interacts with matter. It arises from both natural and man-made sources and has the ability, as a consequence of its interactions with matter, to affect the various organs and tissues within the body. The energy possessed by ionizing radiation is capable of displacing atomic electron bonds and breaking the electron bonds that hold the molecules of matter together resulting in chemical changes, which can lead to harmful effects.

Ionizing radiations are grouped as either **particulate** or **electromagnetic** radiations. Particulate radiations include high energy electrons, neutrons, and protons that produce ionization in matter by direct atomic collisions. There are two principle types of particulate radiation that are associated with radioactive decay, **alpha particles** and **beta particles**. An alpha particle contains two protons and two neutrons and, as a result, is equivalent to a helium nucleus. Alpha particles are emitted from the nuclei of very heavy elements as they undergo radioactive decay. Compared to other types of particulate radiation, alpha particles have great mass and a positive charge. The energy of an alpha particle is transferred over a very short range in matter. In air, alpha particles can travel about 5 cm. As a result, alpha particles from external sources are essentially harmless. Beta particles are identical to electrons with the exception of their origin. Beta particles are emitted from the nuclei of radioactive material, while electrons exist in shells around the nucleus. Beta particles are negatively charged and very light. As a result, they travel farther in matter than alpha particles. Beta particles are capable of traveling approximately 10–100 cm in air.

Electromagnetic radiations include x-rays and gamma rays, which produce ionization in matter by other types of interactions. X-ray and gamma rays are essentially the same with the exception of their origin. Gamma rays are emitted by the nuclei of radioactive materials, while x-rays are man-made in an x-ray tube. For electromagnetic radiation in the medically useful x-ray energy range (<200 keV) the transfer of energy from the photon to matter, resulting in ionization, occurs by processes known as **photoelectric absorption** and **Compton scattering**.

During such interactions with matter, photon energy is transferred by a two-step process. First, the incident photon interacts with an atom causing an electron to be set in motion, which results in kinetic energy being released in the material. Second, the absorption of the released kinetic energy from the electron occurs via excitation and ionization. The excitations and ionizations that occur along the tracks of the charged particles set in motion give rise to biological damage in tissue. The biological damage may be a result of a direct interaction between the charged particle set in motion by the photons, in which cellular macromolecules are directly excited or ionized, or may be a result of an indirect interaction in which the absorption of radiation occurs in a water molecule, producing highly reactive species such as free radicals, which diffuse from the site of origin and subsequently cause biological damage. For x-rays and gamma rays approximately two-thirds of the biological effects on tissue are the result of indirect actions.

Biological Effects of Ionizing Radiation

Exposure to ionizing radiation affects various organs and tissues in the body and may result in a finite probability for radiation-induced disease in persons exposed to the radiation, and in their descendants. Health effects are known to be influenced by radiation characteristics and biological factors and include cancer induction, genetically determined ill health, nonspecific life shortening, developmental abnormalities and degenerative diseases. The effects from the exposure to ionizing radiation may be classified as either **somatic** or **genetic**.

Somatic effects may become evident in the irradiated individual. Such effects are not usually to be expected in individuals exposed in the course of their work in the medical environment. To demonstrate a radiation response in humans within a few days to weeks, the dose must be quite high. Among the somatic effects of radiation are skin erythema, cataracts, and radiation-induced malignancies.

Genetic effects do not produce any significantly observable effect in the exposed individual but may appear in descendants of the exposed individual. They may not be manifest in the children of the exposed individual but may lie dormant for several generations and, eventually, may be eliminated completely from the genetic pool. Such effects result from alterations in the reproductive cells that can lead to defects in the off-spring. Detectable radiation-induced mutations can result if the individual's reproductive cells have been exposed to an appreciable amount of radiation. It is unlikely that any worker in the medical environment would be exposed to ionizing radiation at a level high enough to cause the transmission of appreciable genetic effects.

Among the many factors that will influence the effect of exposure to ionizing radiation are the total dose received, the rate at which the dose was received, the age at exposure, the type of radiation, the sensitivity of the irradiated cells, and the portion of the body that was irradiated.

When x-rays were initially investigated, scientists were unaware of any harmful effects of their use and a number of the early radiation workers suffered injuries that are easily prevented today. Injuries from exposure were reported in Europe within the first year of investigation of x-radiation. In 1904 the first radiation fatality, a radiation-induced cancer, was reported in the United States. Over the next decade blood disorders such as leukemia and anemia, cancerous skin lesions, and cancer deaths

were reported among radiation workers and linked to x-ray exposure. As a result of the high rate of documented radiation-related injuries, the British X-Ray and Radium Protection Committee was formed in 1921 to study ways to reduce radiation exposure to patients and medical personnel.

The goal of radiation protection is to limit human exposure to ionizing radiation to a degree that is reasonable and acceptable in relation to the benefit gained from the activities that involve the exposure, thereby reducing the likelihood of occurrence of somatic and genetic effects.

Sources and Magnitude of Ionizing Radiation Exposure

Everyone is exposed to sources of ionizing radiation. Some individuals will be exposed to a wide variety of such sources, while others will be exposed to only a few. The sources include those of **natural origin** either undisturbed by human activities or that have somehow been affected by human activities and **man-made** sources.

Natural sources include cosmic radiation, terrestrial radiation from naturally occurring radioactive sources in the ground, radionuclides naturally present in the body and inhaled and ingested radionuclides of natural origin, such as radon. Human exposure to these natural sources varies depending on locality and other circumstances. When human exposure to natural sources increases as a result of human's actions, deliberate or otherwise, the natural sources are enhanced.

Man-made sources of radiation result from various man-made materials and devices and include such sources as x-rays and radiopharmaceuticals in medicine, consumer products containing radioactive materials, such as some smoke detectors and static eliminators, nuclear fuel production for power, air travel, and such catastrophic events as atmospheric fallout from nuclear weapons testing and accidents in nuclear power plants.

The magnitude of exposure from these sources for the average member of the United States population has been studied and the results are summarized in Table 8–1 as the average annual effective dose equivalent. Also listed in Table 8–1 is the average annual contribution to the genetically significant dose (GSD). The genetically significant dose to a population is a measure of the average annual gonadal dose to members of the population, adjusted for the expected number of children conceived by each individual after exposure to radiation.

Quantities and Units Relevant To Radiation Protection

Various quantities, units, and radiation dosimetry concepts have been developed and defined to quantify the amount of radiation received by individuals. Historically the quantities and units associated with radiation dosimetry have included the **roentgen (R)**, used for specifying exposure; the **rad** (radiation absorbed dose), used for specifying energy absorbed; and the **rem** (radiation equivalent in man), used for specifying biologically equivalent dose.

Other radiation quantities of importance are the **kerma**, used to describe the kinetic energy released per unit mass; the **air kerma**, used to describe the kinetic energy released per unit mass of air; **integral dose**, used to describe the total radiation energy imparted to matter;

effective dose used to measure the radiation and organ system specific damage in man; and **activity** used to measure the amount of a radioactive material as it undergoes decay.

In 1948, the International Committee for Weights and Measures was charged with developing an international system of units based on the metric system. The committee developed the **Système Internationale d'Unites or SI** units. In recent years the international system of units has been adopted for radiation protection, and within this system of units the older units are no longer applicable. Although the National Council on Radiation Protection and Measurement (NCRP) adopted the SI units for use with ionizing radiation in 1985, traditional units are still very much in use. The following discussion will serve to review the conventional and more familiar units and SI units. Table 8–2 provides conversion between conventional units and SI units.

Exposure

The roentgen (R) represents a unit of exposure in air and was defined as that quantity of x-rays or gamma rays

TABLE 8–1. Annual Effective Dose Equivalent and Genetically Significant Dose in the U.S. Population

Source	Average Annual Effective Dose Equivalent		Average Annual Contribution to the GSD	
	mSv	mrem	mSv	mrem
Natural Sources				
Radon	2.0	200	0.1	10
Other	1.0	100	0.9	90
Occupational	0.009	0.9	≈0.006	≈0.6
Nuclear Fuel Cycle	0.0005	0.05	< 0.005	< 0.5
Consumer Products				
Tobacco	——		——	
Other	0.05–0.13	5–13	≈0.05	<5
Miscellaneous				
Environmental Sources	0.0006	0.06	< 0.001	<0.1
Medical				
Diagnostic x-ray	0.39	39	0.2–0.3	20–30
Nuclear Medicine	0.14	14	0.02	2
Rounded Total	3.6	360	1.3	130

Adapted from NCRP Report No. 93: Ionizing Radiation Exposure of the Population of the United States (Tables 8.1 and 8.2)

TABLE 8–2. Conversions Between Conventional and SI Units

Conventional Unit (Column A)	Conversion Factor (Column B)	SI Unit (Column C)
roentgen	2.58×10^{-4}	coulomb/kilogram
rad	0.01	gray
rem	0.01	sievert
curie	3.7×10^{10}	becquerel

Column A amount multiplied by Column B equals Column C amount.

Column C amount divided by Column B equals Column A amount.

required to produce a given amount of ionization (charge) in a unit mass of air. One roentgen creates 2.08×10^{9} ion pairs per cubic centimeter of air to produce a total ion charge of 2.58×10^{-4} coulomb (C) per kilogram (kg). The roentgen is limited to the measurement of exposure in air only and is not applicable to photons of energy above 3 Mev or to particulate radiations. The roentgen has no direct equivalent or special unit in the SI system of units and is no longer used. Exposure may be expressed directly in C/kg.

Absorbed Dose

The rad was developed as a unit of absorbed energy or dose and is applicable to any material. The rad was defined as 100 ergs of energy absorbed in one gram of absorbing material. In the SI system of units the rad has been replaced by the **gray (Gy)**, which is defined as 1 joule (J) of energy absorbed in each kilogram (kg) of absorbing material. One gray is equivalent to 100 rads; therefore 1 rad equals 10 mGy. This unit is not restricted to air and can be measured in other absorbing materials.

Kerma/Air Kerma

The rad is also a unit of **kerma**, an acronym for **k**inetic **e**nergy **r**eleased in **ma**tter. As radiation passes through matter it interacts and the energy carried by the photons is transformed to kinetic energy of charged particles such

as the electrons in the photoelectric and Compton interactions. The energy imparted directly to the electrons, per unit mass, is the kerma. Some of the kerma may be radiated away as bremsstrahlung if any of these electrons interact with the nuclei of the atoms in the matter. In these instances, kerma and absorbed dose would not be identical. At diagnostic energies, however, practically no brems is produced in the tissues and, as a result, kerma will equal dose. The SI unit for the kerma is the gray.

Air kerma is the kinetic energy released per unit mass of air. X-ray tube outputs and inputs to image receptors are sometimes described in air kerma. An air kerma of 1 cGy (1 rad) corresponds to an exposure of about 1 R.

Integral Dose

The integral dose describes the total amount of energy imparted to matter. It is a product of the dose and the mass over which the energy is imparted. For example, when a patient has a CT scan of the abdomen, the dose per section (irradiated volume) might be 1 rad (10 mGy). Regardless of the number of scan sections, the dose to the irradiated volume would be defined as 1 rad (10 mGy). If the patient has 20 scan sections, the integral dose would be approximately 20 rad (200 mGy).

Equivalent Dose

Different types of radiation, such as alpha and beta particles and neutrons, produce different degrees of biological damage as compared to gamma or x-radiation. To account for the fact that the same absorbed dose of radiation may result in different biological responses for different types of radiation, a unit known as the rem (radiation equivalent man) was developed. The rem is the conventional unit for equivalent dose (H_T). **In NCRP Report No. 116: Limitations of Exposure to Ionizing Radiation (which replaces NCRP Report No. 91), the term equivalent dose replaces the previously used term, dose equivalent (H), in defining dose limits.** These two terms are conceptually different. Dose equivalent (H) is based on the absorbed dose at a "point" in tissue and equivalent dose (H_T) is based on the average absorbed dose in the tissue or organ.

Equivalent dose (H_T,R) is the product of the average-absorbed dose (D_T,R), in a tissue (T) due to radiation (R) and a radiation weighting factor (W_R), previously known as the **quality factor** (Q), which is specific to specific types of radiation and accounts for the biological effectiveness of the specific radiation. The radiation weighting factor for gamma or x-radiation equals one. This means that 1 rad equals 1 rem for gamma or x-radiation. For alpha particles, however, the radiation weighting factor is 20. This means that 1 rad equals 20 rem for alpha particle absorption. In the SI system of units the rem has been replaced by the **sievert (Sv)**, which is defined as the product of the absorbed dose in gray and the radiation weighting factor. One sievert is equal to 100 rem, and 1 rem is equal to 10 mSv.

Effective Dose

Effective dose (E) is the sum of the weighted equivalent doses for all irradiated tissues and organs. It takes into account the fact that not all tissues are equally sensitive to the effects of ionizing radiation. As was seen with equivalent dose and dose equivalent, in NCRP Report No. 116: Limitations of Exposure to Ionizing Radiation, the term effective dose (E) replaces the previously used term, effective dose equivalent (H_E), in defining dose limits.

Since exposure received from ionizing radiation is rarely uniform over the whole body, the concept of effective dose is used to compare the detriment from irradiation of a limited portion of the body with the detriment from irradiation of the entire body and employs weighting factors for the relative risks associated with irradiation of various body tissues. The effective dose is defined as the sum over specified tissues of the products of the equivalent dose in a tissue (T) and the weighting factor for that tissue.

Activity

Activity (A) describes the quantity of radioactive material. It is expressed as the number of radioactive atoms that undergo decay per unit time. The unit of activity has traditionally been the curie (Ci). The curie is defined as 3.7×10^{10} disintegrations per second (dps). One curie is a very large amount of radioactive material. In a typical nuclear medicine procedure, activities from 0.1–30 millicuries (mCi) are used. The SI unit for activity is the becquerel. The becquerel is defined as 1 dps.

Further information regarding international system of units and its application in radiation protection and measurements may be found in **NCRP Report No. 82: SI Units in Radiation Protection and Measurements**. A comparison between SI units and conventional ones is displayed in Table 8–3.

Detection And Measurement of Ionizing Radiation

A number of different dose-measuring devices, known as dosimeters, are employed for detection and measurement of radiation exposure from x-rays. These **dosimeters** may be classified as either **field survey instruments** or **personnel monitoring devices**.

TABLE 8–3. Comparison Between SI and Conventional Units

Quantity	Symbol for Quantity	Expression in SI Units	Expression in Symbols for SI Units	Special Name for SI Units	Symbol Using Special Name	Conventional Unit	Symbol for Conventional Unit	Value of Conventional Unit in SI Units
Activity	A	1 per second	s^{-1}	becquerel	Bq	curie	Ci	3.7×10^{10} Bq
Absorbed Dose	D	joule per kilogram	J/kg	gray	Gy	rad	rad	0.01 Gy
Dose Equivalent	H	joule per kilogram	J/kg	sievert	Sv	rem	rem	0.01 Sv
Exposure	X	coulomb per kilogram	C/kg			roentgen	R	2.58×10^{-4} C/kg

Field Survey Instruments

A number of portable field survey instruments are available for use in radiation detection and measurement. They include the Geiger-Mueller (GM) survey instruments, scintillation detection devices, and ionization chamber instruments. Regardless of the type, field survey instruments should be calibrated at least annually.

Geiger-Mueller Survey Instruments

Geiger-Mueller survey instruments or counters are primarily used to detect the presence of radiation rather than provide exact measurements. A GM counter is a gas-filled detector. It consists of a volume of gas between two electrodes. Ionizing radiation produces ion pairs in the gas that can be collected and measured. GM counters are very efficient at detecting charged particles, such as beta particles, but are relatively inefficient at detecting x- and gamma radiation. GM counters are most commonly used in nuclear medicine as radioactive contamination survey instruments.

Scintillation Detection Devices

Scintillation detectors combine the use of a scintillator with a device that can convert light to an electric signal. Scintillators are materials that emit visible or ultraviolet light when exposed to ionizing radiation. In a scintillation detector, this light is converted to an electric signal and is measured. The most common applications for scintillation detectors are in gamma cameras in nuclear medicine and in some CT scanner detectors.

Ionization Chamber Instruments

Ionization chamber instruments are commonly employed for the measurement of the primary and secondary radiation beam for purposes of evaluation of equipment performance, environmental exposure assessment of scatter and leakage radiation, and for measurement of patient exposure. An ionization chamber works on the principle that when radiation interacts with air electrons, positive ions are produced giving rise to an electrical charge that can be measured.

A typical ionization chamber dosimeter consists of a chamber with a known volume of air and an electrode (Figure 8–1). A small voltage is applied between the elec-

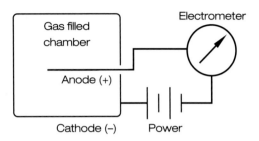

FIGURE 8–1. An ionization chamber dosimeter. The chamber encloses a known volume of air, inside of which a chargeable electrode is positioned to attract electrons freed by the ionization of the gas by the radiation. The difference in the electrode's charge before and after exposure is measured by an electrometer and displayed in radiation units.

trode and the wall of the chamber, so the electrode is positive and the chamber wall is negative. As x-ray photons pass through the chamber they ionize the air. The free electrons from these ionizations are attracted to the positive electrode, where they can be measured with an electrometer. The intensity of the signal that is produced on the electrode is proportional to the radiation exposure that occurred in the air volume of the chamber. This relationship can be displayed on a digital readout in R or C/Kg units. Ionization dosimeters can be designed to measure specific ranges of radiation intensity.

Personnel Monitoring Devices

Individuals who are regularly exposed to ionizing radiation should be provided with personnel monitoring devices to provide an estimate of the exposure received. Personnel monitoring is recommended whenever a possibility exists that an individual will receive more than 1/10 of the recommended dose limit as a result of his or her occupational activities. A personnel-monitoring device measures the quantity of exposure it has received. It is not a radiation protection device. The four most common types of personnel-monitoring devices are the **film badge**, the **thermoluminescent dosimeter** (TLD), **pulsed optically stimulated luminescence (POSL) dosimeter**, and the **pocket dosimeter**.

Film Badges
Film badges are the most commonly used form of personnel-monitoring devices and are usually issued on a monthly basis (Figure 8–2). Two pieces

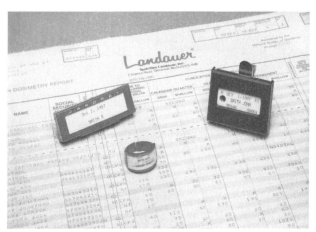

FIGURE 8–2. (Left to right) A typical film badge, thermoluminescent dosimeter ring, and collar badge. *(Courtesy of Tech/Ops Landauer, Inc.)*

of film having different sensitivities to x-rays are contained within a light, tight envelope. This film packet is placed within a holder, which contains a number of different filter elements held in a fixed position with respect to the film. Printed on the front of the film packet is the name of the individual, the beginning date for which the film badge is issued, and other coded information.

When the badge is exposed to ionizing radiation, deposits of silver atoms are distributed in the film emulsion which, upon development, becomes dark in proportion to the degree of radiation exposure received. The resultant optical density can be measured with a densitometer and calibrated to the degree of radiation exposure received.

The filters in the film badge holder provide a means of determining the energy of the incident radiation. Because the absorption of radiation by a specific thickness of given material will depend on the energy of the radiation, the measurement of the relative film densities under the different filters provides a means of estimating the energy of the exposing x-ray beam. Typically copper, cadmium, and aluminum are used as filtering metals.

Film badges are capable of measuring exposures over the range of approximately 10 mrem (0.1 mSv) to 2,000 rem (20 Sv) and are most commonly used to measure the total body exposure of the individual. Readings of less than 10 mrem (0.1 mSv) are generally not detectable and may be reported as minimal (M).

When only one film badge or other personnel-monitoring device is issued it should be worn on the anterior surface of the body between the chest and waist level. When a lead apron is worn and only one film badge or other personnel-monitoring device is issued, it is recommended that it be worn outside the apron at the collar level. Because of the considerable controversy regarding the proper location of the film badge when a lead apron is worn, the local radiation safety officer should be contacted for specific guidance. It is important that all persons wear badges at the same locations.

An additional film badge, usually designated as a whole body badge, may be worn in addition to the collar badge when the potential for significant exposure to the thyroid or eyes exists. This badge is usually positioned near the waist under the lead apron and may be used in conjunction with the collar badge to determine the effective dose. The whole-body badge and collar badge must never be interchanged.

Thermoluminescent Dosimeter (TLD) Badges

Personnel-monitoring devices using thermoluminescent dosimeters are similar in appearance to film badges (Figure 8–2). Instead of using film to measure the radiation exposure, TLD badges contain small chips of a thermoluminescent material, usually lithium fluoride (LiF). When exposed to radiation, a portion of the absorbed energy is stored in the crystal structure of the LiF chips in metastable states. This absorbed energy will remain in these states for long periods of time. If the LiF chips are heated, the absorbed energy is released as visible light. The heating and measurement of the LiF chips are carried out in a device called a reader, and the amount of measured light is proportional to the absorbed radiation dose. TLDs provide approximately the same measurement range as film badges and can be used as whole-body badges or collar badges. Because of their small size, TLDs are commonly used for monitoring exposure to the extremities in the form of ring badges.

Pulsed Optically Stimulated Luminescence (POSL) Dosimeter

A new type of dosimeter that functions much like the TLD is the pulsed optically stimulated luminescence (POSL) dosimeter. The POSL dosimeter measures radiation that passes through a thin layer of aluminum oxide. A laser light is used to stimulate the aluminum oxide, which becomes luminescent in

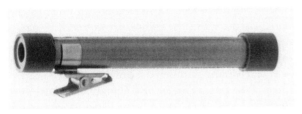

FIGURE 8–3. A pocket ionization chamber. *(Courtesy of Nuclear Associates division of Victoreen, Inc., Carle Place, NY)*

proportion to the amount of radiation exposure it has received.

The POSL dosimeter has distinct advantages over both the film badge or the TLD. It can report doses along a wide range from as low as 1 mrem with a precision of ± 1 mrem. In addition, it can undergo complete reanalysis to confirm the radiation exposure received with no loss of information. It also has excellent long-term and environmental (temperature and humidity) stability. Laudauer,

Inc. offers the Luxel® OSL Dosimeter with a variety of color coding options for both department/series and exchange frequencies. Bimonthly service is available.

Pocket Dosimeter A special type of ionization chamber used for personnel dosimetry is known as a **pocket dosimeter** (Figure 8–3). When irradiated, the radiation ionizes the air in the chamber, which partially neutralizes a previously positively charged electrode (quartz fiber on a wire frame), causing the hairline fiber to move on an exposure scale (Figure 8–4). The amount of ionization and movement of the fiber is proportional to the radiation exposure to the chamber. Such devices are usually charged and read out on a special charger-reader device. Pocket dosimeters are occasionally used for personnel monitoring in situations in which the convenience of an immediate readout is desired (for example, after each procedure in a cardiac catheterization laboratory). However, they provide no permanent record of personnel exposure and are not routinely used.

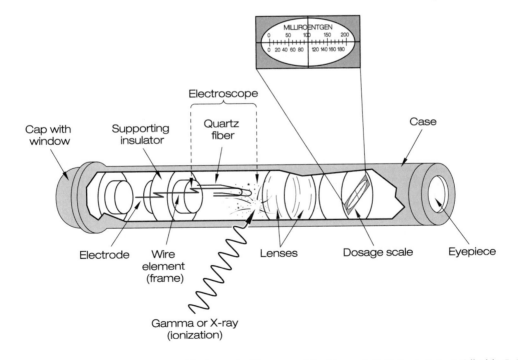

FIGURE 8–4. Cross section of a pocket ion chamber (dosimeter). *(Courtesy of Bushberg, J. T., Seibert, J. A., Leidholdt, E. M., & Boone, J. M. [1994]. The essential physics of medical imaging. Baltimore: Williams & Wilkins.)*

Care of Personnel Monitoring Devices The proper care and handling of personnel monitoring devices is essential to obtaining accurate results. The personnel monitoring device must be worn only by the individual to whom it is assigned, must be worn in the proper location for the prescribed time period, and must be turned in for processing when due.

Both film badge dosimeters and TLD dosimeters may be adversely affected by heat, humidity, mechanical pressure, inadvertent exposure to light, and prolonged delay between exposure and processing. Exposure from the rear or from oblique angles may also result in inaccurate results.

Generally, groups of personnel dosimeters are provided with a control that must be stored in an unexposed area at the facility and returned with the group for processing. This control provides an unexposed level against which the personnel dosimeters are evaluated.

Personnel-monitoring devices should not be worn during medical or dental exams and should never be intentionally exposed to the primary radiation beam. Individuals should be aware of the exposure they receive by reviewing their exposure readings on the reports posted in the facility on a routine basis. Should any aspect of the reported exposure be unclear or cause concern, the individual should seek the counsel of the facility radiation safety officer.

Summary

Exposure to ionizing radiation carries with it both a benefit and a risk. With few exceptions, the diagnostic benefit of a radiologic procedure far outweighs the minimal risk resulting from the x-ray exposure. The information received by the physician from a radiologic examination about the clinical condition of the patient is an essential part of the practice of modern medicine.

Ionizing radiation is any form of radiation that possesses energy capable of displacing atomic electron bonds and breaking the electron bonds that hold the molecules of matter together. The potential biological damage from the ionization process is the reason for the need to understand proper radiation protection practices. Ionizing radiation comes from two major sources: natural background radiation and man-made radiation.

The biological effects of radiation exposure are either somatic, occurring in the individual exposed, or genetic, occurring in the descendants of the individual exposed. It is the responsibility of the radiographer to ensure each patient receives the minimal dose of radiation necessary to produce a diagnostic image. Radiographers must also be properly shielded from unnecessary radiation exposure.

Radiation quantities and units that are important in radiation protection are exposure, absorbed dose, and equivalent dose. The SI units that correspond to these quantities are the coulomb per kilogram (C/kg), the gray (Gy) and the sievert (Sv). The corresponding traditional units are the roentgen (R), the rad, and the rem. Other radiation quantities of importance are the kerma, the air kerma, integral dose, effective dose, and activity.

Various devices are available to detect and measure exposure to ionizing radiation. Portable field survey instruments include the Geiger-Mueller (GM) survey instruments, scintillation detection devices, and ionization chamber instruments. Personnel-monitoring devices include the film badge, thermoluminescent dosimeter, pulsed optically stimulated luminescence dosimeter, and pocket dosimeters.

REVIEW QUESTIONS

1. Explain the differences between alpha and beta particles.

2. Differentiate between somatic and genetic effects.

3. What are the primary sources of ionizing radiation? Give examples of each.

4. What are the three basic quantities of radiation measurement and their associated conventional and SI units?

5. What is the kerma?

6. Describe the function of a GM survey instrument.

7. List the four types of personnel-monitoring devices.

8. Explain the function of the filters in a film badge.

REFERENCES AND RECOMMENDED READING

Bednorck, D. R., Rozenfeld, M., Lanzl, L. H., & Sabau, M. (1981). A protocol for exposure limitations in radiography. *Radiologic Technology. 53*(3) 229.

BEIR V health effects of exposure to low levels of ionizing radiation. (1990). National Academy Press, Washington, DC.

Burhart, R. L., Gross, R. E., Jans, R. G., McCrohen, J. L., Rosenstein, M., & Reuter, F. A., (eds). (1985). *Recommendations for evaluation of radiation exposure from diagnostic radiology examinations.* United States Department of HHS Publication 85–8247.

Bushberg, J. T., Seibert, J. A., Leidholdt, E. M., & Boone, J. M. (1994). *The essential physics of medical imaging.* Baltimore: Williams & Wilkins.

Bushong, S. C. (1997). *Radiologic science for technologists: Physics, biology, and protection* (6th ed.). St. Louis: C. V. Mosby.

Bushong, S. C. (1977). Radiation exposure in our daily lives. *The Physics Teacher.* (March), 135–144.

Curry, T. S., Dowdey, J. E., Murry, R. C. (1990). *Christensen's introduction to the physics of diagnostic radiology* (4th ed.). Philadelphia: Lea and Febiger.

Dowd, S. B. (1994). *Practical radiation protection and applied radiobiology.* Philadelphia: W. B. Saunders.

Elsberry, J. S. (1979). A technique for scatter dose calculations. *Radiologic Technology. 51*(1), 51.

Gibbs, S. J. (1981). Approaches to radiation risk estimation. *The Physical Basis of Medical Imaging.* Editors: Coulam, C. M., Erickson, J. J., Rollo, F. D., Everette, J. A. New York: Appleton-Century-Crofts, 329-342.

Gur, D. & Wald, N. (1986). Probability of causation tables and their possible implications for the practice of diagnostic radiology. *Radiology. 158*, 853-854.

Hall, E. J. (1993). *Radiobiology for the radiologist* (4th ed.). Philadelphia: J. B. Lippincott Company.

Hendee, W. R. (1992). Estimation of radiation risks: BEIR V and its significance for medicine. *Journal of the American Medical Association. 268*, 620-624.

Hendee, W. R. (ed.) (1984). *Health effects of low-level radiation.* Norwalk, CT: Appleton-Century-Crofts.

Hendee, W. R. & Ritenour, R. (1993). *Medical imaging physics* (3rd ed.) St. Louis: C. V. Mosby.

International Commission on Radiation Protection. (1970). *Protection of the patient in x-ray diagnosis publication number 16.* Oxford, England: Pergamon Press, 1970.

Mettler, F. A. & Moseley, R. D. (1985). *Medical effects of ionizing radiation.* Orlando: Grune & Stratton.

Miller, P. E. (1976). Biological effects of diagnostic irradiation. *Radiologic Technology. 48*(1), 11-16.

Morgan, K. Z. (1973). The need for radiation protection. *Radiologic Technology. 44*(6), 385.

NCRP (1990) Report No. 107, *Implementation of the principle of ALARA for medical and dental personnel*, Bethesda, MD: National Council on Radiation Protection and Measurements.

NCRP (1989) Report No. 105, *Radiation protection for medical and allied health personnel*, Bethesda, MD: National Council on Radiation Protection and Measurements.

NCRP (1989) Report No. 102, *Medical x-ray, electron beam and gamma-ray protection for energies up to 50 mev (equipment design, performance and use)*, Bethesda, MD: National Council on Radiation Protection and Measurements.

NCRP (1987). Report No. 93, *Ionizing radiation exposure of the population of the United States*, Bethesda, MD: National Council on Radiation Protection and Measurements.

NCRP (1987). Report No. 91, *Recommendations on limits for exposure to ionizing radiation*, Bethesda, MD: National Council on Radiation Protection and Measurements.

NCRP (1985). Report No. 82, *SI units in radiation protection and measurements*, Bethesda, MD: National Council on Radiation Protection and Measurements.

NCRP (1977). Report No. 54, *Medical exposure of pregnant and potentially pregnant women*, Bethesda, MD: National Council on Radiation Protection and Measurements.

NCRP (1976). Report No. 49, *Structural shielding design and evaluation for medical use of x-rays and gamma rays of energies up to 10 mev*, Bethesda, MD: National Council on Radiation Protection and Measurements.

Noz, M. E. & Maguire, G. Q. (1985). *Radiation protection in the radiologic and health sciences* (2nd ed.). Philadelphia: Lea & Febiger.

Pagel, J. W. (1981). Radiation protection in diagnostic radiology, *The Physical Basis of Medical Imaging*. Editors: Coulam, C. M, Erickson, J. J., Rollo, F. D, & James, A. E. New York: Appleton-Century-Crofts, 303-328.

Radiation exposure from diagnostic radiology exams: General recommendations. (1986). *Radiology Management*. 8(2), 49.

Selman, J. (1983). *Elements of radiobiology*. Springfield, IL: Charles C. Thomas.

Statement from the 1985 Paris meeting of the International Commission on Radiological Protection. (1985). *Radiology*. (September).

Statkiewicz, M. A., Visconti, P. J., & Ritenour, E. R. (1993). *Radiation protection in medical radiography* (2nd ed.). St. Louis: C. V. Mosby.

Stears, J. G., Gray, J. E., & Frank, E. D. (1986). Radiation exposure information. *Radiologic Technology*. 58(1), 31.

Tolan, J. H. (1968). Comments on recent proposals for regulatory control of x-ray exposures. *Radiologic Technology*. 40(3), 124.

Travis, E. L. (1989). *Primer of medical radiobiology* (2nd ed.). Chicago: Year Book Medical Publishers.

Upton, A. C. (1982). The biological effects of low-level ionizing radiation. *Scientific America*. 246(2).

van den Bosch, V. (1987). Radiation effects on the prenatal period. *Canadian Journal of Medical Radiation Technology*. 18(4), 145-148.

Watkins, G. L. (1988). Public health risks from low dose medical radiation. *Radiologic Technolgy*. 59(2), 160.

Wochos, J. F. & Cameron, J. R. (1976). Effect of operator training on patient exposure: An analysis of the NEXT data. *Radiologic Technology*. 48(1), 19-22.

Radiation Protection Procedures for Patients and Personnel

*Röntgen almost from the beginning had conducted all his experiments in his big zinc box. . . .
Then he had added a lead plate to the zinc between the tube and himself, and in doing so he had
unknowingly protected himself completely. With an accurate appreciation of the import of these
unexplained effects, Röntgen foresaw the suffering consequent to the careless handling of the rays.*

Otto Glasser from the biography Dr. W.C. Röntgen

Objectives

Upon completion of this chapter, the student should be able to:

▶ Differentiate between the various advisory groups and regulatory agencies involved in developing radiation protection standards.

▶ Explain the concept of dose limits related to the use of radiation.

▶ Describe the ALARA concept.

▶ Explain the basic principles of reducing exposure to radiation.

▶ Describe techniques used to minimize radiation exposure to patients and personnel.

▶ Discuss the precautions that should be taken to minimize potential fetal exposures.

Advisory Groups And Regulatory Agencies

*A*number of different organizations and agencies are involved in the development of standards for radiation protection and the establishment of regulations for the protection against the hazards that can result from the use of ionizing radiation.

The advisory groups that have shared in the establishment of radiation protection standards include: the **International Commission on Radiological Protection (ICRP)**; the **National Council on Radiation Protection and Measurement (NCRP)**; the **National Academy of Sciences Advisory Committee on the Biological Effects of Ionizing Radiation (NAS-BEIR)**; and the **United Nations Scientific Committee on the Effects of Atomic Radiation (UNSCEAR)**.

The International Commission on Radiological Protection (ICRP) was formed in 1928 and has an international membership, which provides a variety of perspectives on radiologic health issues. In 1929 the ICRP established the National Committee on Radiation Protection and Measurement, which was later chartered by Congress in 1964 as the National Council on Radiation Protection and Measurement (NCRP). The NCRP is a nonprofit organization that is charged with collecting, analyzing, developing, and disseminating in the public interest, information, and recommendations about radiation protection, radiation measurements, quantities, and units. It works cooperatively with the ICRP and other agencies to accomplish its mission.

The National Academy of Sciences Advisory Committee on the Biological Effects of Ionizing Radiation (NAS-BEIR) and the United Nations Scientific Committee on the Effects of Atomic Radiation (UNSCEAR) are two additional advisory groups that study and report on the risks from exposure to ionizing radiation.

In addition to the advisory groups, there are a number of regulatory agencies responsible for protecting the public and occupationally exposed individuals from the effects of ionizing radiation. Regulatory agencies carry the force of law and can inspect facilities, issue fines, and revoke radiation use authorizations. Two such agencies are the **U.S. Nuclear Regulatory Commission (NRC)** and the **U.S. Food and Drug Administration (FDA)**. The U.S. Nuclear Regulatory Commission (NRC) has been given the regulatory authority for special nuclear materials and by-products. In a number of instances, the NRC has entered into agreements with the states to oversee and enforce the regulations. In these "agreement states," it becomes the state's responsibility to enforce NRC regulations. The U.S. Food and Drug Administration (FDA) regulates radiopharmaceuticals as well as the performance and radiation safety requirements of commercial x-ray equipment.

The two primary sources of radiation protection standards in the United States are the Nuclear Regulatory Commission (NRC), which is a U.S. federal agency charged with licensing facilities and controlling the use of radioactive materials, and the National Council on Radiation Protection and Measurements (NCRP), an advisory group that makes recommendations for radiation protection. Both sources are used when setting radiation protection policies and procedures. The NRC regulations are available on the Internet at http://www.nrc.gov/NRC/CFR/PART020/index.html. The NCRP reports are available at http://www.ncrp.com.

Limiting Exposure To Ionizing Radiation

It is important to set limits for the protection of the radiation worker and the general public because of the known biological effects of exposure to ionizing radiation. The primary purposes for establishing dose limits are to limit the risks of **stochastic effects** and to prevent **deterministic effects** (also known as nonstochastic effects). Stochastic effects are those for which no threshold dose of radiation exists, such as cancer and genetic effects. They are random in nature. Regardless of dose, some will experience an effect. As dose goes up, the chance of experiencing an effect also goes up. Deterministic effects such as cataracts, skin erythema, and sterility, are those for which a threshold dose is assumed. As dose increases, the severity of the effect increases. Although the dose has to be high to demonstrate the effect, once that dose is reached, the probability of demonstrating the effect is very high.

For radiation protection purposes, individuals may be divided into two groups. First are those classified as **radiation workers**, who incur, as an occupational risk, a certain likelihood of exposure to ionizing radiation in the course of their normal duties. The second group includes members of the general public.

Radiation workers may be further classified as **occupationally exposed workers** and **occasionally exposed workers**. Occupationally exposed workers are individuals who have a significant potential for exposure to radiation in the course of their employment. Occasionally exposed workers are individuals whose duties may occasionally bring them into areas where radiation exposure may occur. Both occupationally exposed workers and occasionally exposed workers should receive instruction and training regarding hazards of radiation exposure and radiation protection practices.

Dose Limits

Radiation exposure limits pertinent to the protection of radiation workers are known as **dose limits** and are specified for both **whole body** exposure and for exposure to **certain tissues and organs**. Several terms have been used to describe dose limits, including maximum permissible dose, dose equivalent limits, and equivalent dose limits. Prior to 1987, the term maximum permissible dose (MPD) was used to describe dose limits; this is no longer acceptable terminology because no dose is considered permissible.

Dose equivalent limits and cumulative effective dose equivalent replaced MPD and this philosophy was described in NCRP Report No. 91 Recommendations on Limits for Exposure to Ionizing Radiation. In 1993, **NCRP Report No. 116 Limitation of Exposure to Ionizing Radiation** replaced NCRP Report No. 91. This new report follows the same basic framework to dose limits as the previous report but incorporated some changes as provided in ICRP Publication 60. Of particular note is the change in terminology from effective dose equivalent limits (Report No. 91) to effective dose limits (Report No. 116) and dose equivalent limits for tissues and organs (Report No. 91) to equivalent dose limits for tissues and organs (Report No. 116). Equivalent dose (H_T) replaces the previously used term, dose equivalent (H), in defining dose limits. These two terms are conceptually different. Dose equivalent (H) is based on the absorbed dose at a "point" in tissue and equivalent dose (H_T) is based on the average absorbed dose in the tissue or organ.

Currently recommended values for occupational and public dose limits are given in Table 9–1 and reflect the recommendations of the National Council on Radiation Protection and Measurements as put forth in Report No. 116. The effective dose limit for whole body exposure of a radiation worker is 5 rem (50 mSv) per year. Prior to 1987, the NCRP had determined the maximum cumulative whole body dose (MPD) for radiation workers by the formula:

$$H = 5(N-18) \text{ rem}$$

where: H = dose equivalent limit
          N = age in years

Under the new recommendations, the cumulative effective dose (E) limit is age in rem, which is determined in SI units by the formula:

TABLE 9–1. Effective Dose Limit Recommendations

Occupational Exposures		
Effective dose limits		
Annual	50 mSv	(5 rem)
Cumulative	10 mSv x age	(1 rem x age)
Dose equivalent annual limits for tissues and organs		
Lens of eye	150 mSv	(15 rem)
Skin, hands, and feet	500 mSv	(50 rem)
Public Exposures (Annual)		
Effective dose limit		
continuous or frequent exposure	1 mSv	(0.1 rem)
infrequent exposure	5 mSv	(0.5 rem)
Equivalent dose limits for tissues and organs		
lens of eye	15 mSv	(1.5 rem)
skin, hands, and feet	50 mSv	(5 rem)
Embryo-Fetus Exposures (Monthly)		
Equivalent dose limit	0.5 mSv	(0.05 rem)
Education and Training Exposures (Annual)		
Effective dose limit	1 mSv	(0.1 rem)
Dose equivalent limit for tissues and organs		
Lens of eye	15 mSv	(1.5 rem)
Skin, hands, and feet	50 mSv	(5 rem)

Adapted from NCRP Report No. 116: *Limitations of Exposure to Ionizing Radiation*, Table 19.1

where $E = 10 \text{ mSv} \times N$

        E = effective dose limit

        N = age in years

Example: What is the dose limit for a 19-year-old radiation worker, using both the old and new formula?

Answer:

Old: $H = 5(N–18)$ rem

        $H = 5(19–18)$ rem

        $H = 5(1)$ rem

        $H = 5$ rem (50 mSv)

New:

        $E = 10 \text{ mSv} \times N$

        $E = 10 \text{ mSv} \times 19$

        $E = 190$ mSv (19 rem)

Example:

What is the dose limit for a 35-year-old radiation worker, using both the old and new formula?

Answer: $H = 5(N–18)$ rem

Old: $H = 5(35–18)$ rem

        $H = 5(17)$ rem

        $H = 85$ rem (850 mSv)

New: $E = 10 \text{ mSv} \times N$

        $E = 10 \text{ mSv} \times 35$

        $E = 350$ mSv (35 rem)

Irradiation at the upper level of the dose limits is not to be considered as desirable, and in every case efforts to reduce exposures to the lowest possible level should be taken.

Individuals not classified as radiation workers are considered members of the **general public.** For purposes of protection of these individuals, the level of recommended dose limits, exclusive of any exposure received as the result of a medical procedure, has been established as one-tenth of the effective dose limit for radiation workers. That is, 0.5 rem (5 mSv) per year for infrequent exposure and one-fiftieth of the effective dose limit for radiation workers, which is 0.1 rem (1 mSv) per year for continuous exposure. Individuals in education and training have the same effective dose limit (for continuous or frequent exposure) as the general public, that is 0.1 rem (1 mSv).

Nuclear Regulatory Commission (NRC)

The Nuclear Regulatory Commission regulations for radiation protection are known by their Code of Federal Regulations (CFR) No., 10CFR20. Unlike the NCRP, which is an advisory body, the NRC is a U. S. federal government agency and its regulations are law in the United States. NRC licensees were required to implement new standards beginning in 1994. These standards included what is known as the "new" 10CFR20 regulations. The essential changes are shown in Table 9–2.

The most critical of the NRC regulations is the whole body exposure regulation that limits exposure to 500 mSv (50 rem)/year to any organ or 50 mSv (5 rem)/year whole body. As with the NCRP, this regulation has eliminated the old 5(N–18) formula. Also worthy of note are the regulations for exposure to the extremities, lens of the eye, and pregnancy (which is discussed in detail later in this chapter).

Maintaining Exposure As Low As Reasonably Achievable (ALARA)

A basic philosophical principle of radiation protection concerning the use of ionizing radiation emphasizes the need to maintain exposure to ionizing radiation at a level **As Low As Reasonably Achievable** (ALARA), with economic and societal factors being taken into consideration. This premise has been accepted by advisory and regulatory agencies and requires that radiologic personnel take on the responsibility of minimizing the exposure to their patients and any other individuals involved in a radiologic procedure. Implementation of the ALARA principle is achieved by application of the basic principles of radiation protection and a thoughtful approach to all work involving exposure to ionizing radiation.

Protection of Personnel

When radiological procedures are performed, there is a possibility that individuals other than the patient will receive some radiation exposure. While the patient should be the only person exposed to the primary beam, others involved in the procedure may be exposed to radiation scattered from the primary beam or to leakage radiation from the x-ray tube. This occurs particularly during fluoroscopy, mobile examinations, interventional special procedures, and cardiac catheterization. For most radiographic exposures, personnel should be behind protective barriers. Radiologic personnel should not be involved in holding patients who are unable to cooperate during an x-ray exposure. Immobilization devices should be used or, if absolutely necessary, assistance should be requested from the patient's family or friends.

Figure 9–1A & B represent diagrams of two iso-exposure curves that illustrate the percentage of scattered radiation that personnel are exposed to during a single exposure of 20 mAs to a chest phantom. The curves represent the percentage of the exposure to the skin at various distances from the patient using two different kilovoltages (60 kVp and 80 kVp) and two different field sizes (20×20 cm and 28×32 cm). The effect of kVp is illustrated in Figure 9–1A for the transverse plane. The effect of beam restriction (collimation) is shown in Figure 9–1B for the coronal plane. In both instances, an obvious reduction in exposure to scattered radiation occurs as the distance away from a patient increases. In addition, the amount of scatter around a patient is affected to a greater extent by changes in collimation rather than changes in kVp.

Principles of Personnel Exposure Reduction

Reduction of an individual's exposure to ionizing radiation may be accomplished by application of three basic principles: (1) reduce the amount of **time** spent in the vicinity of the radiation source while it is operating, (2) increase the **distance** between the radiation source and the individual to be protected, and (3) interpose a **shielding** material, which will attenuate the radiation from the source. These three basic principles are sometimes referred to as the three cardinal rules of radiation protection.

Time X-ray imaging equipment produces radiation only during the actual exposure used to form the image during a procedure. The time of exposure on a per-image basis is very short (typically much less than 1 second) during radiographic procedures. During fluoroscopic procedures, which are used when dynamic information is required, the x-ray source may be on (usually intermittently) for several minutes to as long as an hour or

TABLE 9–2. Comparison of Requirements of Old NRC Regulation 10CFR20 to New NRC Regulation 10CFR20

	Old 10CFR20	New 10CFR20
Whole body definition	Head, lens of eyes, trunk, gonads, arms above elbow, legs above ankle	Head, trunk, gonads, arms above elbow, legs above knee
Extremities definition	Arms elbows and below, legs ankle and below	Arms elbows and below, legs knees and below
Whole body exposure limits	1.25 rem/calendar quarter **with** maximum 3 rem/qtr **and** 12 rem/yr **if** 5(N-18) not exceeded	Most limiting of: 500 mSv (50 rem)/yr to any organ **or** 50 mSv (5 rem)/yr whole body Note: 5(N-18) is no longer used
Lens of the eye	1.25 rem/qtr, maximum 3 rem/qtr and 12 rem/yr if 5(N-18) not exceeded	150 mSv (15 rem)/yr
Skin of the whole body	7.5 rem/qtr and 30 rem/yr	500mSv (50 rem)/yr
Extremities	18.75 rem/qtr and 75 rem/yr applied to any part of any extremity	500 mSv (50 rem)/yr applied to each extremity
Embryo/fetus/pregnancy		5 mSv/term (0.5 rem or 500 mrem)

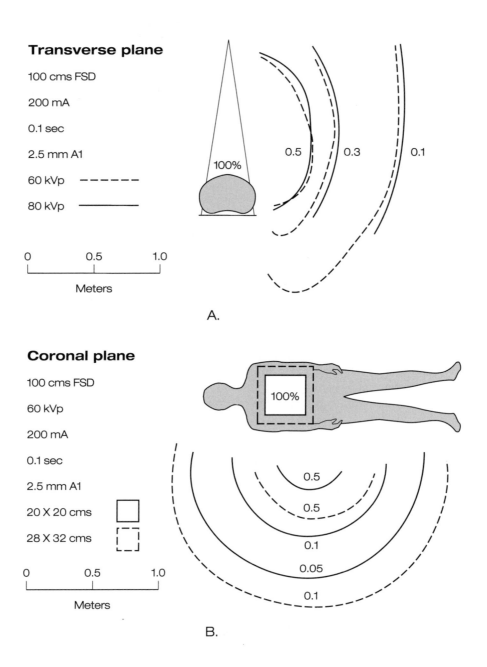

FIGURE 9–1. The iso-exposure curves represent the percentage of the exposure to the skin at various distances from the patient using two different kilovoltages (60 kVp and 80 kVp) and two different field sizes (20 x 20 cm and 28 x 32 cm). The effect of kVp is illustrated in (A) for the transverse plane. The effect of beam restriction (collimation) is shown in (B) for the coronal plane. *(Reprinted with permission from Cartwright, P. [1992]. Distribution and relative intensity of scattered radiation.* Radiography Today. *58[664], 12-13.)*

more. To minimize exposure to radiation, individuals should reduce the amount of time they spend in the vicinity of an operable radiation source. The simplest way to do this is to ascertain whether their presence is needed during the procedure. Whenever possible, individuals should remain behind protective barriers.

Distance

Increasing the distance between the individual and the source of radiation is an effective method to reduce exposure to radiation. As distance from the source of radiation is increased, the radiation level will decrease significantly. Maximizing the distance from an operable source of radiation is a particularly effective method of exposure reduction during mobile radiographic and fluoroscopic procedures.

The amount of exposure reduction can be calculated using the inverse square law, which describes the relationship between distance and radiation intensity. The inverse square law states that the intensity of radiation at a given distance from a point source is inversely proportional to the square of the distance. For example, if the distance between the individual and the source of radiation is doubled, the exposure to the individual will be reduced by a factor of 4 (2^2); if the distance between the individual and the source of radiation is tripled, the exposure to the individual will be reduced by a factor of 9 (3^2). The relationship between distance and radiation exposure is explained in further detail in Chapter 11.

Shielding

Shielding is used when neither time nor distance is effective in achieving the desired degree of reduction in exposure. By interposing any material between the source of radiation and the point at which it is desired to reduce the exposure, a certain reduction in exposure will be achieved. The degree of exposure reduction will depend on the physical characteristics of the material (atomic number, density, and thickness). For fixed x-ray imaging facilities the most common materials are lead and concrete. Such facilities are designed in accordance with specific recommendations (NCRP Report No. 49) depending on the configuration of the equipment, its intended use, and the surrounding area. Additional devices, such as mobile shields, lead-equivalent aprons, and lead-equivalent gloves should be used when it is not possible to take advantage of fixed structural barriers.

Protective Barriers

During the design of fixed x-ray imaging facilities it is necessary to ensure that the layout of the equipment and shielding of the room are such that the exposure to personnel and members of the public within adjacent areas is within the recommended equivalent dose limits. This is accomplished through the use of **structural protective barriers** made of materials having effective x-ray attenuating properties and of thicknesses sufficient to reduce exposures to the desired levels. Commonly used materials include lead sheet, concrete, lead glass, steel, and leaded acrylic.

Protective barriers are classified as either **primary barriers** or **secondary barriers**. Primary barriers can be struck by the primary or useful beam exiting the x-ray tube. Secondary barriers can only be struck by scattered and leakage radiation. The primary beam cannot be directed at secondary barriers. Secondary barriers are always thinner than primary barriers.

The design of structural shielding for x-ray imaging facilities is treated in detail in **NCRP Report No. 49: Structural Shielding Design and Evaluation for Medical Use of X Rays and Gamma Rays of Energies Up to 10 MeV.** Barrier requirements are dependent on the type of equipment, its layout within the room, the occupancy of adjacent areas, and other factors. Such shielding should always be designed by a qualified diagnostic radiological physicist.

Protective Devices

When it is not possible for personnel to remain behind a protective barrier, it is the radiographer's responsibility to ensure that **protective devices** are worn by all personnel, including physicians, nurses, aides, etc. These situations arise frequently during fluoroscopy and some mobile procedures. The most common protective devices are lead aprons and lead gloves. Special devices include leaded glasses and thyroid shields.

During fluoroscopy and mobile radiography, personnel should always wear a protective apron. Lead gloves should also be worn if the hands will be in close proximity to the primary beam. Protective aprons and gloves are usually made of lead-impregnated vinyl within the range of 0.25–1.0 mm of lead equivalency. The greater the lead equivalence, the greater the protective ability and the weight of the item. Aprons vary in weight from a few pounds to over 20 pounds depending on design and lead content. For example, a lead apron that wraps completely around the body, extending from shoulders to knees with a 1 mm lead equivalent, will possess a significant weight. This weight can be a serious consideration if personnel are expected to wear the apron for long periods of time. The protective aprons must possess a minimum of 0.5 mm lead equivalent if the peak energy of the x-ray beam is 100 kVp. Most departments use aprons with 0.5 mm lead equivalent to provide personnel with a balance between protection and weight. Lead gloves usually possess 0.25 mm of lead equivalency.

Protection of the Patient

Proper radiation protection of the patient is achieved through both medical and technical decisions. Medical decisions lie with the patient and are based on the professional judgment of physicians and other practitioners of the healing arts in consultation with the patient.

Technical decisions include a number of factors that affect the amount of radiation a patient receives during a diagnostic x-ray examination. Many of these factors are under the direct control of the radiographer. It is a radiographer's responsibility to understand these factors and to minimize patient exposure while producing a satisfactory diagnostic image.

While it is desirable to minimize the exposure to a patient undergoing a radiologic procedure, it must be kept in mind that the goal of any radiologic imaging procedure is to provide information about the medical condition of the patient to aid in clinical management. Overzealous attempts to reduce patient exposure may significantly compromise the information to be obtained from the examination. Keeping these concepts in mind, the following principles should be applied to minimize exposure to the patient.

Beam Limitation

The size of the x-ray beam should always be restricted to the area of clinical interest and should never exceed the size of the image receptor. Proper collimation not only reduces patient dose but also improves the overall quality of the radiographic image because less scatter radiation is created with smaller field sizes. Ideally, evidence of proper collimation, as demonstrated by an unexposed border on all sides of the radiographic image, should be present.

Technique Selection

Technique factors for a given examination should be selected to minimize dose to the patient. High kVp/low mAs techniques are preferred to decrease patient dose. However, the selected kVp should be chosen so the required contrast in the radiographic image is not compromised as a result of a more penetrating x-ray beam or because of an increase in the amount of scatter radiation reaching the film, which can impair image quality. Tube current and exposure time should be chosen to minimize the degrading effects of anatomical motion. Proper technical factor selection is the responsibility of the radiographer. This decision must take into account the information needed to make a proper diagnosis. It is important to remember that increasing kVp alone does not decrease patient dose but instead will increase patient dose. To reduce patient dose, the increase in kVp must be accompanied by a reduction in mAs to maintain an acceptable film density.

Filtration

Filters are placed at the x-ray port to selectively absorb low energy photons that would be absorbed by the patient and not contribute to the image. These low-energy photons would be absorbed by the patient, resulting in an increase in the patient dose. Specialized filtration is also available. It allows for additional exposure reduction by the selective removal of photons from the beam.

Aluminum is the most common filtering material used and filtration is expressed in terms of the thickness of aluminum equivalency (Al/Eq). The NCRP recommends a minimum total filtration of 2.5 mm Al/Eq for x-ray equipment operating above 70 kVp. When filtration is increased, technical factors do need to be increased to compensate for the reduction in film density associated with the filtration. Despite the need to increase exposure to maintain density, the overall dose to the patient decreases with the use of filtration.

Grids

Radiographic grids are placed between the patient and the image receptor to preferentially absorb scatter radiation. Because grids absorb primary as well as scatter radiation, technical factors must be increased to produce an image of acceptable film density. This increase in technical factors results in an increase in patient dose but image quality is significantly improved. The lowest possible grid ratio consistent with effective scatter removal should be utilized to keep patient dose as low as reasonably achievable.

Gonadal Shielding

Shielding the gonads (ovaries or testes) is especially important to minimize the possibility of any genetic effect on the future children of an exposed individual. Special attention should be paid to shielding the gonads of children and adults of childbearing age.

Proper collimation is important when decreasing gonadal dose, but special gonadal shields should be used any time the gonads are within 4 to 5 cm of the primary beam. The three basic types of gonadal shields are **flat contact shield**s, **shaped contact shields**, and s**hadow shields** (Figure 9–2).

Flat contact shields are usually made of various sizes of lead-impregnated vinyl and are placed between the patient's gonads and the source of radiation. During fluoroscopy, the shield usually needs to be placed under-

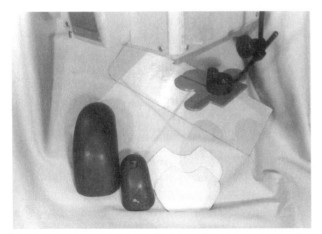

FIGURE 9–2. Gonadal shields: (left to right) flat shield, shadow shield, contact shield.

neath the patient because that is where the source of radiation is most often located. Flat contact shields may need to be secured in place to ensure correct placement for a variety of patient positions.

Shaped contact shields are cup-shaped and designed to enclose the male gonads. These shields provide maximum protection in a number of patient positions.

Shadow shields are mounted to the tube and are placed in the x-ray beam near the collimator. The collimator's light field must be precise for accurate shield placement. The device is adjusted to cast a shadow over the patient's gonads.

Image Receptors

The speed of the image receptor should be chosen to be as high as possible, consistent with the required information of the radiologic procedure. The use of intensifying screens in conjunction with film greatly reduces patient dose by reducing the quantity of x-ray photons needed to create an image. Intensifying screens convert x-ray photons to light photons, which expose the film within the cassette. The speed of the image receptor is influenced by the type of intensifying screen and film. Intensifying screens, which provide efficient absorption of the incident radiation, allow the production of a satisfactory image with less dose to the patient. As the speed of the film/screen system is increased, patient dose is reduced; however, image sharpness is decreased as a result.

Projection

The projection used for a particular exam will have an impact on patient dose to specific body tissues. For example, the lens of the eye receives a greater dose during antero-posterior (AP) projections of the cranium than it does if the postero-anterior (PA) projection is used. Or, a contrast-filled bladder will serve as a gonadal shield for females if the exposure is made with the patient in the AP projection but will not shield the ovaries in the PA projection.

Repeat Radiographs

Any time a radiograph must be repeated, patient dose increases as a direct result of the exposure from the poor radiograph. Radiographers must possess a complete understanding of the entire radiographic process to minimize repeat exposures. Radiographs generally need to be repeated for such reasons as improper exposure factor selection, poor positioning (tube/part/film alignment), poor patient instruction, or improper film processing. Radiographs should only be repeated when the quality of the radiograph compromises the diagnostic information of the procedure. It is important for the radiographer to communicate effectively with the patient and provide the patient with clear instructions during the procedure to minimize the possibility of needing to repeat the exposure.

Patient Exposure Estimates

Estimates of the exposure received by patients undergoing radiographic procedures should be available. These estimates should be developed for the average patient based on standard technique charts and measured exposure characteristics of the radiological imaging equipment. Chapter 13 provides information on calculating the patient exposure for a given procedure and describes ways in which the radiographer can minimize the exposure to the patient.

Equipment

All radiologic imaging equipment should be surveyed periodically by a diagnostic radiological physicist to access its radiation safety characteristics. Such surveys should normally be conducted in conjunction with scheduled preventive maintenance and performance surveys and should be performed at least annually. The results of such surveys should be documented. Any deficiencies should be corrected prior to returning the equipment to clinical service.

Radiation Exposure and Pregnancy

A situation deserving special consideration is the possibility of radiation exposure during the early weeks of pregnancy, generally before the woman is aware of her condition. The dose to the fetus is of concern, particularly in the early stages of development when certain tissues and organs are especially sensitive to radiation. Recent studies, as summarized in the report, BEIR V,

suggest the fetus may be particularly radiosensitive during the period of 8 to 15 weeks post-conception. As a result, care must be taken to reduce radiation exposure to any pregnant individual, including pregnant (or potentially pregnant) patients and pregnant personnel. It is currently recommended by the NCRP that the monthly equivalent dose limit (excluding medical exposure) for the embryo not exceed 0.05 rem (50 mrem, 0.5 mSv) once the pregnancy becomes known.

NCRP Report No. 54, Medical Exposure of Pregnant and Potentially Pregnant Women, discusses the risks associated with fetal exposure: This risk is considered to be negligible at 5 rad or less when compared to other risks of pregnancy, and the risk of malformations is significantly increased above control levels only at doses above 15 rad. Therefore, the exposure of the fetus to radiation arising from diagnostic procedures would very rarely be cause, by itself, for terminating a pregnancy. If there are reasons, other than the possible radiation effects, to consider a therapeutic abortion, such reasons should be discussed with the patient by the attending physician, so that it is clear that the radiation exposure is not being used as an excuse for terminating the pregnancy. (NCRP, 1977)

Pregnant Radiation Worker Exposure Standards

There are two sets of standards that are applied to pregnant radiation workers. These standards include students under the definition of those who are "occupationally" exposed to ionizing radiation because students in radiologic sciences programs are classified as students by occupation, and the exposure occurs during duties in their occupation.

The two standards complement one another. The Nuclear Regulatory Commission (NRC) is a U. S. federal agency charged with licensing facilities and controlling the use of radioactive materials. The National Council on Radiation Protection and Measurements (NCRP) is an advisory group that makes recommendations for radiation protection.

NRC regulations state that the dose equivalent to the embryo/fetus during the entire pregnancy, due to the occupational exposure of a declared pregnant woman, cannot exceed 5 mSv (0.5 rem or 500 mrem). The

NCRP recommends that fetal exposure should be restricted to an equivalent dose limit of 0.5 mSv (0.05 rem or 50 mrem) per month. These two limits are complementary as a normal human gestation spans a 10-month period. Therefore, 0.5 mSv (0.05 rem) for 10 months equals 5 mSV (0.5 rem) for the entire gestational period. The specific citations (which are often referred to in pregnancy policies and state regulations) are NRC regulation 10CFR20.1208 and NCRP Reports #54, #116, and #128 with the primary recommendation issued in Report #116.

Declaring Pregnancy
Pregnant radiation workers are referred to in U. S. federal regulations as "declared pregnant" because a woman has the right to choose whether or not to declare her pregnancy (this was established in a U. S. Supreme Court decision in the case of United Auto Workers vs Johnson Controls). The government currently interprets this as including the right to revoke her declaration at any time. In addition, a female worker can legally declare pregnancy without documented medical proof and there is no limit on how frequently or how long a duration a person can declare she is pregnant.

Although the idea of declaring and undeclaring a pregnancy may sound bizarre, it is legitimate in the light of recent legal decisions that give women the right to choose for their embryo/fetus. This concept requires women to make a decision as to what radiation regulations will be applied to a pregnancy. Therefore, the NRC requires a voluntary declaration of pregnancy to be in writing, dated, and include the estimated month of conception. In addition, **NRC regulation 10CFR19.12 requires that instructions to women assigned to radiation exposure areas must include explanation of the right to declare or not declare pregnancy status as well as requiring that all information in NRC Regulatory Guide 8.13 be discussed.** This mandatory guide has details about the risk of radiation exposure in order to permit women to make an informed decision about declaring a pregnancy. The guide is downloadable from the Internet at http://www.nrc.gov/NRC/RG/08/08-013.html.

ALARA and Pregnancies
It has become common practice to assign declared pregnant women to areas where exposure is likely to be lower. This approach is now being discouraged in compliance with ALARA concepts of keeping all occupational exposure as low as reasonably achievable. The rationale is that any displacement of normal duties places additional radiation exposure burden on fellow workers, both male and female, which they may find unacceptable. Therefore, reassigning declared pregnant women to lower exposure areas causes increased risk to others.

In addition, because most women are not aware of pregnancy until after the most sensitive first trimester has passed, it is very possible that another as-yet-undeclared pregnant woman could be assigned additional time in a high exposure area thus increasing risk to her embryo/fetus at the worst possible time.

Some authors are recommending that if institutions choose to reassign declared pregnant women in opposition to recommended ALARA guidelines, all workers (or students) must clearly understand the ramifications of such a policy. To avoid legal complications it is recommended that all occupationally exposed persons in the institution agree to the policy in writing and that this documentation include specific statements indicating agreement to be placed in higher exposure areas from time to time as necessary to accommodate those women who have declared pregnancy.

The authors of this book recognize the controversial nature of the above recommendations and acknowledge that administrative ethical beliefs about abortion are often linked to pregnancy policies in institutions. However, we believe that radiologic sciences professionals should have a part in the determination of these policies as it is their bodies and future children that are at risk. Informed decisions cannot be made without the information we have supplied above.

The Pregnant Patient
To minimize the possible exposure to an embryo in the earliest days of a pregnancy, a guideline known as the **ten-day rule** was recommended by a number of advisory agencies. This guideline stated that elective abdominal x-ray examinations of fertile women should be postponed until the ten-day period following the onset of menstruation as it would be improbable that a woman would be pregnant during these ten days. Based on the current understanding of radiobiology, this rule is now considered obsolete, primarily because the egg for the next

cycle reaches maximum sensitivity during the 10-day period. The application of this guideline within the radiology department has always proven difficult.

It is now the general belief that postponement of abdominal x-ray examinations is not necessary when the physician requesting the examination has considered the entire clinical state of the patient, including the possibility of pregnancy. The potential pregnancy status of all female patients of childbearing age should always be determined; in the event of known pregnancy, steps should be taken to minimize exposure to the fetus. One way to ensure against irradiating a woman in the early stages of pregnancy is to institute elective scheduling for nonemergency procedures. In many departments, female patients of childbearing ages are asked to provide the date of their last menstrual period (LMP). If there is a concern about a possible pregnancy, the patient's exam may be rescheduled. If a radiologic exam on a pregnant patient is deemed necessary, a diagnostic radiological physicist should perform calculations to estimate the actual fetal dose.

Summary

It is important to set limits for the protection of the radiation worker and the general public because of the known biological effects of exposure to ionizing radiation. Occupational radiation exposure limits pertinent to the protection of radiation workers are known as dose equivalent limits and are specified for both total body exposure and for exposure to certain tissues and organs.

To minimize dose to personnel the basic principles of time, distance, and shielding should be applied. There are two types of fixed x-ray installation protective barriers. Primary protective barriers are designed to protect against the direct exposure of the primary x-ray beam. Secondary protective barriers are designed to protect against exposure from scatter and leakage radiation. When it is not possible for personnel to remain behind a protective barrier, protective devices, such as lead aprons and lead gloves, should be worn.

To minimize patient dose while creating a diagnostic image, the radiographer must understand the factors that have a significant relationship to patient dose, such as beam limitation, technique selection, filtration, grids,

gonadal shielding, image receptors, and repeat radiographs.

Care must be taken to reduce radiation exposure to any pregnant individual, including pregnant (or potentially pregnant) patients and pregnant personnel. It is currently recommended by the NCRP that the equivalent dose limit (excluding medical exposure) for the embryo-fetus not exceed 0.05 rem (0.5 mSv) in any month once the pregnancy becomes known.

REVIEW QUESTIONS

1. What is the annual effective dose limit for whole-body exposure of a radiation worker?

2. What is the cumulative effective dose limit for a 28-year-old radiation worker (in rem and mSv)?

3. Explain the ALARA concept.

4. What are the three basic principles used for minimizing an individual's exposure to ionizing radiation?

5. What is the difference between a primary and secondary protective barrier?

6. How can a radiographer minimize radiation exposure to the patient?

7. What is the equivalent dose limit for the embryo-fetus per month?

8. According to NRC regulations, how does a woman declare herself pregnant?

REFERENCES AND RECOMMENDED READING

Appleton, M. B. & Carr, S. R. (1984). Radiation protection in a neonatal intensive care unit: A practical approach. *Radiography. 50*(592), 137.

Baker, D. G. (1989). How significant are the risks from occupational exposure to ionizing radiation? *Applied Radiology. 18*(9), 19.

Bales, J. & Greening, N. (1991). A practical approach to exposure reduction for imaging staff. *Radiography Today. 57*(652), 14–17.

Barrett, J. (1993). An investigation of radiation dose levels to patients during lumbar spine examinations. *Radiography Today.* 59(675), 19–22.

Beauchemin, R. (1984). Telescopic gonad protector: Analysis and experimentation of a telescopic gonad protector. *The Canadian Journal of Medical Radiation Technology.* 15(1), 39.

Bednorck, D. R., Rozenfeld, M., Lanzl, L. H., & Sabau, M. (1981). A protocol for exposure limitations in radiography. *Radiologic Technology.* 53(3) 229.

BEIR V Health effects of exposure to low levels of ionizing radiation. (1990). National Academy Press, Washington, DC.

Boice, J. D., Mandel, J. S., & Doody, M. M. (1992). A health study of radiologic technologists. *Cancer.* 69, 586–597.

Boone, J. M., & Levin, D. C. (1991). Radiation exposure to angiographers under different fluoroscopic imaging conditions. *Radiology.* 180, 861–865.

Brennan, P. (1995). A dose-reducing radiographic technique in the examination of the pelvis of pregnant women. *Radiography Today.* 61(693), 31–34.

Burhart, R. L., Gross, R. E., Jans, R. G., McCrohen, J. L., Rosenstein, M., & Reuter, F. A., (eds). (1985). *Recommendations for evaluation of radiation exposure from diagnostic radiology examinations.* United States Department of HHS Publication 85–8247.

Bushong, S. C. (1997). *Radiologic science for technologists: Physics, biology, and protection* (6th ed.). St. Louis: C. V. Mosby.

Bushong, S. C. (1984). Policies for managing the pregnant employee. *Radiology Management.* 6(3), 2–7.

Bushong, S. C. (1977). Radiation exposure in our daily lives. *The Physics Teacher.* (March), 135–144.

Butler, P., Thomas, A. W., Thompson, W. E., Wollerton, M. A., & Rachlin, J. A. (1986). Simple methods to reduce patient exposure during scoliosis radiography, *Radiologic Technology.* 57(5), 411.

Butler, P. F. (1985). Chest radiography: A survey of techniques and exposure levels currently used. *Radiology, 533.*

Caprio, M. L. (1980). The pregnant x-ray tech — providing adequate radiation safety for the fetus. *Radiologic Technology,* 52(2), 161.

Cartwright, P. (1992). Distribution and relative intensity of scattered radiation. *Radiography Today.* 58(664), 12–13.

Curry, T. S., Dowdey, J. E., & Murry, R. C. (1990). *Christensen's introduction to the physics of diagnostic radiology* (4th ed.). Philadelphia: Lea and Febiger.

Day, A. (1994). Radiation doses to radiosensitive organs during two different chest radiography techniques. *Radiography Today.* 60(690), 17–20.

Detain, J. (1984). Is it time to question the 10-day rule? *Radiography.* 50(592), 149–150.

Doust, C. (1986). Personal monitoring period for radiographers. *Radiography.* 52(603), 109–112.

Dowd, S. B. (1994). Practical radiation protection and applied radiobiology. Philadelphia: W. B. Saunders.

Dowd, S. B. & Archer, J. (1994). Radiation safety regulations: The evolution and development of standards. *Radiology Management.* 16(1), 39–45.

Elsberry, J. S. (1979). A technique for scatter dose calculations. *Radiologic Technology.* 51(1), 51.

Floyd, C., Baker, A., Lo, J., & Ravin, C. (1992). Measurement of scatter fractions in clinical bedside radiography. *Radiology.* 183(3), 857–861.

Frank, E., Stears, J., Gray, J., Winkler, N. T., & Hoffman, A. D. (1984). Use of the P. A. projection: A method of reducing x-ray exposure to specific radiosensitive organs. *The Canadian Journal of Medical Radiation Technology.* 15(2), 63.

Fry, O. E. & Cesare, G. (1960). Bedside radiography — reduction of patient exposure and orientation of grid cassettes. *Radiologic Technology.* 31(4), 387.

Fung, K. (1994). Lowering patient dose on single-phase x-ray units. *Radiologic Technology.* 66(3), 159–164.

Gibbs, S. J. (1981). Approaches to radiation risk estimation. *The Physical Basis of Medical Imaging.* Editors: Coulam, C. M., Erickson, J. J., Rollo, F. D., & Everette, J. A. New York: Appleton-Century-Crofts, 329–342.

Glaze, S., LeBlanc, A. D., Bushong, S. C. (1984). Defects in new protective aprons. *Radiology,* 217.

Godderidge, C. (1981). A radiology department's response to consumer concerns regarding the hazards of low-dose radiation. *Radiology Management. 4*(3), 1.

Gray, J. E., Stears, J. G., & Frank, E. D. (1983). Shaped, lead-loaded acrylic filters for patient exposure reduction and image—quality improvement. *Radiology.* 825.

Gur, D. & Wald, N. (1986). Probability of causation tables and their possible implications for the practice of diagnostic radiology. *Radiology. 158,* 853–854.

Hall, E. J. (1993). *Radiobiology for the radiologist* (4th ed.). Philadelphia: J. B. Lippincott Company.

Hendee, W. R. (1992). Estimation of radiation risks: BEIR V and its significance for medicine. *Journal of the American Medical Association. 268,* 620–624.

Hendee, W. R. (ed.) (1984). *Health effects of low-level radiation.* Norwalk, CT: Appleton-Century-Crofts.

Hendee, W. R. & Ritenour, R. (1993). *Medical Imaging Physics* (3rd ed.). St. Louis: C. V. Mosby.

Heriard, J. B., Terry, J. A., & Arnold, A. L. (1993). Achieving dose education in lumbar spine radiography. *Radiologic Technology. 65*(2), 97–103.

Hilger, M. T. J. (1983). Radiation exposure to nursing personnel from portable radiographic procedures. *Radiology Management. 6*(2), 16.

Huda, W., Bews, J., Gordon, K., Sutherland, J., Sont, W., & Ashmore, J. (1991). Occupational doses to medical radiation technologists in Manitoba (1978–1988). *Canadian Journal of Medical Radiation Technology. 22*(1), 23–25.

Huda, W. & Gordon, K. (1986). Radiation risks to medical radiation technologists during pregnancy. *The Canadian Journal of Medical Radiation Technology. 17*(3), 121.

Hughes, J. S., Roberts, G. C., Stephenson, S. K. (1983). Occupational exposure in medicine — A review of radiation doses to hospital staff in North West England. *British Journal of Radiology. 56,* 729–735.

International Commission on Radiation Protection. (1970). *Protection of the patient in x-ray diagnosis publication number 16.* Oxford, England: Pergamon Press, 1970.

Irvin, R. (1962). Selective filtration — Effect on patient dose and radiographic quality. *Radiologic Technology. 34*(2), 51.

Jacobi, C. A. (1968). Radiation safety — More than filtration. *Radiologic Technology. 40*(2), 97.

Jadva-Patel, H. (1991). The use of thin metal filters to reduce dose to patients. *Radiography Today. 57*(651), 18–22.

Jankowski, C. B. (1984). Radiation exposure of nurses in a coronary care unit. *The Journal of Critical Care. 13*(1), 55–58.

Jeans, S. P., Faulkner, K., Love, H. G., & Bardsley, R. A. (1985). An investigation of the radiation dose to staff during cardiac radiological studies. *British Journal of Radiology, 58,* 419–428.

Light, M. C., Molloi, S. Y. Yandouo, D. R., Ranallo, F. N. (1987). Scatter radiation exposure during knee arthrography. *Radiology,* 867.

McDormand, C. & Pel, T. (1986). Scoliosis radiography — Let's reduce patient exposure. *The Canadian Journal of Medical Radiation Technology. 17*(1), 37.

Mettler, F. A. & Moseley, R. D. (1985). *Medical effects of ionizing radiation.* Orlando: Grune & Stratton.

Miller, P. E. (1976). Biological effects of diagnostic irradiation. *Radiologic Technology. 48*(1), 11–16.

Milner, S. C. & Naylor, E. (1989). An estimation of doses received by patients in a diagnostic x-ray department. *Radiography Today. 55*(622), 16.

Mitchell, F. (1991). Scattered radiation and the lateral lumbar spine part 1: Initial research. *Radiography Today. 57*(644), 18–20.

Mitchell, F., Leung, C., Ahuja, A., & Metreweli, C. (1991). Scattered radiation and the lateral lumbar spine part 2: Clinical research. *Radiography Today. 57*(645), 12–14.

Mole, R. H. (1984). The 10-day rule: a misnomer. *Radiography. 50*(593), 229–230.

Mole, R. H. (1982). Consequences of pre-natal radiation exposure for post-natal development: A review. *International Journal of Radiation Biology. 42*(1), 1–12.

Mole, R. H. (1979). Radiation effects on pre-natal development and their radiological significance. *The British Journal of Radiology.* 52(614), 89–101.

Morgan, K. Z. (1973). The need for radiation protection. *Radiologic Technology.* 44(6), 385.

NCRP (1998). Report No. 128, *Radionuclide Exposure of the Embryo/Fetus*, Bethesda, MD: National Council on Radiation Protection and Measurements.

NCRP (1994). Commentary No. 9, *Considerations Regarding the Unintended Radiation Exposure of the Embryo, Fetus or Nursing Child*, Bethesda, MD: National Council on Radiation Protection and Measurements.

NCRP (1993). Report No. 116, *Limitation of Exposure to Ionizing Radiation*, Bethesda, MD: National Council on Radiation Protection and Measurements.

NCRP (1990) Report No. 107, *Implementation of the principle of ALARA for medical and dental personnel*, Bethesda, MD: National Council on Radiation Protection and Measurements.

NCRP (1989) Report No. 105, *Radiation protection for medical and allied health personnel*, Bethesda, MD: National Council on Radiation Protection and Measurements.

NCRP (1989) Report No. 102, *Medical x-ray, electron beam and gamma-ray protection for energies up to 50 mev (Equipment design, performance and use)*, Bethesda, MD: National Council on Radiation Protection and Measurements.

NCRP (1987). Report No. 93, *Ionizing radiation exposure of the population of the United States*, Bethesda, MD: National Council on Radiation Protection and Measurements.

NCRP (1987). Report No. 91, *Recommendations on limits for exposure to ionizing radiation*, Bethesda, MD: National Council on Radiation Protection and Measurements.

NCRP (1985). Report No. 82, *SI units in radiation protection and measurements*, Bethesda, MD: National Council on Radiation Protection and Measurements.

NCRP (1977). Report No. 54, *Medical exposure of pregnant and potentially pregnant women*, Bethesda, MD: National Council on Radiation Protection and Measurements.

NCRP (1976). Report No. 49, *Structural shielding design and evaluation for medical use of x rays and gamma rays of energies up to 10 mev*, Bethesda, MD: National Council on Radiation Protection and Measurements.

Nickoli, P. (1993). Exposure reduction through faster speed film-screen systems and a review of ALARA. *Canadian Journal of Medical Radiation Technology.* 24(3), 99–107.

Novitch, M. (1983). Evaluation of radiation exposure in diagnostic radiology examinations. *Radiology Management.* 5(4), 33.

Noz, M. E. & Maguire, G. Q. (1985). *Radiation protection in the radiologic and health sciences* (2nd ed.). Philadelphia: Lea & Febiger.

Omran, H. (1982). Thermoluminescent dosimeters for *in vivo* measurement of radiation exposure and related dose in mammography. *Radiologic Technology.* 53(5), 383.

Osborn, S. B. (1955). Radiation doses received by diagnostic x-ray workers. *British Journal of Radiology.* 28, 650–654.

Pagel, J. W. (1981). Radiation protection in diagnostic radiology, *The Physical Basis of Medical Imaging.* Editors: Coulam, C. M., Erickson, J. J., Rollo, F. D., & James, A. E. New York: Appleton-Century-Crofts, 303–328.

Parkinson, L. (1991). Assessment of dose in computerised tomography. *Radiography Today.* 57(650), 23–28.

Radiation exposure from diagnostic radiology exams: General recommendations. (1986). *Radiology Management.* 8(2), 49.

Raeside, D. E. & Anderson, D. W. (1974). Thermoluminescent dosimetry in the radiological sciences. *Radiologic Technology.* 46(1), 20.

Ragozzino, M. W. (1986). Average fetal depth in utero: Data for estimation of fetal absorbed radiation dose. *Radiology.* 513.

Rossi, R. P., Harnisch, B., & Hendee, W. R. (1982). Reduction of radiation exposure in radiography of the chest. *Radiology.* 144, 909–914.

Rueter, F. G., Conway, B. J., McCrohan, J. L., & Suleiman, O. H. (1990). Average radiation exposure values for three diagnostic radiographic examinations. *Radiology.* 177(2), 341–345.

Selman, J. (1983). *Elements of radiobiology.* Springfield, IL: Charles C. Thomas.

Sholl-Evans, B. (1989). Radiation protection training and information. *Radiography Today. 55*(620), 8.

Shrimpton, P. (1994). Patient dose in CT and recommendations for reduction. *Radiography Today. 60*(683), 9–11.

Shrimpton, P. C. (1989). Monitoring the dose to patients undergoing common x-ray examinations. *Radiography Today. 54*(619), 38.

Starchman, D. & Hedrick, W. (1993). A practical guide for protecting personnel, pregnant personnel, and patients during diagnostic radiography and fluoroscopy. *Radiology Management. 15*(1), 22–30.

Statement from the 1985 Paris meeting of the International Commission on Radiological Protection. (1985). *Radiology.* (September).

Statkiewicz, M. A., Visconti, P. J., & Ritenour, E. R. (1998). *Radiation Protection in Medical Radiography* (3rd ed.). St. Louis: C. V. Mosby.

Stears, J. G., Gray, J. E., & Frank, E. D. (1986). Radiation exposure information. *Radiologic Technology. 58*(1), 31.

Stewart, A. & Kneale, G. W. (1970). Radiation dose effects in relation to obstetric x-rays and childhood leukemias. *Lancet. 1*, 1185–1188.

Tolan, J. H. (1968). Comments on recent proposals for regulatory control of x-ray exposures. *Radiologic Technology. 40*(3), 124.

Travis, E. L. (1989). *Primer of medical radiobiology* (2nd ed.). Chicago: Year Book Medical Publishers.

Tyndol, D. A. & Bedsale, S. M. (1988). Exposure reduction and image quality for pantomographic radiography. *Radiologic Technology. 59*(1), 51.

Upton, A. C. (1982). The biological effects of low-level ionizing radiation. *Scientific American. 246*(2).

Wade, P. (1994). Science and practicalities of patient dose measurement procedures. *Radiography Today. 60*(681), 13–16.

Waldron, L. & Wade, J. (1992). Skin dose reduction as part of a regional x-ray dose assessment programme. *Radiography Today. 58*(659), 9–10.

Warner, R. (1993). Using technique factors to predict patient ESE. *Radiologic Technology. 65*(1), 21–26.

Watkins, G. L. (1988). Public health risks from low dose medical radiation. *Radiologic Technology. 59*(2), 160.

Wesenberg, R. L., Blumhagen, J. D., Rossi, R. P., Hilton, S. W., Gilbert, J. M., & Nedeau, D. J. (1980). Low-dose radiography of children. *Radiologic Technology. 51*(5), 641.

Winkler, N. T. (1969). Minimizing radiation exposure of patients and personnel (screen-film, TFD, filters; shields; grid ratios). *Radiologic Technology. 41*(3), 142.

Wochos, J. F., & Cameron, J. R. (1976). Effect of operator training on patient exposure: An analysis of the NEXT data. *Radiologic Technology. 48*(1), 19–22.

Yoshizumi, T. T., Drummond, K. T., Freeman, J. O., & Mullett, M. (1987). Radiation safety and protection of neonates in radiological exams. *Radiologic Technology. 58*(5), 405.

Young, A. T. (1986). Surface shield: device to reduce personnel radiation exposure. *Radiology,* 801.

The Case of the Double Row of Capsules

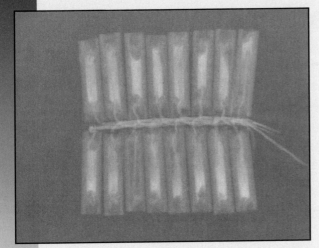

What could possibly produce this image? Special attention to the thin radiopaque lines is helpful.

Answers to the case studies can be found in Appendix E.

CHAPTER 10

Filtration

the bones gleam
out of the dark.
like the ghost of a fern
in stone here
are spine and ribs.

Celia Gilbert, "X-Ray."

OBJECTIVES

Upon completion of this chapter, the student should be able to:

▶ Define filtration, inherent filtration, added filtration, compound filtration, compensating filtration, and total filtration.

▶ Explain the concept of half-value layer equivalency measurements of filtration.

▶ Appraise various types of filters for specific clinical situations.

▶ Describe the effect of filtration on the entire x-ray beam.

*F*iltration is the process of eliminating undesirable low-energy x-ray photons by the insertion of absorbing materials into the primary beam. When inserted properly, filtration permits the radiographer to shape the photon emission spectrum into a more useful beam. Filtration is sometimes called **hardening** the beam because it removes the low-energy (soft) photons (Figure 10–1). The primary reason for filtration is the elimination of photons that would cause increased radiation dose to the patient but would not enhance the radiographic image.

At 20 keV, about 45 percent of the incident photons will penetrate 1 cm of soft tissue but only about 0.0006 percent will penetrate 15 cm. At 50 keV, 3.5 percent of the incident photons (a significant percentage) will penetrate 15 cm. Significant soft-tissue penetration occurs between 30 and 40 keV. Although they contribute to the patient dose, low-energy photons have insufficient energy to exit the patient and make any contribution to the image. Therefore their elimination is desirable.

Measurement

Any material designed to selectively absorb photons from the x-ray beam is called a **filter**. In diagnostic radiology, filtration is typically added between the source and the patient. Aluminum is the most common filter material used, although other materials, such as glass, oil, copper and tin are used or become filters in various instances. **Aluminum is considered the standard filtering material and all filtration can be expressed in terms of the thickness of aluminum equivalency (Al/Eq).** For example, the attachments, mirror and plastic of a collimator might be the equivalent of 0.5 mm of aluminum (Figure 10–2). This would be expressed as 0.5 mm Al/Eq.

Filtration is also expressed in terms of half-value layer. **The half-value layer (HVL) is that amount of absorbing material that will reduce the intensity of the primary beam to one-half its original value.** It is an indirect measure of the total filtration in the path of the x-ray beam. Half-value layers are usually expressed in terms of aluminum filtration equivalency; for example, HVL = 2.0 mm Al/Eq. The federal government specifies the minimum HVLs for all diagnostic x-ray tubes. If the HVL is at the appropriate level, the total filtration in the x-ray tube is adequate to protect the patient from unnecessary radiation.

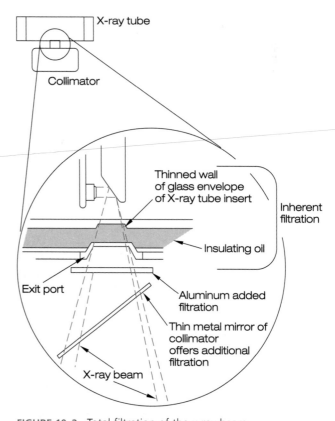

FIGURE 10–2. Total filtration of the x-ray beam.

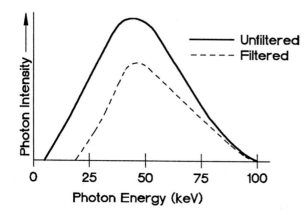

FIGURE 10–1. Effect of filtration on the x-ray beam.

Types of Filtration

Filtration occurs at various points between the x-ray tube and the image receptor. It is either **inherent** in the design of the tube or **added** between the tube and the image receptor.

Inherent Filtration

Filtration that is a result of the composition of the **tube and housing** is often called **inherent filtration** because it is a part of these structures. The thickness of the glass envelope of the tube, the dielectric oil that surrounds the tube, and the glass window of the housing all contribute to the inherent filtration. A typical x-ray tube might have a total inherent filtration of 0.5–1.0 mm Al/Eq. Most of the inherent filtration comes from the window of the glass envelope.

Because of this, mammographic tubes with special molybdenum targets that are designed to produce lower energy photons for soft-tissue imaging often have special beryllium (atomic number 4) windows in the glass envelope to eliminate the majority of the inherent filtration. Beryllium windows can reduce the inherent filtration to 0.1 mm Al/Eq (see Chapter 40).

As tubes age they become gassy, the anode begins to pit and the glass envelope may gain a mild coating of vaporized metal. All these factors will cause an increase in the inherent filtration, thus reducing the tube efficiency. This is the reason why HVL testing of tubes is a recommended quality control procedure for evaluation of tube efficiency and age.

Added Filtration

Any filtration that occurs outside the tube and housing and before the image receptor is considered added. Filtration materials are selected to absorb as many low-energy photons as possible while transmitting a maximum number of high-energy photons. Aluminum, with an atomic number of 13, functions very well as a low-energy absorber.

The collimator device also adds filtration to the beam and is considered to be added filtration. Collimators average 1.0 mm Al/Eq, most of which comes from the silver on the mirror situated in the beam. The mirror is designed to reflect the collimator light to simulate the primary beam field size for positioning purposes. This addition to the inherent filtration is why mammographic units often do not use collimators. The filtering effect would cause absorption of the low-energy photons that are desirable for soft-tissue imaging.

Compound Filtration

A compound filter uses two or more materials that complement one another in their absorbing abilities. Most compound filters are constructed so that each layer absorbs the characteristic photons created by the previous layer. For this reason, compound filters are also referred to as **K-edge filters**. Compound filters place the highest atomic number material closest to the tube and the lowest atomic number material closest to the patient. The final layer is usually aluminum, which has an atomic number of 13.

Although aluminum is the most common filtering material, copper, with an atomic number of 29, functions well for slightly higher energies. When a copper filter is used, it must be backed by an aluminum filter to absorb the 8 keV K-shell characteristic radiation produced by the copper. Copper filters should be at least 0.25 mm thick and backed with a minimum of 1 mm of aluminum.

A good example of a compound filter is the **Thoreaus filter**, used in radiation therapy. This filter combines tin, copper, and aluminum, in that order. Tin has the highest atomic number (50) and is placed first in the beam. Next, a copper filter is added to absorb the 29.3 keV characteristic photons created by the tin. Finally, aluminum is added to the copper to absorb copper's characteristic photons, which would only contribute to increasing patient dose. The 1.5 keV K-shell characteristic radiation produced by the aluminum filter is absorbed in the air between the filter and the patient.

Compensation Filtration

A **compensating filter** is usually designed to solve a problem involving unequal subject densities. The goal is to add an absorber to compensate for unequal absorption within the subject, thus making the overall absorption of the primary beam more equal. This helps in producing a more uniform radiographic film density.

Compensating filters can be made of aluminum, leaded plastic trademarked under the name ClearPb™ or plastic. Even an ordinary saline solution bag can be a useful compensating filter.

The two most popular compensating filters are the **wedge filter** and the **trough filter** (sometimes called a double wedge). The thicker portions of the filter are matched to the less dense patient body parts (Figure 10–3). A wedge filter can be useful for procedures on the thoracic spine, the feet (Figure 10–4) and the lower extremities, particularly during venography and femoral angiography. A trough filter is useful to even the density differences between the mediastinum and the lungs on a chest radiograph.

It is also possible to custom design filters by several methods. Aluminum, ClearPb™ or plastic pieces may be attached by magnets or rods underneath the collimator to permit movement into or out of the primary beam. The advantage of the ClearPb™ is its ability to use the collimator light to project the filter position onto the patient's body. Some plastic filters, such as the boomerang filter, are designed to be placed under the patient. Radiologists may object to the use of compensating filters on the justifiable grounds that they cast artifacts onto the radiographic image.

Explorations have been made into the use of various heavy elements, including some of the rare earths, to utilize K-shell characteristic production to enhance energy ranges that are especially useful. For example, studies have been done using rare earths to increase photon emissions at the energies needed by iodine contrast agents. Difficulties in making these filtration techniques practical have kept them from becoming popular. However, very good results have been obtained for mammography by using a 0.05 mm molybdenum filter and operating the tube at a constant 35 kVp.

Total Filtration

Total filtration is equal to the sum of inherent and added filtration and does not include any compound or compensating filters that may be added later. The thickness of the added filtration varies depending on the anticipated uses of the equipment. The percentage of photons attenuated decreases as photon energy increases, even when filtration is increased (Table 10–1). Note that aluminum filters of 1–3 mm absorb significant percentages of photons below the diagnostic range while permitting the vast majority to pass. The National Council on Radiation Protection and Measurements (NCRP) recommends minimum total filtration levels for diagnostic radiography, as shown in Table 10–2. These filtration levels are commonly used in the United States and correspond to International Council on Radiation

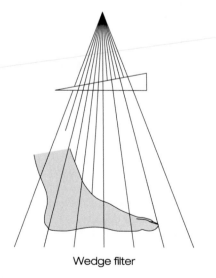
Wedge filter

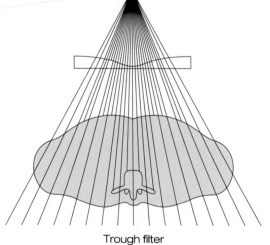
Trough filter

FIGURE 10–3. Compensating filters.

60 kVp	5 mAs	40" SID
No grid	400 RS	

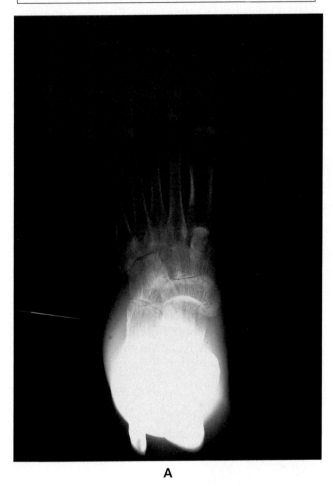

A

60 kVp	5 mAs	40" SID
No grid	400 RS	

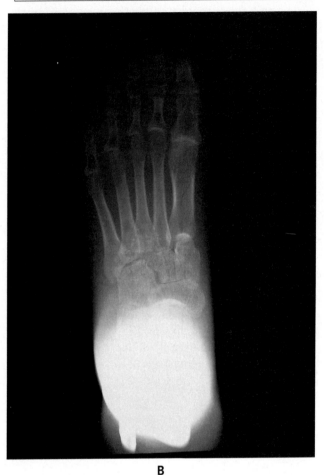

B

FIGURE 10–4. (A) Normal AP foot. (B) The use of a compensating wedge filter for an AP foot.

Protection (ICRP) recommendations. The importance of the reduction in patient dose, as shown in Table 10–3, must not be overlooked.

Effect On Output

Not only does filtration reduce the patient exposure dose by eliminating low-energy photons from the pri-

mary x-ray beam, it also removes a portion of the useful beam. This has a visible effect on radiographic film density. To compensate for the loss of film density **when filtration is increased, technical factors must be increased to maintain the same density**.

Note that in Table 10–3 the decrease in patient dose compares very favorably with the increase necessary to maintain radiographic film density. In other words, although the exposure needs to be increased to maintain

TABLE 10–1. Percent Attenuation of Monochromatic Radiation by Various Thicknesses of Aluminum Filtration

Photon Energy (keV)	Photons Attenuated (%)			
	1 mm	2 mm	3 mm	10 mm
10	100	100	100	100
20	58	82	92	100
30	24	42	56	93
40	12	23	32	73
50	8	16	22	57
60	6	12	18	48
80	5	10	14	39
100	4	8	12	35

Reproduced with permission from Curry, T., Dowdey, J., and Murry, R., *Christensen's Physics of Diagnostic Radiology,* 4th ed. Philadelphia: Lea and Febiger, 1990.

density, there is a greater decrease in overall exposure to the patient.

Beyond 3.0 mm/Al filtration a point of diminishing returns is reached. The reduction in entrance skin exposure (ESE) does not warrant the tube loading increase.

Summary

Filtration is the process of eliminating undesirable x-ray photons by the insertion of absorbing materials into the primary beam. Any material designed to selectively

TABLE 10–2. Recommended Minimum Total Filtration Levels

Operating kVp	Total Filtration
Below 50 kVp	0.5 mm aluminum
50 to 70 kVp	1.5 mm aluminum
Above 70 kVp	2.5 mm aluminum

Adapted by permission from Table 3–1, National Council on Radiation Protection and Measurement. *NCRP Report No. 102, Medical X-Ray, Electron Beam and Gamma-Ray Protection for Energies Up to 50 MeV (Equipment Design, Performance and Use).* Bethesda, MD: NCRP, 1989

TABLE 10–3. Comparison of Patient Exposure With Filtration

Aluminum Filtration in mm	Entrance Skin Exposure in mR	Decrease in Exposure Dose	Increase in Exposure Required to Maintain Same Film Density
60 KVP, 18 CM PELVIS			
none	2,380		
0.5	1,850	22%	14%
1.0	1,270	47%	17%
3.0	465	80%	52%
85 KVP, 18 CM PELVIS			
none	1,225		
0.5	860	30%	0%
1.0	684	44%	12%
3.0	287	77%	34%

From E. Dale Trout, J.P. Kelley, and G.A. Cathey. The Use of Filters to Control Radiation Exposure to the Patient in Diagnostic Roentgenology. *American Journal of Roentgenology* 67:942, 1952.

absorb photons from the x-ray beam is called a filter. Aluminum is the most common filter material used. It is considered the standard filter material and all filtering in diagnostic radiography can be expressed in terms of the thickness of aluminum equivalency (Al/Eq). The half-value layer (HVL) is that amount of absorbing material that will reduce the intensity of the primary beam to one-half its original value.

Filtration occurs at various points between the x-ray tube and the image receptor. It is either inherent in the design of the x-ray tube or added between the tube and the image receptor. Filtration that is the result of the composition of the tube and housing is often called inherent filtration because it is a part of these structures. Any filtration that occurs outside the tube and housing and before the image receptor is considered added. The collimator device adds approximately 1.0 Al/Eq to the beam.

The compound filter uses two or more materials that complement one another in their absorbing ability. A compensating filter is usually designed to solve a problem involving unequal subject density. Two common compensating filters are the wedge and the trough. Total filtration is equal to the sum of inherent and added filtration.

Not only does filtration reduce the patient exposure by eliminating low-energy photons, it also removes a portion of the useful beam and can therefore affect image density.

REVIEW QUESTIONS

1. What is filtration?

2. What is the standard filter material used in diagnostic radiography?

3. Define half-value layer.

4. What is inherent filtration?

5. When more than one filtering material is used, as in a compound filter, how are the materials arranged in relationship to the x-ray source?

6. What are the two most common compensating filters?

7. What is total filtration?

8. How does filtration affect patient dose and beam intensity?

REFERENCES AND RECOMMENDED READING

An inexpensive alternative to compensating filters. (1980). *Radiologic Technology. 52*(2), 206.

Bernier, P. (1982). Clinical application of gadolinium filters in neo-natal radiography. *The Canadian Journal of Medical Radiation Technology. 13*(6), 273.

Burns, C. B. & Renner, J. B. (1994). Molybdenum/aluminum filters perform effectively. *Radiologic Technology. 64*(4), 216-219.

Burns, C. B., Renner, J. B., Gratale, P., Moyle, L. L. (1992). Niobium/aluminum filters reduce patient exposure. *Radiologic Technology. 63*(3), 170-175.

Bushberg, J. T., Seibert, J. A., Leidholdt, E. M., & Boone, J. M. (1994). *The essential physics of medical imaging.* Baltimore: Williams & Wilkins.

Croft, M. J. (1986). Filtration, the answer to the automatic exposure control response problem. *Radiologic Technology. 57*(5), 447.

Cullinan, A. & Cullinan, J. (1994). *Producing quality radiographs.* (2nd ed.). Philadelphia: J. B. Lippincott.

Curry, T. S., Dowdey, J. E., & Murry, R. C. (1990). *Christensen's introduction to the physics of diagnostic radiology* (4th ed.). Philadelphia: Lea and Febiger.

Dendy, P. P. & Heaton, B. (1987). *Physics for radiologists.* Oxford: Blackwell Scientific Publications.

Dilella, D. & Albert, H. (1964). Variable thickness filters for use with 14 x 36 inch film. *Radiologic Technology. 36*(1), 1.

Ekstrand, K. E. (1979). The inverse compensating filter. *Radiology.* 201.

Feczko, P. J. (1983). Compensation filtration for decubitus radiography during double-contrast barium enema examination. *Radiology.* (Dec.), 848.

Geissberger, H. (1966). Wedge-shaped filters for improved radiography of the thoracic vertebrae and the foot. *Medical Radiography and Photography. 42*(1), 6.

Gray, J. E., Stears, J. G., & Frank, E. D. (1983). Shaped, lead-loaded acrylic filters for patient exposure reduction and image-quality improvement. *Radiology. 146*, 825-828.

Hart, J. D., Drake, P. A, & Schmugge, M. L. (1986). Plexiglas filtration in cervicocerebrae. *Applied Radiology. 15*(6), 148.

Howard, C. (1991). How good is the erbium filter? *Radiography Today. 57*(649), 22-26.

Irvin, R. (1962). Selective filtration: Effect on patient dose and radiographic quality. *Radiologic Technology. 34*(2), 51.

Jackson, W. (1976). Filtration in diagnostic radiology. *Radiography. 42*(504), 255.

Jacobi, C. A. (1968). Radiation safety: More than filtration. *Radiologic Technology. 40*(2), 97.

Jadva-Patel, H. (1991). The use of thin metal filters to reduce dose to patients. *Radiography Today. 57*(651), 18-22.

James, N. (1983). High kilovoltage radiography using the Cincinnati filter. *Radiography. 49*(585), 210.

Jenkin, D. *Radiographic photography and imaging processes.* Lancaster: MTP Press.

Johns, H. E. & Cunningham, J. R. (1983). *The physics of radiology* (4th ed.). Springfield, IL: Thomas.

Jones, R. & McKenna, A. (1989). The use of saline as a compensating filter. *Radiologic Technology. 62*(2), 134-138.

Kassebaum, M. K. (1949). The use of compensating filters. *Radiologic Technology. 20*(4), 209.

Kelsey, C. A. (1986). Chest radiographs obtained with shaped filters: Evaluation by observer performance test. *Radiology.* 653.

Kenaga, J. D. (1964). The Bundy compensating filter. *Radiologic Technology. 36*(1), 18.

Kohn, M. L., Gooch, A. W., Keller, W. S. (1988). Filters for radiation reduction: A comparison. *Radiology.* 255.

McEnerney, P. (1951). The value of compensating filters in roentgenography including the double filter technique. *Radiologic Technology. 23*(1), 29.

McFadden, B. (1989). Half value layer calibration. *Canadian Journal of Medical Radiation Technology. 20*(2), 67-74.

National Council on Radiation Protection and Measurements (1989). *NCRP Report No. 102: Medical X-Ray, Electron Beam and Gamma-Ray Protection for Energies Up to 50 MeV (Equipment Design, Performance and Use.)* Bethesda, MD: NCRP.

Seeram, E. (1985). *X-Ray imaging equipment.* Springfield, IL: Charles C. Thomas.

Smith, D. C. & Tidwell, J. (1978). Adjustable sliding aluminum wedge filter: Device for angiographic enhancement. *Radiologic Technology. 49*(4), 459.

Sprawls, P. (1987). *Physical principles of medical imaging.* Rockville, MD: Aspen Publishers.

Stears, J. G., Gray, J. E., Webbles, W. E., & Frank, E. D. (1988). Radiologic exchange (added filtration). *Radiologic Technology. 59*(3), 245-246.

Stears, J. G., Gray, J. E., Webbles, W. E., & Frank, E. D. (1986). The variable filter dial. *Radiologic Technology. 57*(6), 542.

Trout, E. D., Kelley, J. P., Cathey, G. A. (1952). The use of filters to control radiation exposure to the patient in diagnostic roentgenology. *American Journal of Roentgenology. 67*, 946-963.

Uyborny, C. & MacMahon, H. (1984). Foil filters for equalized chest radiography. *Radiology.* 524.

Wilks, R. J. (1981). *Principles of radiological physics.* Edinburgh: Churchill Livingstone.

Wolbarst, A. B. (1993). *Physics of radiology.* Norwalk, CT: Appleton & Lange.

X-ray filter system for exposure reduction. (1987). *Radiologic Technology. 58*(5).

CHAPTER 11

The Prime Factors

X-ray technic, like x-ray equipment, has passed through an evolutionary stage from the beginning, in 1896, to the present time, and the end is not yet in sight.

E. C. Jerman, 1926.

OBJECTIVES

Upon completion of this chapter, the student should be able to:

▶ Explain the relationships between milliamperage (mA), exposure time, mAs and x-ray emission.

▶ State the reciprocity law.

▶ Calculate mAs when given mA and exposure time, mA when given mAs and exposure time, and exposure time when given mAs and mA.

▶ Explain the relationship between kVp and x-ray emission.

▶ State the 15 percent rule.

▶ Calculate the new kVp value needed to maintain density when changes are made in mAs, using the 15 percent rule.

▶ Explain the relationship between distance and x-ray emission.

▶ State the inverse square law.

▶ Calculate x-ray emission (mR) when distance is changed.

▶ Calculate the mAs needed to maintain density when changes are made in distance, using the density maintenance formula.

The Prime Factors

*T*he emission of x-ray photons from an x-ray tube is controlled by a number of factors. Those factors related to tube design and construction have been covered in previous chapters and include tube housing, target material, filtration and voltage waveform. Three factors that affect x-ray emission are under the direct control of the radiographer. These are called the **prime factors**. They are milliamperage-second (mAs), kilovoltage (kVp) and distance (d).

The x-ray beam can be described in terms of both its quantity and its quality. **X-ray quantity** is a measure of the number of x-ray photons in the useful beam. It is also called x-ray output, intensity or exposure. Recall that the unit of measurement of x-ray quantity is the **roentgen (R)**. The factors that directly affect x-ray quantity are milliamperage-second (mAs), kilovoltage (kVp), distance (d) and filtration. **X-ray quality** is a measurement of the penetrating ability of the x-ray beam. Penetrability describes the distance an x-ray beam travels in matter. High-energy x-ray photons travel farther in matter than low-energy photons and are therefore more penetrating. Highly penetrating x-rays are termed hard x-rays and low penetrating x-rays are called soft x-rays. X-ray quality is numerically represented by the **half-value layer (HVL)**. The half-value layer of an x-ray beam is that thickness of absorbing material needed to reduce the x-ray intensity (quantity) to half its original value. The factors that directly affect x-ray quality are kilovoltage and filtration.

The factors that control the quantity and/or quality of x-ray emission are the prime factors and filtration (Table 11–1). Filtration is not something the radiographer controls from exposure to exposure.

Milliamperage-Second (mAs)

Milliamperage (mA) is a measurement of x-ray tube current—the number of electrons crossing the tube from cathode to anode per second. Recall that an ampere is equal to an electric charge of one coulomb flowing through a conductor per second. The coulomb is equal to 6.3×10^{18} electron charges. Therefore, an ampere

TABLE 11–1. Factors Affecting X-Ray Emission

Quantitative Factors	Qualitative Factors
Milliamperage-second	Kilovoltage
Kilovoltage	Filtration
Distance	
Filtration	

equals a flow of 6.3×10^{18} electrons per second and a milliampere would equal 6.3×10^{15} electrons per second. As mA increases so does the number of electrons which are able to cross the tube to reach the x-ray target. **Milliamperage is directly proportional to tube current.** As the mA doubles so does the number of electrons able to cross the tube. The number of electrons reaching the target is also controlled by the length of time the tube is energized. Remember that mA is the number of electrons **per second**. This means that changes in the length of time of exposure will affect the total number of electrons flowing from cathode to anode. X-ray exposure time is measured in **seconds**. Like mA, **exposure time is directly proportional to the number of electrons crossing the tube and is therefore directly proportional to the number of x-rays created**. This is the x-ray quantity.

The number of x-rays that will be created at the target is a product of the number of electrons crossing the tube (tube current) and how long the electrons are allowed to cross (exposure time). **Milliamperage-second (mAs)** is the unit used to describe the product of tube current and exposure time. This simple relationship is described by the equation mA $\times$ s = mAs. Milliamperage-second (mAs) is the primary controller of x-ray quantity. X-ray quantity is directly proportional to mAs. This means that as mAs doubles, x-ray exposure (measured in roentgens) doubles; as mAs triples, x-ray exposure triples and so forth.

If an x-ray control panel is set at 100 mA and 0.05 (1/20) second, the mAs would be 100 $\times$ 0.05 or 5 mAs. If either the mA or the exposure time is doubled, the mAs will double, i.e., 200 mA at 0.05 second equals 10 mAs, as does 100 mA at 0.1 (1/10) second. This means that a number of possible settings on the x-ray control can all yield the same x-ray exposure. For example, 10 mAs can be set using any of the following technical factors:

$$50 \text{ mA} \times 0.2 \quad (1/5) \quad \text{second} = 10 \text{ mAs}$$
$$100 \text{ mA} \times 0.1 \quad (1/10) \quad \text{second} = 10 \text{ mAs}$$
$$200 \text{ mA} \times 0.05 \quad (1/20) \quad \text{second} = 10 \text{ mAs}$$

Obviously, a number of other possibilities exist as well. This relationship can be described in the equation $mA_1S_1 = mA_1S_1$. Because mA and exposure time can be manipulated to achieve the same mAs, **it is best to think in terms of mAs when establishing technical factors**. It is important, for technical factor conversions, that the technologist be able to manipulate the mA and time to arrive at the proper mAs for a particular examination.

Examples: Given the following mA and exposure time values, calculate the mAs.

$$200 \text{ mA} \times 0.083 \text{ second} = \underline{\hspace{1.5cm}} \text{mAs}$$
$$100 \text{ mA} \times 2/5 \text{ second} = \underline{\hspace{1.5cm}} \text{mAs}$$

Answers:

$$200 \text{ mA} \times 0.083 \text{ second} = 16.6 \text{ mAs}$$
$$100 \text{ mA} \times 2/5 \text{ second} = 40 \text{ mAs}$$

Examples: Given the following mAs and mA values, calculate the exposure time.

$$75 \text{ mAs} = 100 \text{ mA} \times \underline{\hspace{1.5cm}} \text{second}$$
$$15 \text{ mAs} = 300 \text{ mA} \times \underline{\hspace{1.5cm}} \text{second}$$

Answers:

$$75 \text{ mAs} = 100 \text{ mA} \times 0.75 \ (3/4) \text{ second}$$
$$15 \text{ mAs} = 300 \text{ mA} \times 0.05 \ (1/20) \text{ second}$$

Examples: Given the following mAs and exposure time values, calculate the mA.

$$mAs = 0.3 \ (3/10) \text{ second} \times \underline{\hspace{1.5cm}} \text{mA}$$
$$mAs = 0.15 \ (3/20) \text{ second} \times \underline{\hspace{1.5cm}} \text{mA}$$

Answers:

$$60 \text{ mAs} = 0.3 \ (3/10) \text{ second} \times 200 \text{ mA}$$
$$75 \text{ mAs} = 0.15 \ (3/20) \text{ second} \times 500 \text{ mA}$$

Density Relationship to mAs

Radiographic density is the degree of blackening of an x-ray film. It is created by deposits of black metallic silver on an x-ray film that has been exposed to light or x-ray and then processed. On the radiographic image, the densities are the result of an x-ray exposure to the film and intensifying screens. Recall that as mAs is increased, x-ray exposure will increase proportionally.

While the relationship between mAs and exposure (mR) is a directly proportional one, the relationship of these two factors to density is much more complex. Density is determined by the amount of silver deposition in the emulsion due to the film type, exposure conditions, exposure (mR) and processing. A DlogE sensitometric curve expresses the relationship between exposure and density, with log relative exposure plotted on the x-axis and density (D) plotted on the y-axis. The relationship between exposure and density determines the shape and position of the DlogE curve for a given film under specific processing conditions. This relationship is described in detail in Chapter 21 Sensitometry.

If the exposure to a film is increased, the density to that film will increase until the point where the film reaches its maximum density (D_{max}). Since density is primarily determined by the amount of exposure a film receives, and since exposure is directly proportional to mAs, **mAs is used as the primary controller of radiographic density**. As mAs increases, x-ray exposure increases proportionally; radiographic density also increases. The direct proportional relationship between mAs and exposure is used to calculate mAs changes necessary to maintain consistent image density when one or more technical factors are altered. By maintaining a specific exposure relative to the speed of the image receptor, consistent image density can be achieved.

The relationship of a film's reaction to exposure was described in 1875 by Bunsen and Roscoe, who studied the reaction of photographic film to light and stated that the reaction of a photographic film to light is equal to the product of the intensity of the light and the duration of the exposure. This concept is known as the **reciprocity law**. When applied to x-rays, the reciprocity law can be restated as the density on an x-ray film should remain unchanged as long as the intensity and duration of the x-ray exposure (controlled by mAs) remains unchanged. This law generally is true for x-ray films exposed using intensifying screens, because most of the film's exposure is from light and not x-rays. The reciprocity law fails for exposures made at extremely short exposure times (less than 1/100 second) or extremely long exposure times (more than a few seconds). Under these circumstances, densities will be somewhat less than the exposures. Reciprocity law failure is not very significant in diagnostic radiology because exposure times are seldom at those extremes.

Radiographic density should remain unchanged as long as the total exposure to the film remains unchanged. If the mAs used to create one image is the same as the mAs used to create a second image of the same structure, then both images should have the same radiographic density. As long as mAs is constant, any combination of mA and exposure time values will create the same density. The radiographs in Figures 11–1A and 11–1B illustrate this point. Remember, accurate results will depend on using equipment that is properly calibrated. Equipment testing is an important part of a quality control program for the radiology department.

Radiographic density will increase to D_{max} when mAs increases and will decrease to near zero when mAs decreases. Either the mA or the exposure time or both may be increased or decreased to cause an increase or decrease in the mAs. The radiographs in Figure 11–1B and Figure 11–1C illustrate this point. When mAs is increased, the radiographic density on the film is increased. The resulting film is darker than the original. If the mAs is reduced by half, the resulting film will be lighter than the original image.

Milliamperage-second (mAs) is the primary controlling factor that will affect the x-ray quantity and radiographic density. The appropriate mAs should be selected to achieve an acceptable radiograph. The technologist is usually in control of the mAs selection. However, the equipment may exert automatic control when the technologist is using an automatic exposure control system, a computerized exposure system, or falling load generators.

Kilovoltage (kVp)

Kilovoltage (kVp) controls both the quantity and quality of the x-ray beam. **Increasing the kilovoltage on an x-ray control panel will cause an increase in the speed and energy of the electrons applied across the x-ray tube.** The space charge compensator corrects for the increase in speed of the electrons to maintain a constant number of electrons/second. The increased energy of the electrons results in the production of x-ray photons with greater energy. As x-ray photon energy increases, the penetrating ability of the photon increases. Kilovoltage affects the **quantity** of the x-ray beam because **more** interactions occur at the target as kVp increases, and it affects the **quality** of the x-ray beam because each electron has more energy, resulting in a beam with greater **penetrability**.

The quantity (intensity) of x-ray photons increases very quickly with increases in kVp. X-ray quantity is **approximately** directly proportional to the square of the ratio of the change in kVp. This means that as kVp is doubled, the amount of x-ray photons increases approximately four times. Although this can be mathematically expressed, this formula would have no practical application because it does not take into account the fact that changes in kVp have a significant effect on the penetrability of the beam.

Density Relationship to kVp

Both the quantity and quality of the x-ray beam will vary significantly with changes in the kilovoltage applied across the x-ray tube. As a result, kVp has a tremendous impact on radiographic density (Figures 11–2A and 11–2B). In addition, because changes in kilovoltage create changes in beam penetrability, kVp is the primary controller of the differences in radiographic densities. This is known as contrast. An increase in kVp causes an increase in penetrability, which will result in an image with less contrast. For the present discussion, the effect of kVp on density will be detailed. Contrast is discussed in Chapter 26.

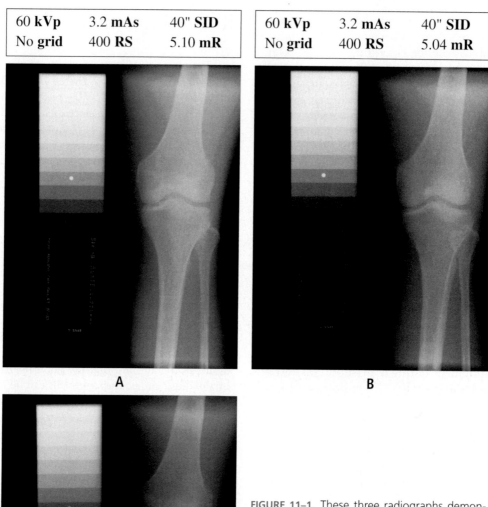

| 60 kVp | 3.2 mAs | 40" SID |
| No grid | 400 RS | 5.10 mR |

A

| 60 kVp | 3.2 mAs | 40" SID |
| No grid | 400 RS | 5.04 mR |

B

C

| 60 kVp | 6.4 mAs | 40" SID |
| No grid | 400 RS | 10.20 mR |

FIGURE 11–1. These three radiographs demonstrate the effect of mAs on radiographic density. Although the mA and time may vary, if the mAs remain unchanged, then radiographic density will be the same. A and B have the same mAs although A was exposed at 80 mA and 0.04 sec, while B was exposed at 160 mA and 0.02 sec. When the mAs is doubled, the exposure to the film doubles (C).

Research was done to determine a practical formula to take into account kVp's effect on both x-ray quantity and quality. This resulted in the **15 percent rule**. The intent of this rule was to provide a guide for radiographers to maintain density. **The 15 percent rule states that an increase in kVp by 15 percent will cause a doubling in exposure, the same effect as doubling the mA or doubling exposure time.** The reverse is also true. If kVp is decreased by 15 percent, exposure will be reduced by one half (Figure 11–2B and Figure 11–2C). Because both the amount and penetrability of x-ray photons increase with increases in kVp, the effect of changes in kVp will vary from low kVps to high kVps. In other words, a smaller change in kVp will have a greater impact on x-ray emission in the lower kVp ranges than in the higher kVp ranges. For example, 15 percent of 40 kVp is 6, while 15 percent of 80 kVp is 12. Exposure will nearly double when kVp is changed from 40 to 46 kVp. At 80 kVp, an increase in 12 kVp is needed to approximately double the exposure.

Example: A radiograph of the pelvis is produced using 25 mAs at 70 kVp. What kVp would be needed to double the exposure?

Answer:
>   15 percent of 70 kVp = 10.5 kVp
>   70 + 10.5 = 80.5 or 81 kVp

Since kVp is expressed as a whole number, answers should be rounded to the nearest whole number.

While kVp has a tremendous impact on radiographic density, **kVp adjustments should not be used to control radiographic density**. The selection of a kVp range for specific radiographic procedures is determined by the desired contrast for the image. This will be discussed in Unit IV.

Distance

The intensity of x-rays varies greatly with changes in distance. Just as the intensity of light from a light bulb will decrease the further one moves from the source, so will x-ray photons spread out from their source at the x-ray tube target. As a result, the x-ray intensity will decrease as the distance from the tube is increased. The measurement of the x-ray intensity is obtained using a dosimeter. X-ray intensity (exposure) is measured in roentgens (R) or, more commonly in diagnostic radiology, in milliroentgens (mR).

From the point of origin of the x-ray beam at the tube target, the beam begins to diverge. The x-ray photons are most concentrated at the target and from there they spread out in all directions. Those photons that exit the tube port constitute the primary, useful beam. As the useful beam spreads and widens, x-ray intensity or quantity begins to diminish. The actual number of photons created remains unchanged but the distribution of the photons varies with the distance. The further from their source, the lower will be the quantity of photons within a given area.

The relationship of x-ray quantity to distance is described in the inverse square law. **The inverse square law states that the intensity of radiation at a given distance from the point source is inversely proportional to the square of the distance.** The inverse square law requires an understanding of some basic rules of geometry. In Figure 11–3 the diverging lines represent the x-ray beam diverging from a collimated source. At a distance of 36 inches (D_1), the x-ray beam covers a square area (abcd). Each side has a given dimension (x) so the area of square abcd would equal x times x or x^2. If the distance is increased to 72 inches (D_2), the sides of the second square (ABCD) are now twice as long, or 2x. The area of square ABCD would be 2x times 2x or $4x^2$. A doubling of the distance has increased the area of the square by four times.

X-ray photons falling in square abcd are spread out over an area four times as large by the time it reaches square ABCD. The number of photons remains the same, but they are now spread over an area four times larger. A dosimeter in square abcd would measure four times more than a dosimeter in square ABCD. For example, if a dosimeter in square abcd measures 100 mR, a dosimeter in square ABCD would measure 25 mR, or four times less.

Thus the intensity or quantity of photons decreases with increased distance for a given area, which is an inverse relationship. More specifically, the relationship is inversely proportional to the square of the distance change. If the distance increases by a factor of three, the intensity would decrease by a factor of 3^2, or nine times.

70 kVp	1.0 mAs	40" SID
No grid	400 RS	4.10 mR

60 kVp	1.0 mAs	40" SID
No grid	400 RS	2.34 mR

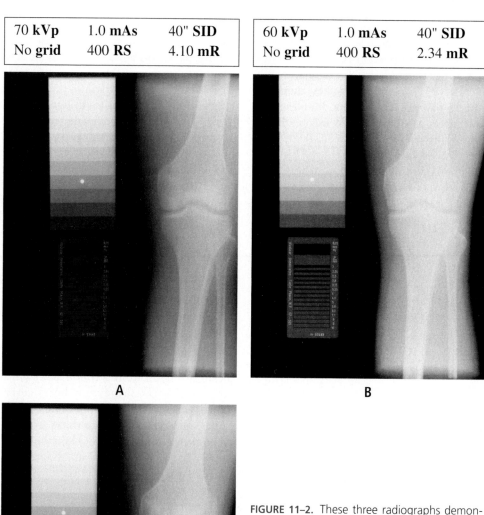

A

B

C

60 kVp	2.0 mAs	40" SID
No grid	400 RS	4.42 mR

FIGURE 11–2. These three radiographs demonstrate the effect of decreasing kVp on radiographic density. A and B show the effect of increasing kVp on density. In C, density is maintained by applying the 15 percent rule.

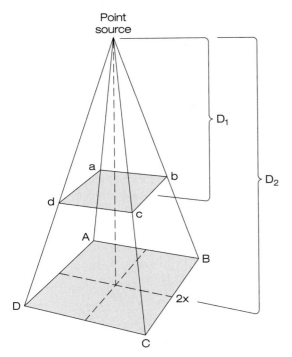

Point
source

D_1

a

b

D_2

d

c

A

B

D

2x

C

FIGURE 11–3. The inverse square law states that the intensity of radiation at a given distance from a point source is inversely proportional to the square of the distance. The lower surface area (ABCD) is twice as far from the source of radiation and is four times (2^2) the surface area of the upper surface area (abcd).

The inverse square law can be used to calculate changes in intensity that occur as a result of changes in distance. The mathematical expression of the law is:

$$\frac{I_1}{I_2} = \frac{D_2^{\,2}}{D_1^{\,2}}$$

where: I_1 = original intensity
I_2 = new intensity
D_1 = original distance
D_2 = new distance

The formula can also be expressed as:

$$I_1 D_1^{\,2} = I_2 D_2^{\,2}$$

In order to calculate any of the four factors, three of the four must be known. The equation can then be rearranged to place the unknown factor alone on one side of the equal sign.

Example: An x-ray exposure of 240 mR is recorded at a distance of 20 inches. If the same technical factors are used, what will the exposure be if the distance is increased to 40 inches?

Answer:

$$\frac{240}{I_2} = \frac{40^2}{20^2}$$

$$I_2 = \frac{240 \times 20^2}{40^2}$$

$$I_2 = \frac{240 \times 400}{1,600}$$

$$I_2 = 60 \ \text{mR}$$

Example: An x-ray exposure of 400 mR is recorded at a distance of 72 inches. If the same technical factors are used, what will the exposure be if the distance is decreased to 40 inches?

Answer:

$$\frac{400}{I_2} = \frac{40^2}{72^2}$$

$$I_2 = \frac{400 \times 72^2}{40^2}$$

$$I_2 = \frac{400 \times 5,184}{1,600}$$

$$I_2 = 1,296 \ \text{mR}$$

The inverse square law should be used when calculating the relationships between distance and x-ray intensity (mR).

Density Relationship to Distance

Since distance has an effect on x-ray intensity (exposure), it will in turn affect radiographic density. **As the distance increases, intensity decreases, which causes a**

decrease in density on the film (Figures 11–4A and 11–4B). The reverse is also true. As the distance decreases, intensity increases, which in turn causes an increase in radiographic density.

A practical application of the inverse square law is found in a formula which is used to compensate for the density changes that occur when distance is changed. The formula is sometimes known as the **density maintenance formula** and is based on the principle of the inverse square law. The density maintenance formula is a **direct square law**. A direct relationship is necessary to compensate for the changes in intensity and density.

Since mAs is the primary controller of x-ray intensity and radiographic density, mAs can be adjusted to compensate for changes in distance. For example, an acceptable chest film results from an exposure taken using four mAs at 100 kVp at a 72-inch distance. A second film must be taken supine at a 36-inch distance. If the same technical factors are used, the inverse square law tells us that when the distance is decreased by a factor of two, the intensity (exposure) will increase by a factor of four. The second film will be too dark if the technical factors are not adjusted. The mAs can be adjusted to compensate for the distance change. The density maintenance formula can be used to determine the compensation necessary for any change in distance (Figure 11–4B and Figure 11–4C). It is a direct square law because mAs should increase proportionally to the square of the change when distance increases, and mAs should decrease proportionally to the square of the change when distance is decreased. In the example above, if the distance decreases by a factor of two (72 inches to 36 inches), the mAs should be reduced by a factor of 2^2, or four. The new mAs would be 1/4th the original, or one mAs. Four mAs at 72 inches will produce the same exposure as one mAs at 36 inches, provided all other factors remain the same.

The density maintenance formula is:

$$\frac{mAs_1}{mAs_2} = \frac{D_1^2}{D_2^2}$$

where: mAs_1 = original mAs
mAs_2 = new mAs
D_1 = original distance
D_2 = new distance

The same formula can be expressed as:

$$mAs_2 = \frac{mAs_1 \times D_2^2}{D_1^2}$$

These formulas have very direct applications to radiography because they provide the radiographer with a means for adjusting mAs to maintain density when changes are made in distance for a given radiographic procedure.

Example: An acceptable radiograph of the abdomen is taken using 25 mAs at 80 kVp at a distance of 40 inches. A second radiograph is requested to be taken at 56 inches. What mAs should be used to produce an acceptable radiograph if the distance is increased to 56 inches?

Answer:

$$mAs_2 = \frac{25 \times 56^2}{40^2}$$
$$mAs_2 = \frac{25 \times 3,136}{1,600}$$
$$mAs_2 = 49 \text{ mAs}$$

Changes in distance will create changes in the x-ray intensity and the radiographic density. The density maintenance formula can be used to compensate for the effect that changes in distance will have on the density of the radiographic image. The radiographs of Figures 11–4A and C demonstrate the application of the direct square law for density maintenance.

Summary

Prime factors are under the direct control of the radiographer and have a significant impact on x-ray photon emission from the tube. The prime factors are milliamperage-second (mAs), kilovoltage (kVp) and distance (d). X-ray emission can be described in terms of both its quantity (amount) and quality (penetrability). X-ray quantity is affected by mAs, distance, kVp and filtration. X-ray quality is affected by kVp and filtration.

Milliamperage-second (mAs) is directly proportional to the number of x-ray photons created in the tube.

60 kVp	2 mAs	36" SID
No grid	400 RS	5.64 mR

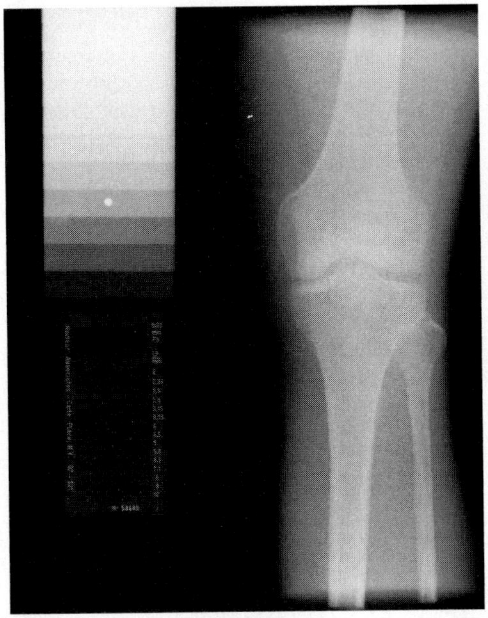

60 kVp	2.0 mAs	72" SID
No grid	400 RS	1.21 mR

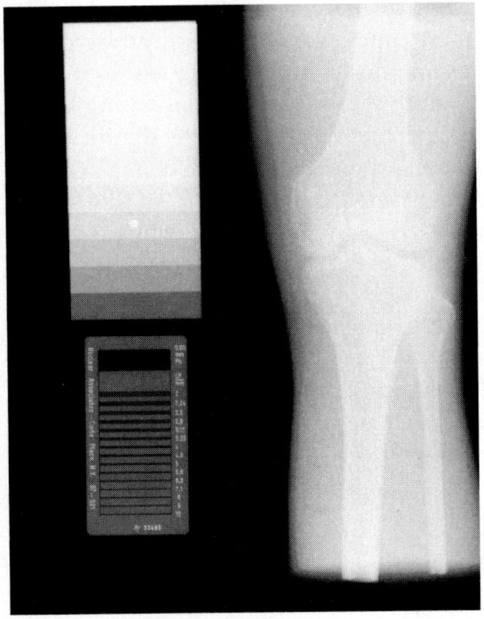

A

B

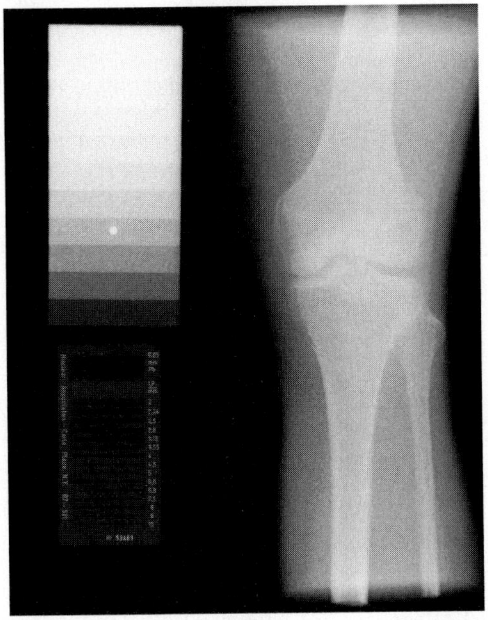

C

60 kVp	8 mAs	72" SID
No grid	400 RS	6.02 mR

FIGURE 11–4. These three radiographs demonstrate the effect of distance on radiographic density. A and B show the effect of increasing distance on density. In C, density is maintained by applying the density maintenance direct square law.

Kilovoltage affects both quantity and quality and its relationship to x-ray emission is not as easily described. Kilovoltage is approximately proportional to the square of the ratio of the change in kVp. Therefore, if kVp is doubled, the x-ray quantity would increase by a factor of four. This does not, however, take into account the increased penetrability of the beam with increasing kVp. As a result, radiographic density is more significantly affected. To maintain exposure with changes in kVp, the 15 percent rule can be applied. The 15 percent rule states that an increase in kVp by 15 percent will cause an approximate doubling of the exposure. To maintain density, if kVp is increased by 15 percent, the mAs must be reduced to one half its original value. The distance from the actual focal spot to the image receptor is the third prime factor. The quantity of x-ray photons is inversely proportional to the square of the distance. As distance increases, exposure will decrease in an inverse proportion to the square of the change in the distance.

REVIEW QUESTIONS

1. What are the three prime factors that affect x-ray emission?

2. What is the unit of measurement for x-ray quantity?

3. Define an ampere.

4. What is the relationship between mAs and radiographic density?

5. What effect does increased kVp have on the speed and energy of the electrons in the x-ray tube?

6. What is the relationship between kVp and radiographic density?

7. State the inverse square law.

8. What is the relationship between distance and radiographic density?

REFERENCES AND RECOMMENDED READING

American Registry of Radiologic Technologists. (1987). Use of 'penumbra' studied. *Radiologic Technology.* 58(1), 74.

Ball, J. & Price, T. (1989). *Chesneys' radiographic imaging.* Oxford: Blackwell Scientific Publishing.

Ball, J. L. & Moore, A. D. (1986). *Essential physics for radiographers* (2nd ed.). Oxford: Blackwell Scientific Publications.

Bushberg, J. T., Seibert, J. A., Leidholdt, E. M., & Boone, J. M. (1994). *The essential physics of medical imaging.* Baltimore: Williams & Wilkins.

Bushong, S. C. (1997). *Radiologic science for technologists: Physics, biology, and protection* (6th ed.). St. Louis: C. V. Mosby.

Carroll, Q. B. (1993). *Fuchs's radiographic exposure, processing, and quality control* (5th ed.). Springfield, IL: Charles C. Thomas Publishers.

Curry, T. S., Dowdey, J. E., & Murry, R. C. (1990). *Christensen's introduction to the physics of diagnostic radiology* (4th ed.). Philadelphia: Lea and Febiger.

Dendy, P. P. & Heaton, B. (1987). *Physics for radiologists.* Oxford: Blackwell Scientific Publications.

DeVos, D. C. (1995). *Basic principles of radiographic exposure* (2nd ed.). Philadelphia: Lea & Febiger.

Eastman Kodak Company, Health Sciences Markets Division. *The fundamentals of radiography* (12th ed.). Rochester, NY: Kodak Publication M1–18.

Eastman, T. R. (1979). *Radiographic fundamentals and technique guide.* St. Louis: C. V. Mosby Co.

Fodor, J. & Malott, J. C. (1992). *The art and science of medical radiography* (7th ed.). St. Louis: Catholic Health Association of the United States.

Fuchs, A. W. (1950). The rationale of radiographic exposure. *Radiologic Technology.* 22(2), 62.

Gifford, D. (1984). *A handbook of physics for radiologists and radiographers.* New York: John Wiley & Sons.

Glasser, O., Quimby, E. H., Taylor, L. S., Weatherwax, J. L., & Morgan, R. H. (1961). *Physical foundations of radiology* (3rd ed.). New York: Paul B. Hoeber Division of Harper & Brothers.

Graham, B. J. & Thomas, W. N. (1975). *An introduction to physics for radiologic technologists.* Philadelphia: W. B. Saunders.

Hay, G. A. & Hughes, D. (1972). *First-year physics for radiographers.* London: Baillierre Tindall.

Hiss, S. S. (1993). *Understanding radiography* (3rd ed.). Springfield, IL: Charles C. Thomas Publishers.

Irfan, A. Y., Pugh, V. I., & Jeffery, C. D. (1985). Some practical aspects of peak kilovoltage measurements. *Radiography. 51*(599), 251–254.

Jerman, E. C. (1926). An analysis of the end-result: The radiograph. *Radiology. 6*, 59–62.

Johns, H. E. & Cunningham, J. R. (1983). *The physics of radiology* (4th ed.). Springfield, IL: Thomas.

Koenig, G. F. (1966). Potential. *Radiologic Technology. 37*(4), 184–198.

Meredith, W. J. & Massey, J. B. (1977). *Fundamental physics of radiology* (3rd ed.). Chicago: Yearbook Medical Publishers.

Morgan, R. H. (1949). An analysis of the physical factors controlling the diagnostic quality of roentgen images: Part V. Unsharpness. *American Journal of Roentgenology and Radiation Therapy. 62*(6), 870–880.

Morgan, R. H. (1946). An analysis of the physical factors controlling the diagnostic quality of roentgen images: Part III. Contrast and the intensity distribution function of a Roentgen image. *American Journal of Roentgenology and Radiation Therapy. 55*(1), 67–89.

Morgan, R. H. (1945). An analysis of the physical factors controlling the diagnostic quality of roentgen images: Part I. Introduction. *American Journal of Roentgenology and Radiation Therapy. 54*(2), 128–135.

Morgan, R. H. (1945). An analysis of the physical factors controlling the diagnostic quality of roentgen images: Part II. Maximum resolving power and resolution coefficient. *American Journal of Roentgenology and Radiation Therapy. 54*(4), 395–402.

Ridgway, A. & Thumm, W. (1973). *The physics of medical radiography.* Reading, MA: Addison-Wesley.

Selman, J. (1994). *The fundamentals of x-ray and radium physics* (9th ed.). Springfield, IL: Thomas.

Sprawls, P. (1990). *Principles of radiography for technologists.* Rockville, MD: Aspen Publishers.

Sprawls, P. (1987). *Physical principles of medical imaging.* Rockville, MD: Aspen Publishers.

Stockley, S. M. (1986). *A manual of radiographic equipment.* Edinburgh: Churchill Livingstone.

Ter-Pogossian, M. M. (1967). *The physical aspects of diagnostic radiology.* New York: Hoeber Medical Division, Harper & Row.

Thompson, M. A., Hattaway, M. P., Hall, J. D., & Dowd, S. B. (1994). *Principles of imaging science and protection.* Philadelphia: W. B. Saunders.

van der Plaats, G. J. (1980). *Medical x-ray techniques in diagnostic radiology* (4th ed.). The Hague: Martinus Nijhoff Publishers.

Wilks, R. J. (1981). *Principles of radiological physics.* Edinburgh: Churchill Livingstone.

Wolbarst, A. B. (1993). *Physics of radiology.* Norwalk, CT: Appleton & Lange.

CHAPTER **12**

X-Ray Interactions

Perhaps no single field of investigation has contributed more to our knowledge of atomic structure than has the study of x-rays.

Arthur H. Compton, preface to the first edition of *X-Rays and Electrons*.

Objectives

Upon completion of this chapter, the student should be able to:

▶ Define attenuation.

▶ Explain the interactions between x-rays and matter in the following:
photoelectric absorption
coherent scattering
Compton scattering
pair production
photodisintegration

▶ Describe the relationship between x-ray interactions and technical factor selections.

X-Ray Interaction with Matter

When an x-ray beam passes through matter, it undergoes a process called attenuation. Attenuation is the reduction in the number of x-ray photons in the beam, and subsequent loss of energy, as the beam passes through matter (Figure 12–1).

Attenuation is the result of x-ray photons interacting with matter and losing energy through these interactions. While some photons will pass through matter and not interact, an x-ray photon can interact with the whole atom, an orbital electron or directly with the nucleus. This will depend on the energy of the photon. Low-energy photons are most likely to interact with the whole atom, intermediate-energy photons generally interact with orbital electrons while very high-energy photons, such as those used for radiation therapy, are capable of interacting with the nucleus. In the diagnostic x-ray range, the interactions are most commonly with orbital electrons.

To fully understand x-ray interactions with matter, it is important to recall the structure of the atom. The center of the atom is a positively charged nucleus containing protons and neutrons. The negatively charged electrons are in orbital paths around the nucleus. The energy required to remove an electron from a shell is termed the binding energy of the shell. The K-shell electrons possess the highest binding energy for a given atom and binding energies decrease progressively for successive shells. Not only is the binding energy characteristic of a given shell, it is also specific to a given atom. K-shell electrons are more tightly bound to the nucleus in high atomic number elements. For example, the binding energy for the K-shell of tungsten (Z = 74) is approximately 70 keV while the binding energy for the K-shell of calcium (Z = 20) is only about 4 keV. The average atom in the soft tissue of the body has an approximate K-shell binding energy of only 0.5 keV. Therefore, **the higher the atomic number of an element, the more energy will be required to remove a K-shell electron from the atom.**

Because electrons that are further from the nucleus are not bound as tightly, they require less energy to remove them from their orbit. Therefore, they possess a greater total energy. Electrons that are closer to the nucleus are bound more tightly and require more energy to remove them from their position. If a free (unbound) electron is assumed to possess a total energy (ability to do work) of zero, then a bound electron would have a total energy of zero minus the binding energy. **The further an electron is from the nucleus, the higher the total energy of the electron will be.** This means that K- shell electrons possess less (more negative) total energy than outer shell electrons. As a result, when an outer shell electron moves into an inner shell, it will release energy equal to the difference between the binding energies of the two shells.

Electrons in the K-shell have the lowest energy total with the highest binding energy, and with each successive shell, **total electron energies increase and binding energies decrease**. These concepts are particularly important to the understanding of x-ray interactions with matter.

There are five basic interactions between x-rays and matter:

1. photoelectric absorption,

2. coherent scattering,

3. Compton scattering,

4. pair production and

5. photodisintegration.

With each of these interactions the x-ray photons either interact and change direction, a process called **scattering**, or are absorbed by the atom. When a photon is absorbed, all of the energy of the photon is transferred to the matter and the photon no longer exists. If a photon interacts and scatters, the photon still exists but usually possesses less energy than before the interaction. Partial energy from the photon is transferred to the matter during the interaction and the lower-energy photon then continues along its new path until again it either interacts and scatters or is absorbed. One photon may scatter several times before it is finally absorbed completely by the matter. The likelihood of one interaction occurring over another varies, depending on the incident photon's energy and the atomic number of the matter. Certain interactions, pair production and photodisintegration, for example, occur only at very high photon energy ranges, while coherent scatter is most predominant in very low photon energy ranges.

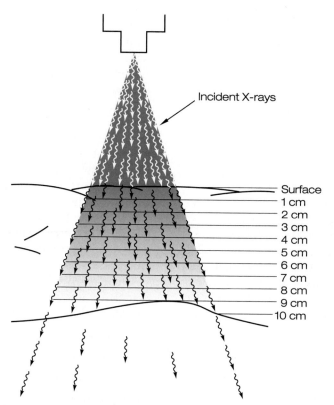

FIGURE 12–1. An x-ray beam undergoes attenuation as it passes through matter.

Photoelectric Absorption

Photoelectric absorption results when an x-ray photon interacts with an inner-shell electron. This interaction is most likely to occur when the incident x-ray photon possesses a slightly greater energy than the binding energy of the electrons in the inner (K or L) shells. The incident photon ejects the electron from its inner shell and is totally absorbed in the interaction (Figure 12–2). The result is an ionized atom, because of the missing inner-shell electron, and an ejected electron, called a **photoelectron**. The photoelectron travels with kinetic energy, which is equal to the difference between the incident photon and the binding energy of the inner-shell electron. This is mathematically expressed in the equation:

$$E_i = E_b + E_{ke}$$

where: E_i = energy of the incident photon
E_b = binding energy of the electron
E_{ke} = kinetic energy of the photoelectron

The incident photon needs an energy which is slightly greater than the binding energy of the electron for the interaction to occur. Since most of the atoms of the body are very low atomic number elements, the binding energies of the K-shell electrons are very low. For example, the K-shell binding energy for carbon is approximately 0.28 keV and oxygen is 0.53 keV. The K-shell binding energies of elements which are important in diagnostic radiology are listed in Table 12–1. Most photoelectric interactions in the body result in the majority of the incident photon energy being given to the kinetic energy of the photoelectron. The photoelectron is matter, not just energy, and therefore will not travel far. It is usually absorbed within 1 to 2 mm in soft tissue. Despite the

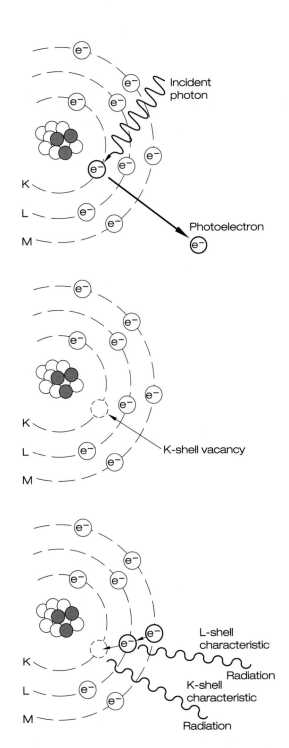

FIGURE 12–2. The photoelectric absorption interaction.

localized absorption, this is still a significant way in which x-ray energy can create biological changes.

The ionized atom is in an unstable state with an inner-shell electron missing. The vacancy is instantly filled by an electron from the L-shell or, less commonly, from an M-shell or free electron. In the vast majority of cases the electron transfers from an outer shell to an inner shell and, as it does, it releases energy in the form of a **characteristic photon**, known as **secondary radiation**. This secondary radiation is produced in the same manner as characteristic radiation is produced at the x-ray target—electron transfer from one shell to another. When it is created at the x-ray target it is considered primary radiation. When characteristic radiation is produced in irradiated matter outside of the x-ray target it is termed secondary radiation. Remember that outer-shell electrons possess a higher energy level than inner-shell electrons. Therefore when an outer-shell electron moves into an inner shell it has excess energy to release. This electron transfer process continues from shell to shell until the atom returns to a normal state and is no longer a positive ion. This process of each shell filling lower shells with a corresponding emission of photons is called a characteristic cascade. The energy of each photon of a **characteristic cascade** will be characteristic of the difference in energy in the two shells between which it dropped.

TABLE 12–1. K-Shell Binding Energies of Radiologically Significant Elements

Atom	Atomic Number	K-shell Binding Energies (keV)
Hydrogen	1	0.016
Carbon	6	0.284
Oxygen	8	0.53
Aluminum	13	1.56
Calcium	20	4.04
Molybdenum	42	20.0
Iodine	53	33.2
Barium	56	37.4
Tungsten	74	69.5
Lead	82	88.0

Because of the predominance of low atomic number elements comprising the human body, the secondary radiation produced is of extremely low energy. Secondary radiation energies are significantly higher for elements such as iodine and barium, which are commonly used as contrast agents in radiology.

There are three basic rules which govern the possibility of a photoelectric interaction:

1. **The incident x-ray photon energy must be greater than the binding energy of the inner-shell electron.** A 30 keV x-ray photon will not be able to remove the K-shell electron from an atom of iodine, which has a binding energy of 33.2 keV, or barium, which has a binding energy of 37.4 keV.

2. **A photoelectric interaction is more likely to occur when the x-ray photon energy and the electron binding energy are nearer to one another.** Of course, the x-ray photon energy must always be greater, but a 40 keV photon is more likely to interact by way of the photoelectric effect with an atom of iodine (K-shell E_b = 33.2 keV) or barium (K-shell E_b = 37.4 keV) than would a 100 keV x-ray photon. As photon energy increases, the chance of a photoelectric interaction decreases dramatically. The actual relationship is expressed as an inverse proportion to approximately the third power of the photon energy (photoelectric effect = $1/(energy)^3$). A significant change is therefore seen in the percentage of photoelectric interactions that will occur when using low kVp techniques versus high kVp techniques. Table 12–2 demonstrates that at 50 kVp, the percent of photon interactions that undergo photoelectric absorption is 50.45 percent with scatter interactions occurring at 49.55 percent. As the kVp increases, the percent of photon interactions by photoelectric absorption decreases. At 130 kVp, photoelectric absorption accounts for only 24.78 percent of the interactions with matter. These concepts become very important to the radiographer when establishing appropriate technical factors for specific body tissues.

3. **A photoelectric interaction is more likely to occur with an electron which is more tightly bound in its orbit.** Binding energies of the electrons are greater in high atomic number elements than in low atomic number elements. In addition, inner-shell electrons have higher binding energies than outer-shell electrons in a given atom. With low atomic number elements, most interactions will occur with the K-shell electron. Because high atomic number elements bind their electrons more tightly, interactions will occur with the K-, L-, and M-shells. In fact, the incident x-ray photon often does not possess sufficient energy to remove a K-shell electron. For example, the K-shell binding energy for lead is 88 keV. X-ray photons below this level are incapable of removing the K-shell electrons but can be absorbed through photoelectric interactions with L- or M-shell electrons. The probability of a photoelectric interaction increases dramatically as the atomic number increases. The relationship is approximately proportional to the third power of the atomic number (photoelectric effect = (atomic number)^3). Since bone has an effective atomic number which is higher than that of soft tissue, photoelectric interactions are more likely to occur in bone than in soft tissue. **It is for this reason that radiography is so spectacularly useful in demonstrating the bones of the body.**

Coherent Scattering

Coherent scatter is an interaction which occurs between very low-energy x-ray photons and matter. It is also called classical scatter or unmodified scatter. There are actually two types of coherent scattering: Thomson scattering and Rayleigh scattering. Thomson scattering involves a single electron in the interaction while Rayleigh scattering involves all of the electrons of the atom in the interaction. Both types have the same basic interaction results.

TABLE 12–2. Percentage of Photon Interactions, Attenutation, and Transmission Characteristics in Soft Tissue Based on Effective Photon Energies

kVp	50	70	80	90	110	130
HVL(mm Al)	1.59	2.11	2.35	2.60	3.12	3.67
Mean Photon Energy (keV)	31.3	40.0	41.1	44.2	49.7	54.5
Effective Photon Energy (keV)	27.0	30.0	31.0	33.0	35.0	38.0
% of Photon Interactions by						
—Scattering (with coherent)	49.55%	62.70%	63.95%	66.70%	69.77%	75.22%
—Photoelectric	50.45%	37.30%	36.05%	33.30%	30.23%	24.78%
% Attenuation						
5 cm Tissue	91.45%	84.28%	83.45%	81.67%	79.70%	76.34%
10 cm Tissue	99.27%	97.53%	97.26%	96.64%	95.88%	94.40%
15 cm Tissue	99.94%	99.61%	99.55%	99.38%	99.16%	98.67%
20 cm Tissue	99.99%	99.94%	99.93%	99.89%	99.83%	99.69%
% Transmission						
5 cm Tissue	8.55%	15.72%	16.55%	18.33%	20.30%	23.66%
10 cm Tissue	0.73%	2.47%	2.74%	3.36%	4.12%	5.60%
15 cm Tissue	0.06%	0.39%	0.45%	0.62%	0.84%	1.33%
20 cm Tissue	0.01%	0.06%	0.07%	0.11%	0.17%	0.31%

Courtesy of Raymond P. Rossi, University of Colorado Health Science Center.

When a very low-energy photon, below approximately 10 keV, interacts with the electron(s) in an atom, it may cause the electron(s) to vibrate at the same frequency as the incident photon. The vibrating or excited atom immediately releases this excess energy by producing a secondary photon which has the same energy and wavelength as the incident photon but which travels in a direction different from the initial photon (Figure 12–3). The result is a scattered photon which possesses the same energy, frequency and wavelength as the initial photon but which is traveling in a different direction. Since there is no energy transferred in the interaction, the atom is not ionized in the process.

Coherent scattering occurs in a very low x-ray energy range which is generally outside the usual range for diagnostic imaging. A very small amount of the scatter radiation reaching the film is produced by this process and, as a result, this interaction has little significance to diagnostic imaging.

Compton Scattering

Compton scattering occurs when an incident x-ray photon interacts with a loosely bound outer-shell electron, removes the electron from its shell, and then proceeds in a different direction as a scattered photon (Figure 12–4). This interaction was described by the American Nobel laureate physicist Arthur H. Compton (1892–1962) in 1922 and is known as the **Compton effect**. Part of the energy of the incident photon is used to remove the outer-shell electron and impart kinetic energy to it. The dislodged electron is called a **Compton or recoil electron**. The photon which exits the atom in a different direction is called a **Compton scattered photon**. It possesses less energy than the incident photon and therefore has a lower frequency and longer wavelength.

The energy transfer in the Compton effect is mathematically expressed in the equation:

$$E_i = E_s + E_b + E_{ke}$$

where: E_i = energy of the incident photon
E_s = energy of the Compton scattered photon
E_b = electron binding energy of the Compton electron
E_{ke} = kinetic energy given to the Compton electron

The incident photon energy is divided between the ejected electron and the scattered photon. The scattered photon retains most of the energy because little energy is needed to eject an outer-shell electron, due to its low binding energy. The scattered photon will continue to interact with atoms until it is eventually absorbed photoelectrically. The recoil electron is available as a free electron to fill a shell "hole" created by another ionizing interaction.

The amount of energy retained by the scattered photon is dependent on the initial energy of the photon and its angle of deflection from the recoil electron. The higher the initial energy of the photon, the greater the energy of the scattered photon. Scattered photons can be deflected at any angle from the recoil electron, just as a cue ball is deflected after it strikes a second ball in a game of billiards. At a deflection of 0°, no energy is transferred because the photon is proceeding in its original direction. As the angle of deflection increases to 180°, more energy is imparted to the recoil electron and less energy remains with the scattered photon (Figure 12–5).

When a scattered photon is deflected back toward the source, it is traveling in the direction opposite to the incident photon. These photons are called **backscatter radiation**. Most photons will scatter in a more forward direction, especially when incident photon energy increases.

In Figure 12–5, the innermost ring represents the highest energy level and the scattered photons are all deflected in a forward direction. The third inner ring

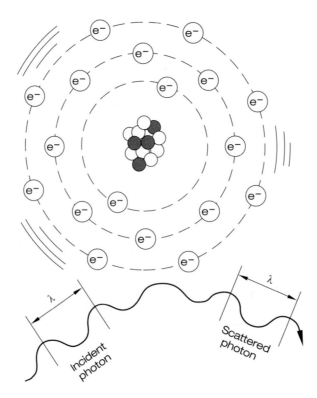

FIGURE 12–3. The coherent scatter interaction.

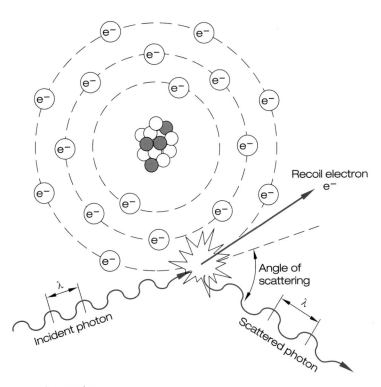

FIGURE 12–4. The Compton scatter interaction.

represents a typical x-ray exposure with an average effective photon energy of 50 keV. While a small number of photons are undergoing backscatter, the majority of the scatter is projected in a forward direction toward the image receptor. For this reason, scatter has a serious impact on image quality.

Scattered Compton photons possess an energy high enough to create a radiation hazard, and to impair image quality. Scatter radiation emitted from the patient is the primary cause of occupational radiation exposure to the radiographer and is therefore the primary reason for wearing protective devices, such as lead aprons and gloves, and for providing protective shielding for the x-ray room. Scatter also adds unwanted density to the radiographic image. These unwanted densities, caused predominantly by scattered photons and less commonly by secondary photons, are called **radiation fog**. Because scatter is coming from all directions, the scattered photons which strike the film place a density on the film which is unrelated to the patient's anatomy. Radiographic grids are devices designed to remove unwanted scatter and improve radiographic image quality.

Pair Production

In a pair production interaction the energy of the x-ray photon is converted to matter in the form of two electrons. For this interaction to occur, a very high-energy photon with an energy of at least 1.02 MeV is required. This is because the energy equivalent of the mass of one electron at rest is equal to 0.51 MeV. During this interaction, a high-energy incident photon comes close to the strong nuclear field and loses all its energy in the interaction. This energy is used to create a pair of electrons, one with a negative charge, a **negatron**, and the other with a positive charge, a **positron** (Figure

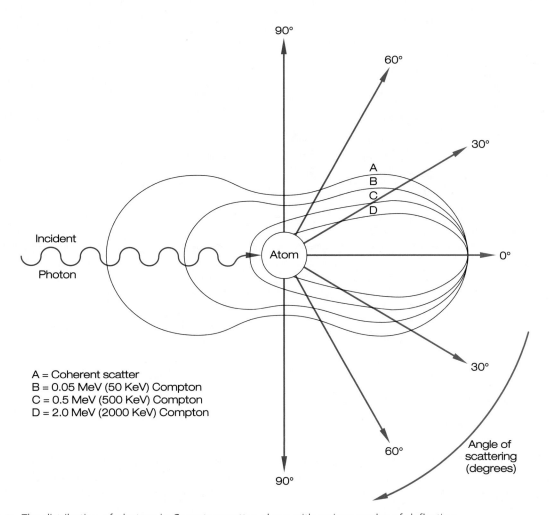

FIGURE 12–5. The distribution of photons in Compton scatter, along with various angles of deflection.

12–6). Since a negative electron is common in nature it is quickly absorbed by other nearby atoms. A positron, because of its unique configuration, with some of the characteristics of a proton, is extremely volatile. It comes to rest and combines with a negative electron nearly instantaneously. When these two particles combine, they disappear and give rise to two photons moving in opposite directions and each possessing energies of 0.51 MeV. This process is called the **annihilation reaction** because matter is being converted back to energy. Pair production requires a minimum incident photon energy of 1.02 MeV but doesn't become a significant interaction until

approximately 10 MeV. Therefore, it does not occur in the diagnostic x-ray imaging range.

Photodisintegration

Photodisintegration is an interaction between an extremely high-energy photon, above approximately 10 MeV, and the nucleus. In this interaction, the high-energy photon strikes the nucleus and all of its energy is absorbed by the nucleus, thereby exciting it. The excited

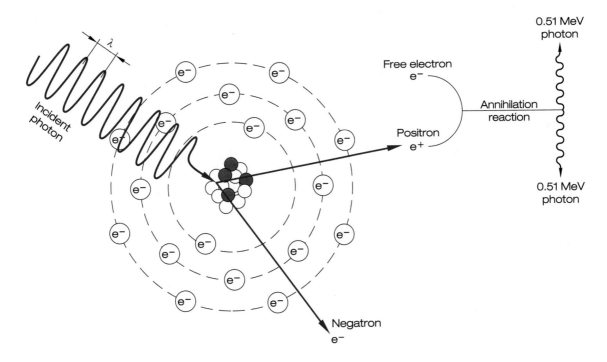

FIGURE 12–6. The pair production interaction.

nucleus responds by emitting a nuclear fragment (Figure 12–7). Because of the high energy level needed to cause this interaction, it is not relevant to diagnostic imaging.

Effect on Technical Factor Selection

Of the five interactions between x-ray and matter, only two have a significant impact on an x-ray image. These two interactions, photoelectric absorption and Compton scattering, must be considered by the radiographer when technical factors are selected.

It is important to remember that in the diagnostic x-ray range the majority of the x-ray beam is attenuated and only a small percentage of photons exit to create the image. Refer to Table 12–2. For a 10 cm tissue exposed at 50 kVp, 99.27 percent of the beam will be attenuated and 0.73 percent of the beam will be transmitted to interact with the image receptor. At 130 kVp, the same

10 cm tissue will attenuate only 94.40 percent of the beam and 5.60 percent of the beam will be transmitted. Obviously, it would be necessary to reduce the overall number of photons (mAs) when the kVp is increased, if the radiographer wants to maintain the same exit dose to the image receptor.

As kVp increases, the total number of photons which are transmitted without interaction increases. This means that the probability of photoelectric and Compton interactions decreases with increasing kVp. A shift does occur, however, in the percentages of photoelectric versus Compton interactions with increased kVp. **The percentage of photoelectric interactions decreases with increased kVp and the percentage of Compton interactions increases with increased kVp.** As a result, as kVp increases, there is an increased percentage of scatter and a decreased percentage of absorption of the attenuated beam. For example, in Table 12–2, for a 5 cm tissue exposed at 50 kVp, 91.45 percent of the beam is attenuated and 8.55 percent is transmitted. At 130 kVp, the same 5 cm tissue will attenuate only 76.34

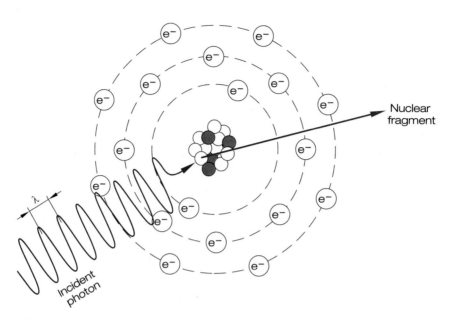

FIGURE 12–7. The photodisintegration interaction.

percent of the beam and 23.66 percent will be transmitted. At 50 kVp, of the 91.45 percent that was attenuated, 50.45 percent of the interactions were photoelectric absorption and 49.55 percent were scatter. At 130 kVp, the overall percent of attenuation decreases (76.34 percent), but most of the interactions are now scatter interactions (75.22 percent) instead of photoelectric absorption (24.78 percent).

In the human body, Compton scattering is the predominant interaction through most of the diagnostic x-ray range. Photoelectric interactions predominate in two circumstances: 1) in the lower-energy ranges (25–45 keV) produced by 40–70 kVp, and 2) when high atomic number elements are introduced, such as the contrast agents iodine and barium. Iodine and barium serve as useful contrast agents because they absorb a greater percentage of the photons through photoelectric interactions. These differences in absorption between the contrast agents and the soft tissues are responsible for creating the visible radiographic image.

Figure 12–8 shows the percent attenuation by photoelectric absorption on the scale on the left and the percent attenuation by Compton scatter on the scale on the right. In the diagnostic x-ray range, for bone and soft tissue, photoelectric absorption predominates at lower energies and then Compton scatter begins to predominate. For high atomic number materials, such as sodium iodine (NaI), barium and lead, photoelectric absorption is the predominant if not exclusive interaction. For this reason, as stated, iodine and barium serve as useful contrast agents and lead serves as a useful material for radiation protection.

When just comparing body tissues, in soft tissue (water) interactions are about 50/50 photoelectric absorption vs. Compton at approximately 26 keV. In bone, interactions are about 50/50 photoelectric absorption vs. Compton at approximately 45 keV (Figure 12–9).

When the photoelectric effect is more prevalent, the resulting radiographic image will possess high contrast. High-contrast images have great differences in densities from white to black, with fewer gray shades in between. This high contrast is the result of the complete absorption of the incident photons without the creation of undesirable scatter to fog the film. High-contrast images can be created by selecting low kVp/high mAs technical factors and through the introduction of contrast agents. In both of these instances, the photoelectric effect will be more predominant. Remember that as the percentage of photoelectric interactions increases so does the absorp-

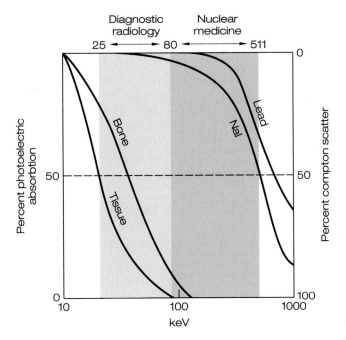

FIGURE 12–8. Percent contribution of photoelectric (left scale) and Compton (right scale) attenuation processes for various tissue as a function of energy. When diagnostic energy photons interact with low Z materials (e. g., soft tissue), the Compton process dominates. *(Reprinted with permission from Bushberg, J. T. et al. [1994]. The Essential Physics of Medical Imaging. Baltimore: Williams & Wilkins.)*

tion of radiation by the patient. This increases the likelihood of biological effects. Therefore, high-contrast, low kVp/high mAs techniques tend to result in higher patient doses.

When Compton interactions prevail, the resulting radiographic image will possess lower contrast. Low-contrast images have very small differences between densities, with more gray shades in between. Low-contrast images can be created by using high kVp/low mAs techniques because Compton interactions predominate as kVp increases. Scatter from Compton interactions is a significant cause of the lower-contrast images. However, low-contrast, high kVp/low mAs techniques tend to reduce patient dose.

Summary

As an x-ray beam passes through matter it undergoes attenuation, which is the reduction in the number of x-ray photons in the beam as it passes through a given thickness of matter. Attenuation is the result of x-rays interacting with matter by way of one of five types of interactions.

The five basic interactions between x-ray and matter are photoelectric absorption, coherent scattering, Compton scattering, pair production and photodisintegration. Only two are significant interactions within the diagnostic range of x-rays. These are photoelectric absorption and Compton scattering. Photoelectric absorption results when an x-ray photon interacts with an inner-shell electron. The incident photon is completely absorbed by the ejection of the electron, which then possesses kinetic energy and is called a photoelectron. The atom is ionized in the process and extremely unstable. The void in the inner shell is filled by the transfer of an electron from an outer shell. As the electron moves into the inner shell it releases a photon, which is characteristic for a given atom. Characteristic photons created in irradiated material by way of the photoelectric effect are called secondary radiation.

Compton scattering is an interaction between an x-ray photon and an outer-shell electron. The incident

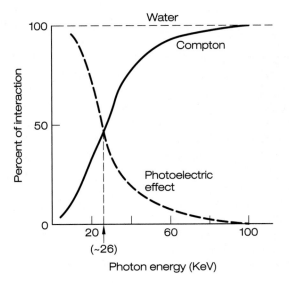

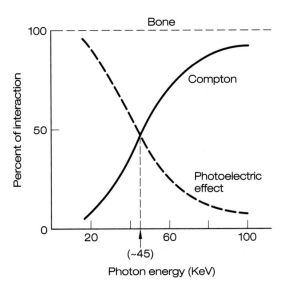

FIGURE 12–9. The relative percentages of photoelectric absorption and Compton scatter in water and bone.

photon ejects the outer-shell electron (Compton or recoil electron). The incident photon loses energy and as a result changes direction or scatters. The scattered photons have sufficient energy to interact again and again. Scatter radiation is the reason for wearing radiation protection devices and for shielding x-ray rooms. Scatter

also adds unwanted densities to the film, which impairs image quality.

Image contrast is affected by the most predominant x-ray interaction. High-contrast images will result when the photoelectric effect is prevalent and low-contrast images will result when Compton scatter is more common. In addition, patient dose is increased when photoelectric interactions prevail. As kVp increases, more photons are transmitted without interaction and patient dose decreases as a result.

REVIEW QUESTIONS

1. Define attenuation.
2. Describe the photoelectric absorption interaction.
3. Describe the coherent scatter interaction.
4. Describe the Compton scatter interaction.
5. What is backscatter?
6. What are the two interactions which have a significant impact on the radiographic image?
7. What type of radiographic contrast will result if the prevalent interaction is photoelectric absorption?
8. What type of radiographic contrast will result if the prevalent interaction is Compton scatter?

REFERENCES AND RECOMMENDED READING

Ball, J. & Price, T. (1989). *Chesneys' radiographic imaging* Oxford: Blackwell Scientific Publishing.

Ball, J. L. & Moore, A. D. (1986). *Essential physics for radiographers* (2nd ed.). Oxford: Blackwell Scientific Publications.

Bushberg, J. T., Seibert, J. A., Leidholdt, E. M., & Boone, J. M. (1994). *The essential physics of medical imaging.* Baltimore: Williams & Wilkins.

Bushong, S. C. (1997). *Radiologic science for technologists: Physics, biology, and protection* (6th ed.). St. Louis: C. V. Mosby.

Compton, A. H. & Allison, H. K. (1935). *X-rays in theory and experiment* (2nd ed.). New York: Van Nostrand.

Curry, T. S., Dowdey, J. E., Murry, R. C. (1990). *Christensen's introduction to the physics of diagnostic radiology* (4th ed.). Philadelphia: Lea and Febiger.

Dendy, P. P. & Heaton, B. (1987). *Physics for radiologists*. Oxford: Blackwell Scientific Publications.

Fewell, T. R. & Shuping, R. E. (1977). Photon energy distribution of some typical diagnostic x-ray beams. *Medical Physics. 4*(3), 187–197.

Gifford, D. (1984). *A handbook of physics for radiologists and radiographers*. New York: John Wiley & Sons.

Glasser, O., Quimby, E. H., Taylor, L. S., Weatherwax, J. L., & Morgan, R. H. (1961). *Physical foundations of radiology* (3rd ed.). New York: Paul B. Hoeber Division of Harper & Brothers.

Graham, B. J. & Thomas, W. N. (1975). *An introduction to physics for radiologic technologists*. Philadelphia: W. B. Saunders.

Hay, G. A. & Hughes, D. (1972). *First-year physics for radiographers*. London: Bailliere Tindall.

Hendee, W. R & Ritenour, R. (1993). *Medical imaging physics* (3rd ed.). St. Louis: C. V. Mosby.

Herman, M. W. (1980). A comparative study of scattered radiation levels from 80 kVp and 240 kVp x-rays in the surgical ICU. *Radiology. 552.*

Johns, H. E. & Cunningham, J. R. (1983). *The physics of radiology* (4th ed.). Springfield, IL: Thomas.

Meredith, W. J. & Massey, J. B. (1977). *Fundamental physics of radiology* (3rd ed.). Chicago: Yearbook Medical Publishers.

Ridgway, A. & Thumm, W. (1973). *The physics of medical radiography*. Reading, MA: Addison-Wesley.

Selman, J. (1994). *The fundamentals of x-ray and radium physics* (9th ed.). Springfield, IL: Thomas.

Sprawls, P. (1990). *Principles of radiography for technologists*. Rockville, MD: Aspen Publishers.

Sprawls, P. (1987). *Physical principles of medical imaging*. Rockville, MD: Aspen Publishers.

Stears, J. G., Gray, J. E., & Frank, E. D. (1990). Radiologic Exchange (scatter radiation). *Radiologic Technology. 61*(3), 221–224.

Ter-Pogossian, M. M. (1967). *The physical aspects of diagnostic radiology*. New York: Hoeber Medical Division, Harper & Row.

Thompson, M. A., Hattaway, M. P., Hall, J. D., & Dowd, S. B. (1994). *Principles of imaging science and protection*. Philadelphia: W. B. Saunders.

Tortorici, M. (1992). *Concepts in medical radiographic imaging*. Philadelphia: W. B. Saunders.

van der Plaats, G. J. (1980). *Medical x-ray techniques in diagnostic radiology* (4th ed.). The Hague: Martinus Nijhoff Publishers.

Wilks, R. J. (1981). *Principles of radiological physics*. Edinburgh: Churchill Livingstone.

Wilson, P. (1977). The interaction of x-radiation and matter. *Canadian Journal of Radiography, Radiotherapy, and Nuclear Medicine. 8*(2), 76–95.

Wolbarst, A. B. (1993). *Physics of radiology*. Norwalk, CT: Appleton & Lange.

CHAPTER 13

Minimizing Patient Dose

I became acquainted very early with the destructive effect of roentgen rays upon living tissue. In fact, it was only a few months after the announcement of Röntgen's discovery that I required medical care for a roentgen burn covering most of the back of one hand.

W. D. Coolidge, "Experiences with the Roentgen-ray tube."

Objectives

Upon completion of this chapter, the student should be able to:

▶ Explain the relationship of entrance skin exposure to other measurement points.

▶ Calculate mR/mAs from a calibration exposure total.

▶ Calculate total entrance skin exposure when given subject part thickness, SID, kVp, mAs and an mR/mAs chart.

▶ Describe typical entrance skin exposures for common radiographic procedures.

▶ Discuss methods of reducing patient dose through effective communication.

▶ Describe various methods of reducing patient dose through effective positioning.

▶ Explain the interrelationship of the prime factors.

▶ Evaluate various exposure factors for the most effective methods of reducing patient dose under various clinical conditions.

▶ Describe an effective method of minimizing patient dose by emphasizing radiation risk factors.

▶ Describe an effective method of maximizing patient diagnostic information by emphasizing radiation benefit factors.

▶ Analyze various approaches to discussing radiation risk versus benefit with patients, physicians and radiologists.

*A*predominant concern of radiographers is how to reduce the radiation dose to the patient. This concern is reflected in every decision made, especially when choosing technique exposure factors. The conscientious radiographer can reduce the patient dose by at least 50 percent in most examinations by choosing appropriate exposure factors.

Although exposure and dose are often used interchangeably, exposure (R) refers to radiation intensity in air, while dose (rad) is a measure of the radiation absorbed as a result of a radiation exposure. Dose is used to identify the irradiation of patients. Exposure (R) is used to calculate entrance skin exposure (ESE) in irradiated patients. Patient dose is usually estimated by conducting phantom experiments.

One of the most important characteristics of the professional is the ability to decide when it is appropriate to tip the radiation benefit versus risk issue in favor of the risk by reducing the patient dose while compromising the diagnostic quality of the image, and when to tip the issue in favor of the benefit by increasing the patient dose while maintaining the diagnostic quality of the image. There are circumstances that dictate when each choice should be made, and this chapter will attempt to lay the foundation necessary to make these decisions.

Estimating Approximate Entrance Skin Exposure

Figure 13–1 illustrates a typical radiographic examination with the exposure indicated at various points. It is obvious that the maximum exposure received by the patient is not at the area of interest but at the skin entrance to the body. This is known as the **entrance skin exposure** and is calculated at the minimum SOD. Note that the minimum SOD is not equal to the SOD of the area of interest and that the entrance skin receives a greater exposure. Although radiobiologists and physicists often discuss organ doses and gonadal doses, the entrance skin exposure is the most common expression

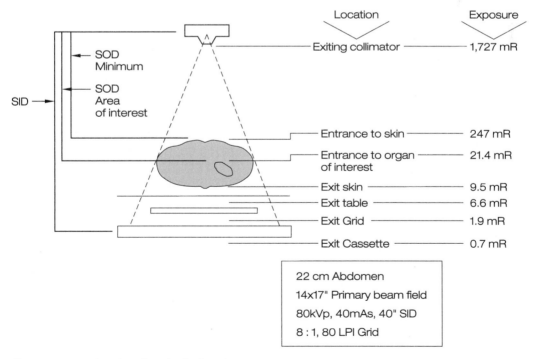

Location	Exposure
Exiting collimator	1,727 mR
Entrance to skin	247 mR
Entrance to organ of interest	21.4 mR
Exit skin	9.5 mR
Exit table	6.6 mR
Exit Grid	1.9 mR
Exit Cassette	0.7 mR

22 cm Abdomen

14x17" Primary beam field

80kVp, 40mAs, 40" SID

8 : 1, 80 LPI Grid

FIGURE 13–1. Exposures at various locations in the imaging process.

to approximate patient exposure because it is safer to assume a maximum effect when attempting to minimize exposure to ionizing radiation.

Diagnostic Radiography mR/mAs Charts

Exposure to patients can be estimated by recording mR/mAs when the x-ray unit is calibrated. This is calculated by recording a reading for any average exposure and then dividing the reading in mR by the total mAs used. The expression mR/mAs represents the formula itself. The mR/mAs measurements are usually recorded for an SID of 40" (100 cm). To estimate the entrance skin exposure, the inverse square law must be applied to determine the exposure for the source-to-entrance skin distance.

The mR/mAs readings vary according to the kVp used, with higher kVp producing greater mR/mAs. Consequently, mR/mAs readings should be recorded for each kVp range within the normal expectations of the unit. A typical mR/mAs chart is shown in Table 13–1.

A quick estimate of entrance skin exposure can be made from this chart, as shown in the example below.

Example: What is the approximate entrance skin exposure for a 20 cm AP abdomen produced at 80 kVp and 20 mAs on the unit for the chart in Table 13–1?

Answer: Table 13–1 indicates that 80 kVp = 3.5 mR/mAs. The exposure required 20 mAs, so the exposure at 100 cm = 3.5 mR/mAs $\times$ 20 mAs and the exposure at 100 cm = 70.0 mR.

TABLE 13–1. A Typical mR/mAs Chart

SID = 40" (100 cm)	
kVp	**mR/mAs**
50	0.9
60	1.7
70	2.5
80	3.5
90	4.5
100	5.6
110	6.9
120	7.9

$$SID = SOD + OID$$
$$100 \text{ cm} = SOD + 20 \text{ cm}$$
$$SOD = 100 \text{ cm} - 20 \text{ cm}$$
$$SOD = 80 \text{ cm}$$

$$\frac{mR_1}{mR_2} = \frac{SOD^2}{SID^2}$$

$$\frac{70 \text{ mR}}{mR_2} = \frac{80 \text{ cm}^2}{100 \text{ cm}^2}$$

$$\frac{70 \text{ mR}}{mR_2} = \frac{6,400 \text{ cm}}{10,000 \text{ cm}}$$

$$mR_2 \times 6,400 \text{ cm} = 70 \text{ mR} \times 10,000 \text{ cm}$$

$$mR_2 = \frac{70 \text{ mR} \times 10,000 \text{ cm}}{6,400 \text{ cm}}$$

$$mR_2 = \frac{700,000}{6,400}$$

$$mR_2 = 109.4$$

Example: What is the total approximate entrance skin exposure for an intravenous pyelogram of a 24 cm abdomen if an AP preliminary scout; 5 min AP; 10 min AP, RPO and LPO; 15 min PA; and 30 min AP radiographs of the abdomen were produced at 70 kVp and 15 mAs on the unit for the chart in Table 13–1?

Answer: Table 13–1 indicates that 70 kVp = 2.5 mR/mAs. Each exposure required 15 mAs, so the approximate entrance skin exposure = 2.5 mR/mAs $\times$ 15 mAs and the approximate entrance skin exposure = 37.5 mR per exposure; 37.5 per exposure $\times$ 7 exposures = 262.5 mR = 0.2625 R.

$$SID = SOD + OID$$
$$100 \text{ cm} = SOD + 24 \text{ cm}$$
$$SOD = 100 \text{ cm} - 24 \text{ cm}$$
$$SOD = 76 \text{ cm}$$

$$\frac{mR_1}{mR_2} = \frac{SOD^2}{SID^2}$$

$$\frac{262.5 \text{ mR}}{mR_2} = \frac{76 \text{ cm}^2}{100 \text{ cm}^2}$$

$$\frac{262.5 \text{ mR}}{\text{mR}_2} = \frac{5{,}776 \text{ cm}}{10{,}000 \text{ cm}}$$

$$\text{mR}_2 \times 5{,}776 \text{ cm} = 262.5 \text{ mR} \times 10{,}000 \text{ cm}$$

$$\text{mR}_2 = \frac{262.5 \text{ mR} \times 10{,}000 \text{ cm}}{5{,}776 \text{ cm}}$$

$$\text{mR}_2 = \frac{2{,}625{,}000}{5{,}776}$$

$$\text{mR}_2 = 454.5$$

Fluoroscopic R/min Charts

Approximate entrance skin exposure for fluoroscopic equipment is measured in R/min. Estimation of approximate entrance skin exposure is calculated in the same manner.

Example: What is the approximate entrance skin exposure for a fluoroscopic examination of the abdomen performed for 5.5 minutes at 110 kVp at 1.7 R/min?

Answer: The exposure required 5.5 min, so the approximate entrance skin exposure = 1.7 R/min × 5.5 min and the approximate entrance skin exposure = 9.35 R = 9,350 mR.

Example: What is the total approximate entrance skin exposure for a fluoroscopic examination of an 18 cm abdomen performed for 7 min and 45 sec at 110 kVp at 1.7 R/min and then followed by an AP, at 10 mAs, left lateral, at 25 mAs, and LPO projection, at 20 mAs, of the stomach at 120 kVp on the unit for the chart in Table 13–1?

Answer: The exposure required 7.75 min, so the approximate entrance skin exposure = 1.7 R/min × 7.75 min and the approximate entrance skin exposure = 13.175 R = 13,175 mR. The total mAs for the three projections = 10 + 25 + 20 mAs = 55 mAs. Table 13–1 indicates that 120 kVp = 7.9 mR/mAs, so the approximate entrance skin exposure = 7.9 mR/mAs × 55 mAs and the approximate entrance skin exposure = 434.5 mR; 13,175 fluoro mR + 434.5 diagnostic mR = 13,609.5 mR = 13.61 R.

$$\text{SID} = \text{SOD} + \text{OID}$$
$$100 \text{ cm} = \text{SOD} + 18 \text{ cm}$$

$$\text{SOD} = 100 \text{ cm} - 18 \text{ cm}$$
$$\text{SOD} = 82 \text{ cm}$$

$$\frac{\text{mR}_1}{\text{mR}_2} = \frac{\text{SOD}^2}{\text{SID}^2}$$

$$\frac{13{,}609.5 \text{ mR}}{\text{mR}_2} = \frac{82 \text{ cm}^2}{100 \text{ cm}^2}$$

$$\frac{13{,}609.5 \text{ mR}}{\text{mR}_2} = \frac{6{,}724 \text{ cm}}{10{,}000 \text{ cm}}$$

$$\text{mR}_2 \times 6{,}724 \text{ cm} = 13{,}609.5 \text{ mR} \times 10{,}000 \text{ cm}$$

$$\text{mR}_2 = \frac{13{,}609.5 \text{ mR} \times 10{,}000 \text{ cm}}{6{,}724 \text{ cm}}$$

$$\text{mR}_2 = \frac{136{,}095{,}000}{6{,}724}$$

$$\text{mR}_2 = 20{,}240 = 20.24 \text{ R.}$$

Typical Entrance Skin Exposure

Numerous studies have been done regarding the exposure delivered to patients during diagnostic radiographic examinations. Diagnostic radiography is by far the greatest source of ionizing radiation exposure for the public. It is estimated that 15 percent of the radiation exposure received by the general public is a result of diagnostic radiographic examinations. Table 13–2 shows the average patient exposure guides for entrance skin exposure as published by the Conference of Radiation Control Program Directors. Within an acceptance range of ±20 percent, this guide is considered to be the standard for current practice in the United States.

Radiography of the lumbar spine, pelvis and hip have the highest ESEs. These examinations deserve special attention from radiographers because careful consideration of the need for the examination, positioning, patient instructions, technical factors and shielding can result in significant reduction in the total dose to the patient.

Flouroscopic systems in the United States are under a limit set by the Food and Drug Administration (FDA) for entrance exposure (kerma in the SI system) at 10 centigrays per minute (10 cGy/min), which is 11.5 R/min. High-level control mode fluoroscopy is limited

TABLE 13–2. Medical Entrance Skin Exposures (ESE) in mR
(Measurements in air with no phantom)

Projection	Patient Thickness (in cm)	Grid	SID (in inches)	ESE in mR 200 speed	ESE in mR 400 speed
Abdomen—AP	23	Yes	40	490	300
Lumbar Spine—AP	23	Yes	40	450	350
Full Spine—AP	23	Yes	72	260	145
Cervical Spine—AP	13	Yes	40	135	95
Skull—LAT	15	Yes	40	145	70
Chest—PA	23	No	72	15	5
		Yes	72	25	15

Reprinted with permission from *Average Patient Guides: 1988.* Conference of Radiation Control Progress Directors, Inc., Frankfort, KY: CRCPD Publication 88–5, 1988.

to an entrance exposure (kerma) of 20 cGy/min, which is 23 R/min.

Reducing Patient Dose With Communication

Radiographers often overlook the importance of gaining the trust and confidence of the patient. This is accomplished by a professional approach that includes technical competence, empathy for the patient and effective communication and questioning skills. When the patient has confidence in the radiographer there is a higher probability that detailed instructions will be followed, which helps to reduce motion and degradation of positioning.

Reducing Patient Dose With Positioning

An effective method of reducing patient dose is through accurate and effective positioning. Avoidance of repeated exposures far outweighs all other methods. However, once positioning skills have been developed to

a degree of competence, several positioning details may further reduce the total dose.

Radiographic Projection

Some organs are especially sensitive to the effects of radiation, for example, the female breast, the kidneys and the lens of the eye. Increased recorded detail and decreased distortion result when the area of interest is placed as close to the image receptor as possible. In most instances a significant reduction in the total dose is achieved because this positioning also places the organ as far from the entrance exposure as possible. For example, a PA chest reduces the dose to the breast, an AP abdomen reduces dose to the kidneys, and a PA skull reduces dose to the lens of the eye. Deviation from these projections should occur only when unusual circumstances dictate an alternate projection.

Immobilization

Proper immobilization is a necessary part of achieving satisfactory recorded detail and diminishing the need for repeat exposures. Elimination of motion and decreased tissue density through compression both contribute to a reduction of patient dose.

Reducing Patient Dose With Technical Factors

The radiographer can significantly reduce the approximate entrance skin exposure to the patient by judicious selection of technique exposure factors. Studies have shown that over 50 percent of repeated exposures are the result of improper technical factor selection. Table 13–3 illustrates the effect each of the major technical factors has on patient dose. In most instances when a technical factor is varied, other factors will be modified to maintain radiographic density. Therefore, the important information is not the direct result of the technical factor change, but the result of compensation to maintain radiographic density or other components of image quality.

Interrelationship of the Prime Factors

The radiation intensity from a diagnostic x-ray unit will vary in a direct relationship with mAs, directly with the square of kVp and inversely with the square of the distance. This total relationship is often expressed as:

$$\frac{(mAs)(kVp)^2}{d^2}$$

At the image receptor the kVp is more likely to be kVp^3 or kVp^4. Although this formula includes only the

TABLE 13–3. Effects of Radiographic Exposure Variables on Patient Dose

	Effect of Patient Dose When:		
		Variable Is Increased but Radiographic Density Is Maintained By Compensating	
Variable	Variable Is Increased without Compensation	with kVp Only	with mAs Only
Kilovoltage	+	NA	−
Milliamperage	+	+	0
Time	+	+	0
Distance			
SID	−	−	0
SOD	−	−	0
OID	+	+	+
Focal spot size	0	NA	NA
Filtration	−	−	+
Field Size	+	varies	varies
Gonadal shielding	−	NA	NA
Subject part density	+	+	+
Grid Ratio	0	+	+
Intensifying screens	0	−	−
Film speed	0	−	−
Film processing			
Developer time	0	−	−
Developer temperature	0	−	−
Developer replenishment	0	−	−

three primary factors, it is useful to understand that they are interrelated and can all be used to influence the total dose.

Kilovoltage Range

When kVp is increased without compensating for other factors, patient dose is increased. Therefore, a decrease in kVp is desired when attempting to reduce patient dose. However, when an increase in kVp is compensated for by a decrease in mAs to maintain radiographic density, a significant reduction in patient dose is achieved. **Selection of the highest possible kilovoltage consistent with image quality is the best method of using exposure factors to reduce patient dose.** With fixed kilovoltage systems, care must be taken to achieve an optimal kVp that is within acceptance limits. Because fixed kVp technique systems tend to utilize higher optimal kVp levels, they usually reduce patient entrance skin exposures. A comparison of approximate ESE levels with the two systems is illustrated in Table 13–4.

Remember that generator phase also has an effect on kilovoltage output. Although an increase in the number of pulses from the generator would seem to increase the patient dose because of the increased average photon energy, there is actually a substantial decrease in patient ESE (from 40 to 60 percent) because of the decrease in the percentage of lower energy photons from the x-ray tube. The lower energy photons tend to be absorbed in the body instead of being transmitted to the image receptor, thus contributing to patient ESE without adding any information to the image receptor. This is clearly shown in Figure 13–2.

TABLE 13–4. Comparison of Approximate Entrance Skin Exposures with Fixed and Variable kVp Technique Systems

Variable—56 kVp, 5 mAs	= 12.8 mR
Fixed—65 kVp, 2.5 mAs	= 9.5 mR
Variable—68 kVp, 40 mAs	= 175.1 mR
Fixed—80 kVp, 20 mAs	= 135.4 mR
Variable—102 kVp, 20 mAs	= 222.0 mR
Fixed—120 kVp, 10 mAs	= 156.3 mR

These examples would produce equivalent radiographic density.

Milliamperage and Time

When mAs is decreased, patient dose is also decreased. When an increase in mAs is compensated by a decrease in kVp, patient dose will increase. An inverse relationship exists between mAs and kVp in maintaining radiographic density. To decrease patient dose, mAs should be maintained at the lowest possible level because there is a direct relationship between mAs and exposure. Because variable kVp technique systems tend to utilize lower kVp levels with higher mAs, the result can be higher average patient ESE than with fixed kVp systems.

Distance

Distance cannot be discussed alone because SID, SOD and OID have differing relationships to patient ESE. When SID or SOD is increased, patient ESE decreases. One study found a 10 percent decrease in patient ESE between an SOD of 40 and 50 inches. When kVp is used to compensate for radiographic density, the ESE will decrease but the use of mAs for compensation will usually increase the total ESE. In most instances, when OID decreases, SOD increases and this will reduce patient ESE. This holds true regardless of whether kVp or mAs is used to compensate for the air-gap contrast and density changes.

Focal Spot Size

Focal spot size has no appreciable effect on patient dose.

Filtration

An increase in filtration will reduce the ESE, even when kVp is compensated to maintain radiographic density. However, when mAs is used to compensate for lost radiographic density, the result is often an increase in the total ESE. This applies only to the small filtration increases used in diagnostic radiography, usually not more than 0.5 mm Al/eq. Any significant increase in filtration (1.0 mm Al/eq or more) would have an overall ESE reduction effect.

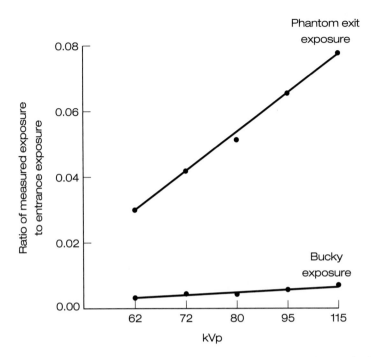

FIGURE 13–2. The effect of kVp on the ratio of measured exposures to entrance exposure. This graph clearly illustrates that increased kVp causes photon energy to be carried through the phantom. (Attenuation is reduced as kVp increases.) The two lines show the relationship of the exit exposure from the phantom compared to the exposure in the Bucky tray. The film density was fixed. *(Reprinted by permission from the American Society of Radiologic Technologists)*

Field Size

When the primary-beam field size decreases, the patient dose also decreases. An increased field size will increase the total dose even when mAs or kVp is adjusted to compensate for radiographic density because a greater tissue area is irradiated. An increase in the primary technical factors is necessary to compensate for lost scatter radiation density when the field size is decreased. Although this appears to increase dose, the elimination of a greater percentage of tissue from the beam is a greater protective method than the increased factors.

Modern x-ray tube collimators utilize two sets of shutters or leaves to eliminate most of the off-focus radiation. When an aperture diaphragm is used instead of a collimator, off-focus radiation can increase the peripheral dose adjacent to the primary beam field.

Gonad Shielding

Gonad shielding is extremely effective in reducing dose to the gonads. There are three major types of gonad shields: flat contact, shadow and shaped contact. Flat contact shields are positioned over the gonads at the skin surface. Shadow shields are positioned in the primary beam immediately below the collimator. Shaped contact shields are worn by the patient to surround the gonads. Gonadal shielding is one of the fine arts of radiography. The radiographer who is competent in the specifics of gonadal anatomy can easily satisfy the concerns of the radiologist or supervisor who has experienced suboptimal shielding that caused repeated exposure to the patient. **Properly placed gonadal shields significantly reduce patient dose while improperly placed gonadal shields can increase patient dose through repeated pro-**

jections. Consequently consistent gonadal shielding becomes a measure of the competency of the radiographer.

Gonadal shields should be used **routinely** for all patients with reproduction capabilities. The only exception to this rule should be projections that require information in the gonadal region. It is critical to locate the exact location of the ovaries or testicles prior to using gonadal shields. Most projections of the pelvic region do not permit the use of gonadal shields. This includes IVP, abdominal, colon, and bony pelvic projections. Hip projections do permit careful gonadal shielding.

Subject Part Density

A decrease in subject part density will decrease scatter production and reduce the patient dose. When compensation for lost scatter is made by increasing mAs or kVp, a reduction in total dose usually holds.

Grids

Using grids result in an increase in patient dose as opposed to non-grid procedures, in order to maintain radiographic density. When the grid ratio is decreased, and radiographic density is maintained by decreases in mAs or kVp, a significant dose reduction can be achieved. The use of a grid of unnecessarily high ratio causes routine increases in patient dose as mAs or kVp is increased to maintain radiographic density.

Intensifying Screens

Using intensifying screens results in a decrease in patient dose as opposed to non-screen procedures, in order to maintain radiographic density. Whenever the screen speed is increased, a significant reduction in mAs or kVp can be achieved while maintaining radiographic density. **The second most effective method of reducing patient dose is to use the highest possible film/screen combination (Table 13–5).**

Film

Using higher speed film results in a decrease in patient dose as opposed to slower speed film, in order to maintain radiographic density. Base plus fog is a factor that should not be related to patient dose reductions. If base

TABLE 13–5. The Effect of Film/Screen Speed on Mean Entrance Skin Exposures

Projection	Chest	Abdomen	Lumbar
100 RS with grid	22.1 mR	553 mR	532 mR
200 RS with grid	14.9 mR	580 mR	813 mR
300 RS with grid	8.1 mR	351 mR	420 mR
400 RS with grid	7.4 mR	350 mR	383 mR

Data from 1987 NEXT survey of hospitals, U.S. Department of Health and Human Services, Food and Drug Administration, Center for Devices and Radiological Health.

plus fog becomes too high, the detrimental effect on image quality will result in repeated exposures. However, a decrease in patient dose can be accomplished when a higher speed film is used and mAs or kVp is reduced to maintain radiographic density. Because higher contrast films also exhibit greater speed, the same effect is achieved with a higher contrast film. Film latitude becomes wider as speed and contrast decrease. Consequently, a narrow latitude film is desirable when attempting to reduce patient dose. This approach requires radiographers to be extremely accurate in selecting technical factors.

Film Processing

The compensations that are required to overcome reductions in developer time, temperature or replenishment can result in unnecessarily high patient dose. Developer time, temperature and replenishment cannot be effectively increased to reduce patient dose. Film processing is a system that must be maintained at an optimal level to ensure satisfactory image quality. Failure to do so can result in increased dose rates, but success in maintaining the system cannot be considered a direct cause of decreased dose.

Discussing Radiation Risk Versus Benefit With Patients

The radiographer is often in the position of discussing radiation risk versus benefit with patients. To the attending physician, and sometimes even to the radiologist, the radiographer must represent the patient's interest in reducing dose. At the same time the radiographer must represent, to the patient, the physician's interest in maximizing diagnostic information. These points of view generally oppose one another. One exception is the use of higher kVp to produce a lower contrast. In this example, patient dose is decreased and the diagnostic information is increased.

Minimizing Patient Dose by Emphasizing Risk

The patient's interest in reducing the total dose must be represented even when the patient does not express such an interest. Some patients even express an opposite interest, as often occurs with minor complaints, such as lung congestion or a sprained ankle, when the patient arrives in the physician's office, a clinic or an emergency room with a request for an x-ray examination. When patients assume this attitude, the physician may prescribe an x-ray examination as a placebo. Most medical ethicists consider the prescription of a procedure for the purpose of deceiving the patient, or a procedure known to be without specific efficacy, to be unethical. This includes unnecessary radiographic examinations, which are known to be potentially detrimental.

In such a situation, the radiographer should perceive an obligation to act in such a way as to eliminate the request for the examination or at least to reduce the number of exposures. Through demonstration of professional competence, the radiographer can obtain the stature necessary to permit consultation regarding modification or elimination of examination requests.

Part of gaining this type of respect is the ability to make well considered judgments on when to advocate reductions in patient dose and when to advocate additional examinations. These judgments require all the radiographer's knowledge of anatomy, physics, radiation biology, positioning, pathology, imaging equipment and, especially, clinical experience. For example, a radiographer should advocate an additional projection of the abdomen when an erect radiograph for an abdominal obstruction series fails to demonstrate the top of both hemidiaphragms. Conversely, the radiographer is acting

professionally when advocating the elimination of separate wrist projections when both hand and wrist examinations have been requested but there is visible trauma only to the hand, the patient has no complaint of wrist pain, and the clinical history does not indicate a high probability of referred stress to the wrist joint.

For examinations that are of questionable need, the radiographer is within professional rights to inform the patient of his or her right to refuse an examination. **Under no circumstances should this be perceived by the radiographer as cause to inform the patient that an examination is not needed or to give a personal opinion regarding medical treatment or diagnosis.** The radiographer must have an introductory background in medical law in order to make judgments of this type. For example, minors, persons who have had their civil rights suspended (such as persons in the custody of law enforcement officers), mentally incompetent persons and some other categories of patients do not have the right to refuse examinations.

The selection of patients for x-ray examinations has been the focus of considerable study, particularly when the chest, lumbar spine and skull are involved. Patients can be divided into asymptomatic and symptomatic groups when determining which should be exposed to radiation. Asymptomatic patients should be examined only when there is significant cause, after considering the incidence and severity of the condition, the detection reliability of the examination, and the usefulness of the examination in treatment. The most common examples of asymptomatic patients are those undergoing screening procedures. Although mass chest and lumbar spine screening are now discouraged, mammography screening is encouraged for women of certain age groups. Symptomatic patients are more likely to require x-ray examination but should fit two major criteria: the examination must be capable of providing the desired information, and the information, even if negative, is expected to contribute to the management of the patient. The radiographer has a responsibility to contribute to these criteria whenever possible, primarily through history-taking. When circumstances that appear to routinely violate these principles are encountered, the radiographer should consider withdrawing from participation in the examinations.

Maximizing Diagnostic Information by Emphasizing Benefit

While advocating a reduction of patient dose, the radiographer must simultaneously impress on the patient the physician's primary concern of maximizing diagnostic information. This includes establishing credibility with the patient by demonstrating competence in answering questions, taking a medical history, manipulating the x-ray equipment, exhibiting a professional demeanor and myriad other details. Established credibility permits the radiographer to convince the patient to follow breathing instructions, endure an additional uncomfortable projection or permit a repeated exposure.

The benefit of radiographic procedures has been an unquestionable aspect of medicine since Röntgen's discovery in 1895. Although this is generally accepted by

TABLE 13–6. Gross Comparison of Relative Radiation Levels*

	Scaled Relative Dose†
Natural background	50–100 chest examinations/year
Diagnostic Radiology	0.1–500 chest examinations/study‡
Nuclear imaging	50–1,000 chest examinations/study¶
Start of acute radiation syndrome	30,000 chest examinations in *one* day
Lethal dose (LD50$_{30}$)	300,000 chest examinations in *one* day
Radiation therapy (small volumes of tissue)	100,000–1,000,000 chest examinations in a few weeks
Ultrasound	This scale does not apply
NMR	This scale does not apply

*Due to differential tissue distributions and sensitivities, such estimates are intended to be rough comparisons (50–100 chest examinations will have different biologic effects from that resulting from 100–200 mrads of natural background).

†1 PA chest examination = 5 millirad average tissue dose in thorax, which corresponds to a whole body equivalent dose of 2 millirads.

‡Dependent on examination types and techniques.

¶Does no properly account for doses received in those tissues in which the radionuclide concentrates.

(Reprinted with permission of Joseph P. Whalen and Stephen Balter, *Radiation Risks in Medical Imaging,* Chicago: Yearbook Medical Publishers, Inc., 1984.)

the public, some patients have a heightened anxiety about exposure, and there are periodic increases in publicity that cause concern over medical radiation exposures. These issues must be addressed by the radiographer as the primary professional contact with the patient. **The radiographer has a responsibility to advocate medically necessary examinations and to assure the patient that the benefit outweighs the risk.**

The primary duty of the radiographer on this issue is to provide the patient with sufficient information to permit the patient to make an informed decision regarding the examination. This can be a very sensitive topic and must be approached in a thorough and professional manner. One of the best accepted methods of providing this information to the patient is through comparison of relative radiation risks. Table 13–6 illustrates comparative risks of chest x-ray examinations to other radiation risks that are common public knowledge. Another effective method of illustrating relative radiation risk is through a catalog of risks, such as the extract shown in Table 13–7.

When a patient requests information about the exact dose for a particular examination, the radiographer has an obligation to attempt to provide that information. However, it is important that the patient have a basic understanding that only an **approximate entrance skin exposure** can be provided. The radiographer should inform the patient that the entrance skin exposure is the maximum exposure and that the actual dose to the area of interest would be significantly less.

The Center for Devices and Radiological Health of the United States Food and Drug Administration has advocated the use of radiation record cards for patients. Proposals have been made for credit card style cards with magnetic record tapes for running totals of approximate entrance skin exposures. There are currently x-ray units available with print-out capability so this information can be given to patients upon request. As the public becomes more informed about the potential risks of medical radiation exposure, additional developments in this arena can be expected.

The patient has the right to refuse radiographic examination. The radiographer is bound by professional duty to respect this right and to advocate it to physicians, including radiologists, if necessary. As long as the patient has the right to refuse treatment, proceeding

TABLE 13–7. Estimated Loss of Life Expectancy Due to Various Causes*

Lifestyle	Estimated Loss in Days
Being unmarried—male	3,500
Cigarette smoking—male	2,250
Being unmarried—female	1,600
Cigarette smoking—female	800
Dangerous job	300
Motor vehicle accidents	207
Alcohol (U.S. average)	130
Accidents at home	95
Average job	74
Radiation job	40
Accidents to pedestrians	37
Safest job	30
Natural radiation	8
Medical x-rays	6
Individual Action	**Estimated Loss in Minutes**
Buying a small car	7,000
Coast to coast drive	1,000
Coast to coast flight	100
Smoking a cigarette	10
Calorie-rich dessert	50
Non-diet soft drink	15
Diet soft drink	0.15
Crossing a street	0.4
Extra driving	0.4/mile
Not fastening seat belt	0.1/mile
1 mrem of radiation	1.5

*Adapted from Cohen and Lee. Reproduced from *Health Physics* 36:707, 1979. Used by permission of the Health Physics Society.

Adapted with permission of Bernard L. Cohen and I-Sing Lee, "A catalog of risks," *Health Physics* 36, 707-722, 1979.

with an examination under protest from the patient may place the radiographer at risk of malpractice action (usually as assault and battery).

Summary

A predominant concern of radiographers is how to reduce the radiation dose to the patient. This concern is reflected in every decision that is made, especially when choosing technique exposure factors. The conscientious radiographer can reduce the patient entrance skin exposure by at least 50 percent in most examinations by choosing appropriate exposure factors.

The maximum dose received by the patient is not at the area of interest but at the skin entrance to the body. This is known as the entrance skin exposure and is calculated at the minimum SOD. Exposure to patients can be estimated by recording mR/mAs when the x-ray unit is calibrated. This is calculated by recording a reading for any average exposure and then dividing the reading in mR by the total mAs used. The expression mR/mAs represents the formula itself. The mR/mAs measurements are usually recorded for an SID of 40" (100 cm). To estimate the entrance skin exposure, the inverse square law must be applied to determine the exposure for the source-to-entrance skin distance. For fluoroscopy, the estimated exposure is calculated in R/min instead of mR/mAs.

Radiographers can reduce dose to the patient through their communication skills, their positioning skills, and through proper selection of technical exposure factors. Technical factors include the kilovoltage, mA, exposure time, distance, filtration, field size, gonadal shielding, subject part density, grids, intensifying screens, film and film processing.

The radiographer is often in the position of discussing radiation risk versus benefit with patients. To the attending physician, and sometimes even to the radiologist, the radiographer must represent the patient's interest in reducing the dose. At the same time the radiographer must represent to the patient the physician's interest in maximizing diagnostic information.

REVIEW QUESTIONS

1. What is the relationship between entrance skin exposure and other measurement points?

2. What is the mR/mAs for a calibration exposure of 80 kVp at 40 mAs that produces a total exposure of 86 mR?

3. What is the total exposure for a patient measuring 26 cm when the SID is 40" for an expo-

sure of 70 kVp and 35 mAs and the mR/mAs at 70 kVp is 2.6 at 40"?

4. How can patient dose be reduced through effective communication?

5. How can patient dose be reduced through effective positioning?

6. What changes should be made in kVp, mA, time and distance if each is the only factor changed to reduce patient dose?

7. What are the variables, other than the prime factors, that can be used to reduce patient dose?

8. What risk factors could be mentioned to answer a patient's inquiry about the dose for an examination?

9. What diagnostic benefits could be mentioned to answer a patient's inquiry about the need for an examination?

10. Describe an approach to discussing radiation risk versus benefit with patients, physicians and radiologists.

REFERENCES AND RECOMMENDED READING

Anderson, P. E., Anderson, P. E., & Van-der-Kooy, P. (1982). Dose reduction in radiography of the spine for scoliosis. *Acta Radiological. 23*, 251–253.

Appleton, M. B. & Carr, S. R. (1984). Radiation protection in a neonatal intensive care unit: A practical approach. *Radiography. 50*(592), 137.

Baker, D. G. (1989). How significant are the risks from occupational exposure to ionizing radiation? *Applied Radiology. 18*(9), 19.

Ball, J. L. (1978). Does high kV reduce the dose? *Radiography. 64*(523), 163.

Barnhard, H. J. (1978). The bedside examination: A time for analysis and appropriate action. *Radiology. 129*, 539–540.

Baxter, A. (1978). Choice of kilovoltage. *Radiography. 64*(524), 196.

Beauchemin, R. (1984). Telescopic gonad protector: Analysis and experimentation of a telescopic gonad protector. *The Canadian Journal of Medical Radiation Technology. 15*(1), 39.

Bednorck, D. R., Rozenfeld, M., Lanzl, L. H., & Sabau, M. (1981). A protocol for exposure limitations in radiography. *Radiologic Technology. 53*(3) 229.

BEIR V health effects of exposure to low levels of ionizing radiation. (1990). National Academy Press, Washington, DC.

Belanich, M. M., Iorio, P., Jonason, R., & Summers, J. (1987). A simple, cost-effective method for determination of entrance skin exposures for Diagnostic Radiology Examinations. *Applied Radiology. 16*, 39–41.

Brown, R. F., Shaver, J. W., & Lamel, D. A. (1980). *The selection of patients for x-ray examinations.* Rockville, MD: U.S. Department of Health, Education, and Welfare, Public Health Service, Food and Drug Administration, Bureau of Radiological Health, HEW Publication (FDFA) 80–8104.

Burkhart, R. L. (1983). *Patient radiation exposure in diagnostic radiology examinations: An overview.* Rockville, MD: U.S. Department of Health, Education, and Welfare, Public Health Service, Food and Drug Administration, Bureau of Radiological Health, HEW Publication (FDFA) 83–8217.

Bushong, S. C. (1999). *Radiation protection in Merrill's Atlas of Radiographic Positions and Radiologic Procedures* (7th ed.) by Philip W. Ballinger. St. Louis: C. V. Mosby, 15–30.

Bushong, S. C. (1977). Radiation exposure in our daily lives. *The Physics Teacher.* (March), 135–144.

Butler, P., Thomas, A. W., Thompson, W. E., Wollerton, M. A., & Rachlin, J. A. (1986). Simple methods to reduce patient exposure during scoliosis radiography, *Radiologic Technology. 57*(5), 411.

Butler, P. F. (1985). Chest radiography: A survey of techniques and exposure levels currently used. *Radiology,* 533.

Cohen, B. L. & Lee, I. (1979). A catalog of risks. *Health Physics. 36*, 707–722.

Collen, M. F. & McClean, P. M. (1983). *Utilization of diagnostic x-ray examinations.* Rockville, MD: U.S. Department of Health, Education, and Welfare, Public Health Service, Food and Drug Administration, Bureau of Radiological Health, HEW Publication (FDFA) 83–8208.

Conference of Radiation Control Program Directors, Inc. (1993). Committee on Quality Assurance in Diagnostic Radiology, *Average Patient Exposure Guides*, Frankfort, KY: Conference of Radiation Control Program Directors, Inc.

Davies, J. & Russell, J. G. B. (1986). Carbon fibre faced cassettes in neonatal radiography: Their use and cost effectiveness. *Radiography. 52*(603), 113.

Dowd, S. B. (1994). *Practical radiation protection and applied radiobiology.* Philadelphia: W. B. Saunders.

Frank, E., Stears, J., Gray, J., Winkler, N. T, & Hoffman, A. D. (1984). Use of the P. A. projection: A method of reducing x-ray exposure to specific radiosensitive organs. *The Canadian Journal of Medical Radiation Technology. 15*(2), 63.

Frank, E. D. (1983). Use of the posteroanterior projection: A method of reducing x-ray exposure to specific radiosensitive organs. *Radiologic Technology. 54*, 343–347.

Gibbs, S. J. (1981). Approaches to radiation risk estimation. *The Physical Basis of Medical Imaging.* Editors: Coulam, C. M., Erickson, J. J., Rollo, F. D., Everette, J. A. New York: Appleton-Century-Crofts, 329–342.

Godderidge, C. (1981). A radiology department's response to consumer concerns regarding the hazards of low-dose radiation. *Radiology Management. 4*(3), 1.

Hall, E. J. (1993). *Radiobiology for the radiologist* (4th ed.). Philadelphia: J. B. Lippincott Company.

Herman, M. W. (1980). A comparative study of scattered radiation levels from 80 kVp and 240 kVp x-rays in the surgical ICU. *Radiology. 134*, 552.

Jankowski, C. B. (1984). Radiation exposure of nurses in a coronary care unit. *The Journal of Critical Care. 13*(1), 55–58.

Joseph, L. P. & Wollerton, M. A. (1984). *Extremity radiography following trauma: An overview.* Rockville, MD: U.S. Department of Health, Education, and Welfare, Public Health Service, Food and Drug Administration, Bureau of Radiological Health, HEW Publication (FDFA) 84–8232.

Light, M. C., Molloi, S. Y., Yandouo, D. R., & Ranallo, F. N. (1987). Scatter radiation exposure during knee arthrography. *Radiology, 867.*

Maillie, H. D., Segal, A., & Lemkin, J. (1982). Effect of patient size on doses received by patients in diagnostic radiology. *Health Physics. 42*, 665–670.

Manny, E. F. & Burkhart, R. L. (1985). *Measurement Techniques for Use With Technique/Exposure Guides.* Rockville, MD: U.S. Department of Health, Education, and Welfare, Public Health Service, Food and Drug Administration, Bureau of Radiological Health, HEW Publication (FDFA) 85–8248.

Manny, E. F., Rudolph, H., & Wollerton, M. A. (1981). *Preemployment low back x-rays: An overview.* Rockville, MD: U.S. Department of Health, Education, and Welfare, Public Health Service, Food and Drug Administration, Bureau of Radiological Health, HEW Publication (FDFA) 81–8173.

McClean, P. M. & Joseph, L. P. (1981). *Plain skull film radiography in the management of head trauma: An overview.* Rockville, MD: U.S. Department of Health, Education, and Welfare, Public Health Service, Food and Drug Administration, Bureau of Radiological Health, HEW Publication (FDFA) 81–8172.

McCullough, E. C. (1976). Exposure requirements in diagnostic roentgenologic procedures. *Applied Radiology.* 95–101.

McGlone, W. E. (1970). Radiation protection of the reproductive organs during radiography of the hip joints. *Radiologic Technology. 41*, 277–279.

Miller, P. E. (1976). Biological effects of diagnostic irradiation. *Radiologic Technology. 48*(1), 11–16.

Milner, S. C. & Naylor, E. (1989). An estimation of doses received by patients in a diagnostic x-ray department. *Radiography Today. 55*(622), 16.

NCRP (1990) Report No. 107, *Implementation of the Principle of ALARA for Medical and Dental Personnel,* Bethesda, MD: National Council on Radiation Protection and Measurements.

NCRP (1989) Report No. 102, *Medical X-Ray, Electron Beam and Gamma-Ray Protection for Energies Up to 50*

Mev (Equipment Design, Performance and Use), Bethesda, MD: National Council on Radiation Protection and Measurements.

NCRP (1987). *Report No. 93, Ionizing Radiation Exposure of the Population of the United States*, Bethesda, MD: National Council on Radiation Protection and Measurements.

Novitch, M. (1983). Evaluation of radiation exposure in diagnostic radiology examinations. *Radiology Management.* 5(4), 33.

Noz, M. E. & Maguire, G. Q. (1985). *Radiation protection in the radiologic and health sciences* (2nd ed.). Philadelphia: Lea & Febiger.

Pagel, J. W. (1981). Radiation protection in diagnostic radiology, *The Physical Basis of Medical Imaging*. Editors: Coulam, C. M., Erickson, J. J., Rollo, F. D., & James, A. E. New York: Appleton-Century-Crofts, 303–328.

Phillips, L. A. (1978). *A study of the effect of high yield criteria for emergency room skull radiography.* Rockville, MD: U.S. Department of Health, Education, and Welfare, Public Health Service, Food and Drug Administration, Bureau of Radiological Health, HEW Publication (FDFA) 78–8069.

Ragozzino, M. W. (1986). Average fetal depth in utero: Data for estimation of fetal absorbed radiation dose. *Radiology.* 513.

Robinson, T., Becker, J. A., & Olson, A. P. (1982). Clinical comparison of high-speed rare-earth screen and par-speed screen for diagnostic efficacy and radiation dosage. *Radiology.* 145, 214–216.

Rosenstein, M. (1988). *Handbook of selected tissue doses for projections common in diagnostic radiology.* Rockville, MD: U.S. Department of Health, Education, and Welfare, Public Health Service, Food and Drug Administration, Bureau of Radiological Health, HEW Publication (FDFA) 89–8031.

Rossi, R. P., Harnisch, B., & Hendee, W. R. (1982). Reduction of radiation exposure in radiography of the chest. *Radiology.* 144, 909–914.

Schrimpton, P. C. (1988). Monitoring the dose to patients undergoing common x-ray examinations. *Radiography Today.* 54, 619.

Shleien, B., Tucker, T. T., & Johnson, D. W. (1977). *The mean active bone marrow dose to the adult population of the United States from diagnostic radiology.* Rockville, MD: U.S. Department of Health, Education, and Welfare, Public Health Service, Food and Drug Administration, Bureau of Radiological Health, HEW Publication (FDFA) 77–8013.

Sholl-Evans, B. (1989). Radiation protection training and information. *Radiography Today.* 55(620), 8.

Shrimpton, P. C. (1989). Monitoring the dose to patients undergoing common x-ray examinations. *Radiography Today.* 54(619), 38.

Skubic, S. E. & Fatouros, P. (1986). Absorbed breast dose: Dependence on radiographic modality and technique and breast thickness. *Radiology.* 263.

Statkiewicz, M. A., Visconti, P. J., Ritenour, E. R. (1993). *Radiation protection in medical radiography* (2nd ed.). St. Louis: C. V. Mosby.

Stears, J. G., Gray, J. E., & Frank, E. D. (1989). Radiologic exchange (dose reduction with 105 mm spot films), *Radiologic Technology*, 60: No. 6, 515–516.

Strategies for reducing health hazards from medical x-rays. (1982). *The Canadian Journal of Medical Radiation Technology.* 13(4), 159.

Travis, E. L. (1989). *Primer of medical radiobiology* (2nd ed.). Chicago: Year Book Medical Publishers.

U.S. Department of Health, Education, and Welfare. (1986). *The Selection of Patients for X-Ray Examinations: Presurgical Chest X-Ray Screening Examinations.* Rockville, MD: U.S. Department of Health, Education, and Welfare, Public Health Service, Food and Drug Administration, Bureau of Radiological Health, HEW Publication (FDFA) 86–8261.

U.S. Department of Health, Education, and Welfare. (1986). *The Selection of Patients for X-Ray Examinations: Skull X-Ray Examination for Trauma.* Rockville, MD: U.S. Department of Health, Education, and Welfare, Public Health Service, Food and Drug Administration, Bureau of Radiological Health, HEW Publication (FDFA) 86–8263.

U.S. Department of Health, Education, and Welfare. (1984). *Nationwide Evaluation of X-Ray Trends (NEXT) - Eight*

Years of Data (1974-1981). Rockville, MD: U.S. Department of Health, Education, and Welfare, Public Health Service, Food and Drug Administration, Bureau of Radiological Health, HEW Publication (FDFA) 84–8229.

U.S. Department of Health, Education, and Welfare. (1983). *The Selection of Patients for X-Ray Examinations: Chest X-Ray Screening Examinations*. Rockville, MD: U.S. Department of Health, Education, and Welfare, Public Health Service, Food and Drug Administration, Bureau of Radiological Health, HEW Publication (FDFA) 83–8204.

U.S. Department of Health, Education, and Welfare. (1981). *Procedures to Minimize Diagnostic X-Ray Exposure of the Human Embryo and Fetus*. Rockville, MD: U.S. Department of Health, Education, and Welfare, Public Health Service, Food and Drug Administration, Bureau of Radiological Health, HEW Publication (FDFA) 81–8178.

U.S. Department of Health, Education, and Welfare. (1980). *The Selection of Patients for X-Ray Examinations: The Pelvimetry Examination*. Rockville, MD: U.S. Department of Health, Education, and Welfare, Public Health Service, Food and Drug Administration, Bureau of Radiological Health, HEW Publication (FDFA) 80–8128.

U.S. Department of Health, Education, and Welfare. (1976). *Specific Area Gonad Shielding: Recommendation for Use on Patients During Medical Diagnostic X-Ray Procedures*. Rockville, MD: U.S. Department of Health, Education, and Welfare, Public Health Service, Food and Drug Administration, Bureau of Radiological Health, HEW Publication (FDFA) 76–8054.

U.S. Department of Health, Education, and Welfare. (1975). *Gonad Shielding in Diagnostic Radiology*. Rockville, MD: U.S. Department of Health, Education, and Welfare, Public Health Service, Food and Drug Administration, Bureau of Radiological Health, HEW Publication (FDFA) 75–8024.

Watkins, G. L. (1988). Public health risks from low dose medical radiation. *Radiologic Technology. 59*(2), 160.

Weatherburn, G. C. (1983). Reducing radiation doses to the breast, thyroid and gonads during diagnostic radiography. *Radiography. 49*, 151–156.

Wesenberg, R. L., Blumhagen, J. D., Rossi, R. P., Hilton, S. W., Gilbert, J. M., & Nedeau, D. J. (1980). Low-dose radiography of children. *Radiologic Technology. 51*(5), 641.

Whalen, J. P. & Balter, S. (1984). *Radiation risks in medical imaging*. Chicago: Yearbook Medical Publishers, Inc.

Winkler, N. T. (1969). Minimizing radiation exposure of patients and personnel (screen-film, TFD, filters; shields; grid ratios). *Radiologic Technology. 41*(3), 142.

Wochos, J. F. & Cameron, J. R. (1976). Effect of operator training on patient exposure: An analysis of the NEXT data. *Radiologic Technology. 48*(1), 19–22.

Yoshizumi, T. T., Drummond, K. T., Freeman, J. O., & Mullett, M. (1987). Radiation safety and protection of neonates in radiological exams. *Radiologic Technology. 58*(5), 405.

Young, A. T. (1986). SURFACE shield: A device to reduce personnel radiation exposure. *Radiology*, 801.

UNIT ▌▌▌

Creating the Image

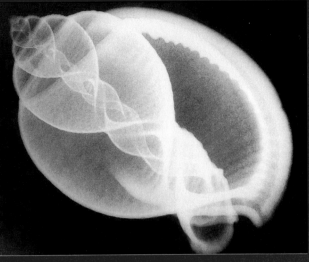

*C*reating the image that appears on the radiograph occupies the majority of the radiographer's time and requires a great deal of skill. The ability of the radiologist to make a diagnosis depends on the radiographer's ability to create a diagnostic quality image. This ability is predicated on a thorough knowledge of the scientific basis by which the image was produced as well as clinical experiences.

This unit introduces the important aspects of **vision and image perception.** Understanding how the information from the radiographic image will be transmitted to the brain of the viewer is critical to understanding exactly how to manipulate the image to maximize the diagnostic information it conveys. Producing quality images requires knowledge of x-ray **beam restriction,** the concept of **the patient as a beam emitter,** the **pathology problem** inherent in many examinations, the proper use of the **grid, radiograph film** and **radiographic processing.** Sensitometry is necessary to evaluate films and monitor their quality, while an understanding of **intensifying screens** and **film/screen combinations** is required to permit minimum patient exposure while maximizing diagnostic information on the film. The diagnostic image is created only when all of these factors are applied with professional skill.

CHAPTER 14

Vision and Perception

She is so tall, so slender, and her bones —
Those frail phosphates, those carbonates of lime —
Are well produced by cathode rays sublime,
By oscillations, amperes and by ohms.
Her dorsal vertebrae are not concealed
By epidermis, but are well revealed.

Around her ribs, those beauteous twenty-four,
Her flesh a halo makes, misty in line,
Her noseless, eyeless face looks into mine,
And I but whisper, "Sweetheart, je t'adore."
Her white and gleaming teeth at me do laugh.
Ah! Lovely, cruel, sweet (radio)graph!

Lawrence K. Russell, Life, 1896.

OBJECTIVES

Upon completion of this chapter, the student should be able to:

▶ Draw a cross-sectional image of a human eye with appropriate anatomical structures identified.

▶ Explain the physiological function of the eye during photopic and scotopic vision.

▶ Discuss the inefficiency of the medical imaging process.

▶ Describe the boundary effect, Mach effect, eye motion, veil glare and the effect of viewing distance on visual perceptions.

▶ State why pattern recognition is the domain of the radiologist.

▶ Discuss the concept of controlling the radiographic image in space.

▶ Apply the concept of three-dimensional thinking to clinical practice.

▶ Identify numerous creative uses of radiography in medicine, technology and art.

Image Perception

*A*t one time or another we have all been fooled by visual misperceptions. A common example is shown in Figure 14–1. Misperceptions of any type can be dangerous in clinical radiography. An important method of overcoming misperception is the elimination of preconceived ideas about an image. A mental erasing of these opinions is necessary to permit high-quality viewing of radiographic images. This is a skill that is cultivated by radiologists until it becomes part of their routine diagnostic procedure. Radiographers observe the diagnostic reporting of images by radiologists with amazement at first, but with increasing confidence as experience adds knowledge about the potential pathological meaning of various radiologic signs. Radiographers should strive toward developing an understanding of the perceptual problems that radiologists encounter when attempting to interpret radiographic images. Through this understanding the radiographer can work toward producing images with patterns that provide maximum assistance to the radiologist in the diagnostic process.

Visual Anatomy

Because radiography depends entirely on images, it is helpful to be introduced to the complexities of visual perception. The mechanics of image perception are

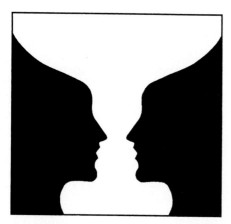

FIGURE 14–1. "The Lady and the Chalice" can be seen either as a pair of black faces in silhouette or as a white vase. This picture was devised by E. Rubin in 1915 and remains popular as a method of demonstrating perceptual differences.

mostly unknown. It is little understood exactly how the eye perceives images and transmits them to the brain. Even less is known about how the brain neurologically processes the information.

The human eye is anatomically designed to gather light, focus it, convert it to nervous impulses and transmit it to the brain for processing. The aqueous humor, cornea, iris and lens gather and focus the light (Figure 14–2). The specialized cells of the retina, especially the fovea centralis (or macula lutea), convert the image to nervous impulses, and the optic nerve transmits the impulses to the brain for processing. With corneal malfunction, such as myopia and hyperopia, the most common problems requiring corrective lenses, a distinct loss of detail is perceived because the incoming light is not properly focused on the retina. This is easily perceived and well-established means are available for correction. Image conversion and processing problems are not as easily perceived and these deserve some elementary study.

Visual Physiology

It is often uncertain whether conversion and processing problems are caused by the light-sensitive cells located in the retina or by mental misperceptions due to neurological processing. Sufficient research has been done at least to outline some of the factors that may cause misperceptions. Understanding that these factors exist and how they can prejudice perception can assist greatly in reducing visual problems.

An excellent example of misperception is the tendency to stare at an object that is difficult to see. Although this may be a good method of mental concentration, it does nothing to improve the visual quality of the image. In fact, it does the opposite. The length of time the human visual system can integrate (acquire information) is only 0.2 second. If the image does not provide enough information to be converted and processed in that time, the visual system will reset itself and reacquire information for the next 0.2 second. Therefore, when insufficient information is provided to the radiologist due to low illumination, excessive film density or distracting reflected light, only an improvement in the quality and quantity of light photons available will improve the visual image. The radiographic film does much to resolve the integration time problem. Because the film emulsion can

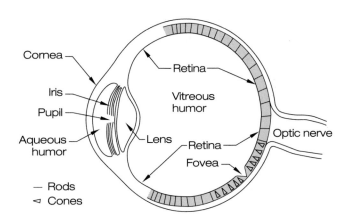

FIGURE 14–2. The human eye.

integrate information for a considerable length of time and then hold that information until processed, it permits the human brain to integrate much more visual information than if the image were viewed as it was acquired from the patient.

Rod and Cone Cells

Human image conversion occurs in the **rod** and **cone** cells located in the retina. Both of these types of cells contain photosensitive pigments that will respond to light by sending an electrical potential to specialized nerve cells. These bipolar cells emit neurological impulses when excited by light photons. The two types of cells are so different in their receiving and sending abilities that neurophysiologists tend to consider them as two separate visual systems. The cells are only about 1 µm in diameter and are concentrated to 100,000 per mm². There are approximately 7,000,000 cones, which are located only at the fovea centralis. There are approximately 120,000,000 rods covering the remainder of the retina.

Photopic Vision

Photopic (daylight) vision is controlled by the cones. Cone cells require relatively bright light to function (a minimum of approximately 100 light photons). Cone cells contain one of three different light-sensitive pigments, each of which is sensitive to a different range of photon wavelength (color of light). The cones are most sensitive to yellow light. Color blindness is a condition that occurs when there is a lack of cones sensitive to a particular color or colors.

Because most of the cones are located at the fovea centralis in high concentration, daylight vision is sharply focused. Therefore **visual acuity** is improved in daylight. The sparse concentration of cones in the retina outside the fovea centralis accounts for poor peripheral vision in daylight. Cones are also able to detect changes in brightness far better than rod cells. This permits much greater recognition of density differences, or contrast, and results in what is called greater **contrast perception** (Figure 14–3).

Scotopic Vision

Scotopic (night) vision is controlled by the rods. Rod cells are sensitive to low light levels (they may respond to as few as fifteen photons) but cannot function in bright light. Rod cells cannot distinguish wavelength, although they are more sensitive to green light. As a result, humans are unable to perceive colors in extremely low light situations. Rod cells function by photosensitization of rhodopsin, also known as "visual purple," because it is most sensitive to blue-green wavelengths. When exposed to vast quantities of light photons, rhodopsin is oversensitized and becomes bleached out. The rod cells then regenerate rhodopsin at the rate of 50 percent each seven minutes. This is the reason a bright light causes temporary blindness in both humans and animals. Because

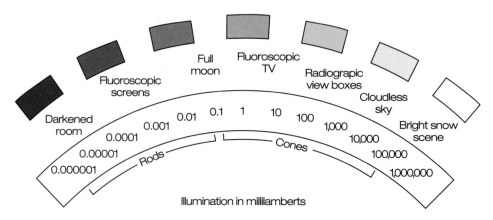

FIGURE 14-3. Human visual ability.

there are no rods in the fovea centralis, dim light vision is entirely peripheral and therefore difficult to bring into sharp focus. In addition, rods are not as concentrated because they are spread over a much greater area than cones. For these reasons, radiologists realize that dim objects are best viewed peripherally. Rods function better when the image information is changing. Slow scanning with an old fluoroscopic unit, night binoculars, or when walking in a dark room will increase visual acuity.

Inefficiency of the Medical Imaging Process

Few radiographers realize exactly how inefficient the entire imaging process is. An early fluoroscopic image study showed that although the x-ray tube was emitting 5,000,000 photons per second per mm^2 amplified over 5,000 times by the fluoroscopic intensification screen, only 65 photons contributed to the final impulses received by the brain. This is a conversion efficiency of 0.00005 percent (1 out of 2,000,000 photons) from the fluoroscopic screen and 0.001 percent (1 out of 100,000 photons) from the tube output.

Threshold Detection

Threshold detection is a visual phenomenon involving the perception of extremely small or faint details. This is more than an issue of the resolution, or fineness of the details, in the image. It also involves minimizing

background density and other artifacts, known as visual noise.

Boundary Effect   A boundary effect occurs because the visual system has difficulty perceiving contrast differences that are distant from one another. When a distinct boundary between various densities can be achieved (this is actually contrast), adjacent differences as small as two percent can be perceived under high illumination (such as a radiographic view box). When the boundary is indistinct, a difference of up to 20 percent may be required. Less intense light levels also affect this perception ability.

There is a rule of thumb in radiography that density changes should be at least 25–33 percent to be visible. This is because two radiographs of differing densities are seen quite distant from one another. If a change of this magnitude formed an adjacent boundary, it would be strikingly apparent. Surrounding densities have an effect on the perception of nearby densities. This results in confusion when judging absolute and relative levels of density and contrast from one image to another.

Another aspect of the boundary effect concerns the length of the boundary line. A subtle density difference along the length of a long boundary may be perceived but when it is shortened the boundary may no longer be perceived. As yet there is no explanation for this phenomenon but radiologists can best observe extremely subtle density differences when they form a long boundary. They may fail to see diagnostic information when density differences are widely separated or form short boundaries. In these instances it is important for the radiographer to attempt to provide better perception through higher contrast.

Mach Effect
Part of the boundary effect may be explained by a phenomenon called the **Mach effect**. The retina contains neural connections that inhibit impulses under certain conditions. One of these conditions is extremely bright light; another is a dramatic change in impulse intensity. The Mach effect occurs when the eye perceives a boundary. Each time there is a change in density there is a change in the intensity of the impulses sent to the brain. When the beginning of the new intensity level is inhibited by the neural connectors, the impulses to the brain are transmitted as shown in the graph in Figure 14–4B. For density differences as shown in the step wedge in Figure 14–4A, the end result is a response as shown in Figure 14–4C. This creates an effect known as **edge enhancement**. Edge enhancement compresses the entire density scale while making the boundary appear more distinct than it really is. For example, in Figure 14–5 many of the lighter density steps appear to be lighter just before the edge of the next darker step. This perceptual illusion is the Mach effect. Although this makes it easier to perceive the edges, radiologists are concerned about the possibility of a small detail being lost because its density is overwritten by edge enhancement. Figures 14–5 and 14–6 have the same light-to-dark scale. Note that the lack of a distinct boundary line causes a difference in perception of the range of visible densities.

Eye Motion
Contrast perception is dramatically increased when the eye uses a scanning motion, as when reading a book. Because the photosensitive cells in the eye can integrate a limited amount of information, eye movement maintains a constantly changing neurological signal, thus avoiding saturation of the optical nerves.

Veil Glare
Veil glare occurs when the intensely bright light from a view box floods the eye directly. This occurs in unexposed areas of the image and between images. The bright light scatters inside the eye and reduces contrast perception, much as Compton scatter does within the patient.

Viewing Distance
Data concerning threshold detection indicate that results change when the viewing distance is changed. This occurs because of the changes in intensity due to the inverse square law and because the physiological processing of the image changes when the angle of the incident light photons changes. In addition, the fovea centralis creates a blind spot at a viewing distance of about nine inches. Therefore, radiologists often vary their viewing distances when addressing areas of perceptual difficulty.

Pattern Recognition
Pattern recognition involves perceiving combinations of details that can be defined and classified toward a

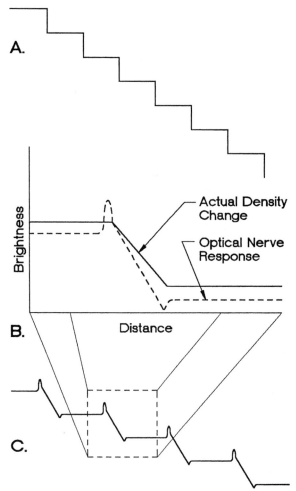

FIGURE 14–4. The Mach effect: (A) actual density differences, (B) comparison of actual density changes to optical nerve response, and (C) optical nerve response from A.

FIGURE 14–5. Optical step wedges. Note the prominent Mach effect through the lighter densities of the upper step wedges.

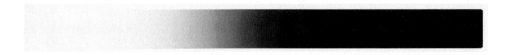

FIGURE 14–6. A continuous gray scale produced with a continuous sloping aluminum step wedge.

diagnosis. This is the area radiologists often study the hardest. Just as it is difficult to identify a picture of a familiar face when it is shown upside down, so it is important that radiologists be presented with images in a routine manner. For example, radiographs are universally viewed as if the viewer were facing the patient (the patient's left is on the viewer's right, etc.).

Pattern recognition involves comparing mental images of patterns — anatomical, physiological, pathological, and histological — to arrive at a diagnostic opinion. Because of the complexities between the visual system and the mental capability to store and recall image patterns from memory, and because of the lack of scientific knowledge about how the brain processes information, pattern recognition is a weak area of research and no data can be provided to help the radiographer assist

the radiologist. Pattern recognition is the true domain of the radiologist, who has the requisite medical knowledge to be competent in this area.

Controlling The Image In Space

One of the challenges to the radiographer is to place the patient so that the area to be imaged is in a position that will enhance the quality of the image. It is helpful to visualize the object of radiographic interest (kidney, scapula, sinus, etc.) as floating in space within the body of the patient. The skill of the radiographer lies in manipulating the object to the correct position in relationship to the x-ray beam and image receptor (film). This is the art of controlling the image in space.

Thinking Three-Dimensionally

The radiographer must be capable of controlling the image in space in an artistic manner. This is one of the critical elements of professionalism. In her book, *Fundamentals of Radiology*, radiologist Lucy Frank Squire encourages us with "An Invitation to Think Three-Dimensionally." This concept is extremely valuable in forming perceptual ability. The experienced radiographer can see an incredible amount of beauty in the radiographs that are produced every day. Just as the barium-coated finger (Figure 14–7) is easily perceived in three dimensions, so are most radiographs viewed in this manner by radiographers. The magnification of structures some distance from the film places them further away in perspective; finely detailed structures seem to move closer, and each image assumes a three-dimensionality usually not noticed by the novice.

Radiographic positioning requires a solid knowledge of the shape and location of skeletal and soft-tissue structures and an indepth understanding of their anatomical relationship to one another. For example, a diagnostic image of the maxillary sinuses can be obtained only after positioning the patient's head so the overlying structures of the cranium do not appear superimposed over the area of interest.

The human body is a three-dimensional object, but radiographic images possess only two dimensions — length and width. Consequently, all radiographic images are missing a critical diagnostic element — the dimension of depth. This can only be compensated for by never settling for a single radiographic view of any structure. **At least two images, as close to 90° angles to one another as possible, are required to view all three dimensions.**

The dimensional views required for all radiographic examinations are **anterior-posterior**, **medial-lateral** and **superior-inferior**. All radiographic images will demonstrate two, but never all three, of these perspectives. For example, a postero-anterior (PA) chest radiograph demonstrates the medial-lateral dimension and the superior-inferior dimension, but not the anterior-posterior dimension. The dimension that describes the entrance and exit of the central ray, which is used to describe the projection, is the dimension not visualized. In situations where superimposition makes PA and lateral projections

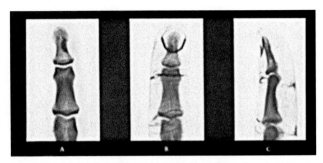

FIGURE 14–7. A three-dimensional effect. *(Reprinted with permission from the publishers of* Fundamentals of Radiology *by Lucy Frank Squire and Robert A. Noveline, Harvard University Press, Cambridge , MA. First edition copyright 1964 by the Commonwealth Fund; second, third, and fourth editions copyright 1975, 1982, and 1988 by the President and Fellows of Harvard College.)*

useless, two oblique positions at 90° angles from one another can be used to achieve the same effect.

An important skill that must be developed by the radiographer is the ability to mentally visualize the changing and moving of overlying anatomical structures from any angle in order to provide an image free of superimposition. Artistic techniques should be understood, such as making exposures while the patient is breathing, thus using patient motion to blur superimposing structures from the image (i.e., to blur ribs from the lateral projection of the thoracic vertebral column).

Radiography As An Art Form

Radiography is an art form. In the century since its discovery it has been used to investigate an incredible variety of animals and objects. Examples of radiography as a technical and purely creative art form abound. Numerous radiographers have not only taken pride in the quality of their clinical abilities but have extended their technical skills into artistic expressions of creativity.

Radiographers can become technically artistic; innovative adaptations of routine procedures should be considered technical artistry. For example, it is technically artistic to reverse routine angles to produce a diagnostic quality acanthio-parietal projection of the skull for a traumatized patient with anterior facial injuries, or to lower the tube and support a film cassette under a wheelchair patient's foot so that it is unnecessary to move a weak patient with a full leg cast onto a radiographic table.

Artistic Radiography

William Conklin, a South Carolina radiographer artist, has achieved national acclaim for his radiography/photography of sea shells (Figure 14–8). Conklin's work has appeared in *National Geographic* and is in the permanent collection of the Smithsonian Institution. Radiography has often been used to produce a unique perspective of flowers, fruit and other plants, as well as of shells and fish.

Nondestructive Testing

The entire industrial radiography field, known as nondestructive testing (NDT) radiography, is unknown to many medical radiographers. The intent of NDT radiography is to assist in the examination and assessment of materials such as castings, welds, etc., through noninvasive techniques.

Biological Research

Radiography has proven an invaluable tool in biological research, not only in medical studies, but also in monitoring animal functions. For example, the study of birds and bats in flight is greatly enhanced by high-speed radiography.

Veterinary Radiography

Veterinary medicine and dentistry also use radiography to accomplish many diagnoses. Figure 14–9, a canary with an egg, is an example of veterinary radiography. This type of radiography is also used in zoos. Radiographers have been called upon to examine all types of animals, from live venomous snakes to passive house pets.

Forensic Radiography

Forensic medicine uses radiography in a wide variety of ways. Grenz rays (5–30 kVp x-rays) are used, as are diagnostic x-rays. Grenz rays are emitted by specially

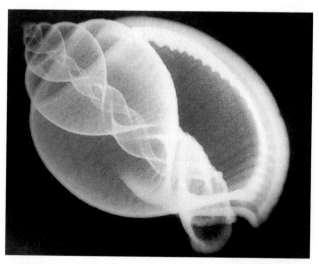

FIGURE 14–8. "Scotch Bonnet," by Willliam A. Conklin, R. T., FASRT. *(With permission of William A. Conklin, Inner Dimension, 1571 Marshall Avenue, Orangeburg, SC 29115)*

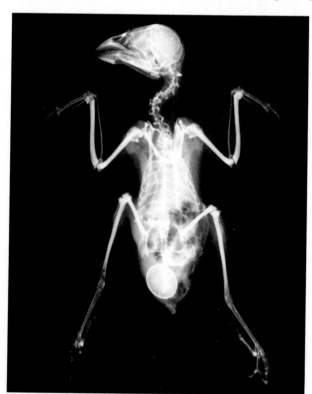

FIGURE 14–9. Canary with an egg. *(Reprinted with permission of the International Society of Radiographers and Technicians from the K. C. Clark Archives, Middlesex Hospital, London, England)*

designed tubes with minimal inherent filtration. They are useful for demonstrating objects as diverse as the ink on money when counterfeiting is suspected, the contents of envelopes and packages, fingerprints and art forgery.

Art Restoration

Grenz ray radiography has also proven useful during restoration of paintings and other art objects. Radiography can detect images under existing paint, frame and canvas construction and different types of paint and brush styles (Figure 14–10A and B).

Archaeological Radiography

Radiography has become a useful archaeological tool, especially in the examination of fragile mummified remains. Numerous reports of such investigations have been published. Most notable in this area is the book *X-Raying the Pharaohs*, in which University of Michigan researchers Harris and Weeks discuss their experiences radiographing the mummies at the National Museum in Cairo. Among their radiographic discoveries were jewelry, diseases, murders, dietary habits and the remains of a baboon that had been assumed to be a royal child (Figure 14–11).

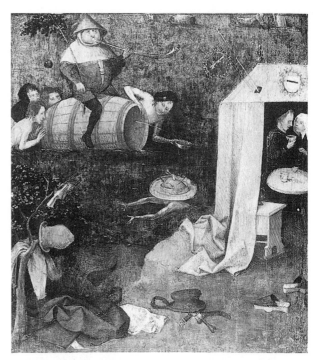

FIGURE 14–10B. "Intemperance" by Hieronymus Bosch. *(Reprinted with permission from Yale University Art Gallery, The Rabinowitz Collection)*

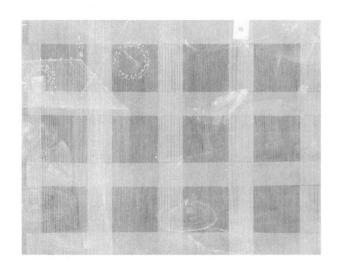

FIGURE 14–10A. A Grenz ray radiograph of a section of "Intemperance" by Hieronymus Bosch. *(Courtesy of Gerald Conlogue, Gulf Coast Community College)*

Poetry

Radiographic images themselves inspire many of us. The physician poet Jack Coulehan was inspired by a chest radiograph to compose this poem:

The Old Man with Stars Inside Him

I look at the X-ray,
a shadow of pneumonia
deep in this old man's chest,
and watch Antonio shake
with a cough that traveled here
from the beginning of life.
As he pulls my hand to his lips
and kisses my hand,
Antonio tells me, for a man
whose death is gnawing at his spine,
pneumonia is a welcome friend
who reaches in between his ribs

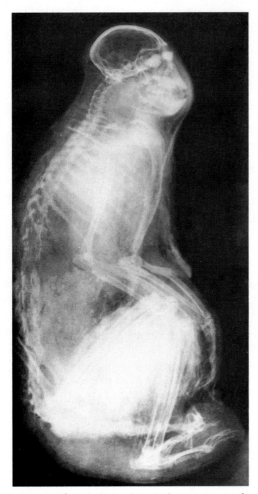 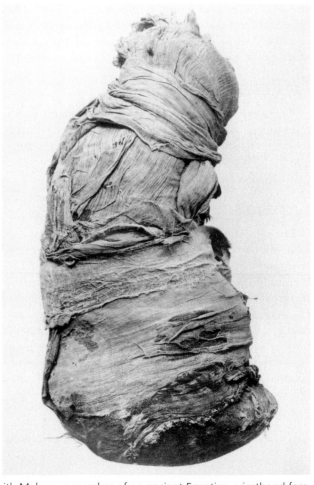

FIGURE 14–11. A female hamadryas baboon mummy found buried with Makare, a member of an ancient Egyptian priesthood family, who was pregnant at the time of her death. *(Reprinted with permission from "X-Raying the Pharoahs," by James E. Harris and Kent R. Weeks)*

without a sound and puff!
a cloud begins to squeeze
so delicately
the great white image of his heart.
The shadow advances
every time Antonio moves —
when a nurse positions his body,
when he takes a sip of ice,
when he shakes with a cough,
moist and diminished.
I see in that delicate shadow
a cloud of gas
at the galaxy's center,

a cloud of cold stunned nuclei
beginning to spin,
spinning and shooting
a hundred thousand
embryos of stars.
I listen to Antonio's chest
where stars crackle from the past
and hear the boom
of blue giants newly caught.
I hear the snap
of white dwarves coughing, shooting.
The second time Antonio
kisses my hand

I feel his dusky lips
reach out from everywhere in space.
I look at the place
his body was
and see inside Antonio, the stars.

Reprinted with permission from Midwest Poetry Review, ©
Jack Coulehan 1988

Summary

Understanding visual perception is an important aspect of clinical radiography. This understanding helps to overcome misperceptions about an image.

The human eye is designed to gather light, focus it, convert it to nerve impulses and transmit it to the brain for processing. Image conversion occurs in the rod and cone cells, which contain photosensitive pigments that will respond to light. Photopic (daylight) vision is controlled by the cones and scotopic (night) vision is controlled by the rods.

Threshold detection is a visual phenomenon involving the perception of extremely small or faint details. The boundary effect occurs because the visual system has difficulty perceiving contrast differences that are distant from one another. When densities are adjacent, small differences can be perceived. Part of the boundary effect can be explained by the Mach effect. When the eye perceives a boundary, a change occurs in the intensity of the impulses sent to the brain. This change in intensity creates an effect known as edge enhancement, which makes the boundary appear distinct. Contrast perception is dramatically increased by eye motion or scanning the image. Veil glare occurs when bright lights, such as a view box, flood the eye. Viewing distance has an effect on threshold detection.

Pattern recognition involves perceiving combinations of details that can be defined and classified toward a diagnosis. It helps the radiologist compare mental images of patterns with medical knowledge.

Radiographers need to think three-dimensionally. Radiographic images possess two dimensions and, as a result, at least two images as close to 90° angles to one another as possible are required to view all three dimensions. It is considered technical artistry when radiographers use innovation to adapt a routine procedure.

Radiography is an art form that has been used to investigate a wide array of animals and objects. It is used in nondestructive testing; biological research, veterinary and forensic radiography; art restoration; archeological radiography; and has even been the subject of poetry.

REVIEW QUESTIONS

1. What is the human eye designed to do?
2. What is the difference between photopic and scotopic vision?
3. Explain the boundary effect.
4. What is the Mach effect?
5. How is pattern recognition used by the radiologist in making a diagnosis?
6. Why is it important for the radiographer to produce two images as close to 90° angles to one another as possible?
7. Name three examples of the use of radiography as an art form.

REFERENCES AND RECOMMENDED READING

Abildgaard, A. & Notthellen, J. A. (1992). Increasing contrast when viewing radiographic images. *Radiology*. *185*(2), 475–478.

Adler, A. M. & Carlton, R. R. (1990). Perceiving the Radiographic Image. *Postgraduate Advances in Radiologic Technology*. Berryville, VA: Forum Medicum.

Adler, A. M. & Carlton, R. R. (1989). Repeating radiographs: Critiquing the Image. *Postgraduate Advances in Radiologic Technology*. Berryville, VA: Forum Medicum.

Adrian-Harris, D. (1979). Aspects of visual perception in radiography. *Radiography*. *45*(539), 237–243.

Arnold, M. (1993). The importance of spatial ability in the selection of student radiographers. *Radiography Today*. *59*(679), 20–22.

Bruce, V. & Green, P. R. (1985). *Visual perception physiology, psychology, and ecology*. London: Lawrence Erlbaum Associates, Publishers.

Carlton, R. R. & McKenna, A. (1989). Repeating radiographs: Setting imaging standards. *Postgraduate Advances in Radiologic Technology.* Berryville, VA: Forum Medicum.

Chester, M. S. (1982). Perception and evaluation of images. *Scientific Basis of Medical Imaging.* Edited by Wells, P. T. N. Edinburgh: Churchill Livingstone.

Cornsweet, T. N. (1970). *Visual perception.* New York: Academic Press.

Curry, T. S., Dowdey, J. E., & Murry, R. C. (1990). *Christensen's introduction to the physics of diagnostic radiology* (4th ed.). Philadelphia: Lea and Febiger.

Davson, H. (1980). *Physiology of the eye* (4th ed.). Edinburgh: Churchill Livingstone.

Dowd, S. B. (1995). *Encyclopedia of radiographic positioning.* Philadelphia: W. B. Saunders.

Fuchs, A. W. (1932). Radiography of the entire body employing one film and a single exposure. *Radiography and Clinical Photography. 10,* 9–14.

Gibbs, S. J., Price, R. R., & James, A. E. (1981). Image Perception, *The Physical Basis of Medical Imaging.* Editors: Coulam, C. M., Erickson, J. J., Rollo, F. D., & James, A. E. New York: Appleton-Century-Crofts, 295–302.

Graham, D. & Thomson, J. (1980). *Grenz rays: An illustrated guide to the theory and practical applications of soft x-rays.* Oxford: Pergamon Press.

Gregg, E. C. (1972). Image manipulation in radiology. *Physics of Diagnostic Radiology.* Editor: Wright, D. J. Rockville, MD: U.S. Department of Health, Education, and Welfare, Public Health Service, Food and Drug Administration, Bureau of Radiological Health, USD-HEW Publication No. (FDA) 74–8006, 282–334.

Hay, G. A. (1982). Traditional x-ray imaging. *Scientific Basis of Medical Imaging.* Edited by Wells, P. T. N. Edinburgh: Churchill Livingstone.

Hendee, W. R. (1989). The perception of visual data. *American Journal of Roentgenology. 152,* 1313–1317.

Hendee, W. R. (1988). The human visual system and its application to perception of radiographic images. *Investigative Radiology. 24,* 25.

Hendee, W. R. (1988). Image analysis and perception. *Textbook of Diagnostic Imaging.* Edited by Putman, C. E. & Ravin, C. E. Philadelphia: W. B. Saunders.

Hendee, W. R. & Ritenour, R. (1993). *Medical imaging physics* (3rd ed.). St. Louis: C. V. Mosby.

Hendee, W. R. & Wells, P. T. N. (1994). *Perception of visual information.* New York: Springer-Verlag.

Hooker, E. Z. (1981). The perceptual domain: A taxonomy for allied health educators. *Journal of Allied Health.* (August), 198–206.

Jaffe, C. C. (1984). Medical imaging, vision, and visual psychophysics. *Medical Radiography and Photography. 60*(1), 1–48.

Jaffe, C. C. (Ed.). (1981). *Second international conference on visual psychophysics and medical imaging.* Piscataway, NJ: IEEE Catalog #81CH 1676–6.

Manning, D. & Cooper, A. (1993). Chest x-ray image quality: Relationships between physical measurements and observer grading. *Radiography Today. 59*(678), 12–15.

Moore, H. D., (Ed.). (1981). *Materials and processes for NDT technology.* Columbus, Ohio: American Society for Nondestructive Testing.

Neisser, U. (1964). Visual search. *Scientific American. 210*(6), 94–102.

Randall, P. A. (1978). Mach bands in cine coronary arteriography. *Radiology. 129,* 65–66.

Richardson, H. D. (1968). *NDT radiography manual.* Washington, DC: U.S. Government Printing Office, U.S. Department of Health, Education, and Welfare.

Rose, A. (1948). The sensitivity performance of the human eye on an absolute scale. *Journal of the Optical Society of America. 38*(2), 196–208.

Schnitzler, A. D. (1973). Image-detector model and parameters of the human visual system. *Journal of the Optical Society of America. 63*(11), 1357–1368.

Squire, L. F. (1982). *Fundamentals of radiology* (3rd ed.). Cambridge, MA: Harvard University Press.

Tuddenham, W. J. (1957). The visual physiology of Roentgen diagnosis. *American Journal of Roentgenology. 78*(1), 116–123.

CHAPTER 15

Beam Restriction

Tell the world to wait
till we set the record straight
x-ray vision
baby, I can see thru you

Moon Martin, Pete Sinfield, and Terry Taylor, "X-Ray Vision,"
from Mystery Ticket.

Objectives

Upon completion of this chapter, the student should be able to:

▶ Identify the factors that affect the amount of scatter radiation produced.

▶ Discuss the primary methods used by radiographers to control the amount of scatter radiation reaching the film.

▶ Explain the purpose and construction of beam-restricting devices.

▶ Compare the advantages and disadvantages of the various beam-restricting devices.

▶ Describe the effect of beam restriction on image quality and patient dose.

Controlling Scatter

Scatter radiation is produced during a Compton inter-action. In this interaction, a primary photon interacts with an outer-shell electron and changes direction, there-by becoming a scattered photon. Scattered photons are not a part of the useful beam and will impair image qual-ity by placing density on the film which is unrelated to patient anatomy. In order to provide the best possible image, the radiographer must try to minimize the amount of scatter radiation reaching the film. **This can best be accomplished by restricting the x-ray beam and by using a grid.** Proper beam restriction will keep the total amount of tissue irradiation to a minimum and has great importance in both improving image quality and reducing patient dose.

As the beam is restricted, fewer primary photons are emitted from the tube and collimator and fewer scat-tered photons are created. Additionally, the decrease in the number of primary photons results in a decrease in the dose to the patient. The only way to improve image quality once scattered photons have been created is to try to decrease the number that are allowed to interact with the film. Grids are devices which are placed between the patient and the film to absorb scatter radiation.

The principle factors that affect the amount of scat-ter produced are 1) kilovoltage and 2) the irradiated material. In order to control the amount of scatter pro-duced, it is important to understand how kilovoltage and the irradiated material affect scatter production.

Kilovoltage

Kilovoltage affects the penetrability of the beam. As kVp increases, fewer photons undergo interaction with matter and more pass through the patient to interact with the film. For the photons that undergo an interac-tion, photoelectric absorption and Compton interac-tions are predominant in the diagnostic x-ray range. Although the total number of photons that undergo interaction decreases with increased kVp, a shift is seen in the percentage of photoelectric versus Compton inter-actions as kVp increases. As the kilovoltage increases, the percentage of x-rays that undergo a Compton interac-tion increases and the percentage of photons that under-go photoelectric absorption decreases. Because Compton interactions create scatter, as kilovoltage increases the percentage of primary photons that will undergo scatter-ing also increases. At the same time, the percentage of primary photons that are absorbed photoelectrically decreases, resulting in a reduction in patient dose.

If kilovoltage is increased with no other change in the technical factors selected for a given exposure, the end result will be an increase in the transmission of photons and therefore an increase in the exit dose from the patient. More radiation will reach the image receptor and the image will be darker. This increase in kilovoltage will also result in an increase in the percent and amount of scatter radiation produced. Table 12–2 illustrates this point. At 50 kVp with a 10 cm tissue, for every 1000 photons, 990 photons (approximately 99 percent) will be attenuated and 10 photons (approximately 1 percent) will be transmitted. Of the 990 attenuated photons, approximately one-half interact by photoelectric absorp-tion and one-half by Compton scatter (495 interactions each). At 130 kVp with a 10 cm tissue, for every 1000 photons, 940 photons (approximately 94 percent) will be attenuated and 60 photons (approximately 6 percent) will be transmitted. Of the 940 attenuated photons, approximately 25 percent (235 photons) interact photo-electric absorption and 75 percent (705 photons) by Compton scatter.

In radiography, the kilovoltage level is selected based predominantly on the size of the part being examined and the radiographic contrast desired for the image. When kilovoltage is increased without any other changes in technical factors, more scatter will result. If, however, the increase in kilovoltage is accompanied by a reduction in mAs to maintain the same exit dose, the overall result will be a decrease in the amount of scatter produced. Overall less photons are needed to create an acceptable image.

An x-ray image is created when some photons pass through the patient unaffected and others are absorbed photoelectrically. This difference is the basis for varying shades of radiographic density. When more photons pass through unaffected, the resulting image has greater den-sity. When more photons are absorbed photoelectrically, the resulting image has less density. Scattered photons from Compton interactions are of no use in demonstrat-ing the structures of interest. They merely add unwanted densities to the film that do not correspond to any particular structure. Much of the overall radiographic density on a film is created by scattered photons. Image quality is improved when the amount of scatter reaching the film is reduced.

Irradiated Material

The amount of scatter created during an interaction is affected by the volume and atomic number of the material being irradiated. The volume of irradiated material is controlled by field size and patient thickness (Figure 15–1).

As the volume of irradiated tissue increases, the amount of scatter increases. Volume increases as the field size increases or as the patient thickness increases. Larger field sizes, such as with 14"×17" (35×43 cm) film, allow for more photons to interact with tissue, thereby creating more scatter. Larger body parts have more tissue to interact with the photons, resulting in greater scatter production. In order to decrease scatter, the smallest possible field size should be used. It is for this reason that beam restriction is an important part of scatter reduction and, of course, of patient protection. Patient thickness cannot be significantly altered by the radiographer, but certain techniques, such as the use of compression bands, can be useful in slightly reducing patient thickness.

The atomic number of the irradiated material also has an impact on the amount of scatter produced because higher atomic number materials have a greater number of electrons within each atom and photons have a greater chance of striking an electron, creating an absorption interaction. Therefore, the higher the atomic number of a material, the greater will be the number of photoelectric absorption interactions and the less scatter. Bone absorbs more radiation and scatters less than soft tissue. For this same reason, high atomic number materials, such as iodine, barium and lead, absorb more radiation through the photoelectric interaction than low atomic number materials do. These photoelectric absorption interactions create the high contrast seen when contrast media are used.

Of the factors affecting the amount of scatter produced, the kilovoltage and the field size are under the direct control of the radiographer. Kilovoltage levels

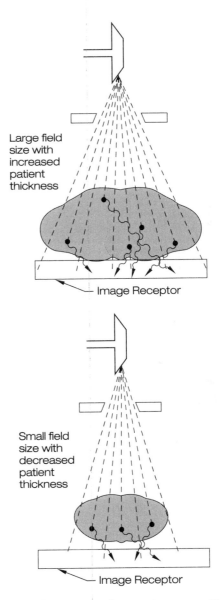

FIGURE 15–1. The amount of scatter increases with increased field size and patient thickness.

must be selected based on the area being radiographed, and the smallest possible field size should always be used. Beam restriction is, therefore, important to image quality. Remember, however, that **when the beam is restricted, less scatter radiation will reach the film and, as a result, technical factors may need to be increased to**

compensate for the reduction in the overall film density. For example, the technical factors used for an AP projection of the abdomen using a 14"×17" (35×43 cm) film would be insufficient to produce a good image of the same patient's gallbladder imaged on an 8"×10" (18×24 cm) film. Technical factors would typically need to be increased 25 to 50 percent to compensate for this type of reduction in the field size.

Beam Restrictors

There are three basic types of beam-restricting devices used to control scatter and reduce patient dose: **aperture diaphragms**, **cones/cylinders** and **collimators**. Each of these devices has advantages and disadvantages which determine how and when they are used in radiography.

Aperture Diaphragm

The aperture diaphragm is a flat sheet of metal, usually lead, with a hole cut in the center and attached to the x-ray tube port. This is the simplest of all beam-restricting devices both in design and in application. Different diaphragms are needed to accommodate different film sizes and different distances. The opening can be made in any size or shape but most are rectangular, square or round. Rectangular diaphragms are most common, to correspond to x-ray film sizes. The size of the opening depends on the desired exposure field, the source to image receptor distance (SID) and the distance from the aperture to the focal spot.

The main advantages in using an aperture diaphragm are its simple design, low cost and ease of use. The principle disadvantage is the increase in **penumbra**, a geometric unsharpness around the periphery of the image. This is the result of the diaphragm's close proximity to the tube port. Penumbra is reduced when the beam restrictor is at an increased distance from the port.

Penumbra is the result of x-ray photons being created in all areas of the focal spot rather than at just a single point. Primary photons diverge from the tube port at varying angles and intersect with the structures of interest at varying angles when creating the image. Reducing penumbra will improve the sharpness of the recorded image edges (Figure 15–2). While the use of different types of restrictors does not alter the sharpness of the internal image details, the further the beam restrictor is from the port, the sharper the edges of the exposed area will be.

Another problem when using an aperture diaphragm is the increase in **off-focus (stem) radiation** reaching the film. This occurs because of the aperture's close proximity to the tube port. Off-focus radiation originates within the x-ray tube but not at the focal spot. Off-focus radiation can result in images, similar to shadows of the patient, beyond the exposed field of radiation (Figure 6–23). These shadows are often believed to be caused by scatter radiation. However, scatter will never create an image of a specific anatomical structure.

The aperture diaphragm was the original type of beam restrictor, but its use is somewhat limited today. Since it is merely a flat sheet of metal with a hole cut in it, no light field is available for use as an aid in positioning. Its primary application is in dedicated equipment, such as for chest radiography, where the field size and the SID do not vary.

Determining the Diaphragm Field Size
When using an aperture diaphragm it may be necessary for the radiographer to determine the size of the projected image on the film. Aperture diaphragms, when used alone, do not provide the radiographer with a light field for viewing the projected image size. To avoid exposing an area larger than necessary, selection of the correct diaphragm and proper SID is critical. The following formula is used to determine the size of the projected image when using a specific aperture diaphragm. This formula is especially useful when a given diaphragm is used at varying distances.

projected image size =

$$\frac{\text{SID} \times \text{diameter of diaphragm}}{\text{distance from focal spot to diaphragm}}$$

Example: A diaphragm is placed 5 inches from the focal spot. The diameter of the opening in the aperture is a 2-inch circle. What would be the projected image size if the SID is 40 inches?

Answer: projected image size =

$$\frac{40 \times 2}{5} = \frac{80}{5} = 16\text{-inch circle}$$

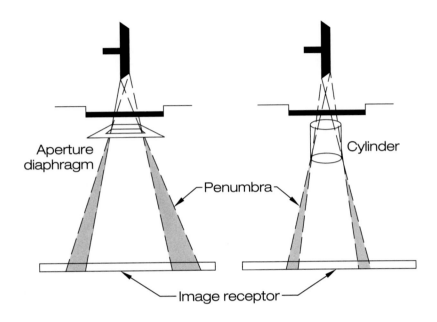

FIGURE 15–2. Penumbra increases as the beam restrictor moves closer to the port. Use of an aperture diaphragm results in greater penumbra than does use of a cylinder.

This same formula can be applied to a rectangular or square diaphragm by substituting length or width for the diameter of the diaphragm.

Cones/Cylinders

Cones and cylinders are essentially circular aperture diaphragms with metal extensions (Figure 15–3). A cone has an extension which flares or diverges, with the upper diameter smaller than the bottom flared end. A cylinder does not flare. Instead, it has the same diameter at the bottom of the extension as it has at the top. A cylinder may be equipped with an extension sleeve which can expand or collapse to vary the degree of beam restriction.

Cones and cylinders are also relatively inexpensive and simple to use. They are most commonly employed in radiography of the skull, spine, gallbladder and breast. The physical weight of a cone sometimes makes it difficult to handle and, when used with a horizontal beam, the weight of the cone may cause the tube to angle slightly, causing cone cutting if the central ray is not checked carefully just prior to the exposure.

Cones, like aperture diaphragms, have the disadvantage of a fixed field size unless they are equipped with an extension sleeve. In addition, flared cones are no better at reducing penumbra along the edges than are aperture diaphragms.

Cylinders, however, do reduce penumbra and off-focus radiation because they provide better beam restriction at a greater distance from the focal spot (Figure 15–2). This is especially true when they are used in conjunction with a collimator, as is most often the case.

Determining the Cone Field Size   Determining the field size for a cone/cylinder involves a method similar to that used with an aperture diaphragm. The following formula can be used to calculate the size of the projected image when using a cone/cylinder.

projected image size =

$$\frac{SID \times lower\ diameter\ of\ cone}{distance\ from\ focal\ spot\ to\ bottom\ of\ cone}$$

Example: The diameter of the lower rim of a cone is 3 inches. The bottom of the cone is placed at a distance 16 inches from the focal spot. What will be the size of the projected image at a 40-inch SID?

Answer: projected image size =

$$\frac{40 \times 3}{16} = \frac{120}{16} = 7.5\text{-inch circle}$$

Collimator

The collimator is the most commonly employed beam restrictor in radiography. Although it is more complex and expensive, the collimator permits an infinite number of field sizes using only one device (Figure 15–4). It also has the advantage of providing a light source for the radiographer as an aid in properly placing the tube and central ray.

A collimator consists of sets of lead shutters at right angles to one another which move in opposing pairs. Each set moves symmetrically from the center of the

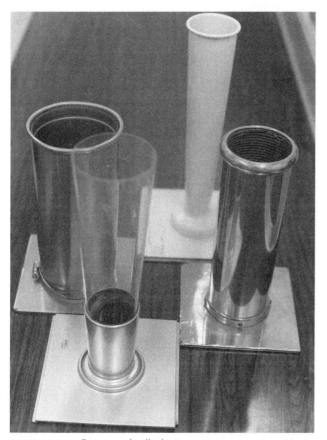

FIGURE 15–3. Cones and cylinders.

field. These lead shutters can be adjusted to correspond to an infinite number of square or rectangular field sizes.

The shutters serve to regulate the field size and, in addition, have two other purposes. The bottom shutters reduce penumbra along the periphery of the beam because of their greater distance from the focal spot. The upper shutters help in reducing the amount of off-focus (stem) radiation reaching the film by absorbing this radiation before it exits the tube.

The collimator offers the radiographer a light field which outlines the exposure field and provides a cross hair to identify the center of the beam. Some units also provide an outline of the automatic exposure control (AEC) chambers' size and location. The light field is provided by mounting a mirror in the path of the x-ray beam at a 45° angle. A light source is then placed opposite the mirror and the light is projected through the collimator. The light source and the x-ray source must be equidistant from one another to ensure that the light field and the x-ray field are the same size. Improper positioning of the mirror or the light can result in improper alignment of the light field to the exposure field. Collimator accuracy should be checked on a regular basis as a part of the department's quality control program.

In the United States it was been required by law from 1974 to 1993 for all fixed radiographic equipment to be equipped with automatic collimators. These devices are known as **positive beam limitation (PBL) devices**. When a cassette is placed in the Bucky tray and secured in position, sensing devices determine the size and placement of the cassette. The sensing devices activate an electric motor which drives the collimator lead shutters into proper position. When operating properly, automatic collimators should leave a small unexposed border on all four sides of the exposed film. However, it is possible to override the PBL devices so that the field size can be controlled by the radiographer.

The use of a collimator results in some filtration of the x-ray beam because the primary beam is passing through the mirror in the collimator. The added filtration is equivalent to approximately 1 mm of aluminum. Because collimators result in increased filtration of the x-ray beam, their use during low-kVp radiography (such as mammography) is restricted.

Proper collimation is the responsibility of the radiographer. Under no circumstances should the exposure

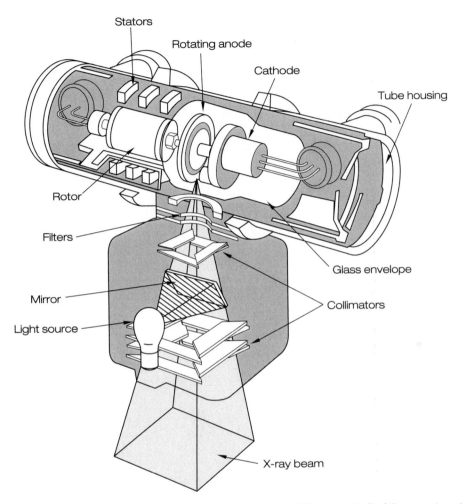

FIGURE 15–4. Schematic drawing of an x-ray tube and collimator. *(Courtesy of Siemens Medical Systems, Inc., Iselin, NJ)*

field exceed the size of the image receptor. Automatic collimation helps to ensure that the exposure field does not exceed the size of the image receptor, but the radiographer should always limit the field to the part being examined. By so doing, image quality can be improved and patient dose can be minimized.

Ancillary Devices

Beam restrictors may be made for a very specific purpose. Ancillary devices are generally designed with a spe-

cial need in mind. Examples include lead blockers and lead masks. These devices are tailored for a specific use during a given procedure. They are designed to restrict the beam to a specific shape for a particular examination.

A lead blocker is simply a sheet of lead-impregnated rubber that can be cut to any size or shape. Placement of a lead blocker on the radiographic table during radiography of the lower spine in the lateral position will help to absorb the scatter that is produced in the soft tissue of the patient's back (Figure 15–5). A lead blocker may also be helpful when placed on the radiographic table above the level of the shoulder during positioning for AP pro-

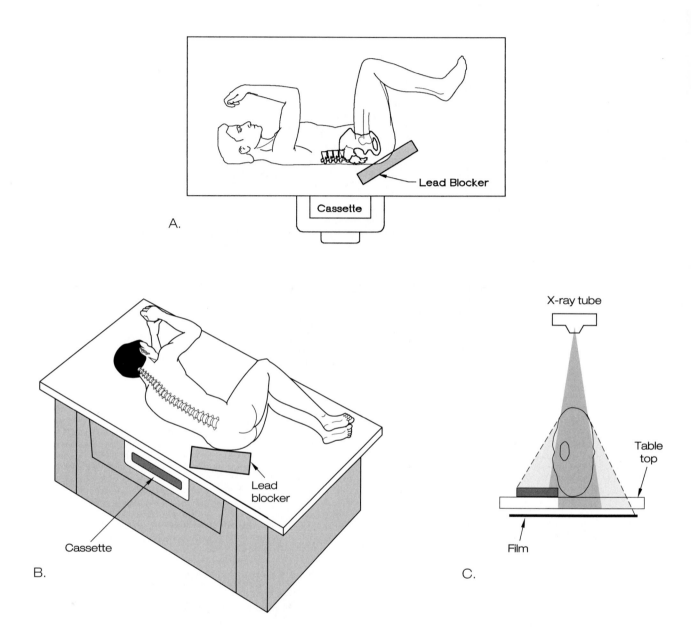

FIGURE 15–5. The use of a lead blocker for radiography of the lower spine (A) bird's eye view, (B) side view of lead blocker absorbing scatter radiation from the patient before it reaches the film, and (C) cutaway view of absorption of scatter.

jections of the shoulder joint. Lead blockers are most helpful when examining large patients, because the amount of scatter increases with increases in the size of the patient.

A lead mask is usually cut to correspond to the particular field size desired and is then secured to the end of the collimator. The most common use of a lead mask is during cerebral angiography. The lead mask helps improve image quality by reducing scatter (Figure 15–6 A & B).

Summary

In order to provide the best possible image, the radiographer must try to control the amount of scatter radiation reaching the film. The principle factors that affect the amount of scatter produced are: 1) kilovoltage and 2) the irradiated material. As kilovoltage increases, the percentage of primary photons that will undergo scattering also increases. As the volume of irradiated tissue increases, the amount of scatter produced is increased. Volume will increase as the field size increases or as the patient thickness increases. The atomic number of the irradiated material also has an impact on the amount of scatter produced. Higher atomic number materials have a greater number of electrons within each atom. Photons have a greater chance of being absorbed by these materials.

There are three basic types of beam-restricting devices that are used to control scatter and reduce patient dose: aperture diaphragms, cones/cylinders and collimators. Each of these devices has advantages and disadvantages which determine how and when they are used in radiography. The collimator is the most commonly employed beam restrictor in radiography because it permits an infinite number of field sizes using only one device. It also has the advantage of providing a light source for the radiographer as an aid in properly placing the tube.

Proper collimation is the responsibility of the radiographer. Under no circumstances should the exposure field ever exceed the size of the image receptor. In addition, the radiographer should always limit the field to the part being examined. By so doing, image quality will be improved and patient dose will be minimized.

REVIEW QUESTIONS

1. Why does beam restriction reduce scatter radiation production?

2. What are the two principle factors that affect the amount of scatter produced?

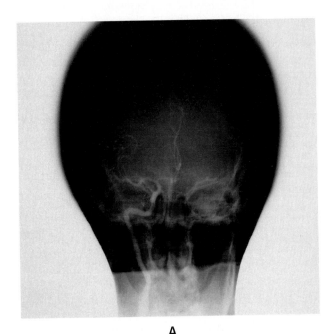

A

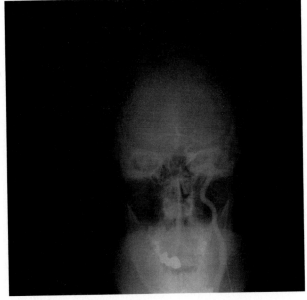

B

FIGURE 15–6A & B. Two radiographs of an AP cerebral angiogram, with and without a lead mask.

3. How does the atomic number of a material affect the amount of scatter produced?

4. What are the three basic types of beam-restricting devices?

5. What is penumbra and how can it be minimized?

6. What is the formula for determining the size of the projected image when using a cone?

7. How is a collimator constructed?

8. What is PBL?

9. How does beam restriction affect patient dose?

REFERENCES AND RECOMMENDED READING

Bushberg, J. T., Seibert, J. A., Leidholdt, E. M., & Boone, J. M. (1994). *The essential physics of medical imaging.* Baltimore: Williams & Wilkins.

Carroll, Q. B. (1993). *Fuchs's radiographic exposure, processing, and quality control* (5th ed.). Springfield, IL: Charles C. Thomas Publishers.

Crooks, H. E. & Ardran, G. M. (1976). Checking x-ray beam field size. *Radiography. 42*(503), 239.

Cullinan, A. & Cullinan, J. (1994). *Producing quality radiographs* (2nd ed.). Philadelphia: J. B. Lippincott.

Curry, T. S., Dowdey, J. E., & Murry, R. C. (1990). *Christensen's introduction to the physics of diagnostic radiology* (4th ed.). Philadelphia: Lea and Febiger.

De Voss, D. (1985). *Basic Principles of radiographic exposure* (2nd ed.). Baltimore: Williams & Wilkins.

Hendee, W. R., Chaney, E. L., & Rossi, R. P. (1977). *Radiologic physics, equipment, and quality control.* Chicago: Year Book Medical Publishers.

Hiss, S. S. (1993). *Understanding radiography* (3rd ed.). Springfield, IL: Charles C. Thomas Publishers.

Lauer, O. G., Mayes, J. B., & Thurston, R. P. (1990). *Evaluating radiographic quality: The variables and their effects.* Mankato, MN: The Burnell Company Publishers.

Mattsson, O. (1955). Practical photographic problems in radiography with special reference to high-voltage technique. *Acta Radiologica. Supplementum 120,* 1–206.

Mitchell, F. (1991). Scattered radiation and the lateral lumbar spine part 1: Initial research. *Radiography Today. 57*(644), 18–20.

Mitchell, F., Leung, C., Ahuja, A., & Metreweli, C. (1991). Scattered radiation and the lateral lumbar spine part 2: Clinical research. *Radiography Today. 57*(645), 12–14.

Rogers, K. D. & Matthers, I. P. (1986). X-ray field collimation in diagnostic radiology. *Radiography. 52*(604), 161.

Seeram, E. (1985). *X-ray imaging equipment: An introduction.* Springfield: Charles C. Thomas.

Thomas, S. R., Freshcorn, J. E., Krugh, K. B., Henry, G. C., Kereiakes, J. G., & Kaufman, R. A. (1983). Characteristics of extrafocal radiation and its potential significance in pediatric radiology. *Radiology. 146,* 793–799.

Thompson, M. A., Hattaway, M. P., Hall, J. D., & Dowd, S. B. (1994). *Principles of imaging science and protection.* Philadelphia: W. B. Saunders.

Wolbarst, A. B. (1993). *Physics of radiology.* Norwalk, CT: Appleton & Lange.

The Case of Lumpy

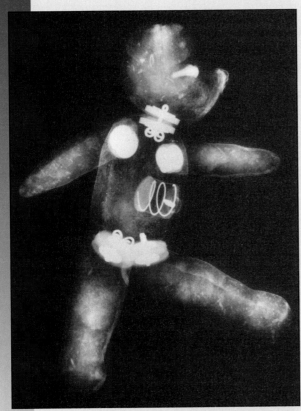

(Reprinted by permission of the International Society of radiographers and Radiological Technicians from the K. C. Clark Archives, Middlesex Hospital, London, England)

What is this lumpy object's name?

Answers to the case studies can be found in Appendix E.

CHAPTER 16

The Patient As A Beam Emitter

. . . the patient . . . would shape up into something that called for attention, his peculiarities, her reticences or candors. And though I might be attracted or repelled, the professional attitude . . . would steady me and dictate the terms on which I was to proceed.

— *William Carlos Williams,* The Autobiography.

Objectives

Upon completion of this chapter, the student should be able to:

▶ Explain the process of attenuation.

▶ Describe the basic composition of the human body.

▶ Describe the effect of the human body on the attenuation of the x-ray beam.

▶ Explain the relationship of the subject (patient) to the density, contrast, recorded detail and distortion of the recorded image.

Attenuation

Attenuation is the reduction in the total number of x-ray photons remaining in the beam after passing through a given thickness of material (Figure 12–1). It is the result of x-rays interacting with matter and being absorbed or scattered. The amount of attenuation is determined by the amount and type of irradiated material. X-rays are attenuated exponentially. This means that they are reduced by a certain percentage for each given thickness of material they pass through. Theoretically, then, the number of x-rays passing through an absorber will never reach zero. This is because each succeeding thickness of material reduces the number of photons by only a fraction of the previous amount.

As an x-ray beam passes through a patient, the beam is attenuated. The thicker the body part being radiographed, the greater the attenuation. In order to provide a sufficient number of x-ray photons for interaction with the film, the original quantity and quality of the photons must be increased with increased body part thickness. The incident beam is significantly altered as it passes through the patient. **The beam emitted from the patient contains the radiologically significant information needed by the radiologist to make a diagnosis.**

Attenuation is also affected by the type of absorber. **Higher atomic number materials (such as lead and barium) attenuate a greater percentage of the beam than low atomic number materials** (such as hydrogen, carbon and oxygen). This is due to the presence of a greater number of electrons with which photons may interact. Bone produces less radiographic density because it attenuates the x-ray beam more than soft tissue. This is predominantly because of the presence of calcium in bone, which has a higher atomic number than the majority of the elements found in the human body. The effective atomic number of the important materials comprising the human body are listed in Table 16–1.

The density of the absorbing material also has an impact on attenuation. **Density is the quantity of matter per unit of volume measured in kilograms per cubic meter.** It describes how tightly the atoms of a given substance are packed together. For example, the molecules in an ice cube are more tightly packed than the same molecules when they are in their liquid state. Bone tissue

is a denser substance than lung tissue. Table 16–1 lists the densities of the important materials comprising the human body. Because density and atomic number affect attenuation, it is important to understand the basic composition of the human body, particularly in terms of the average atomic number and density of the major substances.

The Human Body As An Attenuator

The patient is the greatest variable the radiographer faces when performing a radiographic procedure. The human body is comprised of a variety of organic and inorganic substances. At the atomic level, the body consists primarily of hydrogen, carbon, nitrogen and oxygen. These elements have atomic numbers of 1, 6, 7 and 8 respectively. Calcium, found in concentrated amounts in bones and teeth, has an atomic number of 20.

The composition of the human body determines its radiographic appearance (Figure 16–1). Although human anatomy and physiology are quite complex, when studying the absorption characteristics of the body, four major substances account for most of the variations in x-ray absorption: air, fat, muscle and bone (Figure 16–2).

Air

Air has an effective atomic number of 7.78, which is greater than either fat or muscle. Despite the slightly higher effective atomic number, air has a significantly lower tissue density. As a result, air will absorb fewer

**TABLE 16–1. Basic Substances
Comprising the Human Body**

Substance	Effective Atomic Number	Density (kg/m³)
Air	7.78	1.29
Fat	6.46	916
Water	7.51	1000
Muscle	7.64	1040
Bone	12.31	1650

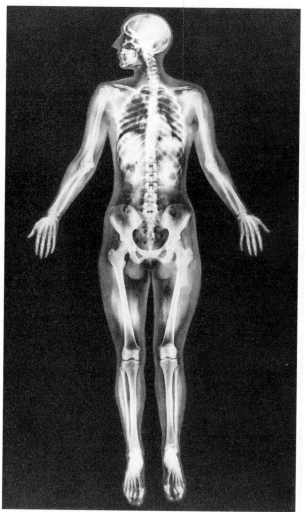

FIGURE 16–1. An antique full-body radiograph. *(Reprinted with permission of the International Society of Radiographers and Radiological Technicians from the K. C. Clark Archives, Middlesex Hospital, London, England)*

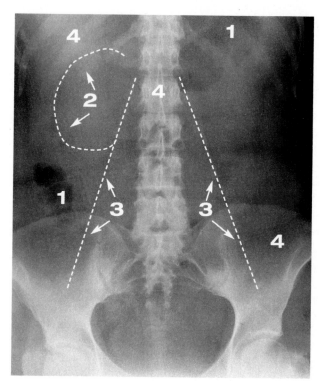

FIGURE 16–2. A radiograph of the abdomen demonstrating (1) air in the stomach and colon, (2) fat around the kidneys, (3) muscle to the right and left of the spine (psoas muscles), and (4) ribs, spine, and pelvis.

photons as they pass through it. Because air absorbs fewer photons than other body substances, more photons reach the x-ray film, thus producing a greater radiographic density. Air is naturally present in the lungs, the sinuses and, in small amounts, in the gastrointestinal tract. On a typical radiograph of the abdomen, air can usually be seen in the stomach and colon.

Fat

Fat is similar to muscle in that they are both among the soft-tissue structures in the body. The soft-tissue structures have effective atomic numbers and tissue densities which are very similar to water's. For this reason, water is sometimes used to simulate soft tissue for experimental purposes. Fat has an effective atomic number which is slightly less than muscle's. In addition, fat has less tissue density than muscle. Muscle cells are more closely packed than fat cells. The amount of fatty tissue varies considerably between patients. While this is also true of muscle tissue, the variations are generally less pronounced and therefore have less effect on the overall attenuation of the beam. On a radiograph of the abdomen, the kidneys can often be outlined because of the perirenal fat capsule that surrounds them.

Muscle

Like fat, muscle is a soft tissue. Muscle, however, has a slightly higher effective atomic number and a greater tissue density than fat. As a result, muscle is a greater attenuator of the beam. On a radiograph of the abdomen, it is often easy to distinguish the psoas muscle on each side of the spine because of the increased absorption of radiation by these muscles.

Bone

The skeletal anatomy is easily seen radiographically because of the calcium content of bone. Calcium has a higher atomic number than most of the elements found in the human body. As a result, bone has the highest effective atomic number of the four basic substances. It also has the greatest tissue density and, as a result, absorbs radiation at a greater rate than any of the soft tissues or air-filled structures. This absorption means that fewer photons will reach the x-ray film and less radiographic density will be produced. On a radiograph of the abdomen, the lower ribs, spine and pelvis are all very easily distinguished because of the increased x-ray absorption that occurs in bone.

The Patient's Relationship to Image Quality

The patient has an impact on all properties affecting radiographic quality: density, contrast, recorded detail and distortion. These are described in detail in Chapters 25–28. The relationships between these factors and the patient (subject) are termed subject density, subject contrast, subject detail and subject distortion.

Subject Density

The various tissues in the human body are responsible for the specific radiographic densities that occur on the film. Recall that radiographic density is the degree of blackening of the x-ray film. Subject density refers to the impact the subject (patient) has on the resultant radiographic density. **Radiographic density will be altered by changes in the amount or type of tissue being irradiated.** In other words, thicker and denser body parts absorb more radiation, thus producing less radiographic density, and vice versa.

Subject Contrast

Radiographic contrast is the difference in densities of a recorded image. The differences in radiographic density are the result of differences in the absorption of the x-ray beam as it passes through the patient. **Subject contrast is the degree of differential absorption resulting from the differing absorption characteristics of the tissues in the body.** Subject contrast is dependent on the specific characteristics of an individual patient's tissues.

When there is little difference in the absorption characteristic of the given body tissues within a part being examined, as in mammography, subject contrast will be low. When there is a greater difference in the absorption characteristics of the body tissues within a part being examined, as in the chest with the lungs, heart, and spine, subject contrast is high.

Subject Detail

One of the primary factors that affects the sharpness or detail of an image is the distance between the structure of interest and the film. Because anatomical structures are located at varying distances from the x-ray film, **the recorded detail of the structures is dependent on their position within the body and also on the body's placement in relationship to the film.** The overall size and placement of the patient has a great impact on the recorded detail. The larger the patient, the greater the distance between the anatomical structures and the film. This results in less sharpness in the recorded details on the film. Conversely, greater sharpness will result when the anatomical part is closer to the film, as is the case with thinner patients. Specific positions have been established to place the anatomical structures of interest in as close proximity to the film as possible. For example, chest radiography is typically performed in the PA projection and in the left lateral position to place the heart closer to the film.

Subject Distortion

Distortion is the misrepresentation of the size or shape of the structure of interest. Because of the way in which certain structures lie within the body, **unless the patient is positioned specifically to demonstrate a particular structure, it may not be accurately represented on the film.** For example, to properly demonstrate the apophyseal joints of the lumbar spine, the patient should be in the oblique position. In the AP projection of the lumbar spine, these joints will be distorted. Distortion, in the form of magnification, also occurs because various anatomical structures sit at varying levels.

Summary

Attenuation is the reduction in the total number of x-ray photons remaining in the beam after passing through a given thickness of material. It is the result of x-rays interacting with matter and being absorbed or scattered. The amount of attenuation will be determined by the amount and type of irradiated material.

The patient is the greatest variable that the radiographer faces when performing a radiographic procedure. The composition of the human body determines its radiographic appearance. When studying the absorption characteristics of the body, four major substances account for most of the variations in x-ray absorption: air, fat, muscle and bone.

The patient has an impact on all the properties that affect radiographic quality: density, contrast, recorded detail and distortion. The relationships between these factors and the patient (subject) are termed subject density, subject contrast, subject detail and subject distortion.

REVIEW QUESTIONS

1. How does atomic number affect attenuation?

2. How does tissue density affect attenuation?

3. What elements comprise the majority of those found in the human body?

4. What are the differences between air, fat, muscle and bone with respect to their attenuation and the resultant radiographic density?

5. How does the patient affect each of the factors of image quality?

REFERENCES AND RECOMMENDED READING

Bower, R. (1989). Stripes in the abdomen. *Radiologic Technology. 60*(6), 511.

Bushberg, J. T., Seibert, J. A., Leidholdt, E. M., & Boone, J. M. (1994). *The essential physics of medical imaging.* Baltimore: Williams & Wilkins.

Carroll, Q. B. (1993). *Fuchs's radiographic exposure, processing, and quality control* (5th ed.). Springfield, IL: Charles C. Thomas Publishers.

Cohen, M. (1971). Attenuation of x-rays in the human body. *Radiography. 37*(436), 88–90.

Curry, T. S., Dowdey, J. E., Murry, R. C. (1990). *Christensen's introduction to the physics of diagnostic radiology* (4th ed.). Philadelphia: Lea and Febiger.

Fuchs, A. W. (1948). Relationship of tissue thickness to kilovoltage. *Radiologic Technology. 19*(6), 287.

Handbook of chemistry and physics. (1989). (69th ed.). Boca Raton, FL: C. R. C. Press.

Hiss, S. S. (1993). *Understanding radiography* (3rd ed.). Springfield, IL: Charles C. Thomas Publishers.

Lindsay, R. & Anderson, J. B. (1978). Radiological determination of changes in bone mineral content. *Radiography. 44*(517), 21–26.

Seeram, E. (1985). *X-ray imaging equipment: An introduction.* Springfield: Charles C. Thomas.

Thompson, M. A., Hattaway, M. P., Hall, J. D., & Dowd, S. B. (1994). *Principles of imaging science and protection.* Philadelphia: W. B. Saunders.

Wolbarst, A. B. (1993). *Physics of radiology.* Norwalk, CT: Appleton & Lange.

The Case of the Injured Animal

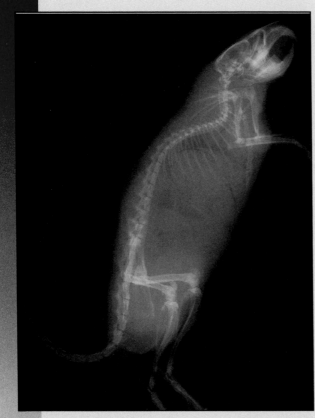

This animal was brought to the radiographic laboratory, dead on arrival. What type of animal is it and what was the cause of death?

Radiograph courtesy of Ron Cramer, Mary Rutan Hospital, Bellefontaine, Ohio.

Answers to the case studies can be found in Appendix E.

CHAPTER 17

The Pathology Problem

*You don't look different
but you have changed
I'm looking through you
you're not the same*

John Lennon and Paul McCartney "I'm Looking Through You," from Rubber Soul.

OBJECTIVES

Upon completion of this chapter, the student should be able to:

▶ Explain the effect that a pathological condition can have on radiation absorption.

▶ Describe the effect of pathology on the radiographic image.

▶ Differentiate between pathological conditions which result in increased attenuation versus those which result in decreased attenuation of the x-ray beam.

▶ Identify pathological conditions which result in an increased attenuation of the x-ray beam.

▶ Identify pathological conditions which result in a decreased attenuation of the x-ray beam.

Pathology and Radiation Absorption

As radiation passes through the patient it undergoes attenuation or absorption of the x-ray photons. The patient is the greatest variable the radiographer faces when trying to select adequate exposure factors for a specific procedure. Attenuation will vary, depending on the thickness and the composition of the patient's tissues. As an added dilemma, the radiographer must also realize that pathological conditions can affect the overall thickness and composition of the patient's tissues. The radiographer must first be aware of the variations between normal body tissues and then be concerned about possible additional variations as a result of a specific disease process.

Pathology is the medical science that is concerned with all aspects of disease, including the structural and functional changes caused by a disease process. Disease will often bring about changes in body tissues that can be viewed radiographically and interpreted by the radiologist. If this were not true, radiography would be of no use in diagnosing disease. These changes may be structural and/or functional in nature and they may or may not have an impact on the degree of radiation absorbed by the patient. Certain diseases can increase or decrease tissue thickness or alter tissue composition (change the effective atomic number or density). When this occurs, the disease will affect the degree of radiation absorption for that specific body tissue. Two common pathologies of the chest demonstrate the differences in radiation absorption (Figure 17–1 A & B). In Figure 17–1A the patient has pneumonia, which causes air-filled lung tissue to fill with fluid. Fluid will absorb more radiation than air. In Figure 17–1B the patient has emphysema. With emphysema, normal lung tissue is destroyed and the air sacs become enlarged. A greater amount of air is then present in the lungs, which results in less attenuation of radiation.

Radiographers must have an understanding of pathology in order to properly select the technical factors for a procedure. Properly reading the x-ray requisition, taking an adequate patient history and close observation of the patient are the essential responsibilities of the radiographer. Fulfilling these responsibilities reduces the need to repeat a film, due to the patient's condition. For example, it may be necessary to adjust the technical factors if a chest x-ray is requested for a patient with emphysema. By taking a good history, the radiographer can determine how long the patient has had the condition and what signs and symptoms the patient has exhibited. By observing signs, such as shortness of breath or prolonged exhalation, the radiographer can assess the extent of the disease. Of course, disease conditions are not always known prior to performing the examination. This is one of the primary reasons a repeat film may be necessary, even though there was no error in judgment on the part of the radiographer. As an individual gains clinical experience, his assessment skills improve and he is able to make better judgments concerning the presence and extent of disease.

If a disease causes the affected body tissue to increase in thickness, effective atomic number and/or density, there will be a greater attenuation of the x-ray beam. As more photons are absorbed by the body tissues, fewer will be available to reach the film to create adequate radiographic density. These diseases are harder to penetrate and are called additive conditions because they require adding to the exposure to achieve the proper density on the film. There is an inverse relationship between additive conditions and radiographic density. This means that when additive conditions are present, radiographic density will decrease as the extent of the disease increases.

If a disease causes the affected body tissue to decrease in thickness, effective atomic number and/or density, there will be less attenuation of the x-ray beam. As more photons are able to pass through the body tissues, more will be available to reach the film to create the radiographic density. These diseases are easier to penetrate and are called **destructive conditions**. They require decreasing the exposure to achieve the proper density on the film. There is a direct relationship between destructive conditions and radiographic density. This means that when destructive conditions are present, the radiographic density will increase as the extent of the disease increases.

A disease influences radiation absorption when it alters the overall number or types of atoms comprising the affected tissue. For example, if a person sprains an ankle, one of the body's responses to the injury is swelling or edema at the site. The ankle becomes

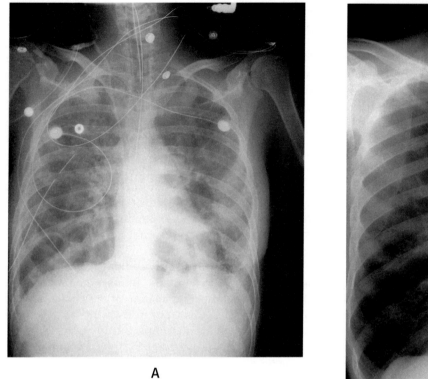

A

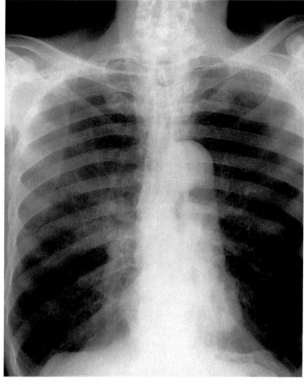

B

FIGURE 17–1. (A) The patient has bilateral pneumonia, resulting in an increase in radiation absorption. (B) The patient has severe emphysema, resulting in a decrease in radiation absorption.

enlarged because there is an increase in blood and serous fluid around the ankle joint. The body tissue increases in thickness, but, in this example, the opacity of the tissue is generally the same. Blood and serous fluid have approximately the same opacity as the soft tissue around the ankle. What is occurring at the molecular and atomic level is an increase, primarily in the number of water molecules (hydrogen and oxygen atoms), which comprise most of blood and serous fluid. If there are more water molecules present around the ankle, a greater number of x-ray photons will interact with that tissue, resulting in increased radiation absorption and decreased exposure to the x-ray film. Technical factors must be increased to compensate for an increase in the thickness of the part. Proper measurement of the body part and

the use of technique charts will ensure that the correct technical factors are selected.

The extent to which a body part is affected by disease will determine if technical factors must be adjusted. For example, no change in technical factors is necessary to visualize a small, localized tumor in the lung, or a small kidney stone. If, however, the tumor is large and diffuse, or the kidney stone causes severe hydronephrosis, adjustments in the technical factors may be required to adequately visualize the pathology (Figure 17–2 A & B). It is important to remember that the degree or extent of the pathology is critical in determining the technical factor adjustments. If the technical factors must be adjusted, the change must be enough to make a visible difference in radiographic density. **To produce a visible difference**

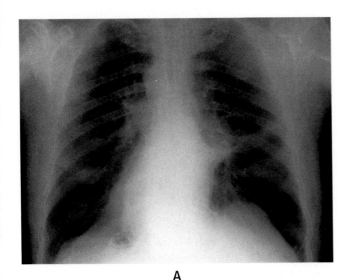

A

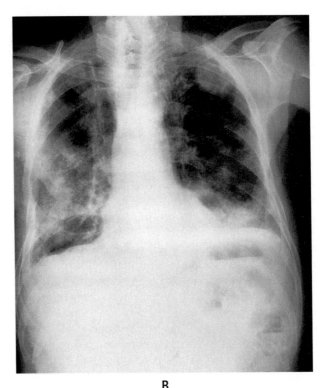

B

FIGURE 17–2. (A) When a tumor is smaller and more localized, there is less need for technical factor adjustments. (B) Tumors that are larger and more diffuse throughout both lungs require greater technical factor adjustments.

requires a minimal change of 25–50 percent in the overall density of the image.

Many diseases do not affect the thickness or opacity of body tissues but can be diagnosed by way of radiography simply because of the structural or functional changes that they produce. These diseases generally do not require an adjustment in the selected technical factors. Examples include ulcers, diverticula and simple fractures (provided there is minimal swelling). There are many diseases that do not affect the thickness or alter the composition of the body tissues and therefore cause no radiographically evident structural or functional changes. These conditions generally do not require radiography; they are usually diagnosed through laboratory testing. Diseases such as diabetes mellitus, anemia and meningitis are examples.

Increased Attenuation (Additive) Conditions

Many disease processes will result in an increase in thickness, effective atomic number and/or density of the body tissue. Recall that the body tissues vary in thickness (the femur is thicker than the humerus) and in composition (bone has a higher effective atomic number and greater tissue density than muscle). These diseases absorb more radiation and require the radiographer to increase technical factors to compensate for the changes in the body tissues. The extent of the disease also plays an important role in technical factor adjustment. The technical factor adjustments will vary, depending upon the degree to which the body tissues are affected. Because of this, each patient will be different and must be examined individually.

No magic formula exists to adjust technical factors to compensate for a pathologic problem. The radiographer must carefully review the requisition, obtain a patient history and then examine the patient. By following these steps, the radiographer can make a judgment concerning the necessary technical adjustment to be made. Experience is particularly valuable in determining the proper changes to be made. As a general rule, additive conditions will require an increase in kilovoltage to adequately penetrate the thicker, more opaque body parts. Remember that an increase of 15 percent in kVp will approximately double the exposure to the film. An increase of 5–15 percent in kilovoltage will compensate for most additive pathologic conditions. Automatic exposure control (AEC) systems will compensate for most pathological changes by adjusting the exposure automatically. However, the compensation will be the result of increased mAs rather than increased kVp.

Some of the common conditions that cause an increase in attenuation and may therefore require an increase in technical factors are outlined. A summary of the conditions is provided in Table 17–1.

Conditions Affecting Multiple Systems

Certain diseases can occur in a wide variety of body systems and, as a result, they may be present in various sites. Whenever an x-ray requisition indicates the presence of any of the following conditions, it may be necessary to increase technical factors for the procedure.

Abscess—an encapsulated infection increases tissue thickness and may alter composition, particularly in the lungs.

Edema—swelling causes an increase in tissue thickness and may alter composition if it occurs in the lungs.

Tumors—an abnormal new growth in tissue results in an increase in tissue thickness and may alter composition, particularly in the lungs or bones or when calcification results.

TABLE 17–1. Summary of Pathology Problems

Increased Attenuation Conditions	Decreased Attenuation Conditions
Multiple Sites	**Multiple Sites**
Abscess	Anorexia Nervosa
Edema	Atrophy
Tumors	Emaciation
The Chest	**The Chest**
Atelectasis	Emphysema
Bronchiectasis	Pneumothorax
Cardiomegaly	
Congestive Heart Failure	
Empyema	
Pleural Effusions	
Pneumoconioses	
Pneumonia	
Pneumonectomy	
Tuberculosis (advanced/miliary)	
The Abdomen	**The Abdomen**
Aortic Aneurysm	Aerophagia
Ascites	Bowel Obstruction
Cirrhosis	
Calcified Stones	
The Extremities and Skull	**The Extremities and Skull**
Acromegaly	Active Osteomyelitis
Chronic Osteomyelitis	Aseptic Necrosis
Hydrocephalus	Carcinoma
Osteoblastic Metastases	Degenerative Arthritis Fibrosarcoma
Osteochondroma	Gout
Paget's Disease	Hyperparathyroidism
Sclerosis	Multiple Myeloma
	Osteolytic Metastases
	Osteomalacia
	Osteoporosis

Conditions of the Chest

The chest is a common site for pathologic conditions and chest radiography is a common diagnostic procedure. It may be necessary to increase technical factors for a procedure whenever an x-ray requisition indicates the presence of any of the following conditions.

Atelectasis—a collapse of the lung results in airlessness of all or part of the lung tissue. This causes lung tissue density to increase.

Bronchiectasis—the chronic dilatation of the bronchi can result in peribronchial thickening and small areas of atelectasis. This causes an increase in lung tissue density.

Cardiomegaly—an enlargement of the heart causes an increase in thickness of the part.

Congestive Heart Failure—when the heart is in failure, the cardiac output is diminished. This results in backward failure, or increased venous congestion in the lungs. Lung tissue density is increased and the heart is enlarged as well.

Empyema—pus in the thoracic cavity causes an increase in tissue density.

Pleural Effusions (Hemothorax, Hydrothorax)—when the pleural cavity fills with either blood or serous fluid, it displaces normal lung tissue. This results in an increased tissue density within the thoracic cavity.

Pneumoconioses—the inhalation of dust particles can cause fibrotic (scarring) changes. When healthy lung tissue becomes fibrotic, density of the tissue increases.

Pneumonia (pneumonitis)—inflammation of the lung tissues causes fluid to fill in the alveolar spaces. Fluid has much greater tissue density than the air normally present.

Pneumonectomy—the removal of a lung will cause the affected side to demonstrate an increase in density since normal air-filled lung tissue is removed.

Pulmonary Edema—when fluid fills the interstitial lung tissues and the alveoli, tissue density increases. This is a typical complication of congestive heart failure.

Tuberculosis (advanced and miliary)—an infection by a mycobacteria causes the inflammatory response, which results in an increase in fluid in the lungs. If the mycobacteria was inhaled, it generally begins as a localized lesion (usually upper lobes), which can spread to a more advanced stage. If the infection reaches the lungs by the bloodstream, it has a more diffuse spread (miliary TB). Increased tissue density results in both advanced and miliary TB (Figure 17–3).

Conditions of the Abdomen

Abdominal conditions usually cause the abdomen to distend. It may be necessary to increase technical factors for a procedure when an x-ray requisition indicates the presence of any of the following conditions. Most technical factor changes, however, will be the natural result of the noted increase in abdominal size when measuring patient thickness.

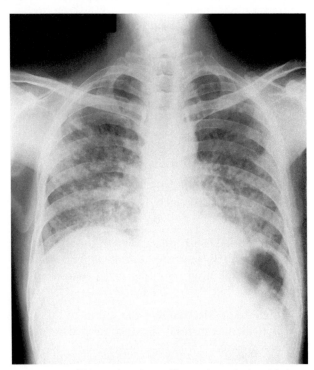

FIGURE 17–3. This patient has miliary tuberculosis with bronchopneumonia. These are both additive conditions, resulting in increased radiation absorption.

Aortic Aneurysm—a large dilatation of the aorta will result in increased thickness of the affected part.

Ascites—fluid accumulation within the peritoneal cavity causes an increase in tissue thickness. The free fluid has a unique "ground glass" appearance radiographically.

Cirrhosis—fibrotic changes in the liver cause the liver to enlarge and ascites can result. The result is an increase in the thickness of the liver and the entire abdomen.

Calcified stones—tones are most commonly found throughout the abdomen in such organs as the gallbladder and the kidney. Calcium may be deposited, which causes an increase in the effective atomic number of the tissue.

Conditions of the Extremities and Skull

Conditions which result in new bone growth are termed osteoblastic. These conditions generally require an increase in technical factors. It may be necessary to increase technical factors for a procedure whenever an x-ray requisition indicates the presence of any of the following conditions.

Acromegaly—an overgrowth of the hands, feet, face and jaw as a result of hypersecretion of growth hormones in the adult will result in an increase in bone mass.

Chronic Osteomyelitis—a chronic bone infection results in new bone growth at the infected site.

Hydrocephalus—a dilatation of the fluid-filled cerebral ventricles causes an enlargement of the head, resulting in an increased thickness.

Osteoblastic Metastases—the spread of cancer to bone can result in uncontrolled new bone growth.

Osteochondroma—a tumor arising in the bone and cartilage will result in an increased thickness of the bone.

Paget's Disease (osteitis deformans)—an increase occurs in bone cell activity which leads to new bone growth. The result is increased bone thickness, with the pelvis, spine and skull most often affected (Figure 17–4).

Sclerosis—an increase in hardening as a result of a chronic inflammation in bone. This increases the density of the bone tissue.

Decreased Attenuation (Destructive) Conditions

Various disease processes can result in a decrease in thickness, effective atomic number and/or density of the body tissue. These conditions cause the absorption of less radiation and require the radiographer to decrease technical factors to compensate for the changes in the body tissues. Recall also that the extent of the disease plays an important role in technical factor adjustment. As a general rule, compensations for destructive conditions can be made by decreasing the mAs. Remember that a decrease of 50 percent in mAs will reduce the exposure to the film by half. A decrease of 25–50 percent

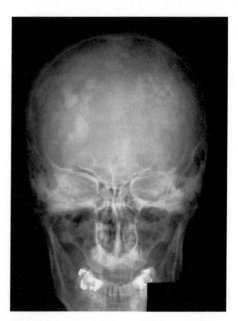

FIGURE 17–4. Paget's disease is an additive condition, resulting in increased radiation absorption.

in mAs will compensate for most of these pathologic conditions. Automatic exposure control (AEC) systems will compensate for most pathological changes by adjusting the exposure automatically.

Some of the common conditions that cause a decrease in attenuation and may therefore require a decrease in technical factors are outlined. A summary of the conditions is provided in Table 17–1.

Conditions Affecting Multiple Sites

Certain diseases can occur in a wide variety of body systems and, as a result, they may be present in various sites. Whenever an x-ray requisition indicates the presence of any of the following conditions, it may be necessary to decrease technical factors for the procedure.

Anorexia Nervosa—a psychological eating disorder which results in an extreme weight loss. Overall body thickness is reduced.

Atrophy—a wasting away of body tissue with diminished cell proliferation, resulting in reduced thickness of a specific part or the entire body.

Emaciation—a generalized wasting away of body tissue, resulting in reduced thickness of the body.

Conditions of the Chest

The chest is a common site for pathologic conditions and chest radiography is a common diagnostic procedure. It may be necessary to decrease technical factors for a procedure when an x-ray requisition indicates the presence of the following conditions.

Emphysema—the overdistention of the lung tissues by air will result in a decrease in lung tissue density.

Pneumothorax—free air in the pleural cavity displaces normal lung tissue and results in decreased density within the thoracic cavity (Figure 17–5).

Conditions of the Abdomen

Abdominal conditions usually cause the abdomen to distend. This distention may be the result of the accu-

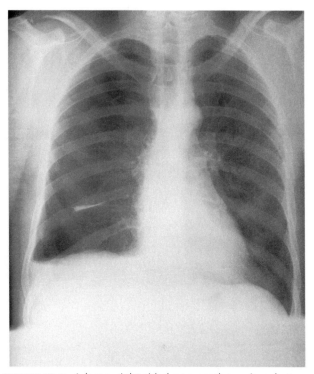

FIGURE 17–5. A large, right-sided pneumothorax is a destructive condition, resulting in decreased radiation absorption.

mulation of fluid (in which case technical factors need to be increased) or air. Distention of the abdomen from air will require a decrease in technical factors. Whenever an x-ray requisition indicates the presence of the following conditions, it may be necessary to decrease technical factors for the procedure because of the presence of air.

Aerophagia—a psychological disorder resulting in abnormal swallowing of air. The stomach becomes dilated from the air and overall tissue density decreases.

Bowel Obstruction—an obstruction in the bowel results in the abnormal accumulation of air and fluid. If a large amount of air is trapped in the bowel, the overall density of the tissues is decreased (Figure 17–6).

Conditions of the Extremities and Skull

Conditions which result in the destruction of bone tissue are termed osteolytic. These conditions result in a

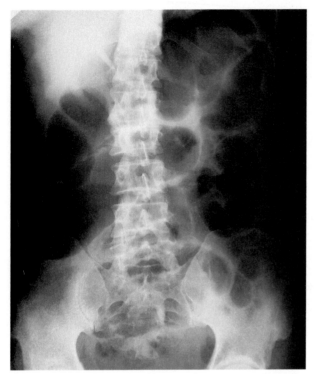

FIGURE 17–6. An obstruction of the large bowel is a destructive condition, resulting in decreased radiation absorption.

loss of bone mass or calcium within the bone. They alter the composition of the bone by decreasing the effective atomic number and/or the tissue density. The result is areas of radiolucency which are easier to penetrate than normal bone. Approximately 50 percent of the bone substance must be lost before changes can be seen radiographically. As a result, these conditions must generally be extensive before technical factor changes are necessary.

Active Osteomyelitis—with a bone infection there is initially a loss of bone tissue (containing calcium), resulting in a decrease in the thickness and composition of the part.

Aseptic necrosis—death of bone tissue results in a decrease in composition and thickness of the part.

Carcinoma—malignancies in bone can cause an osteolytic process, resulting in decreased thickness and composition of the part.

Degenerative Arthritis—inflammation of the joints results in a destruction of adjoining bone tissue, which decreases the composition of the part.

Fibrosarcoma—this malignant tumor of the metaphysis of bone causes an osteolytic lesion with a "moth-eaten" appearance. The result is reduced bone composition.

Gout—during the chronic stages of this metabolic disease, areas of bone destruction result in punched-out lesions that reduce the bone composition.

Hyperparathyroidism—oversecretion of the parathyroid hormone causes calcium to leave bone and enter the bloodstream. The bone becomes demineralized and composition is decreased.

Multiple Myeloma—this malignant tumor arises from plasma cells of bone marrow and causes punched-out osteolytic areas on the bone. Often many sites are affected and reduced bone tissue composition results.

Osteolytic Metastases—when some malignancies spread to bone they produce destruction of the bone, resulting in reduced composition.

Osteomalacia—a defect in bone mineralization results in decreased composition of the affected bone.

Osteoporosis—a defect in bone production due to the failure of osteoblasts to lay down bone matrix results in decreased composition of the affected bone (Figure 17–7).

Summary

The presence of a pathologic condition can greatly affect the degree of radiation absorption. Radiographers must have an understanding of pathology in order to properly select the technical factors for a procedure. Properly reading the x-ray requisition and taking an adequate patient history are essential responsibilities of the radiographer. Fulfilling these responsibilities reduces the need to repeat a film, due to the patient's condition.

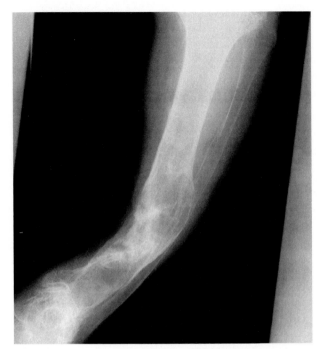

FIGURE 17–7. This patient has a severe bone deformity from a fracture that resulted in chronic osteomyelitis and diffuse osteoporosis. The chronic osteomyelitis is an additive condition (seen around the fracture site) and the osteoporosis is a destructive condition, resulting in a decrease in radiation absorption throughout the remaining bone.

If a disease causes the affected body tissue to increase in thickness, effective atomic number and/or density, that disease will result in a greater attenuation of the x-ray beam. As more photons are absorbed by the body tissues, fewer will be available to reach the film to create adequate radiographic density. These diseases are harder to penetrate and are called additive conditions because they require adding to the exposure to achieve the proper density on the film.

If a disease causes the affected body tissue to decrease in thickness, effective atomic number and/or density, that disease will result in less attenuation of the x-ray beam. As more photons are able to pass through the body tissues, more will be available to reach the film to create the required radiographic density. These diseases are easier to penetrate and are called destructive conditions. They require decreasing the exposure to achieve the proper density on the film.

REVIEW QUESTIONS

1. Why do some pathological conditions affect the attenuation of the x-ray beam?

2. Why is it important that radiographers have an understanding of pathological conditions?

3. What is the relationship between additive conditions and attenuation? destructive conditions and attenuation?

4. Why should the radiographer take a good clinical history and closely observe the patient?

5. Describe how the following additive conditions may affect the radiographic image:

   a. edema

   b. congestive heart failure

   c. pneumonia

   d. ascites

   e. Paget's disease

6. Describe how the following destructive conditions may affect the radiographic image:

   a. atrophy

   b. emphysema

   c. pneumothorax

   d. degenerative arthritis

   e. osteoporosis

REFERENCES AND RECOMMENDED READING

Eisenberg, R. L. & Dennis, C. A. (1994). *Comprehensive Radiographic Pathology* (2nd ed.). C. V. Mosby: St. Louis.

Hiss, S. S. (1993). *Understanding radiography* (3rd ed.). Springfield, IL: Charles C. Thomas Publishers.

Mace, J. D. & Kowalczyk, N. M. (1997). *Radiographic pathology for technologists* (3rd ed.). C. V. Mosby: St. Louis.

Sheldon, H. (1994). *Boyd's introduction to the study of disease* (11th ed.). Philadelphia: Lea and Febiger.

The Case of the White Snakes

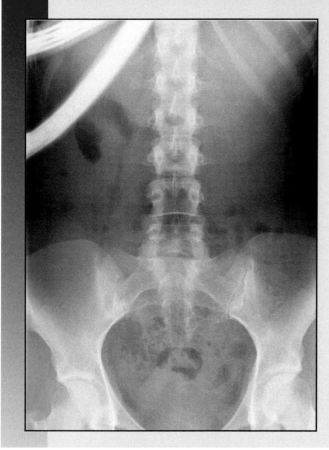

What is the most likely cause of these white, snakelike structures circling the upper corner of the patient's abdomen?

Answers to the case studies can be found in Appendix E.

CHAPTER 18

The Grid

We . . . hope that roentgenologists . . . may become convinced of the serious role played by object-secondary rays, to the end that it will soon be practicable for every roentgenologist to rid himself of their nuisance in his every-day work.

Hollis E. Potter, "The Bucky diaphram principle applied to roentgenography."

OBJECTIVES

Upon completion of this chapter, the student should be able to:

▶ Describe the purpose of the grid.

▶ Explain the construction of a grid, including grid materials, grid ratio, grid frequency and lead content.

▶ Describe the various grid patterns.

▶ Differentiate between parallel and focused grids.

▶ Differentiate between the uses of a stationary and a moving grid.

▶ Explain the process of grid selection for specific radiographic procedures.

▶ Explain the relationship of grid selection to patient dose and radiographic density.

▶ Calculate changes in technical factors to compensate for changes in grid selection.

▶ Describe methods for evaluating the performance of a grid.

▶ Discuss common errors that are made when using a grid and the effects of these errors on the radiographic image.

▶ Describe other scatter reduction methods.

Purpose of the Grid

Agrid is a device which is used to improve the contrast of the radiographic image. It does this by absorbing scatter radiation before it can reach the film. When an x-ray beam passes through the body, one of three things will occur with the primary photons that originated at the target. They will: 1) pass through the body unaffected, 2) be absorbed by the body or 3) interact and change direction (Figure 18–1).

The photons that pass through the body unaffected will interact with the film to create the image. These are the photons responsible for creating the contrast (differences in the densities) on the radiograph. These differences exist because some photons pass through the body while others are absorbed. Absorption of photons occurs as the result of photoelectric interaction. This interaction results in the complete absorption of the primary photon and the production of a secondary photon. The secondary radiation created by this interaction is, with few exceptions, very weak and is quickly absorbed in the surrounding tissues.

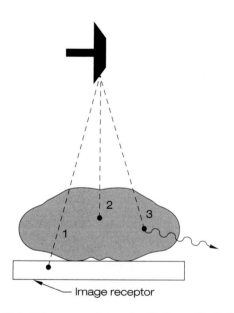

FIGURE 18–1. When x-rays interact with the patient, they will either (1) pass through unaffected, (2) be absorbed, or (3) interact and change direction (scatter).

Primary radiation that interacts and, as a result of this interaction, changes direction is known as scatter radiation. The interaction that produces scatter radiation is known as a Compton interaction. These interactions can result in photons which are strong enough to be emitted by the patient and interact with the film. Since these photons have changed direction they are no longer able to record densities on the film that relate to the patient's anatomy. The densities that they add to the film are of no diagnostic value. Scattered photons add an overall density to the film and, as a result of this overall graying of the image, contrast is lowered. An important point to remember is that the percentage of Compton interactions increases with increased kVp. Therefore, **scatter increases and contrast is further impaired as kVp increases**.

Since the patient is the source of the scatter that is degrading the image, it is logical to assume that the patient will also control the quantity of scatter produced. Scatter increases with increases in the volume of the tissue irradiated and decreases with increased atomic number of the tissue. The volume of tissue that is irradiated is controlled by the thickness of the patient and the exposure field size. While thickness of the patient is predetermined (although it can sometimes be reduced by compression), the field size can be kept to a minimum by collimation. The atomic number of the tissue will also affect the quantity of scatter. The greater the atomic number of the tissue, the less will be the quantity of scatter created. For example, less scatter is produced in bone than in soft tissue, because bone absorbs more photons photoelectrically. This is the result of changes in the number and types of atoms that are present for interaction. In summary, **the amount of scatter radiation increases with 1) increases in patient thickness, 2) larger field sizes, and 3) decreases in atomic number of the tissue**. (This is discussed in further detail in Chapter 15.)

Since a grid is designed to absorb the unwanted scatter radiation, it is necessary to use a grid with thicker, larger body parts and with procedures that require higher kVp techniques. As a general rule, a grid is employed when:

1. body part thickness exceeds 10 cm, and/or

2. kVp is above 60.

A grid is a thin, flat, rectangular device which is made by placing a series of radiopaque lead strips side by side and separating the strips by an interspace material which is radiolucent. The lead strips are of very thin foil and the interspace material is thicker and usually made of aluminum. These strips are then encased in an aluminum cover to protect them from damage.

The very first grid was made in 1913 by the American radiologist Gustav Bucky (1880–1963). Dr. Bucky's first grid consisted of wide strips of lead spaced 2 cm apart and running in two directions, along the length of the film and across the film (Figure 18–2). This crude design created an image of the grid that was superimposed on the patient's image. Despite having to view the anatomy through this checkerboard pattern, the original grid did remove scatter and improve contrast.

In 1920 Hollis Potter (1880–1963), a Chicago radiologist, improved Dr. Bucky's grid design. Dr. Potter realigned the lead strips so they would run in only one direction, made the lead strips thinner and therefore less obvious on the image, and then designed a device (now known as the Potter-Bucky diaphragm) which allowed the grid to move during the exposure. By moving the grid, the lead strips became blurred and were no longer visible on the film. All these improvements resulted in a practical grid device which significantly improved contrast without impairing the view of the patient's anatomy.

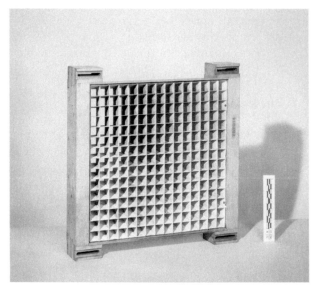

FIGURE 18–2. Dr. Bucky's original grid. *(Reprinted with permission, Smithsonian Institute Photo No. 47022)*

Grid Construction

A wide variety of grids are available today (Table 18–1). The choice of the proper grid for a particular clinical procedure requires an understanding of a grid's function. Grid construction involves the selection of materials, grid ratio and grid frequency.

Grid Materials

A grid is a series of radiopaque strips which alternate with radiolucent interspace strips. These strips are bonded firmly together and then sliced into flat sheets. The radiopaque strips are needed to absorb the scatter radiation and must therefore be made of a dense material with a high atomic number. Lead is the material of choice because it is relatively inexpensive and is easy to shape into very thin foil.

The interspace material must be radiolucent. In other words, it allows radiation to pass easily through it. Several organic and inorganic materials have been tried but only two are commercially available — aluminum and plastic fiber. Ideally, this material should not absorb any radiation. However, in reality, it does absorb a small amount. Aluminum is more commonly used than fiber because it is easier to use in manufacturing and is more durable. Also, because it has a higher atomic number than fiber, it can provide additional absorption of low-energy scatter. With its higher atomic number, aluminum also increases the absorption of primary photons. This can be a disadvantage, especially with low kVp techniques where this absorption would be greater. Fiber interspace grids are preferred when using low kVp techniques where their application can contribute to lower patient dose, such as in pediatric radiography.

Grid Ratio

Grid ratio has a major influence on the ability of the grid to improve contrast. It is defined as the ratio of the height of the lead strips to the distance between the strips (Figure 18–3). This is expressed in the formula:

$$\text{Grid ratio} = \frac{h}{D} \text{ where}$$

$$h = \text{lead strip height}$$
$$D = \text{interspace width}$$

TABLE 18–1. Typical Grid Specifications

Ratio	Linear/ Crosshatch	Focused/ Parallel	Interspace	Lines/Inch	Weight (g/cm²)	Thickness (mm)
15:1	L	F	Al	103	1.74	3.7
15:1	L	F	Al	85	1.64	4.4
12:1	L	F	FIBER	80	1.45	4.4
12:1	L	F	Al	152		1.86
12:1	L	F	Al	103	1.21	3.2
12:1	L	F	Al	85	1.35	3.8
8:1	L	F	FIBER	80	0.96	3.4
8:1	L	F	Al	152		1.34
8:1	L	F	Al	103	0.87	2.3
8:1	L	F	Al	85	0.96	2.8
6:1	L	F	Al	103	0.67	1.9
6:1	L	F	Al	85	0.77	2.3
6:1	L	P	Al	85	0.77	2.3
6:1	C	F	Al	85	1.40	3.8

Specialty Low-ratio Grids					**Purpose**	
4:1	L	F	FIBER	60	Image intensification/Spot filming	
3.5:1	L	P	Al	196	Mammography	
2:1	L	P	Al	196	Mammography	

Example: If the lead strips are 3.0 mm high and are separated by an interspace of 0.25 mm, what is the grid ratio?

Answer:

$$\text{grid ratio} = \frac{3.0}{0.25}$$
$$\text{grid ratio} = 12:1$$

If the height of the grid is a constant, decreasing the distance between the lead strips would result in an increase in the grid ratio. Conversely, if the height of the grid is a constant, increasing the distance between the lead strips would result in a decrease in grid ratio. **An inverse relationship exists between the distance between the lead strips and grid ratio when the height of the grid strips remains the same.**

Higher grid ratios allow less scatter radiation to pass through their interspace material to reach the film. Figure 18–4 demonstrates the effect of grid ratio on the maximum angle possible for a scattered photon to pass through the grid. The higher the grid ratio, the straighter the scattered photon has to be in order to pass through the interspace material. Scattered photons, therefore,

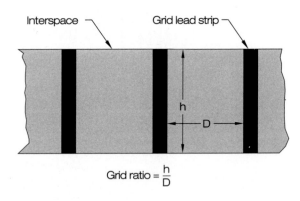

Grid ratio = $\frac{h}{D}$

FIGURE 18–3. Grid ratio is the height of the lead strips divided by the width of the interspace.

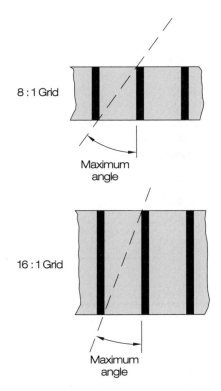

FIGURE 18–4. Grid ratio affects the amount of scatter absorbed by determining the maximum angle of a scattered ray that can get through the grid. The smaller the angle, the less scatter reaches the film.

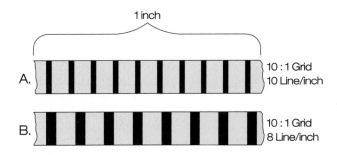

FIGURE 18–5. Grid frequency is the number of grid lines per inch or centimeter. Grids A and B have the same grid ratio, but A has a higher grid frequency than B.

have to be more closely aligned to the direction of the primary photons in order to reach the film. This means that higher grid ratios are more effective at removing scatter. For the same reason, higher-ratio grids require greater accuracy in their positioning and are more prone to grid errors.

Grid Frequency

Grid frequency is defined as the number of grid lines per inch or centimeter. Grids are made with a range in frequency from 60–196 lines/inch (25–78 lines/cm). Most commonly used grids have a frequency of 85–103 lines/inch (33–41 lines/cm). In general, grids with higher grid frequencies have thinner lead strips (Figure 18–5). Very high-frequency grids of approximately 200 lines/inch (80 lines/cm) with very low grid ratios of 2:1 or 3:1 are used in mammography because of the low kVp

techniques and the desire to minimize the possibility of seeing the grid lines on the film.

By combining information about grid ratio and frequency, one can determine the total quantity of lead in the grid. It is the grid's lead content that is most important in determining the grid's efficiency at cleaning up scatter. Lead content is measured in mass per unit area, or grams per square centimeter. In general, the lead content is greater in a grid that has a higher grid ratio and lower grid frequency. **As the lead content of a grid increases, the ability of the grid to remove scatter and improve contrast increases.**

Grid Patterns

Grid strips can be made to run in one or two directions. Grids with lead strips running in only one direction are called linear grids. Grids are also made by placing two linear grids on top of one another so the grid lines are running at right angles. These grids are termed **criss-cross** or **cross-hatched** (Figure 18–6). Dr. Bucky's original grid was made using this pattern.

Linear grids are more commonly used in clinical practice because they can be used when performing procedures that require tube angulation. Linear grids allow the technologist to angle the tube only *along* the long axis of the grid. Angulation *across* the long axis would result in the primary beam being directed into the lead strips. If the primary beam is angled into the lead, the lead will absorb an undesirable amount of primary radiation,

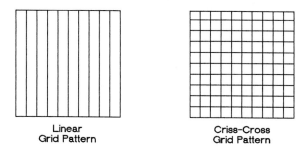

FIGURE 18–6. A linear vs. a criss-cross grid pattern.

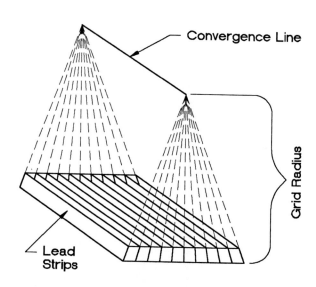

FIGURE 18–7. A focused grid is designed to match the divergence of the x-ray beam. The grid radius is the distance from the face of the grid to the points of convergence of the lead strips.

resulting in a problem known as **grid cut-off**. When criss-cross grids are used, no tube tilt is permitted since any angulation would result in grid cut-off because lead strips are running in both directions.

Grid Types

Grids are manufactured with either a parallel or a focused design. Parallel grids are made with the lead and interspace strips running parallel to one another. This means that if the grid lines were extended into space they would never intersect. Focused grids are designed so that the central grid strips are parallel and as the strips move away from the central axis they become more and more inclined (Figure 18–7).

The focused design results in a grid with lead strips designed to match the divergence of the x-ray beam. If these lead strips were extended, the strips would intersect along a line in space known as the convergence line. The distance from the face of the grid to the points of convergence of the lead strips is called the grid radius. **For the grid to be properly focused, the x-ray tube must be located along the convergence line.** Each focused grid will identify the focal range within which the tube should be located. For example, grids are made with short, medium or long focal ranges, depending on the distance for which they are designed. Short focal range grids (14–18 inches or 36–46 cm) are made for use in mammography; long focal range grids (60–72 inches or 152–183 cm) are used for chest radiography. Focused grids with lower grid ratios allow for greater latitude in the alignment of the tube with the grid. With higher grid

ratios, proper alignment of the grid with the tube is more critical.

Parallel grids are less commonly employed than focused grids and are only available in lower ratios. Because the strips do not try to coincide with the divergence of the x-ray beam, some grid cut-off will occur along the lateral edges, especially when the grid is employed at short SIDs. The parallel grid is best employed at long SIDs because the beam will be a straighter, more perpendicular one (Figure 18–8).

Grid Uses

A grid is used either in a stationary position or mounted in a Potter-Bucky diaphragm to move it during exposure. Most radiology departments have a supply of stationary grids, in various sizes, which can be mounted to the front of a cassette. These are generally made approximately one inch larger than the film size they are intended to cover. Stationary grids are used primarily in portable procedures or for upright or horizontal beam views. Some departments may also purchase a special

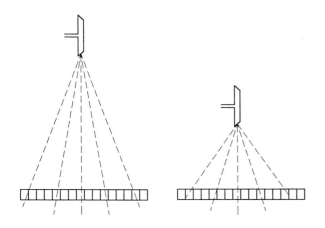

FIGURE 18–8. Parallel grids function best at long, as opposed to short, SID.

cassette with a grid built into it. This design, called a grid cassette, requires reloading the film between exposures using the grid. This may be an inconvenience in situations where multiple films are needed. When grids are used in a stationary fashion, grid lines on the film will usually be noticed on close inspection of the image. This is especially true with low-frequency grids. High-frequency grids, like those used for mammography, have a minimal visual effect.

The most common use of the grid is for procedures using the Potter-Bucky diaphragm (usually called the bucky). This device is mounted below the tabletop of radiographic and radiographic/fluoroscopic tables and holds the cassette in place below the grid. It can move the grid during the exposure so that grid lines will be blurred and therefore not evident on the film. These grids are 17"×17" (43×43 cm), large enough to cover a 14"×17" (35×43 cm) cassette placed either lengthwise or crosswise in the cassette tray.

The direction in which the grid moves is important if it is to accomplish the job of blurring the grid lines. The lead strips of the grid run along the long axis of the table. To blur the lead lines, the grid must move at a right angle to the direction of the lines. This means that it will be moving back and forth across the table and not from top to bottom.

There are two movement mechanisms used today. The movements are described as reciprocating and oscillating. With the reciprocating grid, a motor drives the grid back and forth during the exposure for a total distance of no more than 2–3 cm. With the oscillating grid, an electromagnet pulls the grid to one side and then releases it during exposure. The grid oscillates in a circular motion within the grid frame.

Grid Selection/Conversions

Selecting the best grid to use for a specific radiographic procedure is a complex process. Most procedures which are done with a grid use a moving grid mounted in a table or upright holder. Grid choice must be made in the equipment purchase phase of quality control. Once a grid is selected and mounted in the Potter-Bucky diaphragm, it is not easily changed. Purchase decisions are generally made by the department administrator in collaboration with the radiologist.

Grids absorb scatter and scatter adds density to the film. The more efficient a grid is at absorbing scatter, the less density will be seen on the film. Therefore compensations must be made to increase density. This is generally accomplished by increasing mAs, which in turn results in greater patient dose. The better the grid cleans up scatter, the greater will be the dose given to the patient to achieve adequate density. The amount of mAs needed can be calculated using the following formula:

$$\text{Grid Conversion Factor (GCF)} = \frac{\text{mAs with the grid}}{\text{mAs without the grid}}$$

This formula is referred to as the Bucky factor as well as the grid conversion factor. **Grid-conversion factors (GCF) increase with higher grid ratios and increasing kVp.** Since grids vary in respect to their ratio, frequency and lead content, it would be useful to check the grid conversion factor for each of the common grids used in a department. Table 18–2 offers a guide of grid conversion factors for commonly purchased grids.

Example: A satisfactory chest radiograph is produced using 5 mAs at 85 kVp without a grid. A second film is requested using a 12:1 grid. Using Table 18–2, what mAs is needed to produce a second satisfactory radiograph?

Answer:

$$GCF = \frac{\text{mAs with the grid}}{\text{mAs without the grid}}$$

$$5.5 = \frac{X}{5}\text{mAs}$$

$$X = 5.5 \times 5 \text{ mAs}$$

$$X = 27.5 \text{ mAs}$$

When converting from one grid ratio to another, the following formula is used:

$$\frac{\text{mAs}_1}{\text{mAs}_2} = \frac{GCF_1}{GCF_2}$$

where: mAs_1 = original mAs
mAs_2 = new mAs
GCF_1 = original grid conversion factor
GCF_2 = new grid conversion factor

Example: A satisfactory abdominal radiograph is produced using an 8:1 grid, 35 mAs and 85 kVp. A second film is requested using a 12:1 grid. Using Table 18–2, what mAs is needed to produce a second satisfactory radiograph?

Answer:

$$\frac{\text{mAs}_1}{\text{mAs}_2} = \frac{GCF_1}{GCF_2}$$

$$\frac{35}{X} = \frac{4}{5.5}$$

$$4X = 192.5$$

$$X = 48 \text{ mAs}$$

TABLE 18–2. Grid Conversion Factors

Grid Ratio	60 kVp	85 kVp	110 kVp
No grid	1	1	1
5:1	3	3	3
8:1	3.75	4	4.25
12:1	4.75	5.5	6.25
16:1	5.75	6.75	8

Adapted with permission from *Characteristics and Applications of X-Ray Grids,* Liebel-Flarsheim division of Sybron Corporation, Cincinnati, Ohio.
Approximate values based on clinical tests of pelvis and skull.

Grid Performance Evaluation

The efficiency of a grid in cleaning up or removing scatter can be quantitatively measured. The International Commission on Radiologic Units and Measurements (ICRU) Handbook 89 defines two criteria for measuring a grid's performance: selectivity and contrast improvement ability.

Selectivity

Although grids are designed to absorb scatter, they also absorb some primary radiation. Grids that absorb a greater percentage of scatter than primary radiation are described as having a greater degree of selectivity. Selectivity is identified by the Greek sigma (Σ) and is measured by using the following formula:

$$\text{Selectivity} = \frac{\%\text{ primary radiation transmitted}}{\%\text{ scatter radiation transmitted}}$$

The better a grid is at removing scatter, the greater will be the selectivity of the grid. **This means that a grid with a higher lead content would have a greater selectivity.**

Contrast Improvement Ability

The best measure of how well a grid functions is its ability to improve contrast in the clinical setting. The contrast improvement factor is dependent on the amount of scatter produced, which is controlled by the kVp and volume of irradiated tissue (see Chapter 26). As the amount of scatter radiation increases, the lower will be the contrast and the lower the contrast improvement factor. The contrast improvement factor (K) can be measured using the following formula:

$$K = \frac{\text{Radiographic contrast with the grid}}{\text{Radiographic contrast without the grid}}$$

If K = 1, then no improvement in contrast has occurred. Most grids have contrast improvement factors between 1.5 and 3.5. This means that contrast is 1.5–3.5 times better when using the grid. **The higher the K factor, the greater the contrast improvement.**

Grid Errors

Poor radiographs can result from improper use of the grid. Errors in the use of the grid occur mainly with grids that have a focused design. This is because focused grids are made to coincide with the divergence of the x-ray beam. The tube must be centered to the focused grid and aligned at the correct distance. Additionally, a focused grid has a tube side and a film side based on the angulation of the grid strips. Proper tube/grid alignment is essential to prevent the undesirable absorption of primary radiation known as grid cut-off.

Off-Level

An off-level grid error occurs when the tube is angled across the long axis of the grid strips. This can be the result of improper tube or grid positioning (Figure 18–9). Improper tube positioning results if the central ray is directed across the long axis of the radiographic table. Recall that it is only possible to angle along the long axis of the table with a linear grid and it is not possible to angle at all with a criss-cross grid. Improper grid positioning most commonly occurs with stationary grids being used for mobile procedures or decubitus views. If,

for example, a patient is lying on a grid for a mobile abdominal procedure and the patient's weight is unevenly distributed on the grid, the grid may not be properly aligned to the tube.

An off-level grid error can occur with a focused grid and it is the only positioning error possible with a parallel grid. Care must always be taken when aligning the tube to the grid, especially when using stationary grids, to avoid this error. When this error occurs, there is an undesirable absorption of primary radiation which results in a radiograph with a decrease in density across the entire image (Figure 18–10).

Off-Center

The x-ray tube must be centered along the central axis of a focused grid to prevent an off-center (off-axis or lateral decentering) grid error (Figure 18–11). The center grid strips are perpendicular and become more and more inclined away from the center. This design coincides with the divergence of the x-ray beam from the tube. If the central ray is off-center, the most perpendicular portion of the x-ray beam will not correspond to the most perpendicular portion of the grid. The result is a decrease in film density across the entire film (Figure 18–12).

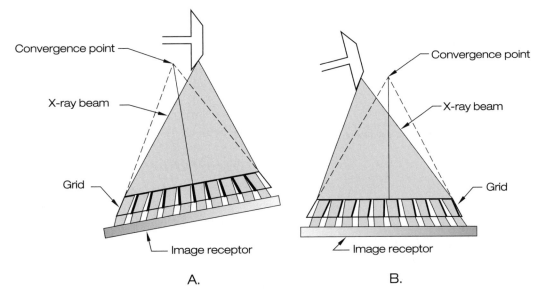

A.   B.

FIGURE 18–9. An off-level grid error can occur with a parallel or a focused grid. A linear grid can be off-level in one direction while a criss-cross grid can be off-level in both directions (across and along the grid).

75 kVp	15 mAs	40" **SID**
15:1 **grid**	400 **RS**	63.4 **mR**

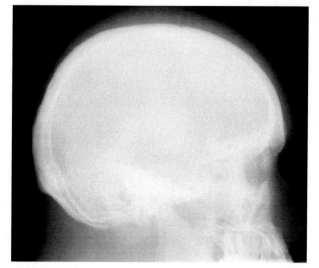

FIGURE 18–10. A radiograph illustrating an off-level grid error.

75 kVp	15 mAs	40" **SID**
15:1 **grid**	400 **RS**	66.1 **mR**

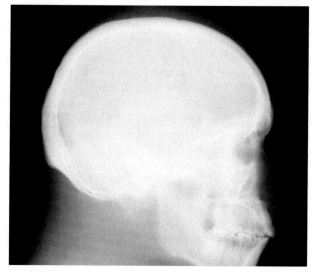

FIGURE 8–12. A radiograph illustrating an off-center grid error.

The greater the degree of lateral decentering, the greater the grid cut-off.

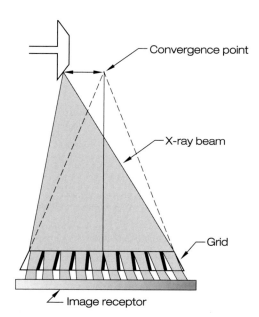

FIGURE 18–11. An off-center grid error.

Off-Focus

A focused grid is made to be used at very specific distances identified as the focal range labeled on the front of the grid. When a grid is used at a distance other than that specified as the focal range, an off-focus error results (Figure 18–13). For example, if a grid has a focal range of 36–44 inches (91–112 cm) and it is used at 72 inches, severe grid cut-off will occur. Off-focus errors result in grid cut-off along the peripheral edges of the film (Figure 18–14). Higher grid ratios require greater positioning accuracy to prevent grid cut-off.

Upside-Down

A focused grid has an identified tube side based on the way the grid strips are angled. If the grid is used upside-down, severe peripheral grid cut-off will occur (Figure 18–15). Radiation will pass through the grid along the central axis where the grid strips are most perpendicular and radiation will be increasingly absorbed away from the center (Figure 18–16). It is important that the technologist check the tube side prior to using a focused grid.

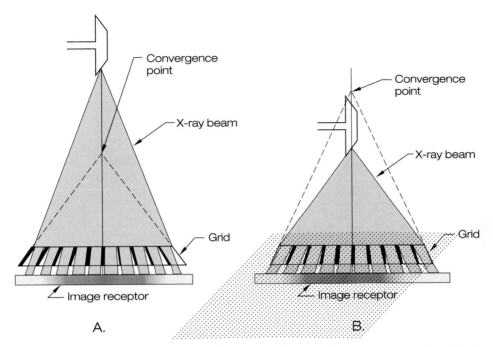

FIGURE 18–13. An off-focus grid error occurs when the grid is used at distances less than or greater than the focal range.

75 **kVp**	15 **mAs**	40" **SID**
15:1 **grid**	400 **RS**	69.3 **mR**

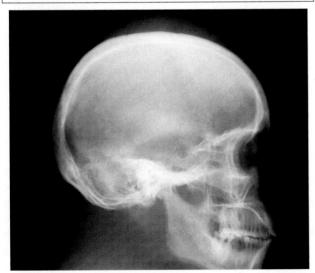

FIGURE 18–14. A radiograph illustrating an off-focus grid error taken at less than the recommended focal range distance.

Other Scatter Reduction Methods

In addition to the use of a grid, there are a number of other methods that can be employed to reduce the amount of scatter reaching the film. Remember, the most important way to improve image quality is to decrease the amount of scatter initially being created. This is best done by restricting the primary beam. Collimating to the size of the area being examined is critical to image quality. Even with the use of close collimation, it is still necessary to reduce scatter reaching the film when radiographing larger body parts or when using higher kVps. The grid is the primary device employed to reduce scatter. The body part may also be compressed to decrease the amount of scatter created. Two other methods that can be used to decrease scatter reaching the film are the air-gap technique and the reverse Kodak X-Omatic™ cassette technique.

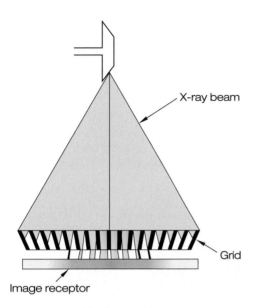

FIGURE 18–15. An upside-down grid error.

75 kVp	15 mAs	40" SID
15:1 grid	400 RS	64.2 mR

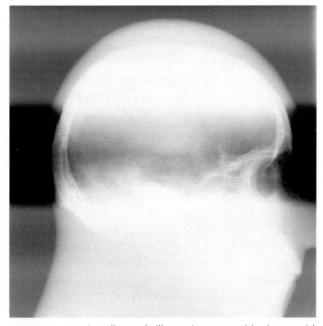

FIGURE 18–16. A radiograph illustrating an upside-down grid error.

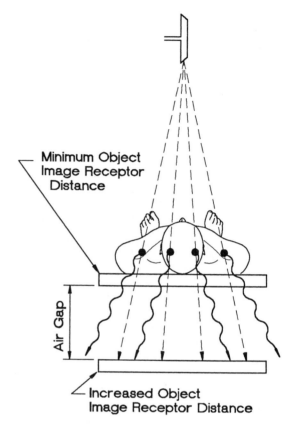

FIGURE 18–17. The air-gap technique reduces the amount of scatter reaching the film.

Air-Gap Technique

The air-gap technique is an alternative to the use of a grid. It has primary applications in magnification radiography and, to a lesser extent, in chest radiography. The technique involves placing the patient at a greater object image receptor distance (OID), thus creating an air gap between the patient and the film. By moving the patient away from the film, the amount of scatter reaching the film will be reduced. As stated earlier, the patient is the source of the majority of scatter. While the same amount of scatter will be created during the exposure, less of the scatter will reach the film if the patient is moved farther away (Figure 18–17). The result is improved contrast without the use of the grid. The primary disadvantage of the air-gap technique is the loss of sharpness that results from increased OID.

Gould and Hale evaluated contrast improvement between the use of a grid and the air-gap technique, showing that a 10-inch (25-cm) air gap has the same degree of clean-up of scatter as a 15:1 grid for a 10-cm body part. This same grid was shown to be more effective at eliminating scatter than the air gap with a thicker (20-cm) body part.

Reverse-Cassette Technique

When performing a procedure that borders between the use of a grid or a nongrid technique, it may be helpful to use a cassette backwards. The Kodak X-Omatic™ cassette may be used in a reverse fashion because the back of the cassette does not contain hinges which would interfere with the image. These cassettes are designed with the front and back made from the same radiolucent material. The only difference between the back and the front of the cassette is a thin sheet of lead foil approximately 0.0006 inches thick, which is located behind the back intensifying screen. This lead is intended to absorb backscatter radiation, which could fog the image.

When the cassette is used in a backwards position, the lead foil will serve as a filter to absorb low energy scattered photons. It functions much like a very low ratio grid. As a result, image contrast can be improved. It should be noted, however, that an increase in technical factors is necessary to compensate for the reduction in radiation reaching the film.

Summary

A grid is a tool used by the radiographer to improve image contrast. Grids are made of lead strips alternating with an interspace material which is usually made of aluminum. Grids are constructed with a specific grid ratio and frequency. The grid ratio and frequency are important in determining the total lead content of the grid. Generally, grids with higher grid ratios and lead content are more efficient at improving contrast. This can be quantitatively studied by measuring the selectivity and contrast improvement ability of the grid.

Grids absorb scatter and scatter adds density to the film. The more efficient a grid is at absorbing scatter, the less density on the film. Therefore compensation must be made to increase density. This is generally accomplished by increasing the mAs, which in turn results in greater patient dose. The better the grid is at cleaning up scatter, the greater is the dose given to the patient to achieve adequate density.

Grids are manufactured in either a linear or criss-cross pattern, with either a parallel or focused design. They can be used in either a stationary manner or may be placed in a device which moves the grid and thereby blurs the grid lines.

Alternatives to the use of a grid are the air-gap technique and the reverse-cassette technique.

REVIEW QUESTIONS

1. Why does a grid improve contrast?

2. As a general rule, when should a grid be used?

3. How is a grid constructed?

4. Define grid ratio.

5. What type of grid pattern has lead strips running in only one direction?

6. How is a focused grid designed?

7. As the ability of a grid to clean up scatter increases, what is the effect on patient dose and radiographic density?

8. How is the contrast improvement of a grid measured?

9. How does an off-level grid error occur?

10. How does the air-gap technique improve contrast?

REFERENCES AND RECOMMENDED READING

Bednarek, D. P., Rudin, S., & Wong, R. (1983). Artifacts produced by moving grids. *Radiology.* (April), 255.

Bushberg, J. T., Seibert, J. A., Leidholdt, E. M., & Boone, J. M. (1994). *The essential physics of medical imaging.* Baltimore: Williams & Wilkins.

Chan, H. P. (1985). Ultra-high-strip-density radiographic grids: A new antiscatter technique for mammography. *Radiology.* (March), 807.

Cullinan, A. & Cullinan, J. (1994). *Producing quality radiographs* (2nd ed.). Philadelphia: J. B. Lippincott.

Curry, T. S., Dowdey, J. E., & Murry, R. C. (1990). *Christensen's introduction to the physics of diagnostic radiology* (4th ed.). Philadelphia: Lea and Febiger.

Doi, K., Frank, P. H., Chan, H. P., Vyborny, C. J., Makino, S., Iida, N., & Carlin, M. (1983). Physical and clinical evaluation of new high-strip-density radiographic grids. *Radiology. 147*(2), 575–582.

Egan, R. L. (1983). Grids in mammography. *Radiology.* (Feb.), 359.

Fry, O. E. & Cesare, G. (1960). Bedside radiography reduction of patient exposure and orientation of grid cassettes. *Radiologic Technology. 31*(4), 387.

Gould, R. G. & Hale, J. (1974). Control of scattered radiation by air gap techniques: Applications to chest radiography. *American Journal of Roentgenology. 122*, 109–118.

Harlow, C. (1993). Off-centering secondary radiation grids. *Radiography Today. 59*(674), 11–13.

Hendee, W. R. & Ritenour, R. (1993). *Medical imaging physics* (3rd ed.). St. Louis: C. V. Mosby.

Heriand, J. & Varma, D. G. K. (1986). A lung opacity caused by grid artifact. *Radiologic Technology. 58*(2), 147.

Hiss, S. S. (1993). *Understanding radiography* (3rd ed.). Springfield, IL: Charles C. Thomas Publishers.

Hufton, A. P., Crosthwaite, C. M., Davies, J. M., & Robinson, L. A. (1987). Low attenuation material for table tops, cassettes, and grids: A review. *Radiography. 53*(607), 17.

Jensen, G. & Scheid, C. (1980). The performance of radiographic grids. *Optimization of Chest Radiography.* Rockville, MD: U.S. Department of Health and Human Services, HHS Publication (FDA) 80–8124.

Lauer, O. G., Mayes, J. B., & Thurston, R. P. (1990). *Evaluating radiographic quality: The variables and their effects.* Mankato, MN: The Burnell Company Publishers.

Potter, H. E. (1931). History of diaphragming roentgen rays by the use of the Bucky principle. *The American Journal of Roentgenology. 25*, 396.

Potter, H. E. (1920). The Bucky diaphragm principle applied to roentgenology. *The American Journal of Roentgenology. 7*, 292.

Seeman, H. E & Splettstosser, H. R. (1955). The effect of kilovoltage and grid ratio on subject contrast in radiography. *Radiology. 64*, 572–580.

Seeman, H. E. & Splettstosser, H. R. (1954). The physical characteristics of Potter-Bucky diaphragms. *Radiology. 62*, 575–583.

Seeram, E. (1985). *X-ray imaging equipment: An introduction.* Springfield: Charles C. Thomas.

Stanford, R. W., Moore, R. D., & Hills, T. H. (1959). Comparative performance of grids in relation to their stated ratio. *British Journal of Radiology. 32*(374), 106–113.

Stears, J. G., Gray, J. E., & Frank, E. D. (1986). Grids are not created equal. *Radiologic Technology. 57*(4), 345.

Stober, E. V. (1951). The term 'ratio' as applied to an x-ray grid. *Radiologic Technology. 23*(3), 180.

Stober, E. V. (1947). Off-distance cut-off. *Radiologic Technology. 19*(3), 111.

Sweeney, R. J. (1977). The use of an inverted Kodak X-Omatic cassette as an improvised grid. *Radiologic Technology. 49*(3), 257–261.

Switzer, D. (1981). The use of grids in diagnostic radiography. *The Canadian Journal of Medical Radiation Technology. 12*(2), 60.

Thompson, M. A., Hattaway, M. P., Hall, J. D., & Dowd, S. B. (1994). *Principles of imaging science and protection.* Philadelphia: W. B. Saunders.

Tortorici, M. (1992). *Concepts in medical radiographic imaging.* Philadelphia: W. B. Saunders.

Trout, E. D., Kelley, J. P., & Cathey, G. A. (1952). The use of filters to control radiation exposure to the patient in diagnostic roentgenology. *American Journal of Roentgenology. 67*(6), 946–963.

Wolbarst, A. B. (1993). *Physics of radiology.* Norwalk, CT: Appleton & Lange.

CHAPTER 19

Radiographic Film

Any discussion relating to the rationale of radiographic exposure should begin with the understanding that the characteristics and the exposure response of x-ray film are the foundations of an exposure system.

Arthur W. Fuchs, from the Jerman Memorial Lecture
at the 1950 Annual Meeting of the American Society of X-Ray Technicians.

Objectives

Upon completion of this chapter, the student should be able to:

▶ Describe the components of radiographic film.

▶ Explain the production of silver halide crystals.

▶ State the purpose of various additives to radiographic film.

▶ Describe latent image formation.

▶ Discuss the differences between direct exposure film, screen film and films for various special applications, such as duplication and subtraction.

▶ Explain the fundamentals of proper film storage and handling.

▶ Identify common radiographic film artifacts.

▶ Discuss automated and daylight loading film systems.

▶ Explain the responsibilities involved in proper radiograph identification.

*P*hotosensitive film remains the most common radiographic image receptor, although modern imaging technology has developed many other receptors (e.g., fluoroscopic screens, and computer-linked detectors). Film was the first image receptor chosen by Röntgen, and it has remained the primary means of recording radiographic images to the present day, although some computer images are now being read for diagnosis without being recorded on film.

Radiographic and photographic film are very similar in nature and both derive from early experiments in recording light images. The discovery of photography cannot be assigned to one person. A permanent photographic process was discovered about 1816 by the French inventor Joseph Nièpce (1765–1833). Nièpce eventually collaborated with the French artist Louis Daguerre (1787–1851), who improved the process and sold it to the French government, which released it to the public in 1839. Simultaneously, between 1835 and 1840, the English photographer William Fox Talbot (1800–1877) developed the now common negative-to-positive process that was given the name photography. Many photographers contributed to the scientific understanding of the process and by the 1850s the process was similar to, although more primitive than, that used today.

Photographic materials are photosensitive, or capable of responding to exposure by photons. Both are sensitive to the wavelengths and energies that comprise most of the electromagnetic spectrum of both light and x-rays (Figure 2–10), although it is possible to manufacture film that is insensitive to portions of the spectrum. Proper use of photosensitive materials requires an understanding of how film is constructed and how the image is formed.

Construction

Diagnostic radiographic film is manufactured by coating both sides of a base material with an emulsion containing photosensitive crystals. Several other materials are also used to improve the performance and permanence of the film. The complete construction of diagnostic radiographic film includes the **base, adhesive, emulsion with crystals and supercoat** (Figure 19–1). The total thickness of the film varies with the manufacturer, from 175 to 300 μm (0.007" to 0.012").

Base

The film base was originally composed of a glass plate. Glass plates coated with emulsion were used in photography from soon after its discovery until World War I (circa 1914) (Figure 19–2). Modern radiography has retained in the professional jargon an old-fashioned term, "flat plate of the abdomen," from this period. Of course, the physician requesting such an image intends

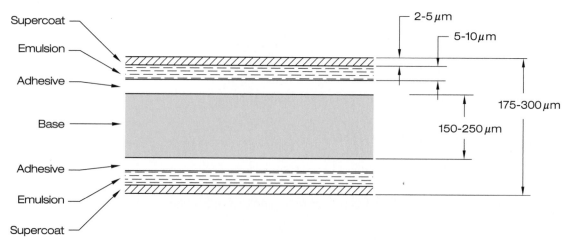

FIGURE 19–1. Cross-sectional view of diagnostic radiographic film.

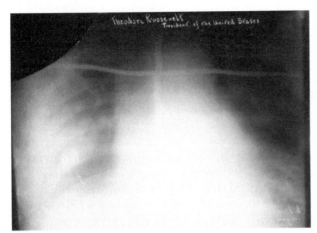

FIGURE 19–2. Glass plate radiograph of Theodore Roosevelt taken at Mercy Hospital in Chicago on October 15, 1912, after he was shot in the chest during an assassination attempt in Milwaukee. *(Reprinted with permission from the American College of Surgeons, Chicago, IL)*

the film base to be of polyester plastic, not a glass plate. Modern plastic bases solved problems such as cut fingers from broken films and strained backs from carrying and filing stacks of heavy radiographs.

During World War I a shortage of the good, optical quality glass needed for the film base caused film manufacturers to switch to cellulose nitrate. Because of its flammable nature (which caused several tragic hospital fires), nonflammable cellulose triacetate was introduced in the 1920s. Modern radiographic film base is polyester, which was introduced in the 1960s by DuPont. It is usually 150–200 μm (0.006″–0.008″) thick.

The film base must be flexible yet tough, stable, rigid and uniformly lucent. It must be flexible to permit easy handling in the darkroom and to make good contact with the cassette pressure pads. It must be stable so that it does not change its dimensions during the heating and immersion in chemicals required for processing. It must be rigid enough to be conveniently placed onto a view box (radiographic illuminator). Most important, it must be uniformly lucent so that it permits the transmission of light without adding artifacts to the diagnostic image.

The film base usually includes a blue dye to tint the film and reduce eyestrain for the interpreting radiologist, thereby increasing the diagnostic accuracy available from the image. The film base is also often coated with a spe-

cial substance to prevent light from one screen crossing over to the other, causing blurring of the image. This reflection of light is called the **crossover effect**. Some manufacturers use an ultraviolet emission from the intensifying screen to reduce the crossover effect. **Halation** is a different effect caused by light being reflected from the air interface on the back of the base material (Figure 19–3). An **antihalation coating** may be applied to the back of single-emulsion film. This coating is designed to absorb the light coming from the emulsion and prevent backscatter, visible light or reflected light from degrading the image. The coating is removed by the processing chemicals to permit light to be transmitted through the film for viewing. Antihalation layers contribute to patient dose and are often used only in extremity systems.

If a single emulsion film is loaded into a cassette with the antihalation coating toward the intensifying screen (the source of the light photons), most of the light will be absorbed. **Single emulsion film must be loaded with the emulsion toward the intensifying screen.** The emulsion side of the film always appears dull, the nonemul-

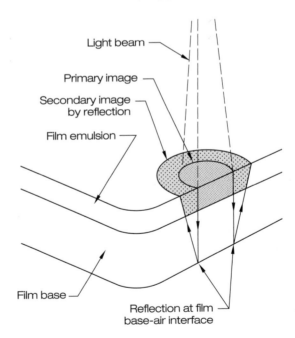

FIGURE 19–3. The halation effect. *(Reprinted with permission of David Jenkins from* Radiographic Photography and Imaging Processes, *MTP Press, Lancaster, England)*

sion side shiny. In addition, single emulsion films have an identifying notch cut in the lower left corner. The mnemonic double L (LL) for the lower left corner makes this easy to remember.

Adhesive

A thin coating of adhesive is applied to the base material before it is coated with the emulsion. This substratum coating is designed to glue the emulsion to the base and prevent bubbles or other distortion when the film is bent during processing or handling, or when it is wet and heated during development.

Emulsion

The emulsion is composed of gelatin in which photosensitive silver halide crystals are suspended. It is spread in an extremely even coating that, depending on the manufacturer, ranges from 5–10 μm (0.0002"–0.0004") of thickness on each side of the base. The purpose of the gelatin is to act as a neutral lucent suspension medium for the silver halide crystals that must be separated from one another to permit processing chemicals to reach them. Gelatin serves as a nonreactive medium through which chemicals can diffuse to reach the silver halides. The gelatin also distributes the crystals evenly over the surface of the film, thus preventing clumping of silver halides that would make one area of the film more photosensitive than another. Additionally, the gelatin must be clear, to permit light to travel through it uniformly, and flexible enough to permit bending without distorting the recorded image. The gelatin that is used for film is of extremely high quality.

The photosensitive agents suspended in the emulsion are silver halide crystals (or grains). The silver halides used in radiographic film are **silver bromide**, **silver iodide** and **silver chloride**. Although the exact formula of each company is a closely guarded trade secret, film manufacturers agree that modern silver halides are 95–98 percent silver bromide, with the remainder usually consisting of silver iodide. This has led to the term **silver iodobromide** as a generic specification of the silver halide crystals.

Because photographic film normally has emulsion on a single side, diagnostic radiographic film is sometimes called **duplitized**, double emulsion or double coated

film. Not all radiographic film is duplitized, though. There are special radiographic films (such as duplication, mammography and fine detail extremity films) that are coated on a single side.

Supercoat

The supercoat is a layer of hard, protective gelatin designed to prevent the soft emulsion underneath from being physically or chemically abused by scratches, abrasions from stacking and skin oils from handling. It is usually designed to be antistatic as well. The supercoat is extremely strong and, when combined with the tough base material, makes it nearly impossible to tear a radiograph. A Chicago phone book would be easier to tear in half than a radiograph unless an edge is cut first.

The only items routinely used during film handling that are capable of permanently damaging the surface of a radiograph are a paper clip and a staple. For this reason, plastic holders or paper film envelopes should always be used to keep radiographs together. Radiographs should not be paper-clipped to reports or requisition orders, and stapled medical records should not be filed in the same envelope with radiographs. To avoid this problem, a properly designed radiograph envelope has a separate compartment for the consultation report.

Manufacturing

Radiographic film is manufactured in four stages: **crystal production**, **ripening**, **mixing** and **coating**.

Crystal Production

Silver-bromide crystal production is accomplished, in total darkness, by combining silver nitrate and potassium bromide in the presence of gelatin. The silver bromide will precipitate out and the potassium nitrate can be washed away as a waste product. The gelatin must be present as a medium to permit the crystals to form. The gelatin functions to limit oxidation and reduce crystal surface energy tension, as well as to facilitate other chemical reactions. This process is described by the formula:

$$AgNO_3 + KBr \rightarrow AgBr \downarrow + KNO_3$$

| silver nitrate | + | potassium bromide | $\rightarrow$ | silver bromide (precipitate) | + | potassium nitrate |

The silver halide crystals are flat and roughly triangular in shape (Figure 19–4). Although different types of film emulsions require different size crystals, they are all very small, about 1 μm (0.00004") on each side. A cubic millimeter contains over half a billion (> 500,000,000) crystals.

The tabular grain process develops flat, tabular crystals two to four times larger that can be more evenly dispersed throughout the emulsion. The advantages of tabular grains include the absorption of a greater portion of the exposing photons, reduced light crossover from one emulsion to the other and reduced silver coating requirements. Tabular grains may also permit 45-second pro-

cessing, but are very sensitive to fluctuations in the developer replenishment rate.

Each crystal is a cubic lattice (or matrix) of silver, bromide and iodine atoms (Figure 19–5). A conventional crystal contains approximately 10^{10} (100,000,000,000) atoms. They are bound together by moderately strong ionic bonds with the silver positive (Ag^+) and the bromine or iodine negative (Br^- or I^-). The crystal structure permits both free silver atoms and free electrons to drift through the lattice. This ability is the key to the formation of the latent image.

It is thought that the halide ions (bromine and iodine) tend to cluster on or near the surface of the crys-

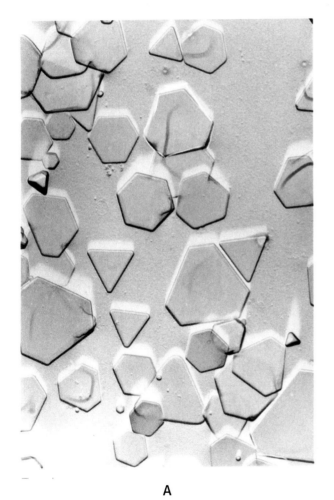

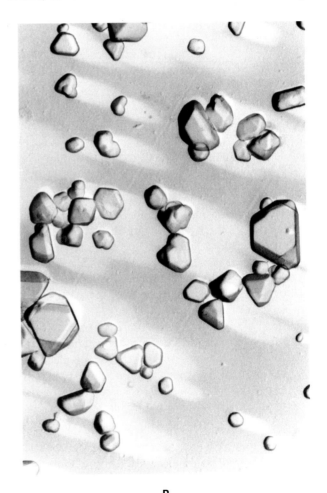

A   B

FIGURE 19–4. Photomicrographs of silver halide crystal. (A) flat triangular tabular crystals (T-grain). (B) conventional crystals. *(Courtesy of Eastman Kodak Company, Rochester, NY)*

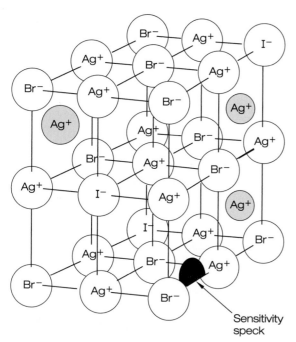

FIGURE 19–5. Cubic lattice arrangement of ions in a silver halide crystal. The surfaces are primarily positive bromine and iodine halides while the interior is primarily positive silver. Note the free silver atom and the sensitivity speck.

tal while the silver ions form the center. This results in silver halide crystals having negatively charged surfaces and positively charged interiors.

The silver halide crystals must have an impurity added, usually gold-silver sulfide, to form **sensitivity specks**. The gold-silver sulfide may adhere to the surface of the crystal or even be partially incorporated into its structure. There can be a few or many specks, but they must be present to provide film sensitivity. During latent image formation the sensitivity specks serve as electrodes to attract the free silver ions. During development the bromide concentrations will serve as ion pumps to assist in the deposition of silver, thus amplifying the image.

Ripening
Ripening is the period during which silver halides are allowed to grow. The size of the crystals determines their total photosensitivity, so the longer the ripening period, the larger the crystals (or grains) and the more sensitive the emulsion. The relationship of crystal size and emulsion thickness to various film factors is shown in Table 19–1. At the proper time, the emulsion

is cooled, shredded and washed to remove the potassium nitrate.

Mixing
The mixing process follows ripening. The shredded emulsion is melted at a precise temperature to properly sensitize the crystals. A number of additives are then mixed into the emulsion. Usually included among these are:

— colored dyes that improve the sensitivity of the silver halides to match the wavelengths of photons that will be striking the emulsion during exposure,

— hardeners to prevent physical trauma,

— bactericides and fungicides to inhibit the growth of these organisms (especially in warmer climates or where water supplies are not chemically treated) and

— antifogging agents to decrease sensitivity to environmental factors, such as heat.

Films are often classified as **panchromatic** or **orthochromatic**, according to their sensitivity to the color of light. **Panchromatic** films are sensitive to all colors while **orthochromatic** films are not sensitive to the red spectrum. This sensitivity is controlled by the dyes that are added during this stage.

Coating
The coating process requires extremely precise and expensive coating equipment. There are only a few factories in the world that can coat emulsions. First the adhesive layer is applied to the base, then the emulsion and finally the supercoat. The emulsion is applied to 40-inch-wide (102-cm) sheets of film which are stored on rolls, cut to size and packaged for the consumer. Standard film sizes are shown in Table 19–2. All film

TABLE 19–1. Relationship Of Film Crystal And Emulsion To Film Factors

	Crystal Size		Emulsion Layer	
	Small	Large	Thin	Thick
Resolution	high	low	high	low
Speed	slow	fast	slow	fast
Contrast	high	low	high	low
Latitude	narrow	wide	narrow	wide

manufacture, packaging, transport, exposure and processing must be accomplished in total darkness.

Latent Image Formation

The photons that reach the emulsion are primarily light photons from the intensifying screens that are in contact with the film. However, x-ray photons are also involved in the production of the image. This deposits energy from the photon within the lattice of the silver halide crystals.

The latent image is the unseen change in the atomic structure of the crystal lattice that results in the production of a visible image. Although there is still much that is unknown about the exact mechanisms that control the formation of the latent image, the theory proposed by Gurney and Mott in 1938 remains almost unchallenged. Their theory accounts for sensitivity specks being essential to the image formation process.

The arrangement of the silver and halide ions, free silver ions and sensitivity specks (Figure 19–5) has been simplified to illustrate the Gurney-Mott theory (Figure 19–6) of latent image formation. The process begins when an incident photon (light or x-ray) interacts with one of the halides (bromine or iodine). The ejected electron is freed to wander and may eventually be attracted and trapped by a sensitivity speck, giving the speck a negative charge. The negatively charged sensitivity speck attracts a free silver ion. The silver ion neutralizes the sensitivity speck (thus resetting the "trap"). This process is known as the ionic stage and is repeated several times until a clump of silver atoms rests at the sensitivity speck. A single incident photon may free thousands of electrons for deposition at sensitivity specks. However, not all freed silver is deposited at sensitivity specks. At least three silver atoms must be deposited for a visible clump of black metallic silver to be formed by chemical development of the image.

Types of Film

The first radiographs were exposed to x-ray photons only. Film is still manufactured for direct exposure, but because it requires a much greater radiation dose, its use

TABLE 19–2. Standard Radiograpic Film Sizes

SI	U.S. Customary
35 × 91 cm	14 × 36 inches
40 × 40 cm	
35 × 43 cm	**14 × 17 inches**
35 × 35 cm	14 × 14 inches
30 × 40 cm	
30 × 35 cm	
28 × 35 cm	**11 × 14 inches**
25 × 30 cm	10 × 12 inches
24 × 30 cm	
24 × 24 cm	9.5 × 9.5 inches
20 × 40 cm	
20 × 25 cm	**8 × 10 inches**
18 × 24 cm	
18 × 43 cm	**7 × 17 inches**
	5 × 12 inches
15 × 30 cm	6 × 12 inches
	6.5 × 8.5 inches

Bold sizes are in routine use at most institutions.

NOTE: In most cases the metric and English sizes are not equivalent; they are similar but not exactly interchangeable.

is severely limited for medical applications. Once the technology had been developed to use the x-rays to produce light at the intensifying screen, the dose reduction resulted in intensifying screen film (usually called screen film) becoming predominant in medical radiography. In addition, numerous special application films have been developed, such as mammography, detail extremity, contact surgical, computer-driven cathode ray tube (CRT), laser exposed, duplication, subtraction, cine and fluoroscopic films.

Direct Exposure or Nonscreen Film

Although used primarily for industrial nondestructive testing (NDT) radiography (Figure 19–7), occasional use of direct exposure film can be justified when extremely fine detail is critical to the diagnostic quality of the image. Because of the extremely high radiation

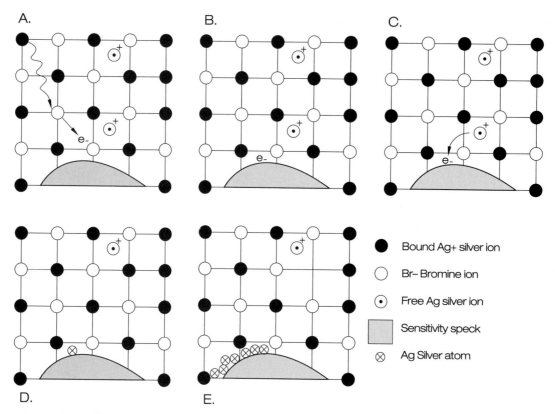

FIGURE 19–6. Latent image formation according to the Gurney-Mott theory.

A — A bromine ion absorbs an incident photon and ejects an electron.

B — The ejected electron is trapped at the sensitivity speck, giving it a negative charge.

C — The negatively charged sensitivity speck attracts a free silver ion.

D — The silver ion neutralizes at the sensitivity speck.

E — Repetition of the process deposits several silver atoms at the sensitivity speck.

exposure that results from the use of nonscreen film, it is unusual to justify its use on living patients. Dental radiography, reconstructive surgery of the hands, biopsy specimen radiography, and forensics are examples of appropriate applications. Direct exposure film has a single emulsion, extremely fine grain silver halide crystals and a much greater silver content. It also requires a much thicker emulsion layer (two or three times that of medical screen film) in order to achieve sufficient sensitivity and still maintain a fine grain. Because of the emulsion thickness, many brands of direct exposure film cannot be processed in automatic radiographic processors and require manual processing.

Intensifying Screen Film

Commonly called screen film, this type of film is available in a wide variety of speeds, contrast ranges, latitudes and resolutions. Each manufacturer has developed specific characteristics for its particular films. Table 19–3 lists the major manufacturers and their trade names to permit identification in clinical situations.

The primary differences are in speed (sensitivity of the silver halides), which is controlled by the size of the crystals and the thickness of the emulsion layer. Contrast, latitude and resolution tend to be linked to speed. Larger crystals and thicker emulsions usually provide lower con-

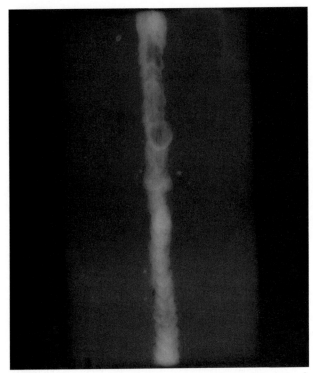

FIGURE 19–7. Industrial nondestructive testing radiograph of a welded joint with a fracture line.

TABLE 19–3. Major Manufacturers Of Radiographic Film And Their Trade Names

Manufacturer	Trade Names
Eastman Kodak	X-Omat, X-Omatic, Lanex, T-Mat
Sterling	Cronex, Quanta
Agfa	Curix, Scopix
Fuji	
Konica	
Ilford	Rapide

trast, wider latitude and less resolution. Screen films are made faster through their double emulsion while a reduction in the silver content has been achieved through more efficient distribution of the silver.

Special Application Films

Most special applications require single emulsion films, although some have a pure gelatin coating on one side to avoid shrinking and curling during processing. **Mammography** and **detail extremity radiography** films have developed as fine-grain films sensitive to a single screen. **Contact surgical radiography** is accomplished with nonscreen film in sterilized plastic packages. **Cathode ray tube (CRT) imaging**, also called video imaging, requires a film that is sensitive to the light emitted by the CRT. Films for CRT are available in blue and green sensitivities as well as orthochromatic for either. They are usually fine grain because patient dose is not a factor when recording CRT images. **Laser films** are directly exposed by the laser used in the imaging camera. Consequently, the film must be sensitive to the color (frequency) of light emitted by the particular camera. The laser light is extremely accurate and because it operates with parallel instead of divergent photons, it produces a near distortion-free image. Fine-grained films are used for this purpose because their exposure is usually not related to the level of patient exposure to radiation, and because the accuracy of the laser image demands a film that can record fine detail.

Duplication film is designed to provide an exact image of the original film. Diagnostic radiographs are actually negatives because they reverse the blacks and whites of the subject (white-bone). Fluoroscopy produces a positive image (black-bone). If an unexposed diagnostic film is laid under a processed film with a good image, a light is turned on for a brief moment and the exposed film is processed, the duplicate film will have densities opposite from the original (i.e., the white-bone image will be converted to black-bone). Duplicating film is pre-exposed to permit it to duplicate the original image (i.e., a white-bone image is recorded as a white-bone image). It is sensitive to the ultraviolet light used in duplicating machines.

Subtraction film is available in two types: subtraction mask film and subtraction film. Subtraction mask film is a fine grain, clear (nontinted) base film designed to reverse the image of a preliminary scout angiogram film. It produces a black-bone image from a white-bone original. It is used during the subtraction process to produce a mask of the scout film. The subtraction film is a different type of film, also fine grain with a clear base, that duplicates the original scout film superimposed over the mask film.

Cineradiography film is 35 mm roll film, exactly like the film used in most single-lens reflex cameras (16 mm roll film is seldom used). It is sensitive to the green light emitted by the fluoroscopic unit. Its primary application is for cardiac catheterization angiography where fine detail is often critical to diagnosis. Cineradiography is an extremely high patient dose technique and therefore should be limited to critical diagnostic areas such as cardiac catheterization.

Fluoroscopic spot filming can be accomplished with screen film but is often done with 70 mm roll film or 105 mm film chips. These films are similar to cineradiography film in that they are sensitive to the green light from the fluoroscope.

Special minimum sensitivity films have been developed for verifying the radiation field during MeV radiation therapy treatments. These films are exposed to massive amounts of radiation.

The Duplication Process

Duplication is the process by which a nearly exact copy, the same size, or miniaturized, is made of a radiographic image. Duplicates arose from the need to share visual information with other institutions, with other hospital departments for educational purposes, and for volume storage and medical legal purposes. Film manufacturers have made duplication relatively easy by producing ready-to-use duplicating film that is processed in automatic processors, and devices for exposing it (Figure 19–8).

Solarization Effect

The solarization effect is a technique from the early days of photography that produces prints by exposure to sunlight. If an ordinary silver halide emulsion is exposed long enough, it will reach the reversal phase and actually lose density.

Duplicating Film

Modern duplicating film has a single emulsion and is presolarized; it is chemically fogged to D-Max by the manufacturer. Therefore, further exposure decreases optical density (OD).

Duplicating film has an average gradient of OD 1.0 to 1.5 and is sensitized to about 359 nm, which is in the ultraviolet range. It is possible to post a simple technique chart by a duplicating unit after a brief trial with duplicating film and a control radiograph.

Various authors have written of techniques used to save overexposure radiographs in order to avoid having to repeat the examination. Diagnostic information from images that are overexposed as much as 75 percent can often be saved via duplication with long exposure times. This technique is limited to original radiographs with a density of OD 3.1 or less.

With some of the faster emulsions now available, the exposure requirements may be so low that the copying unit cannot accurately time them. In these instances, the duplicating system can be slowed down to match the emulsion by blocking part of the unit's ultraviolet tube with blackened film, black electrical tape or by an orange/yellow filter.

Very large institutions and other mass users of radiographic images, such as the military and survey units, often need to reduce the size of images because of limited storage facilities. In these situations a copy-stand device with a roll-film camera can be used. These units use 16 mm to 100 mm photographic roll-film.

The Subtraction Process

Subtraction began as a photographic technique that was used to overcome the superimposition of opacified arteries and various bone structures in lateral cerebral angiograms. Subtraction attempts to remove all densities on the finished image except the opacified vessels. This is accomplished by subduing or subtracting bone densities to a neutral gray, leaving the contrast-medium-filled vasculature in high contrast to the subtracted background.

Procedure

The subtraction procedure is shown in Figure 19–9. It requires:

1. A preliminary scout image without contrast medium.

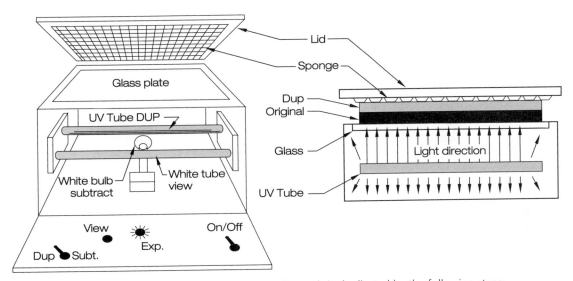

FIGURE 19–8. A radiographic duplication/subtraction unit. A radiograph is duplicated by the following steps:

1. A clean radiograph requiring duplication is placed on the glass plate and centered using the view light control.
2. The view light is switched off. Under safelight, a duplicating film of appropriate size is placed emulsion down on the original radiograph to be duplicated. (Notch in lower left [LL] means the emulsion is facing the operator.)
3. The lid is attached tightly to achieve good film-to-film contact.
4. The timer is set and an exposure is made in the duplicating mode.
5. Both films are removed from the glass plate; the duplicating film is processed, and the original is returned to storage.

Exposure adjustments are made by comparing the duplicate to the original. Because duplicating film is a positive emulsion, exposure adjustments are the opposite of those used for radiographic film. For example, a darker duplicate is produced by decreasing exposure time.

The duplicate image will be slightly less sharp than the original because of the divergence of light as it travels through the two emulsions of the original onto the single emulsion of the duplicate. In addition, the duplicate image will have significantly higher contrast because the slope of the solarized D log E curve is always steeper than with radiographic films. *(Courtesy of Roger Smith, British Columbia Institute of Technology, Vancouver, BC)*

2. A contrast medium image in exactly the same position and with the same technical factors.
3. A special mask and subtraction film.
4. A special subtraction exposure unit installed in a darkroom. (It is possible to perform subtraction on a darkroom bench or with a glass-fronted cassette, using a carefully controlled light source.)

As in all photography, testing is necessary to derive the best results. The density of the mask is the key, since the contrast-medium-injected images should not be repeated. Once a routine is established with fixed techniques, the subtraction procedure exposures should vary little.

Second-Order Subtraction

Second-order subtraction may be used if the first mask is insufficiently dense. The preliminary film is superimposed over the light mask and another mask is produced from the two.

Unsharp Mask Technique

The unsharp mask technique interposes a thick sheet of optical quality glass between the original image and the subtraction film to produce a very blurred mask. The blurred mask can enhance images, particularly for reproduction photography for publication.

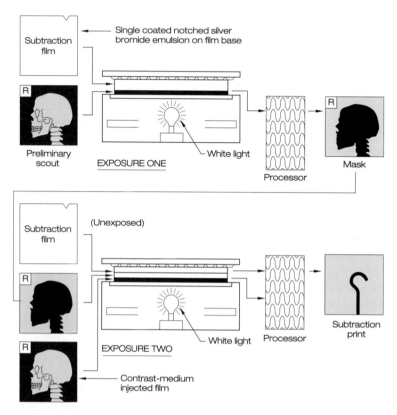

FIGURE 19–9. The subtraction process. A subtracted radiograph is produced by using a duplication/subtraction unit in the following steps. A mask image is produced to subdue or cancel the bone image.

1. Place the preliminary scout radiograph on the glass plate of the duplication/subtraction unit.
2. Under safelight conditions, place an unexposed subtraction mask film emulsion down (notch in LL or UR corner) over the scout radiograph. Close and latch the lid to achieve good film-to-film contact and expose the film in the subtraction mode.
3. Both films are removed from the glass plate; the subtraction mask film is processed and the scout radiograph is returned to storage.
4. The mask is evaluated for sufficient density. Since this is a positive print of the scout radiograph the bones will appear black. Insufficient bone density will not subtract enough density during the subtraction process. Exposure adjustments are made as for diagnostic film (i.e., a darker image is achieved by increasing exposure time).

A subtraction image is produced by selecting the contrast medium radiograph from which a subtraction print is desired and using the following procedure:

1. Place the mask film emulsion up on the glass plate of the duplication/subtraction unit and turn on the view light.
2. Place the contrast medium radiograph over the mask film and align the two images until the maximum subtraction of densities is achieved. Most densities should appear as a uniform density from the combination of the two opposite emulsions with only the contrast medium remaining in high contrast. Secure the alignment of the two images with masking tape.
3. Under safelight conditions, place an unexposed subtraction print film emulsion down (notch in LL or UR corner) over the two aligned films. Close and latch the lid to achieve good film-to-film contact and expose the film in the subtraction mode.
4. All three films are removed from the glass plate; the subtraction print film is processed while the mask film and contrast medium radiograph are returned to storage.
5. The subtraction print film is evaluated for sufficient density and exposure adjustments are made if necessary (i.e., if a darker image is desired the exposure time should be increased). Subtraction print film produces black vasculature. White vasculature can be produced by substituting duplication film for subtraction print film during the final exposure (step 3). *(Courtesy of Roger Smith, British Columbia Institute of Technology, Vancouver, BC)*

Film Storage and Handling

Although often overlooked, the proper storage and handling of film is an important part of radiography. It is not uncommon for a hospital diagnostic radiography department to have an annual film budget of over $1,000,000, and any unit performing radiography quickly discovers that film cost is a considerable budget item. Improper storage and handling of film can be very expensive. More importantly, it can produce film artifacts that compromise image quality. Appendix B (AGFA's Troubleshooting the Radiographic System) details film artifacts and their causes.

Basic Storage and Handling

Attention must be given to the **age** of the film, **heat, humidity, light, radiation and handling**. All film is sold with an expiration date stamped on the box. Photosensitive materials are constantly absorbing photons of both heat and background radiation and, over time, this exposure can reach a level where the fog on the film interferes with image quality. Rotation of new stock must be established to observe expiration dates.

Film should be stored at a temperature of 20°C (68°F) or lower at all times. Professional photographers refrigerate all film, and radiography departments should follow this recommendation. Most radiography departments avoid the problem by arranging film shipments to keep film in storage for only 45 to 60 days. Special application films that must be stored for long periods of time should be frozen. All refrigeration and freezing must be done with the film sealed in moisture-proof containers, as sold by the manufacturer. This essentially arrests the aging process. **Film must be brought to room temperature in advance of use** and before breaking the moisture-proof seal. Failure to do this will destroy the film when atmospheric moisture condenses on the cool film surface, creating waterspot artifacts.

The humidity must be maintained between 30 and 60 percent. Static discharge artifacts are a danger at low humidity, and high humidity causes condensation. A basement area that contains steam, cold water or other fluid pipes and is not included in the building's heating and cooling system is a poor choice for film storage.

All photosensitive materials must be protected from unfiltered light. Because film is sold in light- and moisture-proof packaging, this becomes a problem only with damaged or opened packages. Darkroom safelighting permits film handling with the convenience of limited visibility. All film must be protected from exposure to ionizing radiation. Lead lining of film storage areas will eliminate this problem. Handling of film is often overlooked as a source of problems. **Film should be stored on end**, not flat. Film boxes should be opened carefully, and under no circumstances should a film, paper interleaf or cardboard insert be removed quickly. Abrasion artifacts can occur from quick movement over film and under pressure. Even at the proper humidity, quick movement can cause static discharge with artifact exposure from the resulting light (Figure 3–5). Chemical fumes can also cause film fog. Film should not be stored near cleaning solutions, formaldehyde or other strong chemicals.

Automated Systems

Automatic film handling systems involve a transport mechanism that feeds a single film from a storage unit, transports it into position for exposure between a pair of intensifying screens and then transports it into a processor after exposure. Automatic feed diagnostic units have been marketed successfully. However, in spite of the fact that they save the expense of cassettes, they have not been extremely popular, but automatic feed dedicated chest units have become a standard fixture in high volume departments.

Daylight Systems

Daylight cassette loading systems that can be operated in full light have been available since the 1960s. They have become more common than old-fashioned darkroom systems because they save considerable time as well as eliminate the need for full-time darkroom technicians in busy imaging departments. Daylight systems utilize light-proof units, cassettes with light-proof loading slots or doors, and a light-proof unloading unit connected to a dedicated processor. It is important that radiographers become well acquainted with typical maintenance problems with these units as some systems may be prone to jamming as films are transported from one location to another inside the unit and film processor. Common problems associated with daylight loaders include improper loading of unexposed film into loading cartridges, clogged vacuum outlets or worn loader arms, debris interfering with film transport, and other problems peculiar to specific brands of equipment.

Film Identification

All radiographs should be permanently identified with medical record information. This includes the date of the exposure, the full name of the patient, the institution where the exposure was made, the referring physician, the patient identification number, the examination ordered and any other important information. The identification information is usually added to the film by a light exposure after the radiographic exposure and can be accomplished with a special daylight identification camera and cassette system. It can also be done in the darkroom after the film has been removed from the cassette but before it is processed. Most radiographic cassettes have a lead blocker space in one corner to prevent the film from being exposed to x-rays in that small area. This reserves the space for identification information to be "flashed" by light. This information, like the radiograph, becomes part of the legal medical record and should be treated as such. Additionally, a method of identifying right and left sides of the patient should be required. Many institutions use lead markers, although film punches and blocker placement systems can also be used. The radiographer performing the examination is usually identified through some means; initials or number on a lead marker and signature of accompanying paperwork are common.

Depending upon institutional policy, it may or may not be acceptable to change the identification information if it is recorded incorrectly. Some institutions permit changes to be made with wax pencil, stickers or punches while others require that the radiograph be repeated. The radiographer is nearly always held responsible for recording the identification information correctly.

Summary

Photographic materials are photosensitive, or capable of responding to exposure by photons. Diagnostic radi-

ographic film is duplitized; in other words, the base is coated on both sides with an adhesive, an emulsion with crystals and a supercoat.

The film base is polyester, the adhesive glues the emulsion to the base to prevent distortion during processing or handling, the emulsion is gelatin in which photosensitive silver halide crystals are suspended and the supercoat is a protective layer. An antihalation coating is used to decrease light reflections within the base itself.

Radiographic film is manufactured in four stages: crystal production, ripening, mixing and coating. The silver halides used are silver bromide, silver iodide and silver chloride. The term silver iodo-bromide best describes the silver halides used in radiographic film. They are produced in total darkness by combining silver nitrate and potassium bromide in the presence of gelatin. The silver halide crystals that are produced are flat and roughly triangular in shape. Each crystal is a cubic lattice of silver, bromide and iodine atoms with sensitivity specks. Ripening time determines crystal size and sensitivity. During mixing, additives are included in the emulsion. Panchromatic films are sensitive to all colors while orthochromatic films are not sensitive to red. Coating is the final stage before the film is cut and packaged.

The latent image is the unseen change in the atomic structure of the crystal lattice that results in the production of a visible image. At least three silver atoms must be deposited to form a visible clump of black metallic silver.

Direct exposure or nonscreen film can be used when extremely fine detail is critical although the extremely high radiation exposure requires a careful justification. Intensifying screen film is the most common radiographic film. Films vary in speed, contrast, latitude and resolution. Special application films have been developed for mammography, detail extremity, contact surgical, cathode ray tube (CRT), laser-exposed, duplication, subtraction, cine and fluoroscopic films.

Duplication produces a nearly exact copy of a radiographic image. Subtraction is a process that attempts to better visualize opacified arteries.

Care must be taken in storing and handling film because it is affected by age, heat, humidity, light, radiation and handling. Some of the handling is avoided by automated and daylight systems. All radiographs should be permanently identified with the appropriate medical record information.

REVIEW QUESTIONS

1. What are the primary components of radiographic film?

2. Explain the production of silver halide crystals.

3. What is the purpose of various additives to radiographic film?

4. How is the latent image produced?

5. What are the primary differences between direct exposure film and screen film?

6. Describe the duplication process.

7. Describe the subtraction process.

8. Describe common problems due to improper film storage and handling.

9. What are the radiographer's responsibilities concerning proper radiograph identification?

REFERENCES AND RECOMMENDED READING

Arnold, B., Eisenberg, H., & Bjarngard, B. (1978). Measurements of reciprocity law failure in green-sensitive x-ray films. *Radiology.* 126, 493.

Bruce, G. (1980). Tests to compare two film-materials for use in chest radiography. *Radiography.* 46(547), 170.

Busching, L. W. (1978). Implementing a new x-ray film management system. *Radiologic Technology.* 49(5), 603.

Carroll, Q. B. (1993). *Fuchs's Radiographic Exposure, Processing and Quality Control* (5th ed.). Springfield, IL: Charles C. Thomas Publishers.

Chow, M. F. (1988). The effect of a film's sensitivity to its speed, contrast, and latitude. *The Canadian Journal of Medical Radiation Technology.* 19(4), 147.

Cullinan, A. & Cullinan, J. (1994). *Producing quality radiographs* (2nd ed.). Philadelphia: J. B. Lippincott.

Curry, T. S., Dowdey, J. E., & Murry, R. C. (1990). *Christensen's introduction to the physics of diagnostic radiology* (4th ed.). Philadelphia: Lea and Febiger.

Daniels, C. & Halloway, A. F. (1983). Comparison and variations of the speed of radiographic film. *Radiology.* (Jan), 203.

Davis, L. (1938). *J. B. Murphy: Stormy petrel of surgery.* New York: G. P. Putnam's Sons, 266–268.

Dixon, L. (1979). Two against one — a case for single-sided films. *Radiography.* 45(532), 81.

Doi, K. (1981). Effect of crossover exposure on radiographic image quality of screen-film systems. *Radiology.* (June), 707.

Egyed, M. & Shearer, D. R. (1981). A comparative physical evaluation of four x-ray films. *Radiology Management.* 3(4), 11–20.

Frantzell, A. (1950). The practical roentgenographic importance of reciprocity law failure. *Acta Radiologica.* 34, 6–16.

Fuchs, A. (1956). Evolution of Roentgen film. *American Journal of Roentgenology.* 75, 30–48.

Huda, W., Sourkes, A. M., Loutatzis, M., Watkins, G. B., Ross, C., Halabuza, H., & Rutledge, D. (1987). An intercomparison of Kodak Ortho-G and TMG x-ray film. *The Canadian Journal of Medical Radiation Technology.* 18(3), 105.

Jaffke, R. C. (1957). That versatile non-screen film. *Radiologic Technology.* 29(1), 14.

James, T. H. (1977). *The theory of the photographic process* (4th ed.). New York: Macmillan Publishing.

Jenkins, D. (1980). *Radiographic photography and imaging processes.* Lancaster, England: MTP Press Limited.

Jenkins, D. & Latham, S. M. (1979). The duplication of chest radiographs. *Radiography.* 45(539), 244–248.

Kelsey, C. A. (1983). Anticrossover emulsions evaluated by observer performance tests. *Radiology.* (Jan), 209.

Kim, O., Ahn, M., & Bahk, Y. (1992). Use of film duplicator to lighten dark radiographs. *Radiology.* 184(2), 573.

Kofler, J. & Gray, J. (1991). Sensitometric responses of selected medical radiographic films. *Radiology.* 181(3), 879–883.

Lauer, O. G., Mayes, J. B., & Thurston, R. P. (1990). *Evaluating radiographic quality: The variables and their effects.* Mankato, MN: The Burnell Company Publishers.

Martin, A. J. & Poznanski, A. K. (1977). A simple approach to lightening an overexposed film with a Blue Ray copier. *Radiologic Technology. 49*(1), 39.

Mathias, J. L. & Marquis, J. R. (1976). Radiographic duplication: A simple method of minimizing radiation dosage to the patient. *Radiologic Technology. 48*(3), 293.

McKinney, W. (1988). *Radiographic processing and quality control.* Philadelphia: J. B. Lippincott.

Morgan, R. H. (1946). An analysis of the physical factors controlling the diagnostic quality of roentgen images: Part IV. Contrast and the film contrast factor. *American Journal of Roentgenology and Radiation Therapy. 55*(5), 627–633.

Morgan, R. H. (1944). Reciprocity law failure in x-ray films. *Radiology. 42*, 471–479.

Neblette, C. B. (1962). *Photography: Its materials and processes* (6th ed.). Princeton: Van Nostrand.

Newhall, B. (1964). *The history of photography.* New York: The Museum of Modern Art.

Ramsey, L. J. (1978). Notes on x-ray film speeds. *Radiography. 44*(524), 200.

Rao, G. U. V., Witt, W., Beachley, M. C., Bosch, H. A., Fatouros, P. P., & Kan, P. T. (1981). Radiographic films and screen-film systems. *The Physical Basis of Medical Imaging.* Editors: Coulam, C. M., Erickson, J. J., Rollo, F. D., & James, A. E. New York: Appleton-Century-Crofts.

Roberts, D. P. & Smith, N. L. (1988). *Radiographic imaging: A practical approach.* Edinburgh: Churchill Livingstone.

Rossi, R. P., Hendee, W. R., & Aherns, C. R. (1976). An evaluation of rare-earth screen-film combinations. *Radiology. 121*, 465.

Sanford, L. (1992). The continuing story of film technology. *Radiography Today. 58*(661), 27-29.

Seeram, E. (1985). *X-ray imaging equipment: An introduction.* Springfield: Charles C. Thomas.

Stephenson, G. W. (1990). American College of Surgeons archivist. Personal communication. February 8.

Sweeney, R. J. (1983). *Radiographic artifacts: Their cause and control.* Philadelphia: J. B. Lippincott.

Temme, J. B. & Steiner, P. B. (1988). The case of the intermittent 'film fog'. *Radiologic Technology. 60*(1), 43.

Thompson, M. A., Hattaway, M. P., Hall, J. D., & Dowd, S. B. (1994). *Principles of imaging science and protection.* Philadelphia: W. B. Saunders.

Tortorici, M. (1992). *Concepts in medical radiographic imaging.* Philadelphia: W. B. Saunders.

Wilson, P. (1976). Principles of formation of the latent and developed images. *Canadian Journal of Radiography, Radiotherapy, and Nuclear Medicine. 7*(6), 268–278.

CHAPTER 20

Image Processing

At first it seems to be
a smeared
print: blurred lines and grey flecks
blended with the paper

Margaret Atwood, *"This Is A Photograph Of Me."*

OBJECTIVES

Upon completion of this chapter, the student should be able to:

▶ Explain the process of film development.

▶ Describe the synergistic properties of automatic processor reducing agents.

▶ Identify the primary chemical and its function for each of the developer and fixer agents.

▶ Explain the process of film fixation.

▶ Explain the washing and drying processes of film archiving.

▶ Describe the functions of the subsystems of an automatic processor.

▶ Discuss the design of a radiographic darkroom, including entrances, pass boxes, centralized and decentralized plans and ventilation.

▶ Explain the rationale for the use of silver recovery systems.

▶ Compare the advantages and disadvantages of metallic replacement, electrolytic, chemical precipitation and resin silver recovery units.

*T*he primary purpose of radiographic processing is to deposit enough black metallic silver at the latent image sites to permit a permanent visible image to form. The development of the latent image can be accomplished manually or with automatic processing equipment. Due to the predominance of automatic processors in radiography, manual processing will not be discussed. The process is very similar to automatic processing and any radiographer can apply his knowledge of automatic processing to manual processing with the modifications provided by the manufacturer's information inserts that are packed with the chemicals.

Quality control experts agree that the radiographic film processor is the most sensitive and variable factor in the production of a radiograph. A high percentage of radiographic quality problems can be traced to processor variations or malfunctions. It is the role of the radiographer to monitor the performance of the processor, troubleshoot problems and repair minor malfunctions.

Automatic processing of a radiograph involves four primary steps: **developing**, **fixing** and two archiving steps—**washing** and **drying**. Developing and fixing are accomplished in solutions of numerous chemicals. Archiving involves a two-step process of washing and drying the radiograph for use as a medical record.

Developing

Developing is the first step in processing the film. At this stage silver is deposited at the latent image sites and an image becomes visible. The deposition of silver amplifies the density of the image. Modern x-ray developers are capable of amplifying the image by a factor of 10^8–10^9 within 3 to 4.5 minutes. The silver ions of the latent image are stabilized and more silver is added to the site until a visible silver clump is formed. The primary agents of the developer are two **reducing agents**, although automatic radiographic developer solutions also include an **activator**, **restrainer**, **preservative**, **hardener** and water as a **solvent** (Table 20–1). The action of the developer is controlled by the immersion **time**, solution **temperature** and chemical **activity**.

Reducing Agents

Reducing agents provide electrons to the silver ions attached to the sensitivity specks of the silver halide crystals (the latent image). Silver halides have negative exteriors (where bromine and iodine ions are located) and positive interiors (where silver ions are located). This arrangement effectively prohibits the reducing agent from supplying electrons to the silver ions because the bromine and iodine repel electrons. However, when a sensitivity speck has attracted silver ions, a gate exists through which the interior of the crystal can be supplied with electrons. When a silver ion obtains an extra electron, it is converted to a stable black metallic silver atom. Reduction is actually the process of the reducing agents giving up electrons to neutralize the positive silver ions. This reduction process is illustrated in Figure 20–1.

The secret to the production of the various densities is that the sensitivity speck gate will be larger when more silver ions are deposited at the speck during exposure. A larger gate permits faster reduction of the internal silver atoms. When the reduction process is stopped at the appropriate time, the silver halides have accumulated black metallic silver in proportion to the size of the sensitivity speck gate. This produces a film with varying degrees of blackness. Of course, all silver halides with gates will become totally reduced, and the entire film will appear black if the reducing agents are permitted to work for too long a time, if they work too fast due to high **temperature** or if the solution has too high a **concentration**. The term **chemical fog** is used to describe development when these factors cause unexposed silver halides to be reduced.

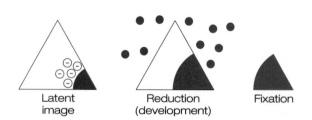

FIGURE 20–1. The reduction of a silver halide crystal through a sensitivity speck gate.

TABLE 20–1. Automatic Radiographic Processing Chemicals and Their Functions

Solution	Time in 90-second Processor	Chemical	Function
Developer	20–25 sec		reduces latent image to visible black metallic silver
reducing agent		phenidone	rapidly produces fine detail shades of gray
reducing agent		hydroquinone	slowly produces heavy densities
activator		sodium carbonate	produces alkaline pH, swells gelatin
restrainer		potassium bromide	decreases reducing agent activity, antifogging agent
preservative		sodium sulfite	controls oxidation, buffer agent
hardener		glutaraldehyde	hardens emulsion, reduces gelatin swelling
solvent		water	dissolves chemicals
Fixer	20 sec		stops reduction and removes undeveloped silver halides from emulsion
clearing agent		ammonium thiosulfate	removes undeveloped silver halides from emulsion
activator		acetic acid	provides acidic pH, stops reduction
hardener		potassium alum	hardens emulsion
preservative		sodium sulfite	maintains pH
solvent		water	dissolves chemicals
Wash	20 sec		removes developing and fixing chemicals
solvent		water	removes excess chemicals
Dry	25–30 sec		removes water and seals emulsion
		hot air	evaporates water and hardens emulsion

Those silver halide crystals that have fewer than three silver atoms on their sensitivity specks are unable to open a gate and remain unreduced (undeveloped). Each reduced silver atom is accompanied by a liberated bromine ion with a negative charge. A bromide ion barrier is created when too many liberated bromine ions are permitted to accumulate. They may produce sufficient charge to repel reducing agents and effectively stop silver halide development. This is the same effect that is achieved by using potassium bromide as a "starter" solution to slow down the hyperactivity of newly mixed developer replenisher solutions. The problem is overcome by replenishment of the developer strength at regular intervals. A freshly cleaned processor may require seasoning by running for 20 to 30 minutes to thoroughly mix the starter solution.

The **reducing agents** used in automatic radiographic processors are **phenidone** (known as P developer) and **hydroquinone** (known as Q developer). **Phenidone quickly reduces silver, enhancing fine detail and subtle shades of gray and works only in areas of light exposure.** It cannot reduce heavily exposed areas. Phenidone replaces the function of metol (often known by the Kodak brand name Elon) in manual processing. **Hydroquinone slowly reduces silver and produces heavy density.** Hydroquinone is ineffective at first but then rapidly increases in action. When the two reducing agents are combined, forming a PQ developer, their reducing ability is greater than the sum of their independent abilities. This is a synergistic phenomenon known as **superadditivity** (Figure 20–2). As can be seen from the graph, phenidone controls the lower part of the curve (the toe) while hydroquinone controls the upper portion (the shoulder).

Oxidation and reduction are opposite processes. When the reducing agent is oxidized, it gives up electrons. Reduction occurs when a silver halide crystal takes one of the electrons and is changed to black metallic silver. The oxidation/reduction process reduces the strength of the developer solution. As developer oxidizes, it changes color, first to a deep amber, then to brown, and finally to a thick, rust red.

Activator

The action of the reducing agents is enhanced by maintaining the developer solution in an alkaline state (around pH 10.0 to 10.5) by using an activator, usually sodium carbonate. Potassium carbonate, sodium hydroxide and potassium hydroxide may also be used. The activator also assists the reducers in reaching the silver halides by causing the gelatin to swell and become more permeable. The activator is caustic and therefore rubber gloves and an apron should be worn when handling developer solutions. Developer solution that is splashed onto clothing and walls is corrosive and should be neutralized with fixer solution or diluted with water.

Restrainer

A **restrainer**, usually potassium bromide, is also added to the developer to restrict the reducing action to those crystals with sensitivity speck gates. It does this by permitting overactive reducers to attack it, instead of unexposed silver halides.

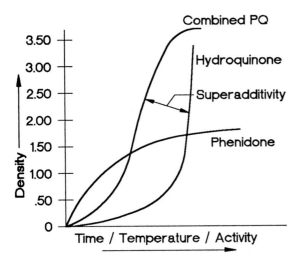

FIGURE 20–2. The superadditivity or synergistic effect of phenidone and hydroquinone combined, as compared to their independent reducing abilities.

Preservative

Sodium sulfite is used as a **preservative** agent to help decrease the oxidation of the reducing agents when they are combined with air. The attraction of air for the reducers is so strong that developer solutions remain effective for only a few weeks after mixing. Common techniques to assist with this problem include floating plastic lids and styrofoam balls to reduce the air-developer interface. This is also a consideration when buying developer solution tanks. Tall, narrow tanks reduce the surface and the oxidation effect. They are more desirable than low, wide tanks. A floating plastic cover or balls (i.e., ping-pong balls) will also reduce the surface area. The tank should not hold more than a two-week supply of solution.

Hardener

Glutaraldehyde is the most common developer solution **hardener**. It controls the swelling of the gelatin to prevent scratches and abrasions to the emulsion during processing. It also maintains uniform film thickness to assist in transport through an automatic processor. Insufficient hardener will cause films to deposit gelatin on processor rollers, which may cause transport and artifact problems for subsequent films. Insufficient hardener may also cause films to exit the processor with moist, softened surfaces. Hot-air drying alone cannot seal the emulsion. Excessive hardener may cause the emulsion to harden prematurely, preventing chemical interactions with the silver halides and trapping moisture in the gelatin.

Solvent

The chemicals are suspended in water as a **solvent**. The water used for mixing chemistry should be filtered to remove impurities (a 5–10 μm filter is recommended). In tropical climates it should be treated to eliminate bacteria and fungus that may find the gelatin emulsion an attractive meal.

Contamination

The developer is the only solution that is dramatically affected by contamination. Only 0.1 percent fixer in a developer tank will destroy the ability of the reducing agents (10 ml in a 2.5 gallon [10 liter] tank). Films processed in contaminated developer appear extremely gray (they exhibit extremely low contrast). Because the fixer tank is adjacent to the developer, it is easy for splashing to occur during quality control and repair procedures. The most common cause of contamination is splashing, which occurs during lifting or replacing the fixer transport rack. Special splash guards are supplied with automatic processors and they should always be used. Developer contamination requires total dumping, washing, refilling and seasoning of the developer tank. Not only is this difficult and time consuming but it also wastes money. When cleaning a processor, the fixer tank should always be filled first. If splashing occurs, it is a simple matter to reclean the developer tank before it is filled.

Evaporation of solutions can also cause contamination. Due to the heat necessary for processing, solutions evaporate and condense on the processor lid. Contamination can occur if fixer condensation drips into the developer tank. Individual evaporation covers for both developer and fixer tanks should be in place at all times. When a processor is shut down, excessive condensation can occur as it cools. To prevent contamination, the processor lid should be propped open whenever the processor is not in use. Splashing or evaporation of developer into the fixer tank does not cause contamination. Developer is regularly carried into the fixer by the films being processed.

Fixing

If a film is exposed to light after development, the unreduced silver halides will open gates and be converted to black metallic silver. This is seen as a slow blackening of the film, which obscures the image. Undeveloped silver halides must be removed from the emulsion to permanently fix the image before exposure to light for viewing. (This was the last reaction to be discovered and delayed development of the photographic process by nearly 25 years.) This important step is accomplished by using a clearing agent that bonds with the unexposed silver halides and removes them from the emulsion. The primary agent of the fixer is the **clearing agent**, although automatic radiographic fixer solutions also include an **activator**, **preservative**, **hardener** and water as a **solvent** (Table 20–1).

Clearing Agent

Nearly all fixer solutions use ammonium thiosulfate as the clearing (fixing) agent (also known by the old-fashioned term "hypo"). Ammonium thiosulfate uses silver in the emulsion to form ammonium thiosilversulfate. Within 5–10 seconds after the clearing agent has begun to function, the film can be exposed to full room light for inspection without damage to the image. If the fixer has not completely cleared the film of unexposed silver halides, the film will have a milky appearance. The **clearing time** is defined as twice the time necessary for the milky appearance to disappear. In a 90-second automatic processor, the clearing time is usually 15–20 seconds.

Activator

Acetic acid is used as the **activator** in the fixer. It maintains an acidic pH (4.0–4.5) to enhance the functioning of the clearing agent. It also serves as a stop bath to keep the reducing agents from continuing to function when the film is immersed in the fixer. Recall that reducing agents function in an alkaline solution. An acidic solution will neutralize and thereby stop the alkaline developing solution from continuing its reduction of the silver halides.

Preservative

The fixer uses the same **preservative** as the developer — sodium sulfite. It dissolves silver from the ammonium thiosilversulfate, thus permitting it to continue to remove silver from the emulsion.

Hardener

The **hardener** in the fixer must function in an acidic environment. Glutaraldehyde is effective only in an alkaline solution, so fixer hardeners are aluminum chloride, chromium alum or potassium alum. The hardener serves the same purpose as glutaraldehyde in the developer — prevention of scratches and abrasions to the emulsion during processing and maintenance of a uniform thickness of the film during transport. Insufficient hardener will cause films to exit the processor with moist, softened surfaces.

Solvent

Water (which should be filtered and treated) is used as the solvent.

Depletion

After a time the fixer solution will become saturated with silver ions from the emulsion. The solution slowly becomes unable to accept additional silver and requires a longer clearing time. Automatic processors constantly replenish the fixer solution to eliminate this problem. The silver ions in the fixer can be reclaimed through various silver recovery processes.

Archiving

The archiving process is composed of two steps: washing and drying. Archiving prepares the film for long-term storage as a medical record by protecting it from deterioration by chemicals, fading and physical forces.

Washing

The **washing** process uses water to remove as much of the fixer and developer solutions as possible. The water temperature should be slightly lower than the other solutions (about 5°F or 3°C lower) because some processors use the water to help control temperature fluctuations in the developer and fixer. The emulsion may reticulate (crack into many pieces) if the temperature is changed too dramatically.

Both fixer and developer solutions contain chemicals that, even in weak concentrations, can damage the image over time. Because most of the developer action is stopped by the acidic pH of the fixer, the main concern is removing the fixer from the emulsion. Failure to provide sufficient agitation or wash time to clear fixer from the film may result in silver stains or a yellowing of the emulsion after a few years.

Warm water will increase the efficiency of the wash. Wash tanks, especially those not made of stainless steel, are susceptible to algae and bacteria growth during periods when the processor is turned off. To eliminate this problem the wash tank should be drained whenever the processor is shut down.

Drying

Drying is done by forcing hot air over both sides of the film as it begins its exit from the processor. The air temperature ranges from 120–150°F (43–65°C). The hot air sets a final hardening to the emulsion and seals the supercoat. Table 20–1 illustrates all of the automatic processing steps, the processing times and the functions of the component chemicals.

Storage

Proper storage is a critical part of the archiving process. The length of time an original radiograph is stored is usually 5–7 years, depending on institutional policies and applicable laws. Films taken of minors and cases involved in litigation may be retained much longer (sometimes permanently). Processed radiographs should be stored at about 70°F (23°C) and 60 percent humidity.

Automatic Processing

Radiographic films were manually processed until Eastman Kodak introduced the first continuous roller automatic processor in 1957. This unit processed a film in 15 minutes and was so large that an overhead winch was required to lift the racks of rollers from the chemical tanks for cleaning. It was a great improvement over manual processing, which required an hour to process and dry a film, and often produced erratic results. Modern processors are much more compact (their racks can easily be lifted by hand) and they process a film in 45–120 seconds (Figure 20–3A).

Automatic processors are complex and utilize several subsystems to completely process a radiograph: the **transport system, dryer system, replenishment system, circulation system and temperature control system**. Table 20–2 illustrates the processor systems and subsystems and their functions. The radiographer should understand the functions of automatic processing systems well enough to diagnose problems that affect image quality. The radiographer should also be capable of basic disassembly of a processor for cleaning or removal of lost or stuck films.

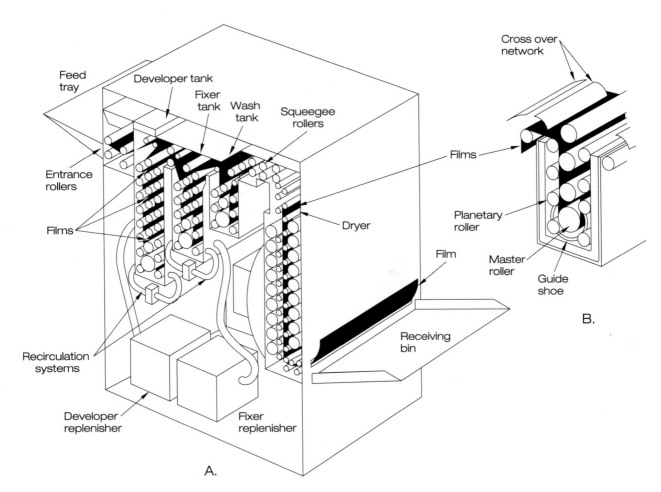

FIGURE 20–3. (A) A modern automatic x-ray film processor. (B) A transport rack and crossover networks in a single tank.

Transport System

The transport system is designed to move a film through the developer, fixer, wash and dryer sections of the processor. As it does this, it controls the length of time the radiograph is immersed in each of the solutions and agitates the chemistry to ensure maximum reaction. The transport system consists of three subsystems: **transport racks**, **crossover networks** and a **drive system.**

Transport Racks
The transport racks consist of three series of rollers designed to move a film through a processing tank (Figure 20–3B). The offset of the three series of rollers provides constant tension to propel the film down into and up out of the processing tank. Note

that the center series of rollers may handle films traveling down and up at the same time. The original processors had difficulty handling films due to shrinking and expansion of the emulsion. The solution temperature, quantity of hardeners and expandability of the emulsion are all designed specifically for automatic processing. Films without these characteristics may not transport through the processor and may even leave artifact causing emulsion deposits on rollers. Single emulsion films are especially difficult because the single emulsion tends to cause the film to curl as it expands and contracts.

Special turnaround equipment is needed to bend and turn a film at the bottom and top of the transport racks. This is accomplished at the bottom of the rack by a com-

TABLE 20–2. Automatic Radiographic Processor Systems and Subsystems

System	Subsystem	Function
Transport		Move film through processor, control immersion time, agitate solutions
	Transport rack	Move film down into and up out of solution tanks
	Crossover network	Turn film down into next tank
	Drive system	Turn rollers
Dryer system		Remove excess water, shrink and seal emulsion
Replenishment system		Replace depleted chemicals in developer and fixer
Circulation system		Stabilize solution temperatures, agitate solutions, mix replenishment chemistry into tank
Temperature control		Maintain solution temperatures

bination of master roller, planetary rollers and guide shoes (deflectors) (Figure 20–3B). The master roller pushes the leading edge of the film against the guide shoes. The guide shoes then force the edge around the master roller with the help of the planetary rollers until it is pointed upwards and can be pulled by the offset rollers. Guide shoes are ribbed to prevent wet films from sticking to a smooth metallic surface. Each transport rack can be lifted from its tank for easy cleaning. The final set of rollers in a transport rack are special squeegee rollers that remove excess solution from the film as it is pulled from each tank.

Crossover Networks
A **crossover network** is used to bend and turn the film when it reaches the top of the transport rack and must be directed down into the next tank or section (Figure 20–3B). Each crossover network operates with a master roller and guide shoes system similar to that in the transport rack. Misaligned guide shoes will scratch the film emulsion as it is driven past. The most common cause of guide shoe misalignment is improper seating of transport racks and crossover networks.

The **entrance rollers** are a special crossover network designed to start the film traveling from the feed tray down into the developer section. These rollers are specially designed with ribs to grip the film and feed it evenly into the first rack. It is important that the entrance rollers grip the film so that it will feed straight through the entire processor. A film that is fed at a slight angle will be driven into the transport gears by the time it travels a distance into the processor.

Always use the guides at each side of the feed tray to align each film as it is fed into the entrance rollers. Films should be fed from alternate sides of the feed tray to avoid excess wear to one side of the transport rollers (i.e., first film right side, second film left side, etc.). **Films should always be fed with the short axis along the feed tray side guide** (Figure 20–4). In some processors the entrance rollers also open a microswitch that activates the replenishment system.

Drive System
The **drive system** consists of a series of mechanical devices designed to turn the numerous rollers in the processor from power supplied by a single motor. The speed of the drive system is usually set to move a film from the entrance rollers to the feed tray (dry to dry) in 45–120 seconds. This speed controls the time the film is immersed in each chemical solution, and slowing or speeding by as little as 2 percent can dramatically affect image quality.

Dryer System
The final stage of processing is drying the film with the **dryer system**. The emulsion of a wet film is sticky and may adhere permanently if brought into contact with another film. The dryer system begins with a series of squeegee crossover rollers removing excess wash water from the surface of the film. The film is then driven

A.

CORRECT: Short side of film against
feed tray guide

B.

WRONG: Long side of film and not
against feed tray guide

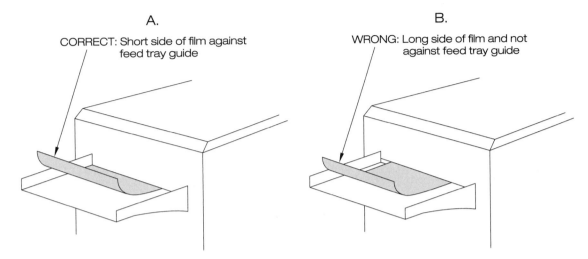

FIGURE 20–4. (A) Proper film feeding. (B) Improper film feeding.

between a double row of slotted, hot forced-air tubes (Figure 20–3A). A high-speed fan draws room air past electric heating coils, producing air at 120–150°F (50–65°C). The film emulsion shrinks and seals dry in a single pass and the film is ready for viewing and storing when it exits the processor. The excess air is returned to the room. This is the primary cause for uncomfortable temperatures in processing areas during hot weather. When damp films exit the processor, the cause is more likely to be in the fixer (depletion or lack of hardener) or wash tank (saturation or insufficient fresh water) than in the dryer section.

Replenishment System

The **replenishment system** replaces chemicals that are depleted through the chemical reactions of processing, oxidation and evaporation. The developer replenisher solution has a different composition than the solution in the processing tank. Because bromides build up in functioning developer, they tend to restrain the activity of the reducing agents on the silver halides. For this reason, developer replenisher lacks sufficient restrainer. A special **starter solution** of acetic acid and potassium bromide (the restrainer) must be added to the replenisher solution when starting a fresh tank of developer. The tank of fresh solution must then be seasoned by running the processor

for 15 to 20 minutes to permit adequate mixing of the solutions.

Volume replenishment is used for high-volume and **flood replenishment** for low-volume units. A volume replenishment system is activated when films enter the processor. The entrance rollers may activate a microswitch or an infrared sensor. In this manner, replenishment of chemical solution strength begins when a film enters the processor and ends when it passes the entrance rollers. This permits replenishment according to the amount of film entering the processor. (A 14" film would replenish solutions more than a 10" film. This is appropriate since it would require more chemistry to process the longer film.) Infrared sensors provide more accurate replenishment as they are capable of sensing not only the length but also the width of the film. A microprocessor can then activate the replenishment pumps for an appropriate length of time. **Flood replenishment** (also called **timed** or **standby** replenishment) is designed for low-volume units where films enter the processor at irregular intervals. The replenishment unit is controlled by a timer that automatically floods the developer and fixer tanks with replenisher solution at a regular interval regardless of the number of films processed.

Although not a replenishment system, a **standby switch** is supplied on many processors. These processors are programmed to shut down some systems when two minutes pass without a film entering the unit. The standby switch usually must be manually activated to bring the entire unit to processing readiness. The standby mode inactivates the entrance rollers so films cannot be fed until the unit is activated.

The replenishment rate can be adjusted so that more fixer is replenished than developer. Although they must be adjusted for specific conditions, procedures and manufacturers' recommendations, developer replenishment rates often range from 4–5 ml per inch (1.5–2.0 ml per cm) of film feed. This is about 55–70 ml per 14-inch (36-cm) length of film. Fixer rates range from 6–8 ml per inch (2.5–3.0 ml per cm). This is about 85–110 ml per 14-inch (36-cm) length of film. Some processors provide a digital display of this information on the front panel.

A replenishment system is designed to pump replenisher solutions from separate storage tanks for the developer and fixer (Figure 20–5). Replenisher tubing usually includes a filter at the exit of the supply tank to collect dirt and sediment. Processors often use dual pumps operated by a single motor. The motor rotates a magnet, which in turn causes magnets in vanes inside the plastic pump bodies to rotate. This system isolates the solutions from each other and the pump motor and makes replacement of pump bodies easy and inexpensive. The replenishment system uses a metering pump, which is more complicated but operates on the same principle.

The storage tanks may be under or adjacent to the processor or, in the case of some large institutions, replenisher may be pumped great distances from a central mixing station. The tanks must be located at a site convenient for the mixing of chemical solutions. A clean area with a drain and corrosive-resistant floor and wall coverings is required.

All mixing should be done strictly according to the manufacturer's recommendations regarding temperature, the proper sequence of additives (for example, solution A, then B, then C, etc.). Always mix additives to water. Adding water to additives will cause splashing of corrosives and a decrease in solution strength. There are occasions when the chemicals react in undesirable ways with one another, the water and air. For example, if hardener is added to fixer replenisher too rapidly, it may precipitate sulfur and aluminum, leaving the solution with insufficient hardener.

Processing solutions are hazardous materials and are covered by several federal agencies in the United States. Since 1986 the Occupational Health and Safety Administration (OSHA), the Environmental Protection Agency (EPA) and the Department of Transportation have all implemented regulations affecting processing chemicals. Users of the chemicals are required to have

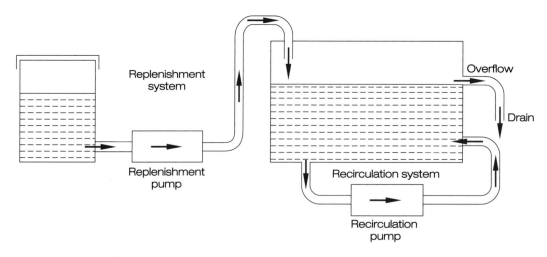

FIGURE 20–5. A typical processor replenishment and circulation system. *(Adapted with permission of David Jenkins from* Radiographic Processing and Imaging Processes, *MTP Press, Lancaster, England)*

material safety data sheets (MSDS) on hand, policies regarding handling, a teaching program and safety equipment, particularly an eyewash station.

Radiographic solutions are not available to the general public in the U.S. When developer solution is mixed on site, the concentrated solution containing hydroquinone and the preservative and activator (usually the first part mixed) has a pH of about 12.0, which is extremely destructive to the eyes if splashed. For this reason, protective eyeglasses should always be worn when mixing solutions. Additionally, hydroquinone can be absorbed through the skin, and glutaraldehyde is a tanning agent that will work on human skin just as it works in leathermaking.

Circulation System

The **circulation system** is designed to **stabilize temperatures, agitate solutions, mix the chemistry and filter** the solutions. Temperatures are maintained in conjunction with the temperature control system. Constant mild agitation of the developer and fixer solutions is required so the chemicals will enter and exit the emulsion. The fresh chemistry added by the replenishment system must be constantly mixed throughout the tanks to avoid overdevelopment, underdevelopment and underfixation. Separate developer, fixer and wash tank circulation systems are required, although a single motor may drive all of the pumps.

Most circulation systems draw chemistry from the bottom ends of the developer and fixer tanks and pump it to the upper ends. Because old chemistry tends to rise in the tank, the excess solution is permitted to overflow from the top of the tank into a drain. In addition, the replenishment pumps usually add fresh chemistry to the upper or middle end of a tank. Some wash systems are made more efficient by the addition of a circulation pump (Figure 20–5). The fixer circulation lines are usually fitted with a 100 μm-wire mesh filter to trap dirt or bits of gelatin that have been washed from films.

The fixer tank overflow has sufficient accumulated silver content to make it financially feasible to attempt to recover as much as possible. **Fixer overflow should be considered toxic and under no circumstances should it be dumped directly into an open drain.**

The wash tank uses a discard circulation system. Constantly recirculated water would quickly become saturated with fixer, which would set up an ionic barrier against additional fixer leaving the emulsion. To prevent this problem from occurring, the wash tank uses a constant flow of fresh water, which is pumped in at the bottom ends of the tank and overflows from the top to a drain. Most manufacturers recommend 4 to 8 liters per minute (1–2 gallons [US] per minute). **It is environmentally unsound to drain wash tank water into sewer lines.** Increasing concern over heavy metal pollution may place liability on persons or institutions responsible for dumping processing chemicals, especially silver. Although expensive, storage of processing overflow and disposal by hazardous materials professionals is advisable.

Temperature Control System

The **temperature control system** maintains all three solutions at compatible temperatures. This is accomplished in conjunction with the circulation system by various methods, depending on the model and manufacturer. A **heat exchanger** is the most common system. It uses a thermostat to heat the developer, since its temperature is the most critical. The developer is then routed through a circulation coil in the bottom of the fixer or wash tank to permit exchange of heat to the fixer by conduction. Developer in a circulation coil does not mix with the fixer or wash water. A 90-second automatic processor will usually require a developer temperature of 92–96°F (33–35°C) while a two-minute processor will operate at 83–86°F (28–30°C).

Cold water processors accept incoming water at cold line temperatures and divert it to the wash tank, where it is heated and stabilized. Some systems require mixing of incoming hot and cold water within a set temperature range. The incoming water is then added to the wash tank, where the temperature stabilizes. Wash tank overflow is diverted to surround the developer and fixer tanks where heat can be conducted through the metal tank wall to maintain solution temperatures. These systems may also use circulation or heater coils in the developer and fixer tanks.

The developer temperature is especially critical. A difference is visible with a fluctuation of only 0.5° (F or C). Some processors provide a digital display of this information on the front panel. The optimal reducing agent temperature is 68°F (20°C) for an immersion time of 4–8 minutes. Much research has been devoted to the formulation of special developer solutions that will produce quality images at temperatures of 92–96°F (33–35°C). These high-temperature developers reduce immersion time to 20–22 seconds, thus permitting 90-second or less processing. Specific developing temperatures vary with manufacturer and can be adjusted with a thermostat. The thermostat is often not easily accessible (sometimes requiring a screwdriver or set screw) to remove the temptation for casual adjustment.

Periodic maintenance of an automatic processor is essential to obtain dependable performance. Since the processor affects the final image produced by nearly all radiographic equipment, and because the unit is often expected to operate 24 hours a day, nonstop, it should have a top maintenance priority.

Darkroom

The darkroom is the light-proof laboratory used for loading and unloading cassettes and feeding film into the automatic processor. Film is twice as sensitive after exposure and must be handled carefully to preserve a diagnostic quality image. An exposed film should be handled in the darkroom with the understanding that mishandling will require a double radiation dose to the patient.

Safelights

Radiographic film is designed to be insensitive to specific wavelengths of orange-red light. This permits the use of low level illumination within this wavelength to make work in the darkroom easier. The amount of light is controlled by the type of filter, wattage of the light source and distance from the working surface. Not all films are insensitive to the same wavelengths. For example, some films designed for rare-earth intensifying screen phosphors require shorter wavelengths (dark red), and some cathode ray tube (CRT) films are sensitive to all light and require total darkness.

Sodium vapor safelights emit an orange-yellow light but their intensity is too high for direct illumination. These safelights must be installed to indirectly illuminate the working area. Installation near the ceiling facing up makes certain that the light loses intensity as it reflects from the ceiling to the working area.

Direct illumination for most radiographic films is possible with a Kodak GBX filter (dark red) over a low intensity (7–15 watt) bulb that is 4 feet (1.25 meters) from the working area. Films that are sensitive only to calcium tungstate phosphor light (blue-violet) may be handled with a Kodak Wratten Series 6B filter (orange-brown) at the same intensity and distance. Light emitting diode (LED) safelights are also available. They emit light in the 660 nm range, use very low power, and last 10 to 15 years. Although they are more expensive, their long life makes them more cost effective.

Too many safelights may result in too great an intensity. A safelight test calculates how long a film may be handled before fogging becomes a problem. Darkroom walls and floor should be light colored to increase the amount of light in the darkroom. If light is safe at its first reflection, it loses intensity and remains safe on additional reflections. When benches and flooring are light colored, it is much easier to locate films and other objects.

Entrance

The darkroom entrance may be of several types. A single door, double interlocking doors, revolving door or light-proof maze may be used. The disadvantage of the single door is that all film must be protected from light, film storage bins must be closed, processor feed tray must be empty, etc., each time the door is opened. The advantage is in space and cost savings. Single-door darkrooms should be equipped with an electric lock on the door that will not open when the film bin is open. This eliminates costly accidental exposure of the entire film bin. The electric lock must open automatically in the event of a power failure. Otherwise, another emergency entrance must be provided for the darkroom. Radiographers and darkroom aides should make it a habit to **always check all film bins before opening a single door entrance**. Double interlocking doors, revolving doors and light-proof mazes permit persons to enter and leave the darkroom without disrupting work in progress.

Pass Box

Film cassettes are passed into the darkroom through a **pass box**, or cassette hatch, which is a light-proof container set in the darkroom wall. Most pass boxes have two sides, one labeled "exposed," the other "unexposed," and both have interlocking light-proof doors. The interlocking doors are designed to prevent both doors from being opened at once, allowing light into the darkroom. A film cassette is taken from the "unexposed" side and the door is closed. The film is then exposed in a radiographic room and returned to the "exposed" side of the pass box. When the door is closed, the darkroom aide may remove the exposed cassette from the pass box, remove and process the film, refill the cassette and return it to the "unexposed" side of the pass box again. This system is very popular because of its speed and convenience.

Plan

A typical darkroom plan is shown in Figure 20–6. This plan has the automatic processor set in the wall between the darkroom and the viewing area. Only the feed tray of the processor extends into the darkroom. The processor is actually located in the viewing area to facilitate periodic maintenance.

When planning a darkroom, one should ensure that the pass boxes and film bins are located where the darkroom aide (who may often be the radiographer) does not have to take steps to reach the processor feed tray. A grounded loading bench should be located directly under each pass box. Grounding of the bench by connecting a wire between the bench top and a well-grounded object (such as a water pipe) reduces the possibility of electrostatic discharge. The film bin should be located under the loading bench.

Darkrooms should be small enough so the darkroom aide does not have to move more than 1–2 steps to perform any operation. A large darkroom is poorly designed and serves no purpose unless other light-proof procedures are routinely performed there (i.e., manual subtraction or duplication, loading specialized cassettes or film holders, etc.).

The darkroom plan should also include a communication system, such as a light-proof speaking grill installed in the door or an intercom. Lighting should be controlled by two separate switches removed from one another. Both full white light illumination (for mainte-

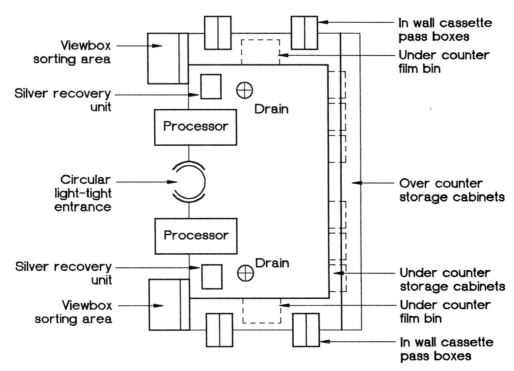

FIGURE 20–6. A typical darkroom plan.

nance and repairs) and safelight illumination (for normal work) should be controlled by a switch. To avoid accidental exposure, the white-light switch should be located higher than the safelight switch (5–6 feet [1.5–1.75 meters] from the floor).

Darkroom ventilation should be a primary concern. Chemical fumes must be vented directly to the outside of the building. Failure to do so can result in toxic fumes being picked up by ventilation systems and delivered to critical areas within a hospital. Most automatic processors have special connections to assist in venting. Good circulation of air from outside the darkroom should also be maintained. Darkrooms in colder climates may also require humidifiers to assure humidity of 40–60 percent during winter months so electrostatic discharge conditions are reduced.

Floor drains are required both inside the darkroom and near the automatic processor outside the darkroom to facilitate maintenance, repairs and daily clean-up. Drains are also a safety precaution against leaks and overflow. They must not be made of copper because processing chemicals will react with copper.

Large departments may use a central processing plan where all films are routed through one or more central darkrooms. These darkrooms are often equipped with two processors. In a compact, well-designed darkroom, an experienced, full time darkroom aide can feed a steady stream of films faster than a single 90-second processor can handle them. Dual processors also permit the darkroom to function even if one is inoperable or undergoing maintenance. Central processing saves the cost of numerous processors and economizes space usage, staffing, etc.

Because of the time required in carrying exposed films to a central darkroom, many large departments utilize a satellite darkroom plan, where single processor darkrooms are placed throughout the department and institution. If a processor is inoperable or undergoing maintenance, the radiographer uses the next nearest darkroom. Satellite processing saves time but is more expensive in equipment, maintenance, facilities and staffing.

Regardless of the plan selected, the area where the processors deposit the finished radiographs should be equipped with benches for handling films and illumination view boxes for viewing them. This area becomes the natural gathering point for the entire radiology department and it is often equipped with computers, telephones, log books, seats, etc., to make it a convenient place to do paperwork and data entry while waiting for radiographs to be processed.

Silver Recovery Systems

As mentioned in the fixer and circulation system sections, sufficient silver is dissolved in the fixer solution to make recovery before discarding feasible from a financial standpoint and to prevent toxic heavy metal pollution of the environment. In the United States the Water Control Act of 1972, Resources Conservation-Hazardous Waste Act of 1976, Clean Water Act of 1984 and Resource Conservation and Recovery Act of 1986 all affect the disposal of heavy metals into the public environment. In essence, these laws require that the best available methods be used to clear silver from fixer overflow solutions prior to disposal. In addition, they limit liquid waste to a toxic level of 5 parts per million (ppm). A permit is required for dumping more than 27 gallons (US) per month into a public sewer and any amount into the ground. Even shipping the waste to a treatment plant requires a permit. Compliance with these regulations is the reason commercial firms are usually employed to handle silver recovery.

The fixer may accumulate silver at the rate of as much as 100 mg/m^2 of film processed. This is well above the dumping limits allowed by law in the United States. In fact, **the fixer is as valuable, if not more valuable, after processing than before**.

About half of the silver in the film remains in the emulsion after processing. The other half is dissolved into the fixer solution. Much of this silver may be removed from the fixer by diverting the overflow through a silver recovery system before discarding. About 5 percent of the silver is carried into the wash tank which, in extremely high-volume circumstances, may also be worth recovery. It is estimated that about 10 percent of the purchase price of film may be recovered, depending on the type of recovery system used and the market price for silver. The cost of recovery will almost always pay for the processing and handling and usually provides a modest financial return to help offset film costs. Silver mining and refining is expensive, and as a result, about half of all silver on the market worldwide comes from recycling.

There are several types of silver recovery units. The most common fixer recovery units are **metallic replacement**, **electrolytic**, **chemical precipitation** and **resin**. All of these units operate by providing electrons that can be used by the silver in the fixer solution to form black metallic silver. They differ in the method by which the electrons are provided and by the process used to refine the metallic silver.

All silver recovery methods require that the fixer sit within the unit for some time to permit the chemical interactions to occur. This **dwell time** is the single most important factor in unit effectiveness. **Agitation** of the fixer solution during this time is also important because it enhances the ability of electrons and silver to contact each other. Finally, the surface area controls the region from which electrons are available or where silver can be deposited.

Metallic Replacement

Metallic replacement units are also called metallic displacement because in these units the fixer acid breaks down the iron in a steel screen or in steel wool and displaces or replaces it with silver. The iron oxides give up electrons for the silver. The metallic silver is precipitated onto the steel. These units are sometimes called silver buckets or cartridges (Figure 20–7). They operate by having the fixer drain into the top, filter through the steel wool or screen, and overflow through a tube connected to the bottom of the container. Metallic replacement buckets are designed for low-volume situations only. They are inefficient as they age and processing is expensive. Fixer overflow from metallic replacement buckets should not be sent to the same drain as the developer overflow. As the steel wool or screen reacts with the fixer, it produces iron oxide, which can form drain-clogging fibers when it reacts with developer.

Electrolytic

Electrolytic units pass a current from a cathode to an anode through the fixer. The ionized silver in the fixer solution is attracted to the negatively charged cathode. It then plates onto the cathode as metallic silver (Figure 20–8). These units are sometimes called cells because

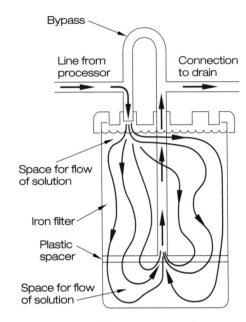

FIGURE 20–7. A metallic replacement silver recovery unit. *(Reprinted courtesy of Eastman Kodak Company)*

they function like a cell in a battery. They are rated according to their recovery capacity (i.e., troy ounces per gallon). They are also classified by their method of agitation, rotating anode, rotating cathode and pumped solution. Electrolytic units are available that will recirculate the fixer for reuse in the processor. Electrolytically processed fixer is deficient in sodium sulfite (the preservative) and this can lead to incomplete fixing. A method of replenishing sodium sulfite must be added when a recirculating fixer system is used. If no silver is present in the fixer, the current will cause the thiosulfate to form sulfur, a smelly process that degrades the quality of the silver plating. This problem can be avoided by using an automatic electrolytic unit that is programmed to increase the current during high volume operation and to reduce it during other periods. **Electrolytic units should not be run when the processor has not been used for a long period of time (such as overnight).** Electrolytic units are designed for moderate and high volume situations and produce easily processed silver flakes (which are chipped from the coated cathode). Most units require regular maintenance because they are

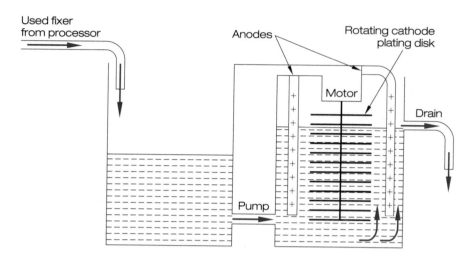

FIGURE 20–8. An electrolytic silver recovery unit.

an electrical hazard. Their electrical components are exposed to moisture, they are prone to short-circuiting and their failure, overuse or underuse may cause hazardous fumes.

Chemical Precipitation

Chemical precipitation units use chemicals (such as zinc chloride and sodium sulfite) that break down in the fixer and release electrons. The metallic silver is heavy enough to precipitate out and fall to the bottom of the tank, where it forms silver sludge. The chemical reactions produce hazardous gasses that are both toxic and explosive. New reagents are available for precipitating extremely large volumes of fixer. Because of the complexity of the process, they are currently used only by commercial silver dealers.

Resin

Resin units use acid to form resin ions. The silver in the solution is attracted to the resin and forms black metallic silver. The resin is then processed to remove the silver.

Monitoring

All silver recovery units must be properly sized for the amount of silver in the fixer. If undersizing is suspected,

a second (**tailing**) unit may be added to process the solution exiting from the first unit. Various types of test strips are available to determine the silver content remaining in the solution as it exits the silver recovery unit. A copper test can be done by dropping a copper penny into the exiting solution. A very light gray coating after 10 seconds is acceptable. A heavy coating indicates too much silver is not being recovered. Correction should begin by checking the function of the existing recovery unit. If it is functioning within acceptable limits, either a larger-capacity recovery unit is needed or a tailing unit should be installed.

Film

The film itself retains half the silver (about 0.1 troy ounce per pound [0.45 kg]) and this can also be recovered. Unexposed (green) film has twice the amount of silver as processed film. However, recycling firms will not pay more for unexposed film. To reclaim the silver, it is recommended that unexposed film be run through a processor to permit the fixer to reclaim half the silver. All scrap film should be saved for recycling, as should all original film when medical files are purged. Because of the weight, space required and value of the silver in radiographs, storage is expensive in hospitals, clinics and physician's offices. When original films are discarded, recycling is a very profitable undertaking.

Summary

The primary purpose of radiographic processing is to deposit enough black metallic silver at the latent image sites to permit a permanent visible image to form. Quality control experts agree that the radiographic film processor is the most sensitive and variable factor in the production of a radiograph. Automatic processing of a radiograph involves developing, fixing, washing and drying.

During development, silver is deposited at the latent image sites and an image becomes visible. The primary agents of the developer are: the two reducing agents, phenidone and hydroquinone; an activator, sodium carbonate; a restrainer, potassium bromide; a preservative, sodium sulfite; a hardener, glutaraldehyde; and water as the solvent. The action of the developer is controlled by immersion time, solution temperature and chemical activity.

Fixing removes the undeveloped silver halides from the emulsion. This is necessary before exposure to light for viewing. The primary agent is the clearing agent, ammonium thiosulfate. Fixer solutions also include an activator, acetic acid; a preservative, sodium sulfite; a hardener, aluminum chloride; and water as the solvent.

The archiving process prepares the film for long-term storage as a medical record. Archiving involves washing the film with water to remove the processing chemicals and drying to harden and seal the radiograph.

Automatic processors utilize several subsystems to completely process a radiograph: 1) the transport system to move a film through the developer, fixer, wash and dryer at a controlled speed; 2) the dryer system to force hot air across the film for drying; 3) the replenishment system to replace chemicals which are depleted through the chemical reactions of processing, oxidation and evaporation; 4) the circulation system to stabilize temperature, agitate solutions, mix the chemistry and filter the solutions and 5) the temperature control system to maintain all three solutions at compatible temperatures.

The darkroom is the light-proof laboratory used for loading and unloading cassettes and feeding them into the automatic processor. Radiographic film is designed to be insensitive to specific wavelengths of orange-red light. Safelights use low-level illumination within this wavelength to make work in the darkroom easier.

Sufficient silver is dissolved into the fixer solution to make recovery before discarding feasible from a financial standpoint and desirable for environmental reasons. The most common types of silver recovery units are metallic replacement, electrolytic, chemical precipitation and resin.

REVIEW QUESTIONS

1. What are the four primary steps in automatic processing?

2. How do the reducing agents, phenidone and hydroquinone, differ in their functions?

3. What is the chemical name and function of the hardener in the developer?

4. What is the purpose of fixing?

5. What are the two steps of the archiving process?

6. How should a film be fed into the automatic processor?

7. Differentiate between volume replenishment and flood replenishment.

8. What is the function of the circulation system in an automatic processor?

9. Under what conditions is direct illumination of a radiographic film safe?

10. How does an electrolytic silver recovery unit operate?

REFERENCES AND RECOMMENDED READING

Anslow, L. (1991). Silver recovery — An evaluation of existing disposal methods in a district general hospital. *Radiography Today. 57*(653), 24–28.

Ball, J. & Price, T. (1989). *Chesneys' radiographic imaging.* Oxford: Blackwell Scientific Publishing.

Bruce, G. (1980). Darkroom safelighting and its effects. *Radiography. 46*(542), 45.

Carroll, Q. B. (1993). *Fuchs's radiographic exposure, processing, and quality control* (5th ed.). Springfield, IL: Charles C. Thomas Publishers.

Chesney, D. N. (1973). Building materials and film fogging. *Radiography. 39*(466), 262.

Cullinan, A. & Cullinan, J. (1994). *Producing quality radiographs* (2nd ed.). Philadelphia: J. B. Lippincott.

Curry, T. S., Dowdey, J. E., & Murry, R. C. (1990). *Christensen's introduction to the physics of diagnostic radiology* (4th ed.). Philadelphia: Lea and Febiger.

Dohms, J. (1992). OSHA safety requirements for hazardous chemicals in the workplace. *Radiology Management. 14*(4), 76–80.

Eastman Kodak Company. (1980). Recovering Silver from Photographic Materials. Rochester, NY: Eastman Kodak Company, Publication No. J–10.

Electrifying artifacts. (1984). *Radiologic Technology. 56*(2), 99.

Film processing. (1978). *Radiologic Technology. 49*(4), 528.

Fodor, J., Malott, J. C., & Sweeny, R. J. (1989). A common artifact. *Radiologic Technology. 60*(4), 325.

Gordon, M. (1988). Chemical hazards in film processing. *International Society of Radiographers and Radiological Technicians Newsletter. 24*(1), 9–12.

Gray, J. E., Winkler, N. T., Stears, J. G., & Frank, E. D. (1983). *Quality Control in Diagnostic Imaging: A Quality Control Cookbook.* Baltimore: University Park Press.

Green, A. & Levenson, G. I. P. (1981). Silver recovery and fixer management: A new approach. *Radiography. 47*(562), 225.

Griffiths, R. (1994). The presence of sulphur dioxide and other toxic fumes within processing environments, and associated health problems. *Radiography Today. 60*(690), 13–16.

Haus, A. G. (Ed.) (1993). *Film processing in medical imaging.* Madison, WI: Medical Physics Publishing.

Jenkins, D. (1980). *Radiographic photography and imaging processes.* Lancaster, England: MTP Press Limited.

Lauer, O. G., Mayes, J. B., & Thurston, R. P. (1990). *Evaluating radiographic quality: The variables and their effects.* Mankato, MN: The Burnell Company Publishers.

Light fog: Picture of a problem. (1984). *Radiologic Technology. 55*(4), 105.

More on artifacts. (1979). *Radiologic Technology. 50*(6), 727.

McKinney, W. (1988). *Radiographic processing and quality control.* Philadelphia: J. B. Lippincott.

Neblette, C. B. (1962). *Photography: Its materials and processes* (6th ed.). Princeton: Van Nostrand.

Newhall, B. (1964). *The history of photography.* New York: The Museum of Modern Art.

Nusbaum, R. C. (1987). Silver reclamation: Management controls maximize yields. *Radiology Management. 9*(3), 42.

Roberts, D. P. & Smith, N. L. (1988). *Radiographic imaging: A practical approach.* Edinburgh: Churchill Livingstone.

Smith, H. S. (1987). Silver recovery trail. *Radiography. 53*(609), 125.

Sprawls, P. (1990). *Principles of radiography for technologists.* Rockville, MD: Aspen Publishers.

Sprawls, P. (1987). *Physical principles of medical imaging.* Rockville, MD: Aspen Publishers.

Suleiman, O. H. (1984). Radiographic film fog in the darkroom. *Radiology.* (April), 237.

Sweeney, R. J. (1983). *Radiographic artifacts: Their cause and control.* Philadelphia: J. B. Lippincott.

Tabar, L. & Haus, A. G. (1989). Processing of mammographic films: Technical and clinical considerations. *Radiology.* 65.

Temme, J. B. & Steiner, P. B. (1988). The case of the intermittent 'film fog'. *Radiologic Technology. 60*(1), 43.

Tortorici, M. (1992). *Concepts in medical radiographic imaging.* Philadelphia: W. B. Saunders.

Turnball, T. (1981). Fixer recycling combines with silver recovery. *Radiography. 47*(557), 115.

van der Plaats, G. J. (1980). *Medical x-ray techniques in diagnostic radiology* (4th ed.). The Hague: Martinus Nijhoff Publishers.

White, J. (1980). Silver recovery: Departmental management approach. *Radiography. 46*(542), 35.

Wilson, P. (1978). Principles of formation of the latent and developed images. *Canadian Journal of Radiography, Radiotherapy, and Nuclear Medicine. 7*(6), 268-278.

Wolbarst, A. B. (1993). *Physics of radiology.* Norwalk, CT: Appleton & Lange.

The Case of the Colon in the Spider's Web

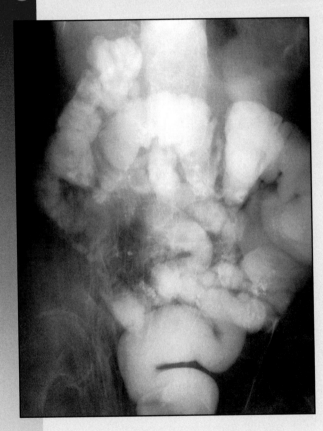

This radiograph of a barium-filled colon has strange vertical lines that seem to enclose the lower GI tract in a web. What is the cause of these lines?

Answers to the case studies can be found in Appendix E.

CHAPTER 21

Sensitometry

You lie on a turning table cold as snow.
Down press the camera's praying-mantis arms,
Avid to embrace your negative below;
Your inner organs light their secret farms
Not even lovers come close enough to know.

Howard Moss, "In the X-Ray Room."

Objectives

Upon completion of this chapter, the student should be able to:

▶ Define sensitometry as it is applied to radiography.

▶ Describe the production of a step wedge on radiographic film through the use of a penetrometer and a sensitometer.

▶ Explain the function of a densitometer.

▶ Estimate the percentage of light transmitted by a radiograph according to optical density logarithms.

▶ Construct a D log E curve from sensitometric data.

▶ State acceptable base-plus-fog and diagnostic range optical density numbers.

▶ Describe the effect of automatic-processor reducing agents on the shape of a D log E curve, especially with relation to speed and contrast.

▶ Define resolution, speed, contrast and latitude.

▶ Explain the effect of silver halide crystal size on image resolution.

▶ Discuss the physical and processing factors that affect film speed.

> ▶ Calculate speed points, speed exposure points and relative speeds from D log E curves.

> ▶ Calculate gamma, gradient point, average gradient and latitude from D log E curves.

> ▶ Analyze D log E curves to determine speed, contrast and latitude relationships.

> ▶ Discuss the relationships between speed, contrast and latitude.

Sensitometry is the measurement of the characteristic responses of film to exposure and processing and is accomplished by exposing and processing a film and then measuring and evaluating the resulting densities. It is primarily the responsibility of the radiographer to use sensitometric methods to evaluate technical factor exposure systems, films, intensifying screens and processing equipment. In addition, sensitometric methods are useful in establishing, evaluating and maintaining technical exposure factor charts and systems, a duty that can be done only by a qualified radiographer.

Sensitometric Equipment

A variety of equipment is necessary to carry out sensitometric procedures. Either a **penetrometer** or a **sensitometer** is required to produce a uniform range of densities on a film. A **densitometer** is required to provide an accurate reading of the amount of light transmitted through the film.

Penetrometer

A **penetrometer** is a series of increasingly thick, uniform absorbers. They are usually made of aluminum steps, although tissue-equivalent plastic is sometimes used (Figure 21–1). A penetrometer is referred to as a **step wedge** because of its shape. It is used to produce a step wedge on radiographic film by exposure to x-rays (Figure 21–2). Because of the vast number of variables in x-ray-generating equipment, the use of a penetrometer is not recommended for quality control monitoring of film processors. However, it is an excellent method for monitoring both x-ray equipment and film/intensifying screen combinations because it reproduces the variables associated with a clinical situation.

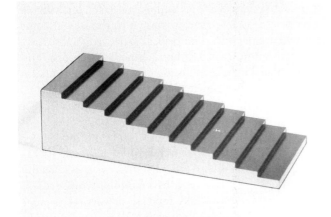
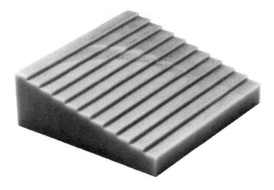

FIGURE 21–1. Two basic types of penetrometers or step wedges: (A) aluminum and (B) tissue equivalent plastic. *(Courtesy of Nuclear Associates Division of Victoreen, Inc., Carle Place, NY)*

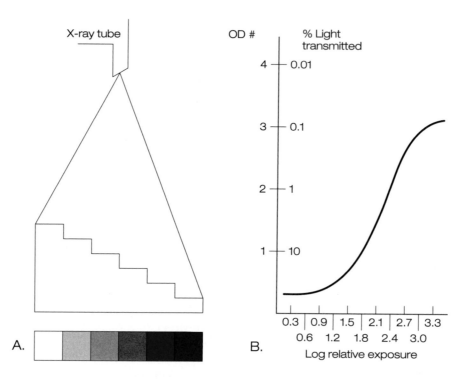

X-ray tube

OD #   % Light
             transmitted

4 ┼ 0.01

3 ┼ 0.1

2 ┼ 1

1 ┼ 10

| 0.3 | 0.9 | 1.5 | 2.1 | 2.7 | 3.3 |
| 0.6 | 1.2 | 1.8 | 2.4 | 3.0 |

Log relative exposure

A.   B.

FIGURE 21–2. A density curve produced from graphing the exposures of a penetrometer exposure. (A) The exposure. (B) The graph.

Sensitometer

A **sensitometer** is designed to expose a reproducible, uniform, optical step wedge onto a film (Figure 21–3). It contains a controlled intensity light source (a pulsed stroboscopic light is best) and a piece of film with a stan-

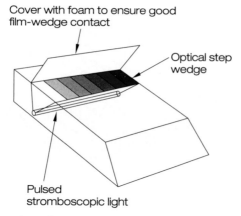

Cover with foam to ensure good
film-wedge contact

Optical step
wedge

Pulsed
stromboscopic light

FIGURE 21-3. A sensitometer.

dardized optical step wedge image (a step tablet). The controlled light source reproduces the same amount of light each time it is triggered. Voltage fluctuations and other factors that might cause the intensity to vary are controlled by circuits that supply an exact quantity of power to a capacitor that discharges to the stroboscopic light when triggered. The optical step wedge absorbs a calibrated amount of this light, leaving a uniform and reproducible "light penetrometer" to expose any film placed in the sensitometer over the optical step wedge. The optical step wedge should not be touched because hands leave a film of oil that interferes with the light intensity.

Optical step wedges (step tablets) are available in 11- and 21-step versions. The 11-step wedges usually increase density 100 percent (by a factor of two) per step. The 21-step wedges usually increase density 41 percent (by a factor of 1.41 times [which is $\sqrt{2}$]) per step. Because the rigid control of the densities produced on the film eliminates other variables, sensitometer produced step wedges are perfect for processor quality control monitoring. Very slight density differences can be detected by sensitometric equipment. When a film is processed, there is a tendency for exhausted reducing agents and bromine ions to be carried backwards on the emulsion as it is driven through the rollers of an automatic processor. For this reason, sensitometric film strips should be fed into automatic processors with either the long axis of the step wedge parallel to the entrance rollers or with the light edge entering the processor first.

Densitometer

A **densitometer** is an instrument that provides a readout of the amount of blackening (density) on a film. A densitometer consists of a calibrated uniform light source, a stage for placing the film to be measured, a light aperture to control the amount of light from the source, a sensor arm with an optical sensor, a readout display and a calibration control (Figure 21–4). Density readings are accomplished by comparing the amount of light emitted by the light source with the amount of light transmitted through the film. To do this, the densitometer must be calibrated before each reading by recording the amount of light the light source is emitting. This is done by pushing the sensor arm so that the sensor is in contact with the light source (this eliminates the inverse square law factor) and by using the calibration control to set the readout display at zero. This cali-

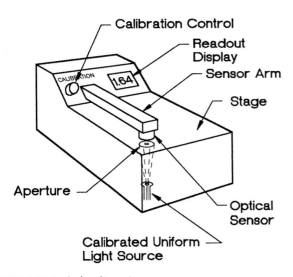

FIGURE 21-4. A densitometer.

brates or **zeroes** the densitometer and prepares it for a reading. When a film is placed on the stage and the sensor arm is pushed down into contact with the film, the densitometer can calculate the difference between the calibration intensity and the intensity of light the film is transmitting. Some densitometers include a filter to negate the blue tint in the film base.

Because films are sensitive to a wide range of exposures, their densities are best visualized if the range is compressed into a logarithmic scale. When using a logarithmic scale with a base of 10, an increment of 0.3 represents a doubling of exposure. This is because the log of 2 is 0.3. The numbers that are displayed by a densitometer are known as **optical density numbers**. They can be expressed with the term OD in front of the number (i.e., OD 1.5). They are calculated using the following formula:

$$OD = \log_{10}\frac{I_o}{I_t}$$

where: OD = optical density number
 I_o = intensity of the incident light
 I_t = intensity of the transmitted light

This formula can be stated as the log of the intensity of the incident light divided by the intensity of the light transmitted through the film. Radiographic film densities range from OD 0.0 to 4.0.

The ability of a film to stop light is termed **opacity**. Opacity is calculated using the following formula:

$$opacity = \frac{I_o}{I_t}$$

where: I_o = intensity of the incident light
 I_t = intensity of the transmitted light

Note that density is the $\log_{10}$ of opacity (density = $\log_{10}$ of opacity). Table 21-1 shows both the opacity and optical density numbers for various percentages of light transmitted within the radiographic film density range of 0.0 to 4.0. For example, if a region of a radiograph has an OD of 1.0, this means only 10 percent or 1/10th of the incident light is transmitted through the radiograph in this region. The opacity of the region would be 10. If the OD number is increased to 1.3, the opacity is doubled (to 20) and the percentage of light transmitted through the film is halved (to 5 percent or 1/20th).

TABLE 21–1. Example Opacities, Optical Density Numbers, And Light Transmission Percentages

Opacity	OD Number	Percentage of Light Transmitted Through Film
1	0.0	100
2	0.3	50
4	0.6	25
8	0.9	12.5
10	1.0	10
20	1.3	5
40	1.6	2.5
80	1.9	1.25
100	2.0	1
200	2.3	0.5
400	2.6	0.25
800	2.9	0.125
1,000	3.0	0.1
2,000	3.3	0.05
4,000	3.6	0.025
8,000	3.9	0.0125
10,000	4.0	0.01

Increments of 0.3 changes in OD numbers represent a doubling or halving of opacity.

The D Log E Curve

Sensitometry is normally shown as a graphic relationship between the amount of exposure and the resultant density on the film (Figure 21–5). The horizontal exposure axis (x axis) is compressed into a logarithmic scale (because of the wide range of densities possible) and the vertical density axis (y axis) is shown as a linear scale. Consequently, the curves are known as Density log Exposure, or **D log E curves**. They are also called **characteristic, sensitometric and Hurter and Driffield (H&D)** curves after the two photographers who first

described the relationships in 1890. The important elements of a typical D log E curve are the base plus fog, toe, straight line portion (gamma), shoulder and maximum density (D_{max}).

The **base plus fog** (b+f) (Figure 21–5A) is the density at no exposure, or the density that is inherent in the film. It includes the density of the film base, including its tints and dyes, plus any fog the film has experienced. Radiographic film base density ranges around OD 0.05–0.10. Processing the film usually adds about OD 0.05–0.10 in fog density. The total base plus fog is seldom below OD 0.10 but should not exceed OD 0.22. Fog may be caused by heat, chemical fumes, light and x-radiation. Over time, the natural amounts of these radiations will produce a slight density that is sometimes called age fog. Most of the fog level will be produced by the processing system. This includes the hyperactivity of the developer solution, primarily caused by the high temperature at which automatic processors operate.

Phenidone is the reducing agent that controls the subtle gray tones early in the development process. This region of the curve is known as the toe (Figure 21–5B) and is predominantly controlled by phenidone.

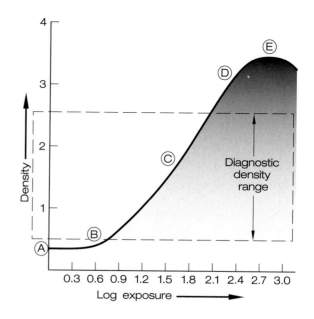

FIGURE 21-5. A typical D log E (characteristic, sensitometric or H&D curve). (A) base plus fog; (B) toe; (C) straight line portion; (D) shoulder; (E) Dmax.

The **straight line portion** of the curve is that portion between the toe and shoulder (Figure 21–5C). It is usually fairly straight because the film is reacting in a linear fashion to exposure in the range of its primary sensitivity, which is in this region. The range of diagnostic densities varies from a low of OD 0.25–0.50 to a high of OD 2.0–3.0. The majority of diagnostic quality information on a radiograph will measure between OD 0.5–1.25. These densities are within the straight line portion of the curve.

Hydroquinone is the reducing agent that controls the heavy black tone later in the development process. This region of the curve is known as the shoulder (Figure 21–5D) and is entirely controlled by hydroquinone.

D_{max} is the maximum density the film is capable of recording (Figure 21–5E). It is the highest point on the D log E curve. It represents the point where all the silver halides have a full complement of silver atoms and cannot accept more. Additional exposure beyond D_{max} will result in less density because silver atoms attached to sensitivity specks will be ionized again, reversing their charge and causing them to be repelled from the speck. This process of **reversal**, or **solarization**, reduces the intensity of the latent image and will produce less density. The true D log E curve is bell-shaped (Figure 21–6). Duplication film is actually film that is preexposed to D_{max} so that additional exposure will cause a reversed, duplicated image instead of a negative one.

Modern film manufacturing techniques permit photochemical engineering of the exact shape of the D log E curve. For example, a film can be engineered for chest radiography that will increase the density of the mediastinal region by enhancing the densities produced for those exposures to the film typical of that region.

Film Characteristics

The primary characteristics of film are classified as **resolution, speed, contrast and latitude**. Sensitometry permits analysis of speed, contrast and latitude within the normal exposure ranges of the film. Extremely long or high-intensity exposure can overload the silver halide crystals and cause a phenomenon known as reciprocity failure. Although films are designed to handle a wide range of exposures, when unusual circumstances require

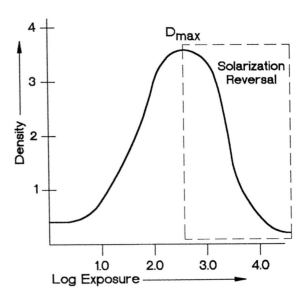

FIGURE 21-6. Solarization or reversal of duplicating film.

large exposures, films may deviate from their expected performance.

Resolution

Resolution is the ability to accurately image an object. It is also called **detail, sharpness, definition and resolving power**. Resolution is measured by the ability to see pairs of lines. The unit of resolution is line pairs per millimeter, expressed as lp/mm.

Film resolution is determined by the **size of the silver halide crystals**. Smaller crystals will darken a smaller area of the film while larger ones will darken larger areas. Information that is smaller than an individual silver halide crystal cannot be visualized. **An inverse relationship exists between film resolution and crystal size** (the smaller the crystals, the higher the resolution; the larger the crystals, the lower the resolution). Silver halide crystals are sometimes called grains, thus the term graininess for poor resolution. Although film graininess can sometimes be seen, radiographic film/screen system resolution is generally controlled by the size of the intensifying screen crystals, not the size of the silver halide crystals in the film emulsion.

Speed

The amount of density (degree of blackening) a film produces for a given amount of exposure is the film **speed**. It is determined by the film's sensitivity to exposure. Speed is controlled by the activity of the phenidone because it affects the toe of the D log E curve. The position of the toe determines how soon the straight line portion will begin, and this indicates the overall speed of the film. Figure 21–7 illustrates the effect of the toe and shoulder on the overall position of the curve.

Film sensitivity is determined primarily by the **size of the silver halide crystals**. However, **the number of sensitivity specks and the thickness of the emulsion layer** also have an effect. Larger crystals will receive more photons because of the greater area they cover. They will also produce more photons than smaller crystals for the same reason. Larger crystals will darken a greater area of the film than smaller crystals with the same exposure. Therefore, **film speed and crystal size are directly related** (the larger the crystals, the faster the film speed; the smaller the crystals, the slower the film speed). **Film**

speed and the number of sensitivity specks are also **directly related** for the same reason.

A thicker emulsion layer will place more crystals in a given area. Each incoming photon may interact with more than one crystal, so when more crystals are stacked on top of one another in the same area, the same number of photons will produce more film density. Therefore, **film speed and thickness of emulsion layer are directly related** (the thicker the emulsion, the faster the film speed; the thinner the emulsion, the slower the film speed).

Screen films are capable of responding to (producing visible densities for) exposures as low as 1 mR and as high as 1,000 mR. In Figure 21–7, film A produces all density levels with less exposure than film B requires for the same density. This demonstrates that film A is more sensitive to exposure, or faster. Film B is less sensitive, or slower.

The **speed point** of a film is that point on the D log E curve where a density of OD 1.0 + b+f is achieved. The American National Standards Institute (ANSI) specifies x-ray film speed as the exposure required to reach OD 1.00. However, many users add base plus fog to this standard. The **speed exposure point** is the log exposure that will produce the speed point for a given film. Film A in Figure 21–7 has a speed exposure point of 1.5, while film B has a speed exposure point of 2.0.

In clinical radiography it is important to be able to adjust technical factors from one film to another. The radiographer must be able to calculate the difference in exposure that will produce a diagnostic quality image on a new film when the proper factors are known for a previous one. In Figure 21–7, film B would require a log exposure of 2.0 to produce OD 1.0. Film A would require a log exposure of 1.5 to produce the same density. The difference in film speed is calculated as:

$$\text{antilog}(\log E_1 - \log E_2)$$

where: $\log E_1$ = log exposure of 1st film
$\log E_2$ = log exposure of 2nd film

Note: The antilog of a number is found by using an antilog table or by entering the number into a scientific calculator and then pressing the INV (inverse) key followed by the LOG key. For calculators without an INV key, review instructions for computing antilogs.

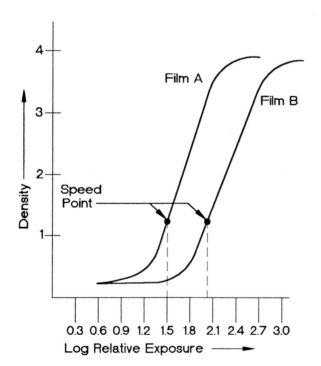

FIGURE 21-7. The effect of film speed on D log E curves.

Example: What is the difference in speed between film A and film B in Figure 21–7?

Answer:

antilog(log E_1 – log E_2) =
  antilog(2.0 – 1.5) =
    antilog(0.5) = 3.16

Film A is 316 percent faster than film B.

Relative speeds have been assigned by film manufacturers to assist radiographers in relating films to one another as they are used in film and intensifying screen combinations (film/screen combinations). Relative film/screen speed can be determined by using the reciprocal of the exposure required to produce a given density:

$$\text{relative speed} = \frac{1}{\substack{\text{exposure in R needed to produce} \\ \text{speed point density (OD 1.0 + b+f)}}}$$

Example: What is the relative speed for a film that requires an exposure of 5 mR to produce the speed point density?

Answer:

$$\text{relative speed} = \frac{1}{\substack{\text{exposure in R needed to produce} \\ \text{speed point density (OD 1.0 + b+f)}}}$$

$$\text{Relative speed} = \frac{1}{5 \text{ mR}}$$

$$\text{Relative speed} = \frac{1}{0.005 \text{ R}} = 200$$

Film speed is affected by immersion **time**, solution **temperature** and chemical **activity**. The immersion **time** in a high-speed automatic processor may be as short as 20–25 seconds. The longer the film is subjected to the chemical action of the developer solution, the greater is the amount of black metallic silver deposited on the latent image sites through the reduction process (Figure 21–8). Film speed is most affected by developer solution **temperature** (Figure 21–9). Only 0.5° will cause a visible change in film density. Higher temperature increases the activity level of the reducing agents in the developer and this produces greater density on the film. High speed automatic processors use high temperatures to permit sufficient development to occur in the 20–25 seconds

the film is immersed in the developer. The chemical activity of the developer solution will also increase the development of density. Film speed is affected when the bromide ion barrier has not formed properly (due to insufficient restrainer or overreplenishment) or when it is too strong (due to excess restrainer or underreplenishment). Determination of the proper time, temperature and activity for a particular developer and film is done by graphing speed, contrast and base plus fog levels for various activity concentrations (Figure 21–10). This is how the manufacturer arrives at the recommended time and temperature for optimal results.

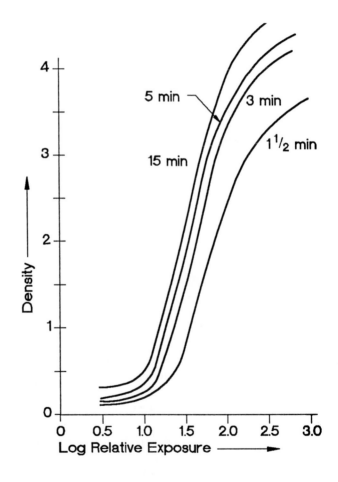

FIGURE 21-8. The effect of developer solution immersion time on film speed.

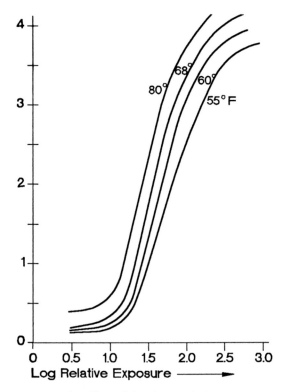

FIGURE 21-9. The effect of developer solution temperature on film speed.

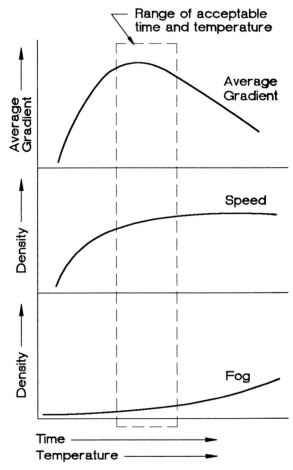

FIGURE 21-10. Determination of optimal development time and temperature for a particular film by comparison of contrast, speed, and base+fog for a particular developer solution concentration.

Contrast

Contrast is the difference between adjacent densities. This concept can be confusing when one tries to understand the difference between density and contrast. There is a relationship between contrast and density because contrast consists of the difference between adjacent densities. For the same film type, **a change in density will affect contrast only when above or below the straight line portion of the D log E curve**.

Contrast is controlled by the level of activity of the hydroquinone. Hydroquinone establishes the shoulder of the D log E curve and the position of the shoulder affects the slope of the straight line portion of the curve (Figure 21–11).

Contrast is defined by the slope of the straight-line portion of the D log E curve, but, because the straight line portion is actually a curve, it is important to define

the point at which the slope is measured. **Gamma** is simply a measure of the slope of the straight line portion of the curve at the speed point (OD 1.0). In practice, a gamma may be read with the speed point in the center, top end or bottom end, as long as all comparative readings are done from the same reference point. Contrast differences cannot be appreciated unless they are measured from identical reference points.

The slope can be read as "rise over run" (Figure 21–12). More sophisticated measurements, such as the trigonometric tangent of the slope, are also used. The slope of any portion of the D log E curve can be calcu-

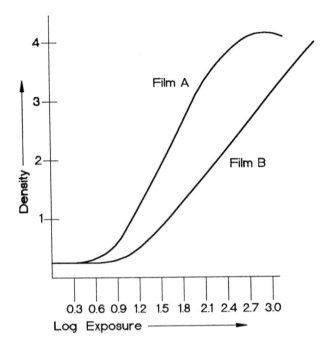

FIGURE 21-11. Comparison of film contrast.

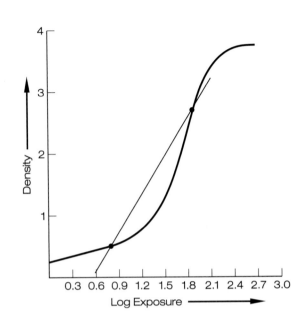

FIGURE 21-12. Average gradient from a D log E curve.

lated and this is known as a **gradient point.** Gradient points must have their OD values stated, e.g., a gradient of 1.75 at OD 0.80. Gradient points are sometimes known by their location: toe gradient, middle gradient and upper gradient. The toe gradient is calculated between OD 0.25 and OD 1.00. The middle gradient is calculated between OD 1.00 and OD 2.00. The upper gradient is calculated between OD 2.00 and OD 2.50. Overall radiographic film contrast is more commonly defined by the **average gradient** of the straight line portion of the D log E curve between OD 0.25 + b+f and OD 2.50 + b+f. Opinions differ on whether b+f should be added to average gradient calculations. The average gradient is calculated as:

$$\text{average gradient} = \frac{\Delta D}{\Delta E} \text{ or}$$

$$\text{average gradient} = \frac{D_2 - D_1}{E_2 - E_1}$$

where: $D_1 = \text{OD } 0.25 + \text{b+f},$
   $D_2 = \text{OD } 2.50 + \text{b+f},$

$E_1 = \text{exposure that produces } D_1$
$E_2 = \text{exposure that produces } D_2$

Note: ΔD is a constant of OD 2.25 (OD 2.50 – 0.25).

Figure 21–13 illustrates the difference between various gradient points and the average gradient. Most radiographic film average gradients are between 2.5 and 3.5.

The important part of the D log E curve is that portion between the toe and the shoulder (the diagnostic range of the film). In this central straight line portion, the density is approximately proportional to the log relative exposure. This is because a straight line will always have a constant ratio. If the slope of the straight line portion is at a 45° angle, the average gradient will measure 1.0. In this example, a doubling of exposure will result in a doubling of the opacity. (Note the term doubling of density is not used because density is a log number. A change of 0.3 in density reflects a doubling or halving of opacity.) **A common misnomer in radiography is that doubling the exposure will double the density.** This is not true for typical radiographic film/screen systems.

Radiographic films have a slope steeper than 45 degrees. In these films, when exposure is doubled, opac-

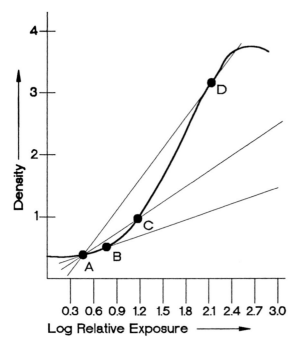

FIGURE 21-13. Average gradient and gradient point calculations from a D log E curve. The slopes of points A-B, A-C, and A-D are quite different.

ity is increased by more than a factor of 2. Because of the steepness of the slope (and the average gradient above 1.0), radiographic films amplify exposure by producing a greater proportion of density per exposure increase. **Doubling the radiographic exposure will produce more than a doubling of radiographic opacity.**

Toe and shoulder gradients are less than a 45° angle (< 1.0) and therefore not only fail to amplify the contrast, but actually decrease it. This is one reason why extremely light or dark areas on radiographs are not acceptable for diagnosis.

A contrast index is often used in quality control to indicate contrast. Because the definition of average gradient depends on comparable densities, when the density itself shifts, a different measure must be established. A contrast index is simply two density points that are subtracted from each other. It gives a measure of the difference between set densities, which represents the contrast. (Contrast is defined at the difference between densities.)

The relationship between density and contrast is complex. To understand how density affects contrast, it is important to realize that the changes in average gradient between the toe and shoulder of the D log E curve are actually changes in contrast. When insufficient or excessive density causes the range of visible densities on the radiograph to change, contrast is affected. For example, the film used for the data in Figure 21–14 achieved a maximum optimal contrast with an OD of 1.2–1.5. For OD measurements above or below this range, contrast is decreased. For radiographic films under most conditions, contrast is maximized when the density range is within the range of diagnostic densities (low of OD 0.12–0.50 and a high of OD 2.0–3.0). When the diagnostic densities are below or above this range, the contrast will be decreased. This occurs because the slope of the range of diagnostic densities has moved into the toe or shoulder of the D log E curve.

The contrast must exist within the diagnostic range of the film if it is to be visualized; in other words, within the straight line portion of the curve.

Latitude

For clinical radiographic purposes, **latitude** is the range of exposures that will produce densities within the diagnostic range (Figure 21–15). Latitude can be recorded as the width of the range of exposures that will produce diagnostic range densities according to the following formula:

$$latitude = E_h - E_l$$

where E_h = OD 2.50 exposure point
          E_l = OD 0.25 exposure point
when E_h = high exposure point
         E_l = low exposure point

Example: What is the latitude for film A in Figure 21–15?

Answer:

latitude = $E_h - E_l$
latitude = 1.8 − 1.1
latitude = 0.7

The latitude for film B can be calculated to be 1.0. Film A has a narrow latitude while film B has a wider latitude. Because a wide latitude film permits considerable varia-

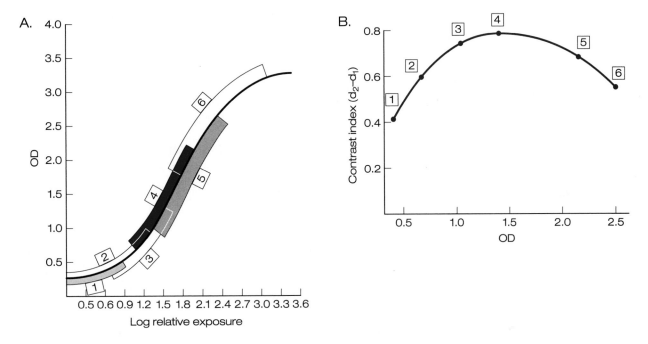

FIGURE 21-14. (A) Density ranges (1-6) from D log E curve of film measured for contrast index. (B) Contrast index for the density ranges (1-6) measured from Figure A. Note that the maximum contrast (range 4) is essentially the straight line portion of the curve. Contrast is decreased for toe and shoulder measurements but is maximized for the straight line portion of the D log E curve (OD 1.2 – 1.5). (Also note that this range corresponds to the speed point [OD 1.2].) *(Courtesy of Charles Burns, MPH, RT(R), University of North Carolina)*

tion in the exposure while still exhibiting densities within the diagnostic range, it is sometimes called a forgiving film. The use of a narrow latitude film for routine radiography requires greater exposure accuracy.

Latitude and contrast are inversely related. As contrast increases, latitude tends to decrease. This affects the overall shape of the D log E curve. Latitude changes whenever there is a change in the average gradient of the D log E curve. Speed could change without altering the average gradient and latitude. A difference in film speed usually results in different contrast and latitude because it is rare for the entire D log E curve to shift the same degree. Usually the toe and shoulder will not shift exactly the same amount and this causes a change in the slope of the straight line portion of the curve (which changes contrast and latitude). The relationships of speed, contrast and latitude to patient dose are listed in Tables 21–2 and 21–3.

Summary

Sensitometry is the measurement of the characteristic responses of a film to exposure and processing. It is accomplished by exposing and processing a film and then measuring and evaluating the resulting densities. Either a penetrometer or a sensitometer is required to produce a uniform range of densities on the film. A densitometer is required to provide an accurate reading of the amount of light transmitted through the film.

Because films are sensitive to a wide range of exposures, their densities are best visualized if the range is compressed into a logarithmic scale. When using a logarithmic scale with a base of 10, an increment of 0.3 represents a doubling of exposure. This is because the log of 2 is 0.3.

Sensitometry is normally shown as a graphic relationship between the amount of exposure and the resultant

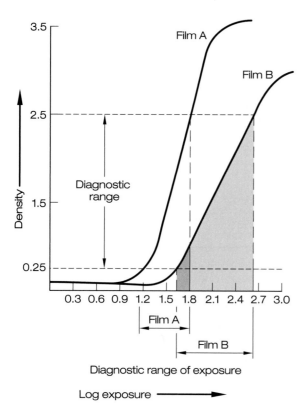

FIGURE 21-15. Comparison of film latitude. The range of relative exposure is indicated for each film.

TABLE 21–2. Relationship Between Contrast, Latitude, and Patient Dose

Contrast	Latitude	Patient Dose
high	narrow	high
low	wide	low

TABLE 21–3. Relationship Between Speed and Patient Dose

Speed	Patient Dose
slow	high
fast	low

thickness of the emulsion. Relative speeds have been assigned by film manufacturers to assist radiographers in relating films to one another as they are used in film/screen combinations. Contrast is the difference between adjacent densities. It is defined as the slope of the straight line portion of the D log E curve. Latitude is the range of exposures that will produce densities within the diagnostic range. As contrast increases, latitude tends to decrease.

REVIEW QUESTIONS

1. What is the purpose of sensitometry?

2. Explain the design of a penetrometer.

3. Why is a logarithmic scale used for describing optical densities?

4. Describe the five important elements of the D log E curve.

5. What is the relationship between film resolution and the size of the silver halide crystals?

6. What is the relationship between film speed and emulsion layer thickness?

7. State the formula for relative speed.

8. How is the average gradient calculated?

9. What is the relationship between contrast and latitude?

density on the film. The horizontal axis (exposure) of the graph is compressed into a logarithmic scale and the vertical axis (density) is a linear scale. Consequently, the curves are known as Density log Exposure or D log E curves. They are also called characteristic, sensitometric and Hurter and Driffield (H&D) curves. The important elements of the D log E curve are the base plus fog, toe, straight-line portion (gamma), shoulder and maximum density (D max).

The primary characteristics of film are resolution, speed, contrast and latitude. Resolution is the ability to accurately image an object and is measured by the ability to see line pairs. The amount of density a film produces for a given amount of exposure is the film speed. The film speed is determined by the size of the silver halide crystals, the number of sensitivity specks and the

REFERENCES AND RECOMMENDED READING

Agfa-Gevaert. *Sensitometry*. Mortsel, Belgium: Agfa-Gevaert N.V.

Carroll, Q. B. (1993). *Fuchs's radiographic exposure, processing, and quality control* (5th ed.). Springfield, IL: Charles C. Thomas Publishers.

Chow, M. F. (1988). The effect of a film's sensitivity to its speed, contrast, and latitude. *The Canadian Journal of Medical Radiation Technology. 19*(4), 147.

Eastman Kodak Co. *Sensitometric properties of x-ray films*. Rochester, NY: Eastman Kodak Company Radiography Markets Division.

Fuji. *X-ray sensitometry*. Tokyo: Fuji Photo Film Co., Ltd., Medical X-Ray Products Technical Handbook.

Gray, J. E., Winkler, N. T., Stears, J. G., & Frank, E. D. (1983). *Quality control in diagnostic imaging: A quality control cookbook*. Baltimore: University Park Press.

Haus, A. G. (Ed.) (1993). *Film processing in medical imaging*. Madison, WI: Medical Physics Publishing.

Jenkins, D. (1980). *Radiographic photography and imaging processes*. Lancaster, England: MTP Press Limited.

Kofler, J. & Gray, J. (1991). Sensitometric responses of selected medical radiographic films. *Radiology. 181*(3), 879–883.

McKinney, W. (1988). *Radiographic processing and quality control*. Philadelphia: J. B. Lippincott.

Rao, G. U. V., Witt, W., Beachley, M. C., Bosch, H. A., Fatouros, P. P., & Kan, P. T. (1981). Radiographic films and screen-film systems. *The Physical Basis of Medical Imaging*. Editors: Coulam, C. M., Erickson, J. J., Rollo, F. D., & James, A. E. New York: Appleton-Century-Crofts.

Roberts, D. P. & Smith, N. L. (1988). *Radiographic imaging: A practical approach*. Edinburgh: Churchill Livingstone.

Rossi, R. P., Hendee, W. R., & Aherns, C. R. (1976). An evaluation of rare-earth screen-film combinations. *Radiology. 121*, 465.

Sprawls, P. (1990). *Principles of radiography for technologists*. Rockville, MD: Aspen Publishers.

Sprawls, P. (1987). *Physical principles of medical imaging*. Rockville, MD: Aspen Publishers.

Stears, J. G., Gray, J. E., & Frank, E. D. (1986). Sensitometry necessity. *Radiologic Technology. 57*(5), 442.

Thompson, M. A., Hattaway, M. P., Hall, J. D., & Dowd, S. B. (1994). *Principles of imaging science and protection*. Philadelphia: W. B. Saunders.

Tortorici, M. (1992). *Concepts in medical radiographic imaging*. Philadelphia: W. B. Saunders.

Wolbarst, A. B. (1993). *Physics of radiology*. Norwalk, CT: Appleton & Lange.

CHAPTER 22

Intensifying Screens

I decided to try a combination of Edison's fluorescent screen and the photographic plate. . . . The combination succeeded even better than I had expected. A beautiful photograph was obtained with an exposure of a few seconds. That was the first x-ray picture obtained by that process during the first part of February 1896.

Autobiography of M. Pupin, From Immigrant to Inventor.

Objectives

Upon completion of this chapter, the student should be able to:

▶ Explain the purpose of radiographic intensifying screens.

▶ Describe the function of each layer of an intensifying screen.

▶ Evaluate the desirability of phosphor materials according to atomic number, conversion efficiency, spectral emission and fluorescence.

▶ Describe luminescence.

▶ Analyze the effect of phosphor crystal size, layer thickness and concentration on intensifying screen resolution.

▶ Explain the effect of film/screen contact on resolution.

▶ Describe how to remedy quantum mottle.

▶ Classify intensifying screens according to intensification factor, descriptive rating and relative speed number.

▶ Describe the effect of K-shell absorption edges on intensifying screen efficiency.

▶ Describe the components of a radiographic cassette.

▶ Describe the proper cleaning and care of radiographic cassettes and screens.

▶ Evaluate film/screen combinations for specific clinical uses.

*I*ntensifying screens are used to amplify the incoming x-ray beam and reduce patient radiation dose. Introduced in 1896 by the American inventor Thomas Edison (1847–1931), intensifying screens produce large quantities of light photons when struck by x-rays. In this manner they intensify the latent imaging power of the beam, even though less than 33 percent of the x-ray photons that strike the cassette interact with the intensifying screen. Over 99 percent of the latent image is formed by this light, with less than one percent contributed by x-ray photons. This permits a great reduction in the amount of radiation necessary to produce a diagnostic quality image. Intensifying screens are normally used in pairs with duplitized film, although there are specialized cassettes that are designed for a single screen with single emulsion film.

Construction

Intensifying screens are composed of radiolucent plastic, coated with phosphors that will emit light when struck by x-ray photons. They are designed to be mounted in pairs inside the top and bottom of a light proof cassette so that a sheet of radiographic film can be sandwiched tightly between them. A screen consists of **a base, a reflective layer, a phosphor layer and a protective coat** (Figure 22–1).

Base

The **base** is usually made of polyester plastic 1 mm thick, although cardboard and metal have been used. Its requirements are similar to those for a film base. It must be flexible yet **tough**, rigid, chemically **inert** and uniformly radiolucent. It **must be flexible** to permit it to achieve good contact with the film. It must be rigid enough to stay in place in the top and bottom of a cassette. It must be chemically inert so that it does not react with the phosphor and interfere with the conversion of x-ray photons to light. It also must not react with air or chemicals in a manner that would cause discoloration. Discoloration filters and changes the wavelengths of the light emitted by the screen by absorbing wavelengths that could be used to create the radiographic image. Because films are designed to be most sensitive to the particular wavelength of light emitted by the screen, discoloration may require more light, and consequently more patient radiation dose, to form the latent image. Most important, base material must be uniformly radiolucent so that it permits the transmission of x-ray photons without adding artifacts to the diagnostic image.

Reflective Layer

The base material is not transparent to light. In fact, a special layer of reflective material, such as magnesium oxide or titanium dioxide, about 25 μm thick, is used to reflect light toward the film. When a phosphor is struck by an x-ray photon, it will emit light isotropically (in all directions) (Figure 22–2A). When a reflective layer is added (Figure 22–2B) nearly twice as much light is reflected toward the film. This increase in light striking the film assists in creating the latent image and decreases the radiation dose to the patient.

Light that is emitted at a large angle from the direction of the incident x-ray photon will have a slightly longer wavelength. Some intensifying screens use dyes in

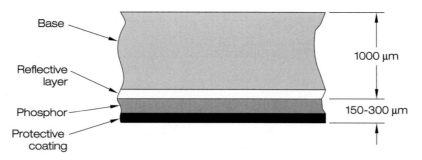

FIGURE 22-1. Cross-sectional view of a typical radiographic intensifying screen.

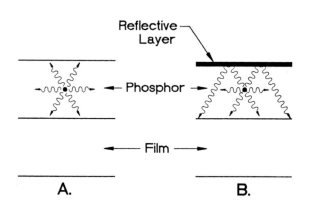

FIGURE 22-2. Intensifying screen reflective layer redirection of isotropic light emission to film.

the reflective layer to selectively absorb this longer-wave-length light. This assists in reducing the scattering of light that would decrease the resolving ability of the screen. Scattered light of this type causes a large area of penumbra, which reduces the sharpness of the image.

Phosphor Layer

The active layer of the intensifying screen is the **phosphor** layer. Phosphors are materials that are capable of absorbing the energy of an incident x-ray photon and then emitting light photons. Röntgen discovered x-rays when he observed the luminescence of the phosphor barium platinocyanide from a piece of cardboard in his laboratory. This phosphor layer varies from 150–300 μm, depending on the speed and resolving power of the screen.

Protective Coat

A coating of protective plastic about 25 μm thick is applied on top of the phosphor layer. The coating protects the phosphor layer from abrasions and stains during the loading and unloading of films. Fingernails and jewelry are the prime trauma to screens in the darkroom. Although the protective coating will prevent scratching of the phosphor layer during normal handling, repeated trauma can remove the coating. When intensifying

screens are scratched, phosphor crystals may be removed, creating unexposed white line artifacts on the radiographic image.

Phosphors

Phosphors must have a high **atomic number**, high **conversion efficiency**, **appropriate spectral emission** and **minimal phosphorescence**.

Atomic Number

A high **atomic number** is desirable to increase the probability of an incident x-ray photon interaction. Because x-ray photons are of high energy, a high atomic number is required to permit photoelectric and Compton interactions.

Conversion Efficiency

The ability of the phosphor to emit as much light per x-ray photon interaction as possible is a measurement of the screen speed. As this **conversion efficiency** increases, the radiation dose to the patient decreases. A typical conversion efficiency would produce 1×10^3 light photons per incident 50 keV x-ray photon for a rare-earth screen.

Spectral Emission

The **spectral emission** is an indication of the precise wavelength of light emitted by the phosphor. It is important that the spectral emission match the sensitivity of the film to ensure maximum latent image formation.

Luminescence

Luminescence is the ability of a material to emit light in response to excitation (usually by increased outer-electron-shell energy levels). Because of the narrow energy band within which these interactions occur, luminescent materials emit light with wavelengths that are characteristic of the particular luminescent material. This results in light emissions of a characteristic color. **Fluorescence and phosphorescence are the two types of luminescence.** Fluorescence occurs when the light is emitted within the time it takes an electron to complete one orbit of the affected shell electrons (within one nanosecond). Phosphorescence occurs when the light is emitted for a period longer than that necessary for one orbit of the affected shell electrons. In other words, **fluorescence is instantaneous emission while phosphorescence is delayed emission**, sometimes considerably delayed. Phosphorescence occurs when the phosphor continues to emit light after the incident x-ray photon energy has dissipated. Maximum fluorescence and minimal phosphorescence are desirable because delayed emission of light may permit the film to be removed from the cassette before the maximum latent image formation has occurred. Additionally, if another film is loaded into the cassette it may be faintly exposed to a previous image.

Delayed phosphorescent emission is called **screen lag or afterglow** and is common in older intensifying screens with exhausted phosphors. The normal life of intensifying screen phosphors is five to seven years. All intensifying screens must be replaced routinely. As screens age, their phosphors decrease in activity. Because of this, it is highly recommended that all screens in a particular working area be replaced simultaneously. For example, all radiographic rooms serviced by a single darkroom should have the screens replaced at the same time. This assures the radiographer that all cassettes contain intensifying screens of approximately the same activity level.

A simple demonstration of phosphor activity is achieved by darkening an x-ray room and observing the light emitted by intensifying screen phosphors when an exposure is made. Observations of this type can be made through leaded glass and from behind leaded walls. The light emissions can be varied by using screens of different phosphors, different ages and exposures of different mAs and kVp levels. Roughly 50,000 photons per mm^2 must exit the object being examined to produce a radiographic image. The intensifying screens must produce enough light from these photons to create the latent image in the film emulsion.

Several phosphors have been used in radiography since Röntgen's discovery: zinc sulfide, barium lead sulfate, calcium tungstate ($CaWO_4$) and a family of hybrid rare earths including gadolinium, lanthanum and yttrium. Calcium tungstate was used by Edison and it predominated as the best phosphor until the late 1970s, when the rare earths were introduced. Rare earths now predominate.

Rare Earths

Rare earths have become popular as phosphor materials because they have greater absorption abilities, intensification factors and conversion efficiency. Calcium tungstate screens have an x-ray-to-light conversion efficiency of about five percent, as compared to rare-earth conversion efficiencies of 15–20 percent. The rare-earth screens use phosphors with atomic numbers of 57–71. These elements are known as rare earths because they are difficult to isolate, although more common than cobalt in nature. Currently, gadolinium and lanthanum are being used in compounds with activators and other chemicals (Table 22–1). The primary reason rare-earth phosphors have gained widespread acceptance is because they offer increased speed while maintaining resolution, when compared to similar speed calcium tungstate screens. Their cost is greater but radiographers are increasingly choosing the expense over the patient dose required when using calcium tungstate screens. Phosphor technology has outstripped advancements in other radiographic equipment. Some rare earths are so fast tubes have insufficient time to produce enough mAs to prevent quantum mottle, automatic exposure control minimum reaction times are too long to avoid erratic densities, and reciprocating grids are not fast enough to prevent grid lines from being imaged. These factors must be considered when using extremely fast rare-earth screens (film/screen combinations above RS 500).

TABLE 22–1. Rare-earth Intensifying Screen Phosphors with Manufacturer and Trade Name

Rare Earth	Primary Emission Color	Manufacturer	Trade Name
gadolinium oxysulfide	green	Kodak	Lanex
gadolinium oxysulfide	green	3M	Trimax
gadolinium oxysulfide	green	Fuji	
lanthanum oxybromide	blue	Agfa-Matrix	
lanthanum oxybromide	blue	Du Pont	Quanta III
lanthanum oxybromide	blue	Ilford	Rapide

Characteristics

Intensifying screens exhibit the same types of characteristics as films. Consideration must be given to screen **resolution, speed, contrast and latitude**.

Resolution

Resolution is the ability to accurately image an object. Intensifying-screen resolution is controlled by the size of the phosphor crystals, the thickness of the layer and the concentration of the crystals, exactly as silver halide size and distribution affect film resolution (Figure 22–3). Smaller crystals and a thinner layer increase resolution but decrease screen speed. Larger crystals and a thicker layer decrease resolution but increase screen speed (Figure 22–4). **Phosphor crystal size and layer thickness are both inversely related to resolution and directly related to screen speed.** A greater concentration of crystals will increase both resolution and screen speed. Phosphor concentration is directly related to resolution and screen speed. Intensifying screen phosphor crystals are much larger than the silver-halide crystals in the film emulsion. In radiographic film and intensifying screen combinations **the screen resolution always predominates over the film resolution**.

Measurement The naked eye can resolve about 10–20 lp/mm. Direct exposure nonscreen radiographic film can resolve up to 100 lp/mm, detail speed screens about 15 lp/mm, par speed screens about 10 lp/mm and high speed screens about 7 lp/mm.

Film/Screen Contact One of the most common screen resolution problems is caused by poor contact between the film and the intensifying screen in the cassette (Figure 22–5). Poor film/screen contact also

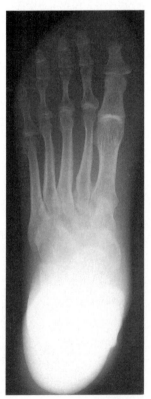

60 kVp
5 mAs
40" SID
No grid
100 RS
10.7 mR

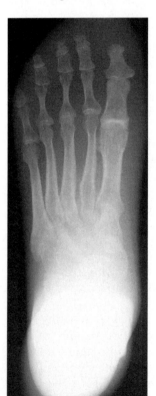

60 kVp
0.8 mAs
40" SID
No grid
600 RS
1.74 mR

FIGURE 22-3. The effect of intensifying screen resolution on image quality: (A) fine detail intensifying screens; (B) high speed intensifying screen.

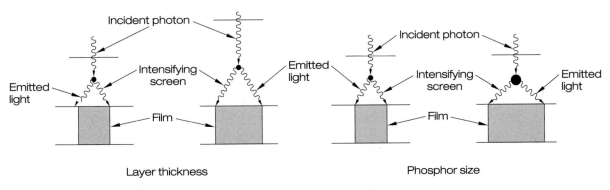

FIGURE 22-4. The effect of intensifying screen phosphor layer thickness and crystal size on film resolution.

decreases the image density. There are numerous possible causes of poor film/screen contact, including foreign objects in the cassette and warped or damaged cassettes.

Quantum Mottle

Each phosphor crystal emits light that exposes a corresponding area of silver-halide crystals in the film emulsion. When insufficient phosphor crystals emit light to expose a coherent expanse of film, the resulting image will appear grainy (Figure 22–6). Quantum mottle is caused by an insufficient quantity of photons striking the intensifying screen. Although film graininess may appear mottled, radiographic mottle is nearly always a result of intensifying screen quantum mottle. The radiographer controls the quantity of photons with the mAs setting, so an increase in this factor will eliminate quantum mottle. Fluoroscopic tubes normally operate at very low mA levels. For this reason, quantum mottle is more commonly seen in fluoroscopy.

Speed

The speed or sensitivity of the intensifying screen is determined by the same factors that control resolution. Increasing phosphor size and layer thickness increases speed. An increase in phosphor concentration also increases speed. In addition, there are factors that affect speed but not resolution. As kVp is increased, the efficiency of the intensifying screen will also increase. **An increase in kVp will cause an increase in screen speed.** Intensifying screen phosphors have relatively high atomic numbers, so higher kVp will increase the probability of light producing interactions within the phosphors. **Temperature** increases (over 100°F [38°C]) will decrease screen speed significantly. This is usually of concern only in extremely hot climates or during outdoor radiography.

Screen Speed Classifications

Three casual systems of classifying intensifying-screen speed have devel-

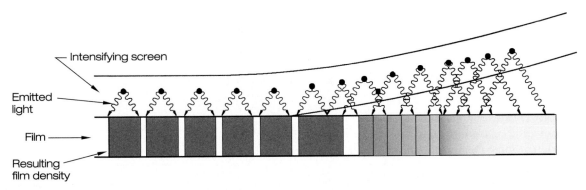

FIGURE 22-5. Poor resolution and increased image density due to loss of film/screen contact.

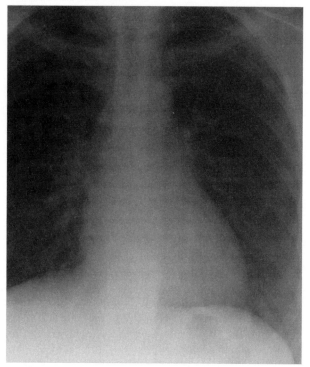

FIGURE 22-6. Quantum mottle.

oped: **the intensification factor, descriptive rating and relative-speed number.**

The most accurate factor that measures the speed or sensitivity of an intensifying screen is the **intensification factor**. It is a measurement of the amplification of the image that occurs due to the screen's ability to convert x-ray photons to light. It is directly related to the conversion efficiency of the phosphor. It is calculated as:

$$\text{intensification factor} = \frac{D_n}{D_s}$$

where: D_n = exposure in mR nonscreen
D_s = exposure in mR with screens

Most radiographic intensifying screens are also classified with a **descriptive rating** of either **high speed**, **par speed** (**also called universal or medium speed**) and **fine detail** (**high resolution**). Some manufacturers use their own descriptive terms and many of these are trademarks.

The most useful rating of intensifying screens is the **relative speed**. Relative speed is expressed with par speed

screens and film being arbitrarily assigned a relative speed (RS) number of 100 as a control point. High speed screens are usually rated RS 200–1,200 while fine detail screens are usually rated RS 20–80.

K-shell Absorption Edge

Calcium tungstate screens will absorb about 20–40 percent and rare-earth screens will absorb about 50–60 percent of the incident beam. These percentages vary depending upon the keV level of the incident photons. Nearly 100 percent of the absorption occurs through photoelectric interactions. Because photoelectric interactions produce characteristic photons, when the incident x-ray photons match the K-shell binding energy of the phosphor, there is a dramatic increase in characteristic production within the screen. This is the **K-shell absorption edge** (Figure 22–7). The K-shell edges for screen phosphors can result in a dramatic increase in light emission. This causes problems for the radiographer who uses a variable kVp technical factor system. If the kVp selected happens to be on or slightly above the K-shell edge, a slight decrease in kVp can cause a tremendous decrease in light emission, greatly reducing film density, instead of the slight decrease intended. In the reverse situation, if the original kVp happens to be slightly below the K-shell edge and a slight increase is desired, if the increase activated the K-shell peak, the resulting increase in density might be excessive. On a repeated examination, these situations could require third exposures. Table 22–2 provides the K-shell edges for the most common phosphors. **The kVp level**

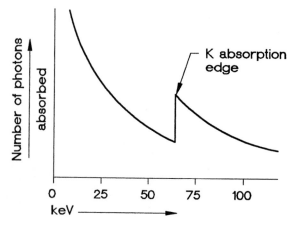

FIGURE 22-7. The K-shell edge effect for calcium tungstate phosphors.

TABLE 22–2. K-Shell Edges
for Intensifying Screen Phosphors

Phosphor	K-shell Edge	Atomic Number
lanthanum	39 keV	57
gadolinium	50 keV	64
tungsten	70 keV	74

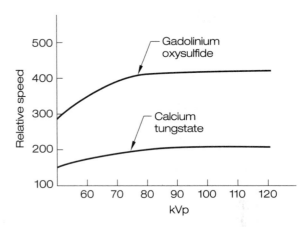

FIGURE 22-9. The approximate kVp dependence of the relative speed of calcium tungstate and gadolinium-oxysulfide intensifying screens. *(By permission of John Stears, Joel Gray, and Eugene Frank, Mayo Foundation, Rochester, MN)*

should not be varied around screen-phosphor K-shell edges. Note that the K-shell edges are stated in keV levels. About 5 to 6 percent higher kVp levels would be required to produce the maximum number of K-shell edge-level photons for single-phase generators.

The reason rare-earth phosphors are more efficient is because they take advantage of the increased absorption of x-ray photons after the K-shell edge. Figure 22–8 compares the absorption of both calcium tungstate and rare-earth phosphors. The range of increased efficiency due to the K-shell edge is highlighted. This increased efficiency range is approximately 35–70 keV (roughly equivalent to 40–75 kVp). However, there is not a linear relationship when comparing the speed of calcium-tungstate and rare-earth phosphors (Figure 22–9). Therefore it is important not to assume that one set of intensifying screens is twice or half as fast as another

across the entire kVp range. Especially at lower kVps, this relationship may not hold true.

Asymmetrical Screens Extremely efficient intensifying screens may require that they be used as matched pairs. When the conversion efficiency is very high, significantly more light is emitted by the top screen than the bottom one. To compensate for the top side of the film being overexposed and the bottom underexposed, the top screen may be thinner to equalize the light emission between the screens. These types of screens are provided with labels for top and bottom. If they are installed improperly, a significant loss of screen speed results.

Contrast and Latitude

Intensifying screen contrast and latitude are insignificant factors because most phosphors have a relatively linear conversion efficiency except for their K-shell edges. Film contrast and latitude are much more critical because of the nonlinear shape of the D log E curve. A slight improvement in screen contrast is achieved by the use of antihalation crossover dyes in the screens, but their use remains primarily with film base and emulsion. However, the effect of intensifying screens on image contrast is so slight as to be negligible.

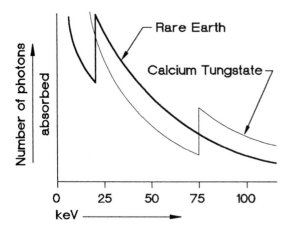

FIGURE 22-8. The increased efficiency range of rare-earth phosphors due to the K-shell edge effect.

Cassettes and Holders

Cassettes and holders are designed to create a portable, light proof case for film, to utilize the intensifying screens to best advantage and to attenuate the residual x-ray beam as much as possible (Figure 22–10). A wide variety of sizes and types of cassettes are available. Originally, direct exposure film was exposed in a cardboard holder, which is simply a light proof container. Today there are numerous specialty cassettes available, such as curved cassettes and cassettes designed for specialty equipment, such as panoramic facial units.

Characteristics

The front of the cassette must be uniformly radiolucent to eliminate artifacts, rigid to provide good support for body parts and lightweight. The intensifying screens are attached to the inside of the front and back of the cassette. At least one must be mounted on a foam pressure pad to provide good contact between the screens and the film. The back must be rigid and lightweight and may also include a sheet of lead foil to reduce the residual beam and absorb backscatter. Backscatter is a significant problem with large body parts, especially in hypersthenic chest and abdomen examinations. It is caused when the incident beam is of such magnitude that enough backscatter is produced from behind the cassette to form a second image (Figure 22–11). The lead sheet must be minimal in cassettes designed to be used with automatic exposure controls (AECs).

Extremely low-attenuation graphite carbon fiber materials are sometimes used for cassettes, grid interspaces and tables when low-energy photons may be carrying critical information. Computed tomography and angiography tables, grids and cassettes are examples. Although expensive, graphite can reduce attenuation by up to 50 percent and permits a corresponding reduction in patient dose.

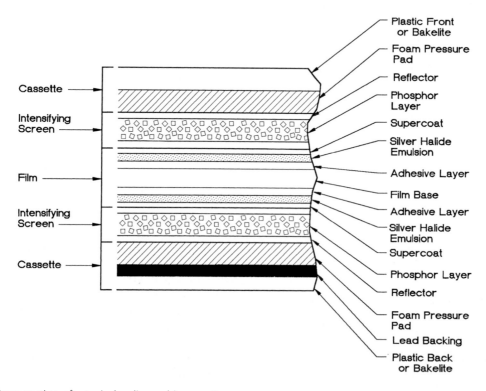

FIGURE 22-10. Cross section of a typical radiographic cassette.

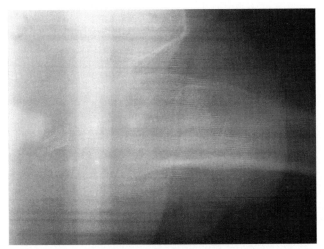

FIGURE 22-11. Backscatter forming an image of a cassette hinge. This resulted from lack of collimation, which permitted the remnant beam to strike a wall and backscatter through the back of the cassette onto the film. *(Courtesy of Eugene Frank, Mayo Foundation, Rochester, MN)*

Eastman Kodak introduced the X-Omatic™ cassette (Figure 22–12) in the 1970s. This cassette was a significant improvement in film-screen contact, beam attenuation and weight. X-Omatic™ cassettes are manufactured with a slight curve, thus causing squeegeeing of air as they are closed and eliminating the air pockets that cause poor film/screen contact. The cassettes are made of lightweight plastic with excellent radiolucent qualities. A thin sheet of lead foil in the back of the cassette is designed to eliminate residual scatter. The lead foil absorbs sufficient scatter to permit the cassette to be used backwards as a no-line grid. Specialized mammography cassettes are available with polystyrene fronts for low attenuation and thin sides to permit film edges to demonstrate chest wall tissues.

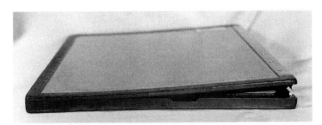

FIGURE 22-12. The Eastman Kodak X-Omatic ™ cassette.

Care

Loading and Storage

When loading cassettes, the tops should never be fully open in order to prevent dust and condensation from accumulating and to prevent the formation of the artifacts they cause on the radiograph. The cassette top should be opened slightly; 2–3 inches or 6–8 cm is enough for the experienced darkroom technician to unload and load any cassette.

Cassettes should be stored on end like a book and empty of film. Because of the frequency of cassette use, nearly all radiography departments observe the first recommendation, but not the second.

Cleaning

Intensifying screens and cassettes should be cleaned regularly. They must not be cleaned with tap water or any cleaning solution not specifically designed for intensifying screens. Most commercial firms offer an electrostatic cleaning solution that will not leave mineral stains, will not become sticky (resulting in damage when screens stick to film or to one another after cleaning) and discourages static electricity that could discharge and expose film.

The proper procedure for cleaning intensifying screens is to unload the cassette in the darkroom and then use unsterile 1" × 1" or 2" × 2" gauze sponges to apply an electrostatic cleaning solution liberally to the screen, working in strokes from side to side across the cassette. The procedure should then be repeated at right angles to the first series of strokes and followed by using dry sponges to remove excess liquid. **Never close a wet cassette** as the screens may adhere to one another, permanently damaging their surfaces. Set the damp cassettes in a clean location until they dry thoroughly (an x-ray table top is ideal). The cassettes may be reloaded in the darkroom and returned to use.

Artifacts

A loaded cassette that is stored near heat, bright sunlight, or in an ionizing radiation area may fog the film as the heat, light, or ionizing radiation activates the screen phosphor slightly. Always store cassettes away from any type of radiation.

A white spot (low density) represents an area where an artifact blocked the transmission of light between the screen and film or prohibited the ionizing radiation from activating the intensifying screen. Pitted screens or dust on the film or screen in the cassette are common causes of white spots. Cleaning the screens will often remove the artifacts.

Poor contact between the film and screens can produce lack of detail. A screen contact quality control test may be performed to verify the artifact diagnosis, but often the cassette and screens must be discarded.

Summary

Intensifying screens produce large quantities of light photons when struck by x-rays, thereby amplifying the incoming x-ray beam and reducing patient radiation dose. Over 99 percent of the latent image is formed by light from the screens, with less than one percent being contributed by x-ray photons.

An intensifying screen consists of a base, reflective layer, phosphor layer and protective coat. The base is usually made of polyester plastic and serves to hold the phosphor layer. The reflective layer is added to increase the amount of light reaching the film. The phosphor layer is the active, light emitting layer of the screen and the protective coat protects the phosphor layer from abrasions.

The phosphors used in intensifying screens must have a high atomic number, high conversion efficiency, appropriate spectral emission and minimal phosphorescence. Luminescence is the ability of a material to emit light in response to excitation. The two types of luminescence are fluorescence and phosphorescence.

A variety of phosphor materials have been used in radiography. The most popular of the phosphors are the rare earths.

Intensifying screens exhibit the same characteristics as film: resolution, speed, contrast and latitude. Resolution and speed are affected by phosphor crystal size, layer thickness and the concentration of the crystals. Contrast and latitude are relatively insignificant factors.

Cassettes and holders are designed to create a portable, light proof case for the film, to utilize the intensifying screens to best advantage and to attenuate the residual x-ray beam as much as possible. Cassettes should never be fully open when loading and unloading film. Both cassettes and intensifying screens should be cleaned regularly.

REVIEW QUESTIONS

1. How do intensifying screens reduce patient dose?

2. What are the four basic components of an intensifying screen?

3. What characteristics should an intensifying screen phosphor possess?

4. What is the difference between fluorescence and phosphorescence?

5. What is the relationship between resolution and phosphor crystal size, layer thickness and phosphor concentration?

6. What is quantum mottle?

7. What is the difference between calcium tungstate screens and rare-earth screens in terms of x-ray beam absorption?

8. What is the purpose of a cassette?

REFERENCES AND RECOMMENDED READING

A cassette problem. (1986). *Radiologic Technology. 57*(3), 247.

Ardran, G. M., Crooks, H. E., & James, V. (1969). Testing x-ray cassettes for film-intensifying screen contact. *Radiography. 35*(414), 143.

Ball, J. & Price, T. (1989). *Chesneys' radiographic imaging.* Oxford: Blackwell Scientific Publishing.

Buchanan, R. A. (1972). An improved x-ray intensifying screen. *The Institute of Electrical and Electronics Engineers Transactions on Nuclear Science. 19*, 81-86.

Burgess, A. E. & Hicken, P. (1982). Comparative performance of x-ray intensifying screens. *Radiology.* (May), 55.

Bushberg, J. T., Seibert, J. A., Leidholdt, E. M., & Boone, J. M. (1994). *The essential physics of medical imaging.* Baltimore: Williams & Wilkins.

Carroll, Q. B. (1993). *Fuchs's radiographic exposure, processing, and quality control* (5th ed.). Springfield, IL: Charles C. Thomas Publishers.

Cullinan, A. & Cullinan, J. (1994). *Producing quality radiographs* (2nd ed.). Philadelphia: J. B. Lippincott.

Curry, T. S., Dowdey, J. E., & Murry, R. C. (1990). *Christensen's introduction to the physics of diagnostic radiology* (4th ed.). Philadelphia: Lea and Febiger.

Damascelli, B., Garbagnati, F., Ceglia, E., Milella, M., Spagnoli, I., & Certo, A. (1984). Rare-Earth screens and angiography. *Applied Radiology. 13*(3), 105.

Davies, J. & Russell, J. G. B. (1986). Carbon fibre faced cassettes in neonatal radiography: Their use and cost effectiveness. *Radiography. 52*(603), 113.

DeSmet, A. A. (1981). Evaluation of a new rare-earth screen for skeletal radiography. *Radiology.* (Nov), 542.

Doi, K., Loo, L., Anderson, T. M., & Frank, P. H. (1981). Effect of crossover exposure on radiographic image quality of screen-film systems. *Radiology. 139*, 707-714.

Franji, S. M. & El-Khoury, G. Y. (1981). Applications of double-screen roentgenography. *Applied Radiology. 10*(1), 59.

Fuchs, A. W. (1956). Evolution of Roentgen film. *The American Journal of Roentgenology and Radium Therapy. 75*(1), 30-48.

Fuchs, A. W. (1947). Edison and roentgenology. *The American Journal of Roentgenology and Radium Therapy. 57*(2), 145-156.

Gray, J. E., Winkler, N. T., Stears, J. G., & Frank, E. D. (1983). *Quality control in diagnostic imaging: A quality control cookbook.* Baltimore: University Park Press.

Hiss, S. S. (1993). *Understanding radiography* (3rd ed.). Springfield, IL: Charles C. Thomas Publishers.

Hollis, K. D. (1975). Rare-earth phosphor intensifying screens. *Radiography. 41*(491), 249.

Hufton, A. P., Crosthwaite, C. M., Davies, J. M., & Robinson, L. A. (1987). Low attenuation material for table tops, cassettes, and grids: A review. *Radiography. 53*(607), 17.

Jenkins, D. (1980). *Radiographic photography and imaging processes.* Lancaster, England: MTP Press Limited.

Keefe, D. D. & De Brusk, D. (1980). A systematic approach toward rare-earth imaging. *Applied Radiology. 9*(6), 105.

Kodera, Y., Doi, K., & Chan, H. (1984). Absolute speeds of screen-film systems and their absorbed-energy constants. *Radiology. 151*, 229-236.

Lam, R. W. & Price, S. C. (1992). Pitfalls of rare earth imaging: Conquering the three Ps. *Radiologic Technology. 63*(4), 248-251.

Lauer, O. G., Mayes, J. B., & Thurston, R. P. (1990). *Evaluating radiographic quality: The variables and their effects.* Mankato, MN: The Burnell Company Publishers.

Lawrence, D. J. (1977). Kodak X-omatic and Lanex screens and Kodak films for medical radiography. *Medical Radiography and Photography. 53*(1), 2.

McKinney, W. (1988). *Radiographic processing and quality control.* Philadelphia: J. B. Lippincott.

Morgan, R. H. (1953). Roentgenoscopic screen intensification. *Radiologic Technology. 25*(2), 80.

New screen speed convention. (1986). *Radiologic Technology. 58*(1), 73.

Nickoli, P. (1993). Exposure reduction through faster speed film-screen systems and a review of ALARA. *Canadian Journal of Medical Radiation Technology. 24*(3), 99-107.

Olson, A. & High, M. (1981). Performance of automatic exposure controls when used with rare-earth intensifying screens. *Radiology.* (Aug.), 491.

Pritchard, C. & Hufton, A. (1976). The use of rare-earth intensifying screens in obstetric radiography. *Radiography. 42*(493), 14.

Riihimaki, E. J. (1982). Improvement of x-ray intensifying screen efficiency of special design of the screen. *Radiology.* (Feb.), 229.

Roberts, D. P. & Smith, N. L. (1988). *Radiographic imaging: A practical approach.* Edinburgh: Churchill Livingstone.

Sackett, M. H. (1977). Caution: Speed ahead - rare earth imaging systems. *Radiologic Technology. 48*(5), 537.

Schmidt, R. A. (1983). Evaluation of cassette performance: Physical factors affecting patient exposure and image contrast. *Radiology.* (March), 801.

Shearer, D. R. & Moore, M. M. (1986). Lag in radiographic imaging systems: Simple methods for evaluation. *Radiology. 159*(1), 259-263.

Sklensky, A. F., Buchanan, R. A., Maple, T. G., & Bailey, H. N. (1974). Quantum utilization in x-ray intensifying screens. *The Institute of Electrical and Electronics Engineers Transactions on Nuclear Science. 21*, 685-691.

Skucas, J. & Gorski, J. (1980). Application of modern intensifying screens in diagnostic radiology. *Medical Radiography and Photography. 56*(2), 25-36.

Sprawls, P. (1990). *Principles of radiography for technologists.* Rockville, MD: Aspen Publishers.

Sprawls, P. (1987). *Physical principles of medical imaging.* Rockville, MD: Aspen Publishers.

Stears, J. G., Gray, J. E., & Frank, E. D. (1987). New intensifying screens — twice the speed? *Radiologic Technology. 58*(4), 345-346.

Sturm, R. E. & Morgan, R. H. (1949). Screen intensification systems and their limitations. *The American Journal of Roentgenology and Radium Therapy. 62*(5), 617-634.

Sweeney, R. J. (1983). *Radiographic artifacts: Their cause and control.* Philadelphia: J. B. Lippincott.

Sweeney, R. J. (1977). The use of an inverted Kodak X-Omatic cassette as an improvised grid. *Radiologic Technology. 49*(3), 257-261.

Thompson, M. A., Hattaway, M. P., Hall, J. D., & Dowd, S. B. (1994). *Principles of imaging science and protection.* Philadelphia: W. B. Saunders.

Tortorici, M. (1992). *Concepts in medical radiographic imaging.* Philadelphia: W. B. Saunders.

Trout, E. D. & Kelley, J. P. (1973). The effect of the temperature of intensifying screens on radiographic exposure. *Radiologic Technology. 45*(2), 70-72.

van der Plaats, G. J. (1980). *Medical x-ray techniques in diagnostic radiology* (4th ed.). The Hague: Martinus Nijhoff Publishers.

Venema, H. W. (1979). X-ray absorption, speed, and luminescent efficiency of rare earth and other intensifying screens. *Radiology. 130*, 765-771.

Vyborny, C. J. (1980). Relative efficiencies of energy to photographic density conversions in typical screen-film systems. *Radiology.* (Aug.), 465.

Wilson, P. (1977). Principles of intensifying screens in image formation. *Canadian Journal of Radiography, Radiotherapy, and Nuclear Medicine. 8*(3), 134-140.

Wolbarst, A. B. (1993). *Physics of radiology.* Norwalk, CT: Appleton & Lange.

The Case of the Line in the Stomach

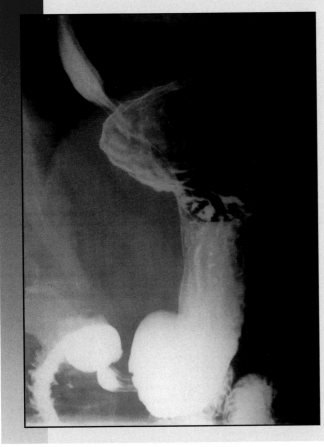

Although barium has been used to coat this stomach for the air contrast study, an odd line appears at its midpoint. What is causing the line?

Answers to the case studies can be found in Appendix E.

CHAPTER 23

Film/Screen Combinations

Mr. Edison has discovered . . . tungstate of calcium . . . [with which] you can see other people's bones with the naked eye. . . . On the revolting indecency of this there is no need to dwell. But what we seriously put before the attention of the Government is that the moment tungstate of calcium comes into anything like general use, it will call for legislative restriction of the severest kind.

Pall Mall Gazette, March 1896.

OBJECTIVES

Upon completion of this chapter, the student should be able to:

▶ Relate the emission spectra of various intensifying screens to specific types of radiographic film.

▶ Explain radiographic film/screen combination relative speed numbering systems.

▶ Calculate relative speed conversions from one film/screen combination to another.

▶ Describe various methods of measuring resolution, including a basic description of line pairs per millimeter, line spread function and modulation transfer function.

▶ Relate film/screen contrast to latitude.

▶ Determine appropriate film/screen combinations for various clinical situations.

*R*adiographic film and intensifying screens are designed to complement each other and to produce the highest quality image with the lowest patient radiation dose. Film and screens must be matched to each other to achieve diagnostic quality images. If the screens have been designed to emit a specific wavelength, then the film must be designed to have enhanced sensitivity to the same wavelength. **Mismatching of film and screens often increases patient dose.**

Emission Spectra

The spectral emissions of intensifying screen phosphors and radiographic films are shown in Figure 23 – 1. Note that blue sensitive film will not respond to most of the wavelengths emitted by the rare-earth phosphors. However, green sensitive film is more sensitive to the entire range of phosphor emissions, including the yellow-green wavelengths. Note also that green sensitive film is not quite as sensitive to the blue-violet wavelengths as the blue sensitive film. The spectral emission colors for various brands of intensifying screens are shown in Table 22–1.

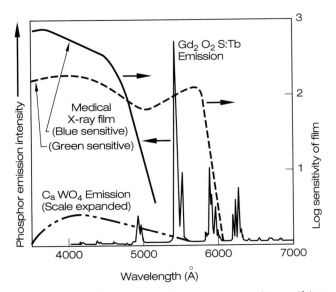

FIGURE 23-1. Light sensitivity of various films and intensifying screens. Note that blue sensitive screens are not sensitive to the major rare-earth light emissions. *(Reprinted with permission from Robert A. Buchanan, "An improved x-ray intensifying screen." IEEE Transactions on Nuclear Science © 1971 IEEE)*

The appropriate film/screen combination for a specific clinical situation must be selected based on the combined qualities of the film and the screen. Clinical selection cannot be accomplished by evaluating film and intensifying screens separately. The qualities that must be considered are **speed**, **resolution**, **contrast** and **latitude**. Film/screen combination relationships are the same as the interrelationships of these factors for film (see Tables 21–2 and 21–3). The most common decision that must be made when selecting film/screen combinations is image resolution versus patient dose.

Characteristics

The important characteristics of film/screen combinations are **speed, resolution, contrast and latitude.**

Speed

The speed of an imaging system depends on the **thickness of the layer** of phosphor or silver halide, the **crystal/phospher** size and the **efficiency** of the crystal/phospher in emitting (in the case of intensifying screens) or capturing (in the case of silver halides) photons.

Commercial firms use relative speed (RS) numbers to rate film/screen combinations. The numbers are not quantitative and represent no units. They are based on a relative value of 100 for calcium tungstate intensifying screens used with a medium contrast and latitude blue sensitive film. This was the standard film/screen combination known as par or medium speed before the advent of rare-earth screens (Table 23–1). Each manufacturer tends to calibrate film/screen combinations to its own brand of calcium tungstate medium-speed standard. However, it has been suggested that the base RS 100 be calibrated equal to 1.28 mR to produce the film speed point (OD 1.00 + base + fog). **Relative speed numbers are usually established at 70–80 kVp, with 80 kVp preferred.** When kVp values below 70 or above 100 are used, RS numbers may be less consistent. Therefore the relationship between the RS number and the sensitivity of the film/screen combination is established by the following formula:

$$\text{Sensitivity in mR} = \frac{128}{\text{RS}}$$

TABLE 23–1. Typical Radiographic Intensifying Screen Comparisons

Intensifying Screen	Typical Relative Speed When Combined With Appropriate Film	Approximate lp/mm	Minimum Receptor Activation Dose
calcium tungstate detail	50	8	2 mR
calcium tungstate par speed	100	5.5	1 mR
rare earth detail	100	8	1 mR
rare earth par speed	200	5.5	0.4 mR
rare earth high speed	400	4.5	0.2 mR

Table 23–2 shows the relationship of RS number to the sensitivity in mR to produce the film speed point.

Relative speed (RS) numbers are accurate enough to be used by radiographers to convert exposure technique settings from one situation to another. The formula for converting mAs from one relative speed to another is:

$$\frac{mAs_1}{mAs_2} = \frac{RS_2}{RS_1}$$

where: mAs_1 = old mAs
  mAs_2 = new mAs
  RS_1 = old relative speed
  RS_2 = new relative speed

TABLE 23–2. Relationship Between Relative Speed Number and Exposure Sensitivity

RS Number	Exposure Sensitivity in mR
1200	0.10
800	0.16
400	0.32
200	0.64
100	1.28
50	2.56
25	5.00
12	10.00

The most common problem is to determine a new mAs for use with a relative speed that is different from the one for which an acceptable technique is known. To determine a new mAs, the following version is used:

$$mAs_2 = \frac{RS_1 \times mAs_1}{RS_2}$$

Example: What is the proper mAs for use with a 400 RS system when technical factors of 80 kVp and 50 mAs produce an acceptable image with a 200 RS system?

Answer:

$$\frac{mAs_1}{mAs_2} = \frac{RS_2}{RS_1}$$

$$\frac{50}{mAs_2} = \frac{400}{200}$$

$$mAs_2 \times 400 = 50 \text{ mAs} \times 200$$
$$mAs_2 \times 400 = 10{,}000 \text{ mAs}$$

$$mAs_2 = \frac{10{,}000 \text{ mAs}}{400}$$

$$mAs_2 = 25 \text{ mAs}$$

Example: What is the proper mAs for use with a 250 RS system when technical factors of 80 kVp and 50 mAs produce an acceptable image with an 800 RS system?

Answer:

$$\frac{mAs_1}{mAs_2} = \frac{RS_2}{RS_1}$$

$$\frac{50}{mAs_2} = \frac{250}{800}$$

$$mAs_2 \times 250 = 50 \ mAs \times 800$$

$$mAs_2 \times 250 = 40,000 \ mAs$$

$$mAs_2 = \frac{40,000 \ mAs}{250}$$

$$mAs_2 = 160 \ mAs$$

Film/screen combinations are available from RS 20 to RS 1,200 (Table 23–3). An RS combination of 400 is the most common compromise between patient and resolution in hospital settings. Although not an absolute relationship, for the most part higher RS numbers reduce patient dose, decrease latitude and decrease resolution. Film/screen combinations to RS 1,800 have been produced but are not available due to unacceptable image quality.

Resolution

Recorded detail, sharpness and resolution are measured as **line pairs per millimeter** (**lp/mm** or cycles per mm), **line spread function (LSF)**, and **modulation transfer function (MTF).**

Line Pairs Per Millimeter
Line pairs per millimeter, or cycles per millimeter, measures the minimum size and space between objects that can be visualized on the final image.

Line Spread Function
The line spread function (LSF) measures the ability of a film/screen system to accurately measure the boundaries of an image. It is calculated by using a microdensitometer to measure the ability of the image receptor to record a line from a 10 μm wide beam of radiation. A typical film/screen system might display density from a 10 μm line over 600–800 μm.

Modulation Transfer Function
The modulation transfer function (MTF) provides the best measurement of the resolving ability of a film/screen combination. It measures the information lost between the subject and the image receptor. There are no units of MTF. The MTF is determined primarily by the amount of light diffusion that occurs between the screens and the film. The MTF is primarily controlled by the chemical composition of the screen, phosphor size, thickness of the phos-

phor layer, absorbing dye and, most important, by film/screen contact. Therefore MTF is a function of the screens because the resolving power of film is far superior to that of the intensifying screens. The intensifying screens impose the resolution limitations on the film/screen system.

The MTF is sometimes presented as a formula:

$$MTF = \frac{Recorded \ Detail \ (Resolution)}{Available \ Detail \ (Resolution)}$$

A perfect MTF would be 1.0. Therefore MTFs are less than 1.0 because more information cannot be recorded than what is available. An MTF curve plots MTF against resolution (lp/mm) (Figure 23–2). Faster film/screen combinations exhibit an obvious decrease in resolution when compared to the detail combinations.

Contrast

Contrast is primarily the contrast of the film, although intensifying screens, especially the rare earths, also exhibit contrast. The effect of higher contrast that is achieved when lower kVp can be used due to higher speed screens is often overlooked. In addition, the rare-earth phosphors often exhibit slightly higher contrast.

Latitude

The film/screen system latitude is primarily dependent upon the latitude of the film, which is directly related to the contrast. Narrow latitude film/screen systems exhibit high contrast. High speed film/speed systems tend to have lower resolution (decreased detail).

Selecting Film/Screen Combinations

The selection of appropriate film/screen combinations requires consideration of the various film and screen characteristics. For example, Figure 23–3 illustrates the differences between two types of screens and three types of film. The radiographs on the left were produced with detail screens while those on the right were produced with high speed screens. The top row of radiographs were produced with a general-purpose film, the

TABLE 23–3. Manufacturer's Relative Speed/Film Combinations

AGFA RELATIVE SPEED FILM/SCREEN COMBINATION CHART (GREEN SYSTEMS)

FILM sensitivity/speed/contrast/latitude	SCREEN				
	Curix® Ortho Fine	Curix® Ortho Medium	Curix® Ortho Regular	Curix® Ortho Fast	Curix® Optos H
Curix® Ortho HT-G green/low/high/narrow	100	250	400	700	not recommended
Curix® Ortho HT-L green/low/medium/wide	100	250	400	700	not recommended
Curix® Optos H green/low/low/wide	not recommended	not recommended	not recommended	not recommended	400

AGFA RELATIVE SPEED FILM/SCREEN COMBINATION CHART (ULTRA VIOLET (BLUE) SYSTEMS)

FILM sensitivity/speed/contrast/latitude	SCREEN		
	Curix® Ultra Detail	Curix® Ultra Rapid	Curix® Ultra Super Rapid
Curix® HC-S ultraviolet/high/high/narrow	200	400	600
Curix® HC-SL ultraviolet/high/medium/wide	200	400	600
Curix® HC-U ultraviolet/medium/low/wide	not recommended	250	350

AGFA RELATIVE SPEED FILM/SCREEN COMBINATION CHART (MAMMOGRAPHY SYSTEMS)

FILM sensitivity/speed/contrast/latitude	SCREEN	
	HD	HD S
Curix® HC-S green/high/high/narrow	100*	140*

*Internal reference only: mammography speeds are relative to HDR-C film with HD screens being defined as 100 speed.

Continued

TABLE 23–3. Manufacturer's Relative Speed/Film Combinations

STERLING RELATIVE SPEED FILM/SCREEN COMBINATION CHART (GREEN SYSTEMS)

FILM sensitivity/speed/contrast/latitude	SCREEN
	Quanta V
Cronex 8 OR Cronex Ortho TG green/low/high/narrow	400
Cronex 8L OR Cronex Ortho TL green/low/low/wide	400

STERLING RELATIVE SPEED FILM/SCREEN COMBINATION CHART (BLUE SYSTEMS)

FILM sensitivity/speed/contrast/latitude	SCREEN		
	Quanta Detail	Quanta Fast Detail	Quanta III
Cronex 7L OR Cronex 10L blue/low/low/wide	50	100	400
UltraVision UV-G OR Cronex 4 blue/low/high/narrow	100	200	800
UltraVision UV-L OR Cronex 4L blue/low/high/narrow	100	200	800
Cronex 7 OR Cronex 10T blue/high/high/narrow	200	400	not recommended

FUJI RELATIVE SPEED FILM/SCREEN COMBINATION CHART (GREEN SYSTEMS)

FILM sensitivity/speed/control/latitude	SCREEN			
	Kyokko GF-1	Kyokko GM-1	Kyokko GH-1	Kyokko GX-1
RXO-G green/low/high/narrow	100	200	400	800
HR-G green/low/high/narrow	100	200	400	800
RXO-L green/low/low/wide	100	200	400	800
HRC green/low/low/wide	100	200	400	800
HRH green/high/high/narrow	not recommended	400	800	not recommended

Continued

TABLE 23–3. Manufacturer's Relative Speed/Film Combinations

FUJI RELATIVE SPEED FILM/SCREEN COMBINATION CHART (BLUE SYSTEMS)

FILM sensitivity/speed/contrast/latitude	SCREEN	
	Kyokko Special	Kyokko Super Special
RX blue/low/high/narrow	300	500
RXL blue/low/high/narrow	300	500
RXS blue/high/low/wide	600	1000
RXG blue/high/high/narrow	600	1000

KODAK RELATIVE SPEED FILM/SCREEN COMBINATION CHART (GREEN SYSTEMS)

FILM sensitivity/speed/contrast/latitude	SCREEN			
	Lanex® Fine	Lanex® Medium	Lanex® Regular	Lanex® Fast
T-Mat G green/low/high/narrow	80	300	400	600
T-Mat L green/low/low/wide	80	300	400	600
T-Mat S green/low/high/narrow	80	300	400	600
T-Mat H green/high/high/narrow	not recommended	400	600	1000

KODAK RELATIVE SPEED FILM/SCREEN COMBINATION CHART (BLUE SYSTEMS)

FILM sensitivity/speed/contrast/latitude	SCREEN	
	X-Omatic® Fine	X-Omatic® Regular
Xktamat G blue/low/high/narrow	20	50

Continued

TABLE 23–3. Manufacturer's Relative Speed/Film Combinations

KONICA RELATIVE SPEED FILM/SCREEN COMBINATION CHART (GREEN SYSTEMS)

FILM sensitivity/speed/contrast/latitude	SCREEN			
	KF	KM	KR	KS
MG-SR green/low/high/narrow	100	300	400	600
MGH-SR green/low/high/narrow	100	300	400	600
MGL-SR green/low/low/wide	100	300	400	800
MGC-SR green/low/low/wide	not recommended	300	400	not recommended
MGV-SR green/high/high/narrow	150	400	600	800

This table illustrates only the combinations available when both film and screen are ordered from the same manufacturer. There are other manufacturers of film and intensifying screens and some manufacturers listed in this table make additional films. Film manufacturers should always be consulted prior to attempting to create a film/screen combination for clinical use to assure that current information is considered. Film and screen names change with advancements in manufacturing technologies. These charts are provided as examples based on information available at the time of publication. Film manufacturers' technical information with laboratory verification by the authors were used to establish comparable classifications in this table. The authors are aware that manufacturers and other radiologic researchers' data may differ slightly due to laboratory conditions. The authors welcome comments and modifications of this chart. Forward comments to Rick Carlton, Box 910, Arkansas State University, State University, AR 72404-0910, rcarlton@crow.astate.edu.

middle row with a wide-latitude film and the bottom row with a high-contrast film. The exposure factors were adjusted to maintain a consistent density. Variations in resolution can be seen by comparing the resolution tools from the right column with those from the left. Variations in contrast can be seen by comparing the number of steps visible on the penetrometer from the top, middle and bottom rows.

Clinical Choices

Film and intensifying screen manufacturers publish film/screen combination charts that compare all possible combinations of their films and intensifying screens. These charts often highlight the RS numbers and provide commentary on appropriate clinical uses and the

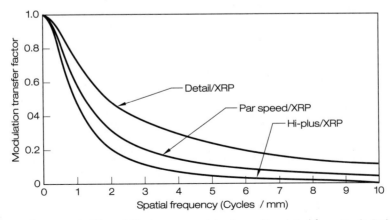

FIGURE 23-2. MTF versus lp/mm for several different film/screen combinations. *(Reprinted from Kunio Doi,* MTF's and Wiener Spectra of Radiographic Screen-Film Systems. *HHS Publication FDA 82-8187)*

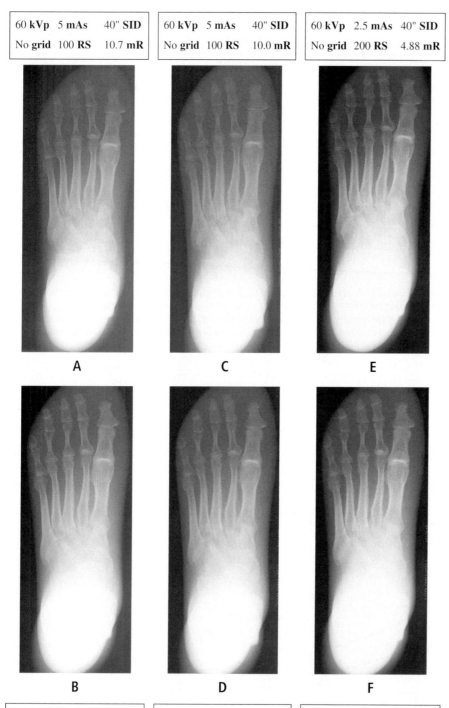

| 60 **kVp** 5 **mAs** 40" **SID** |
| No **grid** 100 **RS** 10.7 **mR** |

| 60 **kVp** 5 **mAs** 40" **SID** |
| No **grid** 100 **RS** 10.0 **mR** |

| 60 **kVp** 2.5 **mAs** 40" **SID** |
| No **grid** 200 **RS** 4.88 **mR** |

A   C   E

B   D   F

| 60 **kVp** 0.8 **mAs** 40" **SID** |
| No **grid** 600 **RS** 1.74 **mR** |

| 60 **kVp** 0.8 **mAs** 40" **SID** |
| No **grid** 600 **RS** 1.66 **mR** |

| 60 **kVp** 0.4 **mAs** 40" **SID** |
| No **grid** 1200 **RS** 0.88 **mR** |

FIGURE 23-3. Differences between two types of screens and three types of film. The radiographs on the top were produced with detail screens while those on the bottom were produced with high speed screens. Radiographs A and B were produced with a general purpose film; C and D with a wide latitude film; and E and F with a high contrast film.

image quality factors (speed, resolution, contrast and latitude).

Various types of intensifying screen phosphors are more efficient at various kVp levels (Figure 23–4). These factors must be considered when selecting combinations for various clinical situations. The primary advantages and disadvantages of rare-earth film/screen combinations are shown in Table 23–4.

The objectives of high-quality images and reduced patient dose are well within the focus of modern film/screen combination technology. However, this depends considerably on the appropriate choice of film/screen combination for specific clinical situations.

Angiography

Rare-earth film/screen combinations were immediately recognized for their value in angiographic studies. The advantage of decreased patient dose while maintaining image resolution is obvious when short exposure times are critical at the same time that numerous exposures are required, resulting in high total exposure. Because angiography produces high subject contrast between injected vessels and surrounding tissues, quantum mottle noise is less of a problem than in other studies.

TABLE 23–4. Advantages and Disadvantages of Rare-earth Film/Screen Combinations

Advantages	Disadvantages
Reduced patient dose	Increased quantum mottle noise
Reduced staff dose	Increased cost
Increased tube life	kVp influences efficiency
Use of lower power generators	
Reduced patient motion	
Reduced kVp (while maintaining contrast)	
Reduced mA (while maintaining focal spot size)	

Gastrointestinal and Urologic Radiography

Both gastrointestinal and urologic examinations are procedures in which high subject contrast permits the use of high speed rare-earth film/screen combinations.

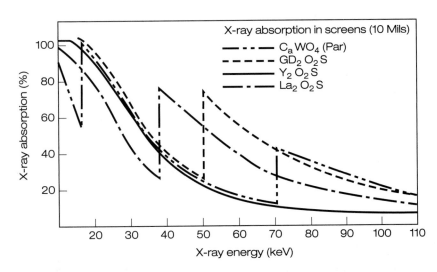

FIGURE 23-4. Absorption efficiency of various intensifying screen phosphors. Note that although rare earths are significantly more efficient between 40 and 70 keV, calcium tungstate is slightly more efficient above 70 keV. (*Reprinted with permission from A. F. Sklensky, R. A. Buchanan, T. G. Maple, and H. N. Bailey, "Quantum utilization in x-ray intensifying screens."* IEEE Transactions on Nuclear Science © *1974 IEEE*)

High subject contrast often permits higher quantum mottle noise ratios without objectionable interference with the diagnostic information of the image.

Abdominal Radiography

Faster calcium tungstate or slower rare-earth systems have been suggested for abdominal radiography because of low subject contrast, which requires reducing quantum mottle noise.

Skeletal Radiography

Skeletal examinations are usually divided into extremity examinations, in which detail film/screen combinations are very desirable due to the subtle differences that provide clues to some pathologies. Pelvic and lumbar examinations present totally different problems because of large subject thickness and the less subtle nature of regional pathologies.

Chest Radiography

High kVp chest radiography (> 100 kVp) is achieved more efficiently with calcium tungstate film/screen combinations than with rare earths.

Pediatric Radiography

Pediatric examinations are also prime candidates for higher-speed film/screen combinations because large portions of the body are often included within the primary-beam field, effects of the radiation exposure will be carried longer and motion is the primary imaging problem for the radiographer.

Summary

Radiographic film and intensifying screens are designed to complement each other and to produce the highest quality image with the lowest patient radiation dose. To accomplish this, film and screens must be matched to each other, especially with regard to their emission spectra. Mismatching of film and screens increases patient dose.

The qualities that must be considered in a film/screen combination are speed, resolution, contrast and latitude.

The most frequent decision that must be made when selecting film/screen combinations is image resolution versus patient dose.

Commercial firms use relative speed (RS) numbers to rate film/screen combinations. The formula for converting mAs from one relative speed to another is:

$$\frac{mAs_1}{mAs_2} = \frac{RS_2}{RS_1}$$

Recorded detail, sharpness and resolution are measured as line pairs per millimeter (lp/mm or cycles per mm), line spread function (LSF), and modulation transfer function (MTF). Contrast is primarily the contrast of the film, although intensifying screens, especially the rare earths, also affect contrast. The film/screen system latitude is primarily dependent upon the latitude of the film. The selection of appropriate film/screen combinations requires consideration of the various film and screen characteristics and of the clinical situation for which they are to be used.

REVIEW QUESTIONS

1. What are the emission spectra of calcium tungstate and rare-earth intensifying screens?

2. What is the formula used to calculate a relative speed conversion from one film/screen combination to another?

3. What are the three methods of measuring resolution?

4. How is film/screen contrast related to latitude?

5. What clinical situation(s) would justify the use of a detail speed film/screen combination?

6. What clinical situation(s) would justify the use of a high speed film/screen combination?

REFERENCES AND RECOMMENDED READING

Ball, J. & Price, T. (1989). *Chesneys' radiographic imaging.* Oxford: Blackwell Scientific Publishing.

Braun, M. & Wilson, B. C. (1982). Comparative evaluation of several rare-earth film-screen systems. *Radiology. 144,* 915.

Burgess, A. E. & Hicken, P. (1982). Comparative performance of x-ray intensifying screens. *Radiology.* (May), 55.

Bushberg, J. T., Seibert, J. A., Leidholdt, E. M., & Boone, J. M. (1994). *The essential physics of medical imaging.* Baltimore: Williams & Wilkins.

Bushong, S. C. (1997). *Radiologic science for technologists: Physics, biology, and protection* (6th ed.). St. Louis: C. V. Mosby.

Carroll, Q. B. (1993). *Fuchs's radiographic exposure, processing, and quality control* (5th ed.). Springfield, IL: Charles C. Thomas Publishers.

Cullinan, A. & Cullinan, J. (1994). *Producing quality radiographs* (2nd ed.). Philadelphia: J. B. Lippincott.

Curry, T. S., Dowdey, J. E., & Murry, R. C. (1990). *Christensen's introduction to the physics of diagnostic radiology* (4th ed.). Philadelphia: Lea and Febiger.

Cohen, G. (1984). Dose efficiency of screen-film systems used in pediatric radiography. *Radiology.* (July), 187.

Damascelli, B., Garbagnati, F., Ceglia, E., Milella, M., Spagnoli, I., & Certo, A. (1984). Rare-earth screens and angiography. *Applied Radiology. 13*(3), 105.

DeSmet, A. A. (1982). An evaluation of screen-film combinations for detail skeletal radiography. *Radiology. 143,* 259.

DeSmet, A. A. (1981). Evaluation of a new rare-earth screen for skeletal radiography. *Radiology.* (Nov.), 542.

Doi, K., Holje, G., Loo, L., & Chan, H. (1982). *MTF's and Wiener spectra of radiographic screen-film systems.* United States Department of Health and Human Services, Public Health Service, Food and Drug Administration, Bureau of Radiological Health: HHS Publication FDA 82-8187.

Doi, K., Loo, L., Anderson, T. M., & Frank, P. H. (1981). Effect of crossover exposure on radiographic image quality of screen-film systems. *Radiology. 139,* 707-714.

Eastman Kodak Company. (1976). *Image insight 3: Screen imaging.* Rochester, NY: Eastman Kodak Company, Publication M3-71.

Goodman, D. A., Wells, C. A., & Weston, P. J. (1977). An evaluation of some screen film combinations for use in radiography of the extremities. *Radiography. 43*(515), 253.

Gratal, P., Burns, C., & Murray, J. (1987). Advantages of a 400 speed image receptor system for cast radiography. *Radiologic Technology. 58*(5), 401.

Haus, A. G. & Cullinan, J. E. (1989). Screen film processing systems for medical radiography: A historical review. *Radiographics. 9*(6), 1203-1224.

Higashida, Y., Frank, P. H., & Doi, K. (1983). High-speed, single-screen/single-emulsion film systems: Basic imaging properties and preliminary clinical applications. *Radiology.* (Nov.), 571.

Hiss, S. S. (1993). *Understanding radiography* (3rd ed.). Springfield, IL: Charles C. Thomas Publishers.

Jenkins, D. (1980). *Radiographic photography and imaging processes.* Lancaster, England: MTP Press Limited.

Kodera, Y., Doi, K., & Chan, H. (1984). Absolute speeds of screen-film systems and their absorbed-energy constants. *Radiology. 151,* 229-236.

Lam, R. W. & Price, S. C. (1992). Pitfalls of rare earth imaging: Conquering the three Ps. *Radiologic Technology. 63*(4), 248-251.

Lawrence, D. J. (1977). Kodak X-omatic and Lanex screens and Kodak films for medical radiography. *Medical Radiography and Photography. 53*(1), 2.

Le Page, J. R. & Trefler, M. (1983). The use of high-speed film/screen combinations to improve diagnostic image quality. *Radiology. 147,* 265.

McKinney, W. (1988). *Radiographic processing and quality control.* Philadelphia: J. B. Lippincott.

New screen speed convention. (1986). *Radiologic Technology. 58*(1), 73.

Ovitt, T. W., Moore, R., & Amplatz, K. (1975). The evaluation of high-speed screen-film combinations in angiography. *Radiology. 114,* 449.

Rao, G. U. V. & Fatouros, P. P. (1978). The relationship between resolution and speed of x-ray intensifying screens. *Medical Physics. 5,* 205-208.

Rao, G. U. V., Fatouros, P. P., & James, A. E. (1978). Physical characteristics of modern radiographic screen-film systems. *Investigative Radiology. 13*, 460.

Rao, G. U. V., Witt, W., Beachley, M. C., Bosch, H. A., Fatouros, P. P., & Kan, P. T. (1981). Radiographic films and screen-film systems. *The Physical Basis of Medical Imaging.* Editors: Coulam, C. M., Erickson, J. J., Rollo, F. D., & James, A. E. New York: Appleton-Century-Crofts.

Rossi, R. P., Hendee, W. R., & Aherns, C. R. (1976). An evaluation of rare-earth screen-film combinations. *Radiology. 121*, 465.

Rucker, J. L. (1980). Rare-earth screen/film combinations and a quality-control program. *Applied Radiology. 9*(4), 57.

Sackett, M. H. (1977). Caution: Speed ahead — rare earth imaging systems. *Radiologic Technology. 48*(5), 537.

Shearer, D. R. & Moore, M. M. (1986). Lag in radiographic imaging systems: Simple methods for evaluation. *Radiology. 159*(1), 259-263.

Sprawls, P. (1990). *Principles of radiography for technologists.* Rockville, MD: Aspen Publishers.

Sprawls, P. (1987). *Physical principles of medical imaging.* Rockville, MD: Aspen Publishers.

Stears, J. G., Gray, J. E., & Frank, E. D. (1987). New intensifying screens — twice the speed? *Radiologic Technology. 58*(4), 345-346.

Stears, J. G., Gray, J. E., & Frank, E. D. (1987). Selecting the best screen-film combination. *Radiologic Technology. 58*(3), 239-242.

Taylor, K. W., McLeich, B. P., Hobbs, B. B., & Hughes, T. J. (1980). Selection of screen-film combinations. *The Canadian Journal of Medical Radiation Technology. 11*(3), 154.

Thompson, M. A., Hattaway, M. P., Hall, J. D., & Dowd, S. B. (1994). *Principles of imaging science and protection.* Philadelphia: W. B. Saunders.

Thompson, T. T. (1985). *A practical approach to modern imaging equipment* (2nd ed.). Boston: Little, Brown and Company.

Thompson, T. T. (1974). Selecting medical x-ray film. *Applied Radiology. 3*, 47-51.

Thornbury, J. R., Fryback, D. G., Patterson, F. E., & Chiavarini, R. L. (1978). Effect of screen-film combinations on diagnostic certainty: Hi-plus/RPL versus Lanex/Ortho G in excretory urography. *American Journal of Roentgenology. 130*, 83.

Tortorici, M. (1992). *Concepts in medical radiographic imaging.* Philadelphia: W. B. Saunders.

U.S. Department of Health, Education, and Welfare, Food and Drug Administration. (1976). Bureau of Radiological Health. *First Image Receptor Conference: Film/Screen Combinations.* Washington, DC: HEW Publication (FDA) 77-8003.

Venema, H. W. (1979). X-ray absorption, speed, and luminescent efficiency of rare earth and other intensifying screens. *Radiology. 130*, 765-771.

Vyborny, C. J. (1980). Relative efficiencies of energy to photographic density conversions in typical screen-film systems. *Radiology.* (Aug.), 465.

Wolbarst, A. B. (1993). *Physics of radiology.* Norwalk, CT: Appleton & Lange.

The Case of the Missing Lower Pelvis

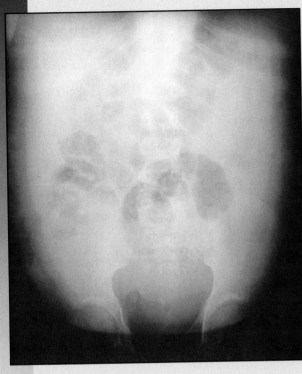

For some unexplained reason, this patient's lower hips and pelvis disappeared. Why?

Answers to the case studies can be found in Appendix E.

UNIT **IV**
Analyzing the Image

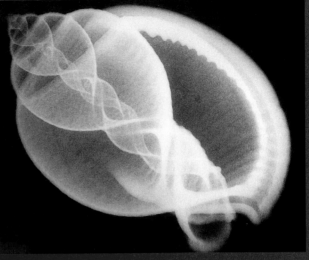

*T*he ability of the radiographer to analyze the image brings his or her professional skills to the highest levels possible. The process of analyzing demands a thorough knowledge of the scientific basis by which the image was produced as well as a significant amount of clinical experience. When these skills are applied to a problem-solving technique, the process of diagnosis results. The radiographer diagnoses the image exactly as the physician diagnoses pathology. This unit is designed to provide the analytical abilities in both diagnosis and treatment that make the radiographer an image expert.

Before attempting to diagnose the quality of the image, it is important that the radiographer understands **establishing imaging standards,** including a diagnostic problem-solving technique. Then it is important to explore each of the properties which affect radiographic quality in depth to examine their controlling and influencing factors, their effect on the appearance of the image, how to assess them, and how to make adjustment properly. Separate chapters on **density, contrast, recorded detail,** and **distortion** explore these elements. When a diagnostic process is applied to all of the properties together, an artistic skill in image evaluation results. A system that utilizes this process is presented as the **art of film critique.**

Finally, it is the responsibility of the radiographer to monitor and evaluate the performance of all radiographic equipment. This is accomplished through the process of **quality management.**

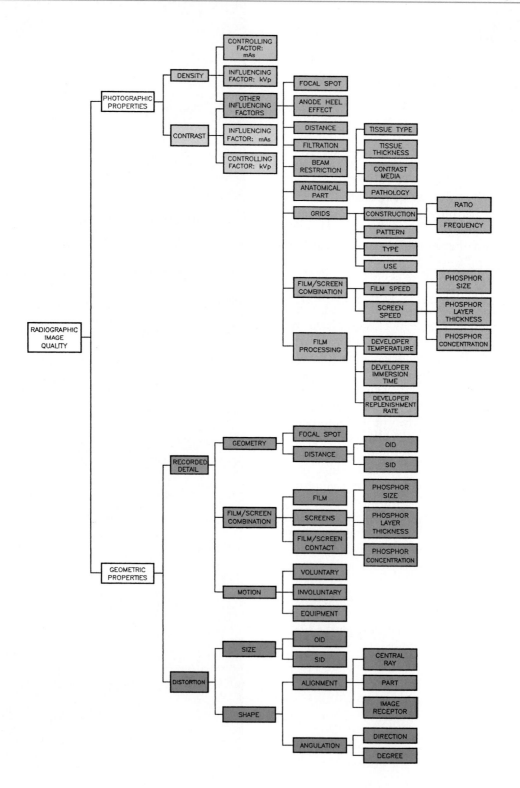

CHAPTER 24

Establishing Imaging Standards

[a] requirement of radiography when it is to be practiced as a personal art is the deliberate deviation from "average values." The practice of deviating from average values, settings, measurements, etc. is the mark of the successful professional man in almost any field, and is the principle reason for the esteem he enjoys in his community. His services are sought because he knows how and when to deviate from a standard solution of a problem.

Gerhart S. Schwarz, M.D., inventor of the XVS Unit-Step Radiography System.

Objectives

Upon completion of this chapter, the student should be able to:

▶ Describe the pyramid problem of geometrical progression as it relates to radiographic image quality.

▶ Apply the four steps of the diagnostic process to a clinical imaging problem.

▶ Explain how image acceptance limits may fluctuate due to various external factors.

Professional Imaging Standards

Just as all professionals are expected to adhere to the technical and ethical standards of their field, so radiographers are expected to establish personal imaging standards which satisfy the diagnostic needs of the radiologist and the quality needs of the supervisor. Additionally, they must not violate the personal ethical standards of radiation protection and patient care. Everyone makes mistakes, but professionals are able to correct their mistakes by using a careful analytical process to determine exactly what went wrong. In radiography, emphasis must be placed on learning how to look at images critically.

The Pyramid Problem

A major roadblock in overcoming complex problems such as establishing imaging standards is sometimes called the **pyramid problem**. An acceptable radiograph is the result of a multitude of factors, including technical factor selection, subject density, contrast, pathology and film processing. Unfortunately, some factors can act upon each other, thus creating a pyramid of problems for the radiographer. When many factors are acting upon each other, the result is an astronomical number of possibilities.

The Analytical Process

Diagnosing and Treating the Image

Anyone working in a clinical setting quickly becomes acquainted with the process of medical diagnosis. Determining the cause of a problem is a fascinating process. Most medical professionals would welcome an opportunity to participate in this process but they are restricted by law. In fact, the *Scope of Practice of the American Registry of Radiologic Technologists* states "under no circumstances (shall a radiographer) give out oral or written diagnoses." However, the diagnosis of technical problems in the imaging process requires the same skills that a physician uses in medical diagnosis.

Physicians are experts in the science of anatomy and physiology. Radiologists are physicians who are expert in the art of diagnosing through anatomical images as well. But even radiologists are not trained in the finer points of creating and analyzing the image. In this area the radiographer is the true professional expert. The diagnosis and treatment of image quality is the domain of the radiography profession and radiographers are eminently qualified to practice this art and science.

The Diagnostic Process

A knowledge of the diagnostic process is necessary for the radiographer to diagnose and treat the image. The secret to solving any pyramid problem is a careful and meticulous breakdown of the whole into individual parts. The difference between being good and being great is often only a matter of attention to detail. Taking time to break down and analyze technical problems permits proper diagnosis to occur. When properly followed, the diagnostic process makes the treatment clear. Diagnosis involves the highest level of mental acuity. It requires the use of the skills of analysis, synthesis and evaluation to solve complex problems. A diagnostic problem-solving strategy includes four major steps.

Narrowing the Search Field   The first phase involves **narrowing the search**. Experts begin with a review of the entire image to avoid premature narrowing. During this review a search is made for anything that is different from a diagnostic quality image. When differences are noticed a pattern is sought, especially when there is more than one cue. These cues focus attention on a suspicious area, thus narrowing the search. An example would be a film that looks light, gray and blurred. An inexperienced radiographer might jump to the conclusion that the image was too light and there was motion. However, an expert radiographer might notice additional cues, such as the loss of detail confined to a small region and proper film density in other areas.

Hypothesis Activation   The second phase requires that the cues be used to **seek hypotheses**. An effort is made to formulate a hypothesis that will explain all the cues. Cues that do not fit the hypothesis should be held in reserve. In the example, the inexperienced radiographer might hypothesize that too little radiation was used and that the patient was breathing. The expert would realize that many hypotheses could account for the image, including several cases of "too little radiation," such as insufficient kVp, mA or time, excessive distance and improper film, screens or processing. They would also include several explanations for a blurred image, such as poor film/screen contact, increased object-to-image receptor distance and tube motion, as well as the patient motion hypothesis.

Information Seeking   The next phase demands that the hypotheses be tested by **seeking more information**. When stumped, radiographers should use general questioning to produce more cue information. It may be necessary to shift focus to other possible solutions when new cues are discovered. In the example, the novice radiographer might ask the patient if she held her breath. When the patient answers "yes," the novice radiographer might not believe her, rather than reject the hypothesis of patient motion. The expert, on the other hand, might notice during the questioning of the patient that her breast was superimposed over the area of interest. This additional cue could be used to return to the image. A new look at the film might show that the light grayness was confined to the breast region.

Hypothesis Evaluation   The last phase of the diagnostic process is the **evaluation of the final hypothesis**.

It is critical that the hypothesis used resolves the greatest amount of cue data. At this point the radiographer should be able to predict the solution to the problem. The inexperienced radiographer would apply the "too little radiation and patient motion" hypothesis and increase the mAs while watching the patient closely. The expert radiographer would conclude that the most likely hypothesis was increased subject density, decreased subject contrast and poor film/screen contact. The expert would then ask the patient to move the breast aside and use a different cassette with good film/screen contact. Of course, the expert would produce a diagnostic quality image. The novice would be left with a darker film of even poorer quality than the first one.

Remember, however, data shows that novices often do surprisingly well when using the diagnostic process. Diagnosing ability can be improved by:

1. Remembering that cues are not a diagnosis;
2. Being careful to separate observations from inferences;
3. Not jumping to conclusions at the first cue;
4. Looking for competing hypotheses;
5. Trying each cue with each hypothesis;
6. Validating the hypothesis with questioning, when possible;
7. Ruling out hypotheses one by one;
8. Being cautious of premature closure;
9. Being tentative in the diagnosis until experienced; and, most important,
10. **Being confident in your expert knowledge.**

Acceptance Limits

Knowing how to diagnose an imaging problem is not helpful until the knowledge can be applied to radiographic quality analysis. This application involves establishing and adhering to quality imaging standards.

Graphing Acceptance Limits

The main goal must be to fix the limits of the radiographs that will be accepted against those that will not. This is much easier to understand by looking at the concept of acceptance limits graphically. The quality (in density and contrast) of all the radiographs produced by a technologist over a period have been graphed in Figure 24–1.

Although the radiographer's goal is to always produce a diagnostic quality image, suboptimal radiographs are often accepted for diagnosis. There are many reasons for this practice, the most important being the knowledge that the prime cause of increased patient radiation dose is repeated exposure. Radiologists do not expect textbook results on every patient. They do, however, have the right to expect the radiographer to provide an image that permits them to see all the structures critical to their diagnosis. Figure 24–2 shows where a typical radiologist might draw the line on dark or low and light or high films. The important thing to remember is that if the radiographer, supervisor, radiologist or other physician determines that an image is not acceptable, **it is outside the acceptance limits of quality**. When this occurs, the radiographer is obligated to analyze the image and make a proper decision on what factor or factors caused the error. The technique and procedure must then be adjusted to bring the unacceptable film back to the **perfect center** of diagnostic quality.

Striving for Perfection

Too often there is a tendency to correct only enough to obtain a passable image (Figure 24–3). **All corrections**

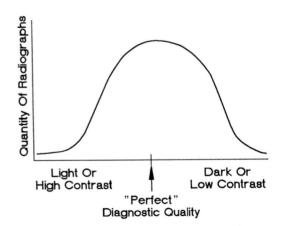

FIGURE 24-1. Radiographic image quality distribution curve. Note that the curve is skewed to the dark side. Standard practice dictates that a dark or low contrast image is always preferable to one that is too light or high contrast.

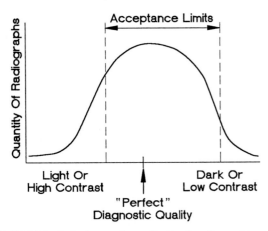

FIGURE 24-2. Typical acceptance limits of radiographic quality.

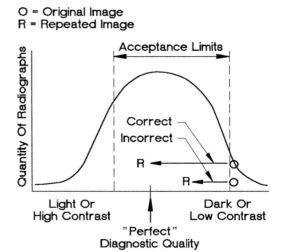

FIGURE 24-3. Correcting image quality.

should strive for perfection. Attempting to get by with minimal adjustments contributes to a negative image of the profession. The best radiographer can miscalculate and produce a poor image once, but competency is questioned when a radiographer is repeatedly unable to correct mistakes. The true professional completes the meticulous analysis by making a competent adjustment and achieves near perfection each time an exposure must be repeated.

Factors Affecting Acceptance Limit Curves

It is interesting to consider the factors that may affect the shape of the acceptance limit curve. Figure 24–1 is skewed to the dark or low contrast side because these errors are more acceptable than light or high contrast mistakes. A bright light is capable of revealing information that is obscured on a dark film. However, when a film is too light there is no method to see information that is not present in the emulsion. There are many other factors that can modify the shape of the acceptance curve. When acceptance limits are very narrow, a high repeat rate occurs (Figure 24–4). However, if the radiographers are not producing many perfect films, the repeat rate will remain high (Figure 24–5) even when acceptance limits are very wide.

An interesting phenomenon has been observed over the years in many radiology departments. When a radiograph is hovering near the acceptance limits for the department, radiographers will often attempt to have it

approved by a radiologist known to have wide acceptance limits. Departmental acceptance limits are simply a composite of the limits imposed by each radiologist, supervisor and radiographer in the department. Narrow acceptance limits may cause radiographers to produce more films near perfect center, thus changing the curve shape, as shown in Figure 24–6.

Conversely, wide limits may permit radiographers to become careless and produce fewer films near perfect center, thus changing the curve shape, as shown in Figure 24–5. Many factors can change the shape of the

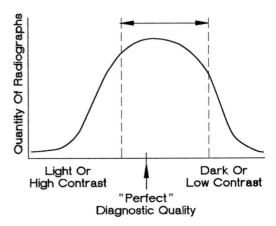

FIGURE 24-4. Narrow acceptance limits may produce a high repeat rate.

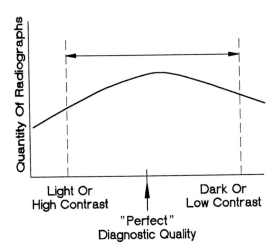

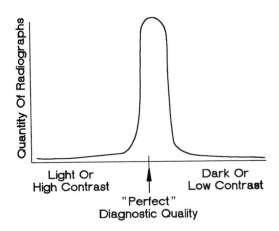

FIGURE 24-7. Ideal acceptance limits.

FIGURE 24-5. Wide acceptance limits may produce a high repeat rate by permitting radiographers to become careless and produce fewer films near perfect center.

image quality curve. Among them are the positioning and technical abilities of the radiographer, the quality standards of everyone involved in the imaging chain, the condition of the equipment, the stress level of the department and on and on. Awareness of these factors, combined with high professional standards, can help one's personal curve appear as in Figure 24–7.

Practical Considerations

In actual clinical practice the achievement of a diagnostic quality image the first time is not as hard as it might at first appear. Each factor must be varied within set limits to see a noticeable change in the image. It is important not only to learn the rules pertaining to image quality but to be sure they are used in clinical practice. The real problem is in learning **to make large enough changes to cause visible differences** on the film. Radiographers who are unsure of their ability often make timid changes that cannot be seen in the repeat radiograph. When a decision is made to repeat a procedure (and doubly expose the patient), a change large enough to bring the image to the center of diagnostic quality must be made. Shifting the image from just outside the acceptance limits to just inside them is inexcusable. As professionals, radiographers must always strive toward perfection.

Summary

Professional imaging standards can be established by overcoming the pyramid problem. Evaluating imaging problems is the true professional expertise of the radiographer. The analytical process of diagnosis is appropriate for use in solving these problems. The diagnostic process involves narrowing the search field, hypothesis activation, information seeking and hypothesis evaluation.

The concept of acceptance limits is helpful in understanding how repeated radiographs must be corrected. All repeated radiographs should strive for perfection by attempting to reach the "diagnostic quality" center of the

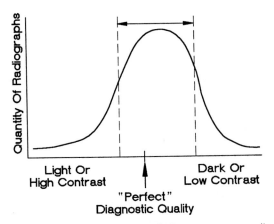

FIGURE 24-6. Narrow acceptance limits may cause radiographers to produce more films near perfect center.

acceptance limit curve. When a decision is made to repeat a procedure, a change large enough to bring the image to the center of diagnostic quality must be made.

REVIEW QUESTIONS

1. What is the pyramid problem?

2. What are the four steps in the diagnostic problem solving strategy?

3. What is the purpose of a cue in narrowing the search?

4. When is an image determined to be outside acceptance limits?

5. Why are acceptance limit curves skewed to the dark side?

REFERENCES AND RECOMMENDED READING

American Registry of Radiologic Technologists. (1987). Article I, Section D. *Rules and Regulations As Revised August 1987*. Minneapolis: American Registry of Radiologic Technologists.

Berman, L., De Lacey, G., Twomey, E., Twomey, B., Welch, T., & Eban, R. (1985). Reducing the errors in the accident department: A simple method of using radiographers. *British Journal of Radiology. 290*, 421-422.

Bowman, S. (1991). Introducing an abnormal detection system by radiographers into an accident and emergency department: An investigation into radiographers' concerns about the introduction of such a system. *Research in Radiography. I*(I), 2-20.

Carlton, R. R. (1992). Another dimension of quality assurance in radiology. *Introduction to Radiologic Technology* (3rd ed.). Editors: Gurley, L. T. & Callaway, W. J. St. Louis: C. V. Mosby, 149-166.

Carlton, R. R. & McKenna, A. (1989). Repeating radiographs: Setting imaging standards. *Postgraduate Advances in Radiologic Technology*. Berryville, VA: Forum Medicum.

Carnevali, D. L., Mitchell, P. H., Woods, N. F., & Tanner, C. A. (1984). *Diagnostic reasoning in nursing*. Philadelphia: J. B. Lippincott.

Carroll, Q. B. (1993). *Evaluating radiographs*. Springfield, IL: Charles C. Thomas Publishers.

Cheyne, N., Field-Boden, W., Wilson, I., & Hall, R. (1987). The radiographer and the front line diagnosis. *Radiography. 53*(609), 114.

Cullinan, A. & Cullinan, J. (1994). *Producing quality radiographs* (2nd ed.). Philadelphia: J. B. Lippincott.

Cullinan, J. E. (1981). A 'perfect' chest radiograph — or a compromise? *Radiologic Technology. 53*(2), 121.

Dowd, S. B. (1995). *Encyclopedia of radiographic positioning*. Philadelphia: W. B. Saunders.

Edwards, J. & Bowman, S. The expanding role of the radiographer. *Radiologic Science and Education. 1*(1), 14-20.

Goldman, L. W. (1977). Effects of film processing variability on patient dose and image quality. *Second Image Receptor Conference: Radiographic Film Processing: Proceedings of a Conference held in Washington, DC, March 31-April 2, 1977*. Rockville, MD: U.S. Department of Health, Education, and Welfare, Public Health Service, Food and Drug Administration, Bureau of Radiological Health, HEW Publication (FDA) 77-8036, 55-63.

Hendee, W. R. & Ritenour, R. (1993). *Medical imaging physics* (3rd ed.). St. Louis: C. V. Mosby.

Milne, A. (1982). When the radiographer knows but is not allowed to tell. *Radiography News*. (April).

Mumford, L. C. (1980). Radiographic quality 'a seminar'. *The Canadian Journal of Medical Radiation Technology. 11*(1), 10.

Prior, J. A., Silberstein, J. S., & Stang, J. M. (1981). *Physical diagnosis: The history and examination of the patient*. St. Louis: C. V. Mosby.

Singer, B. H. (1971). The aesthetic method in radiographic exposure. *Radiologic Technology. 42*(6), 411.

Swinburn, K. (1977). Pattern recognition for radiographers. *The Lancet*. (March 20).

CHAPTER 25

Density

Radiographic density and contrast are closely related, but by a careful study of the radiograph they may be readily differentiated and each brought under control.

Ed. C. Jerman, The Father of Radiologic Technology.

OBJECTIVES

Upon completion of this chapter, the student should be able to:

▶ Identify density as a prime component of the photographic properties controlling visibility of detail of radiographic image quality.

▶ Define density.

▶ Describe the effects of density changes on image appearance.

▶ Describe the process of evaluating image density.

▶ Explain why mA and time are the controlling factors of density.

▶ Explain how each influencing factor affects image density.

▶ Assess radiographic density on various radiographic images.

▶ Recommend appropriate adjustments to compensate for variation in the controlling and influencing factors that affect image density.

Assessing Density

*D*ensity is one of the two photographic properties that comprise visibility of detail. Visibility of detail refers to the fact that the radiographic image is visible to the human eye only because sufficient density (and contrast) exists to permit the structural details to be perceived. **The density of the radiographic image is the degree of overall blackening from the black metallic silver deposited in the emulsion** and is the easiest of the prime technical factors to evaluate and adjust. Unless otherwise specified, the term density refers to radiographic density.

The physical concept of density has been discussed in detail in previous chapters (particularly in Chapter 21, Sensitometry). In this chapter the concept of density is approached in an artistically professional manner aimed at diagnosing the image. The art of radiography is a clinical one and must be practiced as such. It is extremely important that this information be used in a clinical setting concurrently with its study.

The major consideration in assessing density is verification that proper densities are visible throughout the anatomical area of interest on the radiograph. Of course, these densities must be well within the range of human visibility (usually OD 0.25–2.50). Much of this ability to verify proper densities is a result of clinical experience (Figure 25–1). It is obvious that the proper density for lung tissue is not as great as the proper density for the thoracic spine, even though they are both thoracic structures. Common sense and a trained professional eye are the primary tools of the radiographer when evaluating density. The ability to assess density is a result of continued conscientious evaluation of images during clinical experiences. The radiographer who becomes professionally interested in the process of diagnosing the image quickly gains and refines this ability.

Information is recorded on a radiograph that is too dark but may not exist at all on a radiograph that is too light. The dark radiograph has received too many photons and, as a result, has recorded too much information. A bright light or computerized optical scanner can eliminate the excess information and reveal details within the range of human visual ability. This is not the case with a radiograph that is too light. The light radiograph has not received the information in the first place and is not

A

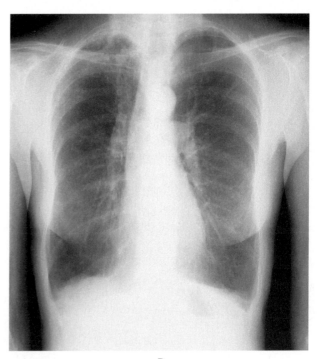

B

FIGURE 25-1. Clinical experience in assessing density: (A) Although this image is not acceptable for the clavicle, it is a diagnostic quality image of the acromio-clavicular joints, (B) Although this image is not acceptable for the thoracic spine, it is a diagnostic quality image of the chest.

capable of being manipulated to reveal details that were never recorded. Consequently, **whenever a choice must be made between excess and insufficient density, the wise decision is always the choice that will produce the darker image**.

Effects on Image Appearance

The effects of mAs and the other influencing factors on image density are not exact because of the multiple variables that are part of the imaging system. Many of the variables affect the density of the image in a nonlinear fashion under some conditions. For example, the typical D log E curve is only somewhat linear in the straight line portion. If exposure conditions push into the toe or shoulder regions of the curve, dramatic density changes can be seen. Similarly, density changes can sometimes be seen from only a slight non-linearity in the intensifying screen phosphor response curve, the film silver halide response, the thermionic emission of the x-ray tube filament, etc.

Fortunately, these variables have a statistical tendency to balance one another. But in cases where conditions cause a majority of the variables to increase or decrease exposure a total of more than 30 percent, an unexpected change in image density may become visible. Even when unexpected density changes exceed the 30 percent necessary to become visible, they seldom place the image outside the acceptance limits.

Factors Affecting Density

A wide variety of factors affect radiographic density (Figure 25–2). These factors are classified as either **controlling** or **influencing** factors. The controlling factor should be used as the principle method for adjusting for insufficient or excessive radiographic density.

Milliampere-Seconds as the Controlling Factor

While the relationship between mAs and exposure is a direct proportional one, the relationship of these two factors to density is much more complex. Density is determined by the amount of silver deposition in the emulsion due to the film type, exposure conditions, exposure (mR) and processing. A D log E sensitometric curve expresses the relationship between exposure and density, with log-relative exposure plotted on the x axis and density (D) plotted on the y axis. The relationship between exposure and density determines the shape and position of the D log E curve for a given film under specific processing conditions. This relationship is described in detail in Chapter 21. Recall that density is the $\log_{10}$ of opacity and opacity is the relationship of incident light to transmitted light. For example, if a region of a radiograph has an OD of 1.0, only 10 percent or 1/10th of the incident light is transmitted through the radiograph in this region. The opacity of the region would be 10. If the OD number is increased to 1.3, the opacity is doubled (to 20) and the percentage of light transmitted through the film is halved (to 5 percent or 1/20th). Increments of 0.3 changes in OD numbers represent a doubling or halving of opacity.

The important part of the D log E curve is that portion between the toe and the shoulder (the diagnostic range of the film). In this central straight line portion, the density is approximately proportional to the log relative exposure. This is because a straight line will always have a constant ratio. If the slope of the straight line portion is at a 45° angle, the average gradient will measure 1.0. In this example, a doubling of exposure will result in a doubling of the opacity. (Note the term doubling of density is not used because density is a log number. A change of 0.3 in density reflects a doubling or halving of opacity.) **A common misnomer in radiography is that doubling the exposure will double the density.** This is not true for a typical radiographic film/screen system.

If the exposure to a film is increased, the density to that film will increase to a point. Since density is primarily determined by the amount of exposure a film receives, and since exposure is directly proportional to mAs, **mAs is used as the primary controller of radiographic density**. As mAs increases, x-ray exposure increases proportionally and radiographic density also increases (Figure 25–3). The direct proportional relationship between mAs and exposure is used to calculate mAs changes necessary to maintain consistent image density when one or more technical factors are altered.

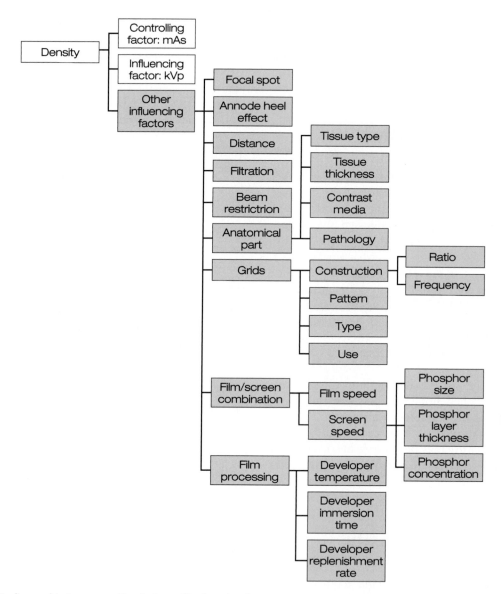

FIGURE 25-2. Radiographic image quality: factors affecting density.

By maintaining a specific exposure relative to the speed of the image receptor, consistent image density can be achieved.

When applied to x-rays, the reciprocity law can be restated to say the density on an x-ray film should remain unchanged as long as the intensity and duration of the x-ray exposure (controlled by mAs) remains unchanged. Remember that the reciprocity law fails for extremely short (less than 0.01 second) or long (more than a few seconds) exposure times. Within the range of normal radiographic exposures, it can become a factor in special situations (such as pediatric extremities or high-speed angiography).

Density should remain unchanged as long as the total exposure to the film and all other conditions remain unchanged. If the mAs used to create one image is the

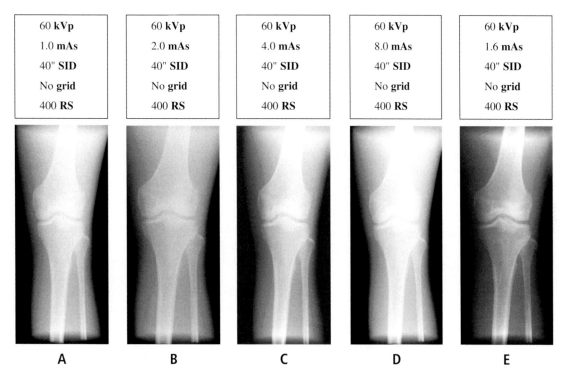

60 kVp	60 kVp	60 kVp	60 kVp	60 kVp
1.0 mAs	2.0 mAs	4.0 mAs	8.0 mAs	1.6 mAs
40" SID	40" SID	40" SID	40" SID	40" SID
No grid	No grid	No grid	No grid	No grid
400 RS	400 RS	400 RS	400 RS	400 RS
A	B	C	D	E

FIGURE 25-3. The effects of mAs change on exposure. Images A-D demonstrate the effect of increasing mAs. Each image is double the mAs of the previous one. Image E represents a 20 percent decrease in mAs from image B.

same as the mAs used to create a second image of the same structure, then both images should have the same radiographic density. As long as mAs is constant, any combination of mA and exposure time values will create the same density. This was demonstrated previously by the radiographs in Figure 11–1. Of course, accurate results depend on using equipment that is properly calibrated and maintained through an effective quality control program.

The control of radiographic density in most instances rests with the radiographer. An appropriate mAs setting may be selected from a technique chart developed for the particular x-ray unit in use. An automatic exposure system will control the time but the mA and the exact density setting will be decided by the radiographer. Computerized exposure systems will provide a suggested technique setting which can then be modified. Other variables, such as generator phase or falling loads, may also affect the final decision. The experienced radiographer will adapt the suggested mAs setting for the indi-

vidual patient. Experience and study of various body habitus, pathologies, positioning and equipment quickly provide the radiographer with clinical knowledge that can be used for these adjustments.

The minimum change necessary to cause a visible shift in density is 30 percent of mAs, or any other influencing factors that would equal this change. Various authors over the years have set the minimum for a visible density change at values between 25 and 35 percent of mAs. Although studies of vision have demonstrated that some people can detect changes in density as small as one percent, this level of perception is not possible when viewing a complex clinical image with many widely separated densities. Some trained professionals, such as radiologists and radiographers, can perceive as small a change as 10 percent on a radiograph but this is extraordinary. In clinical practice a change as small as 30 percent is seldom justified. A comparison between Figures 25–3B and E illustrate a 20 percent change in mAs. This change is difficult to see and would not compensate for improper density.

A radiograph must be outside the acceptance limits to require repeating the exposure. All acceptance limits permit some degree of variation — at least 30 percent too light or too dark. In these instances the radiograph would have to be significantly more than 30 percent darker or lighter than a diagnostic quality image.

The general rule of thumb for mAs changes is to make adjustments in increments of doubles or halves. For example, a repeated film that is too light at 10 mAs should be repeated at 20, 40 or 80 mAs, depending on the circumstances. Of course, determining which circumstances require 20 mAs, which require 40 mAs, and which require 80 mAs is something that is acquired only through experience and further study. Figures 25–3 illustrate the doubling and halving rule.

Regardless of variations in equipment output, anatomy, physiology or pathology, the idea is to adjust the intensity to permit the same amount of radiation to reach the film, thus creating the same density. From this perspective, the art of radiography does not look especially difficult. However, many other factors are yet to be added to the simple task of determining appropriate density.

One clinical practice that should be avoided is attempting to adjust density by increasing or decreasing "a step in time." Due to wide variation in x-ray unit controls, "a step in time" may be a 10 percent change on one unit but a 20 percent or even 30 percent change on another. In fact, time stations are often not linear on the same unit. This makes the "step in time" rule dangerous because of its inconsistency. In addition, in many instances "a step in time" will not even accomplish a visible density change.

Essentially, if the radiograph does not require doubling or halving of the exposure, it seldom requires repeating. Exceptions to this rule are special studies where a fine adjustment of barely 30 percent is crucial to demonstrating a small vessel or pathological condition. The radiographer will often adjust his or her technique chart by a 30 percent margin, but will seldom subject the patient to a second exposure for such a minor change. Making exposure adjustments should be a case of taking bold action (at least doubling or halving) or taking no action at all.

Kilovoltage as an Influencing Factor

Kilovoltage alters the intensity of the beam reaching the image receptor in two ways. Kilovoltage controls the energy and, therefore, the strength of the electrons striking the target of the x-ray tube for any given mAs. More important, kilovoltage controls the average energy of the x-ray photons produced at the anode target. Therefore, a change in kilovoltage alters the intensity of the beam when the mAs and other factors remain the same. Kilovoltage also affects the production of scatter radiation. Because of this, a change in kilovoltage alters the intensity of the beam after it enters the subject (or object) but before it forms the image.

Both the quantity and quality of the x-ray beam will vary significantly with changes in kilovoltage. As a result, kVp has a tremendous impact on radiographic density. Research has been done to determine a practical formula which takes both the quantity and quality factors into account. The primary finding is that there are too many variables to be quantified into a reliable formula. A visible change in density can usually be detected with a 4–5 percent change in kVp in the lower ranges (30–50 kVp), but an 8–9 percent change is required in the middle ranges (50–90 kVp), and a 10–12 percent change in the higher ranges (90–130 kVp).

Because the radiographer must have a method of using kilovoltage to adjust and compensate for density changes, the rough guide known as the **15 percent rule** has been developed. The 15 percent rule is used as a guide to maintain the same density when kilovoltage changes, as follows:

A 15 percent increase in kilovoltage causes a doubling of exposure to the film. A 15 percent decrease in kilovoltage causes a halving of exposure to the film.

Example: A radiograph of the elbow is produced using 4 mAs at 60 kVp. What kVp would be required to halve the exposure to the film?

Answer:

60 kVp $-$ (60 kVp $\times$ 15%)
60 kVp $-$ (60 kVp $\times$ 0.15)
60 kVp $-$ (9 kVp) $=$ 51 kVp

The 15 percent rule is somewhat accurate within the range of 60 to 100 kVp. Of course, this does not include the entire diagnostic radiography range, which may run from 30 to 150 kVp. The percentage of kVp required to halve the exposure to the film is always greater as the kVp increases. This is primarily due to the increased scatter radiation produced at higher kilovoltages. However, the greatest variable in the production of scatter is the thickness of the part. Therefore, density is increased when radiographing a thick subject (Figure 25–4). Consequently, a 20 percent rule may be more accurate when radiographing a 5 cm wrist, while a 15 percent rule may be more accurate when radiographing a 20 cm abdomen. Another factor which has a mathematical effect on the 15 percent rule is the starting kVp. The percentage change for doubling or halving decreases slightly as the starting kVp increases. In actual fact, **the 15 percent rule may vary from a 15 percent rule to a 25 percent rule** within the diagnostic radiography range of kVps and the diagnostic range of radiographic film densities. The 15 percent rule is commonly applied by radiographers because it can be used without produc-

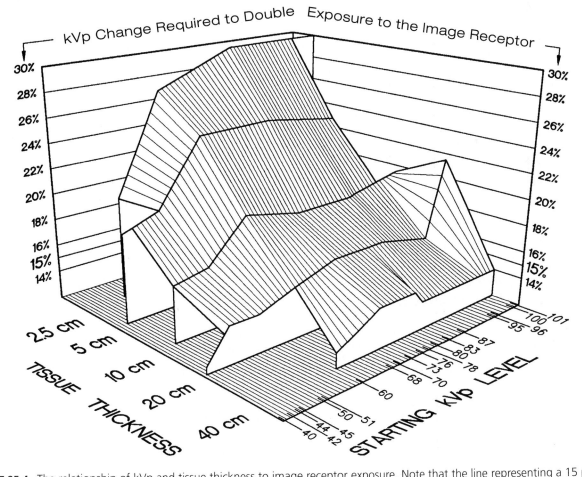

FIGURE 25-4. The relationship of kVp and tissue thickness to image receptor exposure. Note that the line representing a 15 percent increase in kVp is not within the range of some part thicknesses and kVps used in routine diagnostic radiography. It is apparent that the 15 percent rule is not a constant and must be applied with careful consideration of other factors, especially tissue thickness and starting kVp. (*Data extracted from "Kilovoltage Conversion in Radiography" The X-Ray Technician, 31: 373-379, 436, 1960 by Gerhart S. Schwartz with permission of the American Society of Radiologic Technologists. Graphics courtesy of Chris Innskeep, Lima Technical College.*)

ing images outside the acceptance limits. However, understanding the variability of the rule will do much to increase awareness of potential problems when radiographing extremely large or small objects, or with unusually low or high kVp settings. Changing kilovoltage is the primary method of changing image contrast. **Consequently, the 15 percent rule will always change the contrast of the image.** When a contrast change is desirable, the 15 percent rule is a useful method of maintaining density. However, when only a density change is desired, the 15 percent rule should not be used because it causes a contrast change as well. When density changes are desired, the method of choice is to vary the mAs because it is the controlling factor for density.

The configuration of the generator is another important consideration in how kVp affects density. The total number of higher energy photons in the x-ray tube emission spectrum is controlled by the amount of ripple in the waveform. For example, a single-phase, two-pulse (1φ2p) waveform has a significantly lower average photon energy than a three-phase, twelve-pulse (3φ12p) waveform, resulting in less density (see Chapter 7).

Compensation for the configuration of the generator is most commonly accomplished by considering only the phasing and number of pulses. Conversion factors have been developed for these compensations (Table 25–1).

TABLE 25–1. Conversion Factors Effect of Generator φ on Image Density

When Converting Generator Phase From:	To:	To Maintain Image Density, Multiply mAs by a Conversion Factor of:
1φ2p	3φ6p	0.6
1φ2p	3φ12p/high frequency	0.5
3φ6p	1φ2p	1.6
3φ6p	3φ12p/high frequency	0.8
3φ12p/high frequency	1φ2p	2.0
3φ12p/high frequency	3φ6p	1.2

Derived from DuPont Bit System, 10th edition, E.I. DuPont Nemours, Inc., Wilmington, DE.

Example: If 80 kVp and 20 mAs produce a satisfactory image on a 1φ2p unit, what mAs should be used with the same patient and examination on a 3φ12p unit?

Answer:

mAs × conversion factor
20 mAs × 0.5 = 10 mAs

Other Influencing Factors

Focal Spot Size Larger focal spots utilize a greater incident electron stream than small focal spots. Most manufacturers carefully compensate for this effect by adjusting the actual mA at the filament for dual-focus tubes. The actual mA received by the filament when set at 100 mA for a large focal spot is less than the actual mA received when set at 100 mA for a small focal spot. There should be no difference between large and small focal spots when the unit has been calibrated properly. However, this effect may differ by the 30 percent necessary to alter image density in an improperly calibrated unit.

Large focal spots tend to bloom more at higher milliamperages and may occasionally reach a point where they alter image density. Blooming occurs with large milliamperages because the incident electron beam is not as easily focused by the focusing cup. It is rare for blooming to cause a visible density difference.

Because properly calibrated units will not exhibit image density changes when focal spots are changed, differences of this type should be reported as a quality control procedure. If density differences are perceived due to focal spot blooming, replacement of the tube may be indicated.

Anode Heel Effect The anode heel effect alters the intensity of radiation, and therefore the density, between the anode and cathode ends of the x-ray tube. Depending on the angle of the anode, this effect can cause a density variation of up to 45 percent between the anode and cathode ends of the image. Image density is always greater at the cathode end. The anode heel effect is more pronounced when the collimator is open wide than when it is closed because a greater portion of the peripheral beam, and therefore a greater portion of the intensity difference, reaches the image receptor when the collimator is wide open. The anode heel effect is also more significant when using extremely small angle anodes (12° or less).

When the anode heel effect becomes apparent, it can be minimized or converted to an advantage. It is minimized by collimating the beam and eliminating as much of the intensity difference at the periphery as possible. If a given film size is required (i.e., 14 × 17") collimation may be achieved by using a greater SID.

The anode heel effect may be converted to an advantage in examinations of objects with greater subject density at one end than at another. The advantage is utilized by placing the portion of the object with the greatest subject density toward the cathode end of the tube. This utilizes the greater intensity for the greater subject density and leaves the lesser intensity of the anode end of the tube for the lesser subject density. The anode heel effect can often be used to advantage in a number of examinations (Table 25–2).

Distance (SID and OID) **Source-to-image receptor distance (SID)**, also known as focus-to-film distance (FFD), **alters the intensity of the beam reaching the image receptor, according to the inverse square law. The inverse square law affects exposure in inverse proportion to the square of the distance.** This is represented by the formula:

$$\frac{I_1}{I_2} = \frac{D_2^{\,2}}{D_1^{\,2}}$$

where: I_1 = old intensity
I_2 = new intensity
$D_1^{\,2}$ = old distance squared
$D_2^{\,2}$ = new distance squared

The law states that the intensity varies inversely with the square of the distance.

The inverse square law formula expresses the change in intensity when the distance changes. For example, as distance increases, radiation intensity and radiographic density decrease. However, the most common situation in radiography is a need to maintain an acceptable density while changing the distance. To maintain density, mAs (or an influencer) must be changed to compensate for the density change. The **density maintenance formula** is used for this purpose. This formula is based on the

TABLE 25–2. Projections That May Use the Anode Heel Effect to Advantage

Projection	Body Part To Be Placed Toward	
	Cathode End of Tube	Anode End of Tube
Femur (AP/lateral)	hip	knee
Lower leg (AP/lateral)	knee	hip
Humerus (AP/lateral)	shoulder	elbow
Forearm (AP/lateral)	elbow	wrist
Thoracic spine (AP)	abdomen	neck
Thoracic spine (lateral)	neck	abdomen
Lumbar spine (AP/lateral)	pelvis	abdomen

inverse square law but is reversed to a direct square law because mAs must increase when distance increases, and vice versa, in order to maintain density.

$$\frac{mAs_1}{mAs_2} = \frac{D_1^{\,2}}{D_2^{\,2}}$$

where: mAs_1 = original mAs
mAs_2 = new mAs
$D_1^{\,2}$ = old distance squared
$D_2^{\,2}$ = new distance squared

Example: If a satisfactory density is obtained with 20 mAs at 72", what mAs will be required to maintain the same density at 40"?

Answer:

$$\frac{mAs_1}{mAs_2} = \frac{D_1^{\,2}}{D_2^{\,2}}$$

$$\frac{20 \; mAs}{mAs_2} = \frac{72^2}{40^2}$$

$$\frac{20 \; mAs}{mAs_2} = \frac{5,184}{1,600}$$

$$mAs_2 = \frac{20 \; mAs \times 1,600}{5,184}$$

$$mAs_2 = \frac{32,000}{5,184}$$

$$mAs_2 = 6.2 \; mAs$$

It is more useful when algebraically changed to solve for the new mAs, which is the most common factor that must be calculated in clinical practice:

$$mAs_2 = \frac{mAs_1 \times D_2^2}{D_1^2}$$

Example: If a satisfactory PA chest radiograph is made at 72" with 4 mAs, what mAs will be required at 56"?

Answer:

$$mAs_2 = \frac{mAs_1 \times D_2^2}{D_1^2}$$

$$mAs_2 = \frac{4 \ mAs \times 56^2}{72^2}$$

$$mAs_2 = \frac{4 \ mAs \times 3,136}{5,184}$$

$$mAs_2 = \frac{12,544}{5,184}$$

$$mAs_2 = 2.5 \ mAs$$

The density maintenance formula is only accurate within a moderate acceptance range. **The nonlinearity of some components in the imaging system (such as developer activity, intensifying screen phosphor emission and film silver halide response) makes it impossible to exactly quantify the relationship between radiation beam intensity and density.**

Table 25–3 illustrates the mAs change factors for the most common distances employed in radiography. The vast majority of diagnostic radiography today is done at 40" to 72". In addition 56", which is halfway between 40" and 72", is useful in mobile radiography when circumstances do not permit either of the two preferred distances. A useful rule of thumb for doubling and halving distances can be derived from this table by considering the 30 percent range necessary to produce a visible density difference in the image:

Use only the distances 40", 56" and 72". When increasing distance, double the mAs for each change. When decreasing distance, halve the mAs for each change. For example, halve the mAs when changing from 72" to 56" and

TABLE 25–3. mAs Change Factors For Approximate Density Maintenance When Distance Changes

To calculate the new mAs, multiply the old mAs by the factor in the corresponding to the distance change.

	New Distance				
Old Distance	36" 90 cm	40" 100 cm	48" 120 cm	56" 140 cm	72" 180 cm
36" (90 cm)	—	1.23	1.77	2.42	4.00
40" (100 cm)	0.81	—	1.44	1.96	3.24
48" (120 cm)	0.59	0.69	—	1.36	2.25
56" (140 cm)	0.41	0.51	0.73	—	1.65
72" (180 cm)	0.25	0.31	0.44	0.60	—

halve it again when changing from 56" to 40".

Distance doubling and halving will bring density within roughly 50 percent of the original density and usually within image acceptance limits. This is only a rough rule of thumb for clinical practice. The exact conversion factors will produce much better mAs estimates.

Object-to-image receptor distance (OID), also known as object-to-film distance (OFD), has an effect on image density. The air-gap technique uses an increased OID to prevent scatter radiation from reaching the image receptor. This scatter radiation would normally cause a visible decrease in density when radiographing large patients. In most instances, OID variations are insufficient to cause visible density changes.

Filtration
Filtration and its ability to alter beam intensity affect density. All types of filtration—inherent, added and total—alter density. Density decreases when filtration is increased.

X-ray units are calibrated with inherent, added and total filtration in place. When added filtration is changed, which is rare, a half-value layer calculation should be made to permit adjustment of mAs or other factors to maintain density. When compensating filtration is used, density must be established for both filtered and unfiltered regions. As with any other density problem, this is a matter of measurement of part size and clinical experience.

Beam Restriction

Restricting the beam, collimating, or reducing the primary beam field size reduces the total number of photons available. This reduces the amount of scatter radiation and therefore reduces the overall density of the image.

Scatter production is dramatically increased with large anatomical part size and high starting kVp levels (Figure 25–4). Therefore, these two factors also determine when compensation must occur for beam restriction. However, the effect of beam restriction on density depends on how much scatter reaches the image receptor, not how much scatter is produced. Some of the scatter that is produced, especially in very large patients or when using high ratio grids, may not reach the image receptor and therefore will not affect the density. For example, a high efficiency grid may be capable of removing as much as 95 percent of the scatter, leaving very little to affect image density.

Technical factor compensation for changes in density is required only under the following circumstances:

- **large anatomical part**
- **high kilovoltage**
- **low grid efficiency**
- **nongrid examinations**

Figure 25–5 demonstrates that only extremely small beam restrictions (4"×4" or smaller) when used with no grid or a low efficiency grid require mAs compensation to maintain image density. **The compensation necessary in mAs for the effect of beam restriction on image density is less than 30 percent (a visible density difference) for nearly all images produced with grids at 8"×10" or larger beam sizes** (Figure 25–6).

Anatomical Part

Because the patient is the prime attenuator of the beam, the anatomical part being examined has a great deal of influence on the density on the film. The amount of attenuation is dependent on the thickness and type of the tissue being radiographed. The tissue type is affected by the average atomic number and the density (quantity of matter per unit volume) of the tissue. The use of contrast media will alter the average

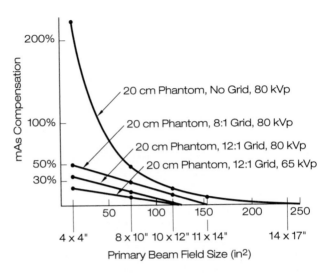

FIGURE 25-5. The effect of beam restriction on mAs compensation required to maintain image density. (Courtesy of Charles Burns, University of North Carolina, Chapel Hill, NC)

atomic number of the tissue and can affect density. Pathology can alter tissue thickness and/or type.

There is an inverse relationship between tissue thickness/type and radiographic density. In other words, as tissue thickness, average atomic number of the tissue, and/or tissue density increases, radiographic density decreases. **This is not a linear relationship** because of the multitude of variations in tissue composition. Depending on the type of contrast media or the type of pathology, an inverse or a direct relationship may exist.

Adjustments for changes in the anatomical part depend on the radiographer's ability to assess the tissue thickness and tissue type while also considering the pathology and the use of contrast media. This ability is achieved only through clinical experience. Technique charts are designed to compensate for most changes in tissue thickness and type. Radiolucent contrast media (such as air) will increase radiographic density, while radiopaque contrast media (such as barium and iodine) will decrease radiographic density. Pathology can have either an additive or a destructive effect. Additive conditions decrease density while destructive conditions increase density.

A special problem related to part thickness occurs whenever severe tube angles (more than 15°) are used. The geometry of a severe tube angle causes a significant

85 kVp	1.0 mAs	40" **SID**
12:1 **grid**	400 **RS**	29.8 mR

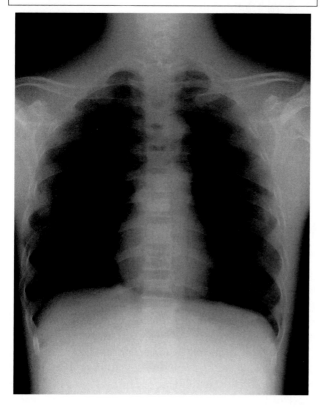

85 kVp	1.0 mAs	40" **SID**
12:1 **grid**	400 **RS**	31.6 mR

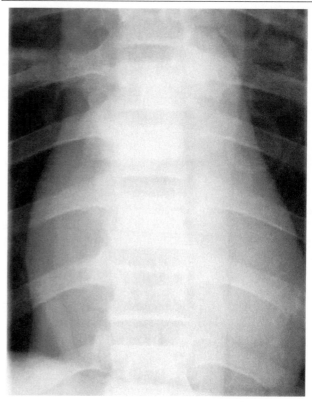

FIGURE 25-6. The effect of beam restriction on density. Although both radiographs were produced at the same technical factors, A was collimated to 14″ x 17″ while B was collimated to 4″ x 8″.

difference in tissue thickness between the edges of the image (Figure 25–7). Measurement of body parts for angles must occur at the central ray to average these differences. However, in some instances more than a 30 percent exposure difference may occur between the central ray and both ends of the image (more than a 60 percent difference between the ends of the image). Careful consideration of technical factors and use of the anode heel effect, when possible, may prevent some of these problems.

Casting materials present during orthopedic radiography affect the thickness of the anatomical part. Casting materials differ somewhat in composition but they attenuate the beam in a manner very similar to normal tissue attenuation. **Adjustments for cast materials should be made for the increased thickness of the body part exactly as if an uncasted part of the same size were being radiographed.** No adjustment should be made for the casting material itself.

Grids Grids absorb scatter which would otherwise add density to the film. The more efficient the grid, the less the density. Grids with high ratios, low frequency and dense interspace material; moving grids and improperly used grids (incorrect focal distance, etc.) all reduce density.

Compensation for varying grid ratios is generally accomplished by increasing mAs. The amount of mAs needed can be calculated using the grid conversion factors (see Table 18–2). Changes between grids, which is

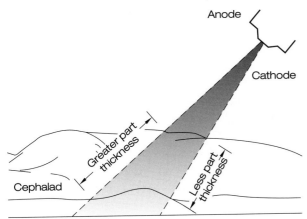

AP Sigmoid colon

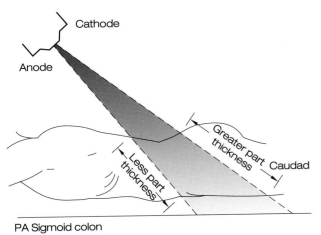

PA Sigmoid colon

FIGURE 25-7. The effect of severe tube angle on density. Note the changes in part thickness from the superior to inferior edges of the primary beam field.

the most common clinical problem, are accomplished by using the following formula:

$$\frac{mAs_1}{mAs_2} = \frac{GCF_1}{GCF_2}$$

where: mAs_1 = original mAs
mAs_2 = new mAs
GCF_1 = original grid conversion factor
GCF_2 = new grid conversion factor

Because the primary purpose of a grid is the improvement of contrast, compensating for density changes by varying the kVp is not recommended because it may change the contrast in the opposite direction, thus negating the reason for using the grid in the first place.

Film/Screen Combination

Both film and intensifying screens alter density. When the intensifying screen phosphors convert x-ray photons to the light photons that will expose the silver halides in the film, they attenuate the intensity of the light that has become the imaging beam. When the silver halide crystals in the film emulsion form latent image centers, they establish the physical foundation for the black metallic silver that is the definition of density. Relative speed (RS) numbers are the most useful parameters for intensifying screen combinations.

Relative speed (RS) numbers have been developed by manufacturers to permit easy adjustment of technical factors when changing film/screen combinations (see Chapter 23). As relative speed increases, the amount of exposure required to maintain the same density decreases. Compensations for changes in relative speed can be made by adjusting mAs because exposure is directly proportional to mAs. Density can be maintained by using the following formula:

$$\frac{mAs_1}{mAs_2} = \frac{RS_2}{RS_1}$$

where: mAs_1 = old mAs
mAs_2 = new mAs
RS_1 = old relative speed
RS_2 = new relative speed

Of course, the relative speed conversion formula may also be algebraically expressed as:

$$mAs_2 = \frac{RS_1 \times mAs_1}{RS_2}$$

Example: What is the proper mAs for use with an 80 RS system when technical factors of 55 kVp and 5 mAs produce an acceptable image with a 200 RS system?

Answer:

$$\frac{mAs_1}{mAs_2} = \frac{RS_2}{RS_1}$$

$$\frac{5}{mAs_2} = \frac{80}{200}$$

$$mAs_2 \times 80 = 5 \ mAs \times 200$$

$$mAs_2 \times 80 = 1,000 \ mAs$$

$$mAs_2 = \frac{1,000 \ mAs}{80}$$

$$mAs_2 = 12.5 \ mAs$$

Film Processing The condition of the film processing solutions can dramatically alter density. Establishment of density, contrast and base plus fog parameters for the film processing system is part of the quality control program. Ascertaining that film processing density, contrast and base plus fog values are within parameters can remove film processing as a density factor.

Density will increase when the developer solution temperature increases, immersion time increases or replenishment rates increase. Density will decrease when the above factors decrease, as well as when contamination decreases solution strength.

Summary

Density is one of the two photographic properties that comprise visibility of detail. Visibility of detail refers to the fact that the radiographic image is visible to the human eye only because sufficient density (and contrast) exists to permit the structural details to be perceived. The density of the radiographic image is the degree of overall blackening from the black metallic silver deposited in the emulsion.

When mAs is decreased, the resulting film density will be decreased and vice versa. The effects of mAs and the other influencing factors on density are not exact because of the multiple variables that are part of the imaging system.

A wide variety of factors affect radiographic density. These factors are classified as either controlling or influencing factors. The controlling factor is mAs and it should be used as the principle method for adjusting for insufficient or excessive radiographic density. The influencing factors include kilovoltage, focal spot size, anode heel effect, distance, filtration, beam restriction, anatom-

TABLE 25–4. Effect On Density When Factors Are Changed

+	= increases density
−	= decreases density
Ø	= negligible effect

Controlling Factor
+	Increasing milliamperage-seconds
−	Decreasing milliamperage-seconds

Influencing Factors
+	Increasing kilovoltage
−	Decreasing kilovoltage
+	Increasing number of pulses in the generator waveform
−	Decreasing number of pulses in the generator waveform
Ø	Focal spot size
Ø	Anode heel effect
−	Increasing distance
+	Decreasing distance
−	Increasing filtration
+	Decreasing filtration
−	Increasing beam restriction/collimation
+	Decreasing beam restriction/collimation
−	Increasing anatomical part thickness or tissue type
+	Decreasing anatomical part thickness or tissue type
+	Using radiolucent contrast media
−	Using radiopaque contrast media
−	Additive pathological conditions
+	Destructive pathological conditions
−	Increasing grid ratio
+	Decreasing grid ratio
+	Increasing film/screen combination relative speed
−	Decreasing film/screen combination relative speed
+	Increasing film processing developer time, temperature and/or replenishment rate
−	Decreasing film processing developer time, temperature and/or replenishment rate

ical part, grids, film/screen combination and film processing.

When the controlling or any of the influencing factors are altered, some change in density will occur. However, with some of the factors, the effect is often negligible. Table 25–4 illustrates the effect on density when the various factors are changed.

REVIEW QUESTIONS

1. Define radiographic density.

2. What is the controlling factor of radiographic density and how does it affect it?

3. How are density adjustments made for changes in kilovoltage?

4. How do the inverse square law and the density maintenance formulas differ from one another?

5. How do variations in the anatomical part affect density?

6. What are the relationships to density of grid ratio, frequency, interspace material and grid use?

7. What is the relationship to density of relative speed for film/screen combinations?

8. How does film processing affect density?

REFERENCES AND RECOMMENDED READING

Bauer, R. G. (1970). High kilovoltage chest radiography with an air gap. *Radiologic Technology. 42*, 10–14.

Bierman, A. & Boldingh, W. H. (1951). The relation between tension and exposure times in radiography. *Acta Radiologica. 35*, 22–26.

Bloom, W. L., Hollenbach, J. L., & Morgan, J. A. (1965). *Medical radiographic technic* (3rd ed.). Springfield, IL: Charles C. Thomas Publishers.

Bryan, G. J. (1970). *Diagnostic radiography: A manual for radiologic technologists.* Baltimore: Williams & Wilkins.

Cahoon, J. B. (1961). Radiographic technique: Its origin, concept, practical application and evaluation of radiation dosage. *The X-Ray Technician. 32*, 354–364.

Carlton, R. R. & McKenna, A. (1989). *Repeating radiographs: Setting imaging standards, Postgraduate Advances in Radiologic Technology.* Berryville, VA: Forum Medicum.

Carroll, Q. B. (1993). *Evaluating radiographs.* Springfield, IL: Charles C. Thomas Publishers.

Carroll, Q. B. (1993). *Fuchs's radiographic exposure, processing, and quality control* (5th ed.). Springfield, IL: Charles C. Thomas Publishers.

Chow, M. F. (1988). The effect of a film's sensitivity to its speed, contrast, and latitude. *The Canadian Journal of Medical Radiation Technology. 19*(4), 147.

Clark, K. C. (1953). An introduction to high-voltage technique. *Radiography. 19*, 2–33.

Cullinan, A. & Cullinan, J. (1994). *Producing quality radiographs* (2nd ed.). Philadelphia: J.B. Lippincott.

Distance — technique relationship of angulated projections. (1980). *Radiologic Technology. 52*(3), 301.

DuPont Company Photosystems & Electronic Products Department. *Positioning and Exposure Guide for General Radiography.* Wilmington, DE: Publication R–53806–1.

Eastman Kodak Company. (1980). Health sciences markets division. *The Fundamentals of Radiography* (12th ed.). Rochester, NY: Kodak Publication M1–18.

Eastman, T. R. (1975). Technique charts: The key to radiographic quality. *Radiologic Technology. 46*, 365–368.

Eastman, T. R. (1973). Measurement: The key to exposure with manual techniques. *Radiologic Technology. 45*, 75–78.

Eastman, T. R. (1969). Chest technique through body habitus. *Radiologic Technology. 41*, 80–84.

Eastman, T. R. *The radiographic technique guide.* Wilmington, DE: DuPont deNemours, Inc. Photo Products Department Publication A–99101.

Epp, E. R., Weiss, H., & Laughlin, J. S. (1961). Measurement of bone marrow and gonadal dose from the chest x-ray examination as a function of field size, field alignment, tube kilovoltage and added filtration. *British Journal of Radiology. 34*, 85–100.

Files, G. W. (1952). *Medical radiographic technique.* Springfield, IL: Charles C. Thomas Publishers.

Files, G. W. (1935). Maximum tissue differentiation. *The X-Ray Technician. 7*, 17–24+.

Fuchs, A. W. (1958). *Principles of radiographic exposure and processing.* Springfield, Illinois: Charles C. Thomas Publishers.

Fuchs, A. W. (1950). The rationale of radiographic exposure. *The X-Ray Technician. 22*, 62–68, 76.

Fuchs, A. W. (1949). Control of radiographic density. *The X-Ray Technician. 20*, 271–273, 291.

Fuchs, A. W. (1948). Relationship of tissue thickness to kilovoltage. *The X-Ray Technician. 19*, 287–293.

Fuchs, A. W. (1947). The anode 'heel' effect in radiography. *Radiologic Technology. 18*(4), 158.

Fuchs, A. W. (1940). Balance in the radiographic image. *The X-Ray Technician. 12*(3), 81–84, 118.

Funke, T. (1966). Pegged kilovoltage technic. *Radiologic Technology. 37*, 202–213.

Geiger, J. (1960). The heel effect. *Radiologic Technology. 32*(1), 55.

General Electric Company Medical Systems Department. *How to Prepare an X-ray Technic Chart.* Milwaukee: Publication 4301A.

Gratale, P., Wright, D. L., & Daughtry, L. (1990). Using the anode heel effect for extremity radiography. *Radiologic Technology. 61*(3), 195–198.

Gratale, P., Turner, G. W., & Burns, C. B. (1986). Using the same exposure factors for wet and dry casts. *Radiologic Technology. 57*(4), 325-328.

Hiss, S. S. (1993). *Understanding radiography* (3rd ed.). Springfield, IL: Charles C. Thomas Publishers.

Jenkins, D. (1980). *Radiographic photography and imaging processes.* Lancaster, England: MTP Press Limited.

Jerman, E. C. (1928). *Modern x-ray technic.* St. Paul: Bruce Publishing.

Kebart, R. C. & James, C. D. (1991). Benefits of increasing focal film distance. *Radiologic Technology. 62*(6), 434–441.

Lauer, O. G., Mayes, J. B., & Thurston, R. P. (1990). *Evaluating radiographic quality: The variables and their effects.* Mankato, MN: The Burnell Company Publishers.

Mattsson, O. (1955). Practical photographic problems in radiography. *Acta Radiologica. Supplementum 120.* 1–206.

Morgan, J. A. (1977). *The art and science of medical radiography* (5th ed.). St. Louis: Catholic Hospital Association.

Schwarz, G. S. (1961). *Unit-step radiography.* Springfield, IL: Charles C. Thomas Publishers.

Schwarz, G. S. (1960). Kilovoltage conversion in radiography. *The X-Ray Technician. 31*, 373–379, 436.

Schwarz, G. S. (1959). Kilovoltage and radiographic effect. *Radiology. 73*, 749–760.

Seeman, H. E. (1968). *Physical and photographic principles of medical radiography.* New York: Wiley & Sons.

Thompson, M. A., Hattaway, M. P., Hall, J. D., & Dowd, S. B. (1994). *Principles of imaging science and protection.* Philadelphia: W. B. Saunders.

Tortorici, M. (1992). *Concepts in medical radiographic imaging.* Philadelphia: W. B. Saunders.

United States War Department. (1941). *Technical manual: Roentgenographic technicians,* TM 8–240, July 3.

Williams, W. A. (1956). Radiographic effect formula: Its practical application. *The X-Ray Technician. 28*, 1–6, 67.

Wilsey, R. B. (1921). The intensity of scattered x-rays in radiography. *American Journal of Roentgenology. 8*, 328-338.

The Case of the Animal with the Large Calcified Tumor-Like Mass

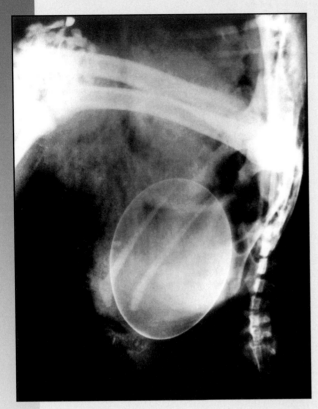

What is the huge mass in the lower abdomen of this animal?

Answers to the case studies can be found in Appendix E.

(Reprinted by Permission of the International Society of Radiographers and Radiological Technicians from the K.C. Clark Archives, Middlesex Hospital, London, England.)

CHAPTER 26

Contrast

The conclusion drawn from these experiments was that there was no mystery — that, other things being equal, contrast was determined solely by the voltage used. . . .

W. D. Coolidge, "Experiences with the Roentgen-ray tube."

Objectives

Upon completion of this chapter, the student should be able to:

▶ Identify contrast as a prime component of the photographic properties controlling visibility of detail of radiographic image quality.

▶ Explain the various terms used to describe contrast.

▶ Define radiographic contrast and the factors that affect it.

▶ Describe the factors that affect image receptor (film) contrast.

▶ Describe the factors that affect subject contrast.

▶ Describe the effect of fog on image contrast.

▶ Describe the effects of contrast changes on image appearance.

▶ Determine the technical factor changes necessary to achieve optimal contrast.

▶ Assess radiographic contrast on various radiographic images.

▶ Recommend appropriate adjustments to improve contrast under various conditions.

▶ Explain why kilovoltage peak is the controlling factor of contrast.

▶ Explain how each influencing factor affects image contrast.

Assessing Contrast

Contrast is one of the two photographic properties that comprise visibility of detail. Visibility of detail refers to the fact that the radiographic image is visible to the human eye only because sufficient contrast (and density) exists to permit the structural details to be perceived. **Radiographic contrast is the difference between adjacent densities.** It can be mathematically evaluated as the percentage or ratio of the differences between densities. These differences can range from clear white through various shades of gray to black.

Because contrast consists of various densities, a thorough knowledge of the factors that control density is a prerequisite to understanding it. Although contrast must be considered an independent factor, the fact that it is composed of densities makes it very difficult to separate it from the evaluation of overall density. Any change in overall density will affect contrast. This makes contrast the most difficult of the prime technical factors to evaluate and adjust.

Describing Contrast

When the differences between adjacent densities that comprise contrast are great, the image is described as high contrast. The result is fewer discernible shades of gray. Conversely, when the differences are minimal, the image is described as low contrast. This produces more discernible shades of gray. Figure 26–1F has the fewest shades of gray and therefore has the highest contrast.

In Figure 26–1A–F, there are progressively less discernible shades of gray. Figure 26–1A has the lowest contrast image. This is analogous to a gray scarf on a gray coat, which has low contrast, versus a black scarf on a white coat, which has high contrast. Table 26–1 summarizes the relationships between the various terms used to describe contrast.

As the differences between adjacent densities increase, there are fewer shades of discernible gray and the contrast is increased. Increasing contrast produces a high contrast image. As the differences between adjacent densities decrease, there are more shades of discernible gray and the contrast is decreased. Decreasing contrast produces a low contrast image.

TABLE 26–1. Relationship Between Terms Used To Describe Contrast

High Contrast	Low Contrast
Few shades of gray	Many shades of gray
Increased contrast	Decreased contrast
Low kVp	High kVp
Short scale contrast	Long scale contrast

The term "good contrast" is often applied to high contrast, but this is a misnomer and should be avoided because high contrast is not necessarily the most desirable. In fact, in most instances low contrast provides more information. Low contrast provides more differences in density even though the difference between densities is less. As long as the differences remain within the visible range of densities, low contrast provides more diagnostic information. Figures 26–2A and B are good examples of how high contrast fails to provide all the information that is obtained from a low contrast image.

Contrast is a psychovisual perception. In other words, the psychological effects of the relationships between the densities produce a visual perception that we call contrast. The perception problem is greater because not only do individuals have different physiological visual abilities, but individual background experiences also affect the final perception. Perhaps it would be better to think of contrast in terms of an individual's "contrast sensitivity."

Although high contrast images may be perceived as more pleasing to the untrained eye, radiographers and radiologists realize that, although the lower contrast image is not as dramatic in its presentation, it often demonstrates more information. Without contrast there would be no image because all densities would appear identical. More information is visible simply because more densities are present, thus forming more possibilities for contrast differences.

Scale of contrast is the number of useful visible densities or shades of gray. Short scale contrast refers to an image that demonstrates considerable or maximal differences between densities and has a minimal total number of densities. Conversely, long scale contrast refers to an image that demonstrates slight or minimal differences

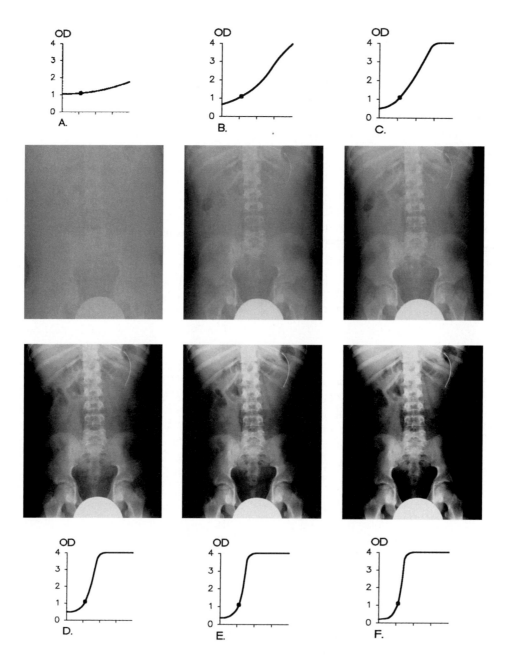

FIGURE 26-1. Pure contrast changes in a digital abdomen image produced with a fixed density point. These computerized images vary only in contrast as shown in the accompanying D log E curves. From A-F the contrast curve becomes steeper and shorter, but the density point does not move up or down. C is considered optimal contrast for a diagnostic image. *(Computed radiography images courtesy of Bruce Long, Indiana University Medical Center, Indianapolis)*

between densities but has a maximal total number of densities (Figure 26–3). **Short scale contrast is also called high contrast, or increased contrast, while long scale contrast is called low contrast, or decreased contrast.**

The advent of computerized digital processing has made it useful to sometimes describe contrast as **physical** and **visible**. Physical contrast is the total range of density values recorded by the image receptor. It is the maximum contrast possible and is the most accurate representation of the varying intensities present in the x-ray beam after it has passed through the subject. Visible contrast is the total range of density values that can be perceived by the human eye in a single image. It is a portion of the physical contrast and comprises the information from which diagnosis is made. Computers allow radiographers access to the entire range of densities available. Radiographers manipulate the physical contrast available into the visible range to produce the diagnostic image.

Manipulating Contrast

The image receptor records many densities that cannot be seen by the human eye. Depending on the desired contrast, the recorded densities are compressed or expanded to form a range of visible densities. This can be accomplished by changes in the film's D log E curve, adjustments in kVp, or by the use of a computer. Compression or expansion of the range of densities separates the physical contrast that is actually recorded by the image receptor from the visible contrast that can be perceived by the viewer on a single image.

Radiographic Contrast

Radiographic contrast is the total amount of contrast acquired from both the anatomical part and the film. These are described as **subject and image receptor** (film) contrast, respectively.

Image Receptor (Film) Contrast

Image receptor (film) contrast is the range of densities that the image receptor is capable of recording. Mathematically, this is expressed as the slope of the D

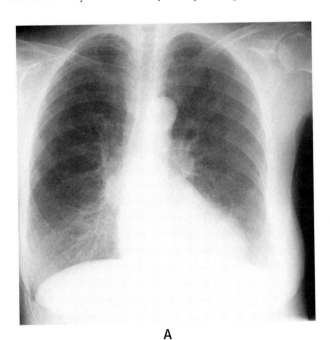

A

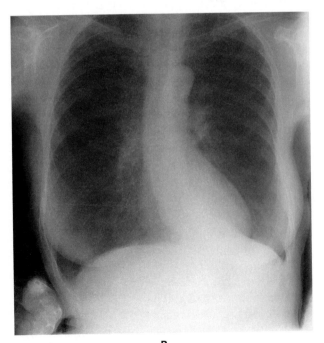

B

FIGURE 26-2. High and low contrast (A) Chest radiograph produced using 80 kVp. (B) Chest radiograph of same patient using 110 kVp.

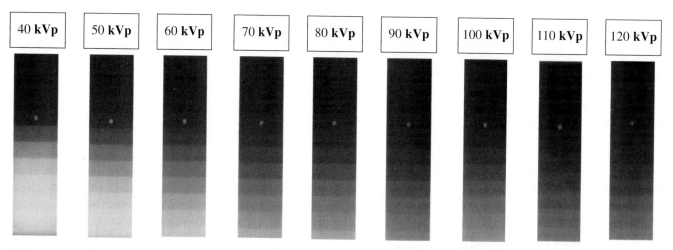

FIGURE 26-3. Variations in scale of contrast. The number of shades of gray, the scale or range of contrast, increases as kVp increases.

log E curve. Film contrast depends on four factors: the use of **intensifying screens, film density, the D log E curve, and processing**.

Intensifying Screens

Intensifying screens create an inherently higher contrast image. Although the exact reason is unknown, contrast is always lower for a film exposed to x-rays only than it is for the same film exposed to light from intensifying screens. It is most likely related to the way in which the film responds to the x-ray photons. The D log E curve changes dramatically when a film designed for exposure by light is exposed directly to x-rays. Changing screen speed has a negligible effect on contrast.

Film Density

Film contrast also changes with changes in film density. The exact effect is shown in Figure 26–4. There is an optimal range of densities that permits contrast to be visualized at a maximum. Excessive or inadequate density decreases contrast. This is especially true in the toe and shoulder regions of the curve. If the kVp remains constant, mAs and distance will determine the actual value of exposure, thereby determining the location of the exposure on the log relative exposure axis of the curve. If a film is exposed correctly, the film densities will fall within the visible range of the D log E curve. If the exposure places the developed densities on the toe (an underexposed film) or shoulder (an overexposed film), the slope is not as steep, resulting in a decrease in contrast (Figure 26–5).

D log E Curve

The primary determinant of the shape of the D log E curve is the physical composition of the film emulsion. As the slope of the curve becomes steeper, contrast is increased. For example, in Figure 26–6, film A possesses higher contrast than film B. Because of the steeper slope of the curve, the visible den-

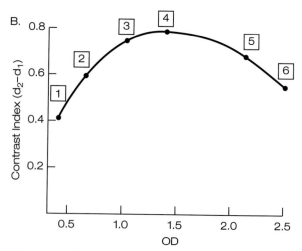

FIGURE 26-4. Contrast index for the density ranges (1-6). Note that the maximum contrast (range 4) is essentially the straight line portion of the curve. Contrast is decreased for toe and shoulder measurements but is maximized for the straight line portion of the D log E curve (OD) 1.2-1.5. (Also note that this range corresponds to the speed point [OD 1.2].) *(Courtesy of Charles Burns, MPH, RT(R), University of North Carolina)*

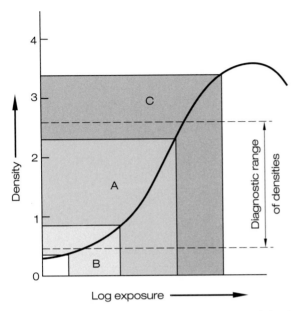

FIGURE 26-5. The effect of film density on contrast. (A) When the film is correctly exposed, the densities fall within the visible range. (B) An underexposed film occurs when the exposure places the developed densities into the toe. (C) An overexposed film occurs when the exposure places the developed densities into the shoulder. The decrease in contrast of underexposed and overexposed films occurs because the slope is not as steep in the toe and shoulder.

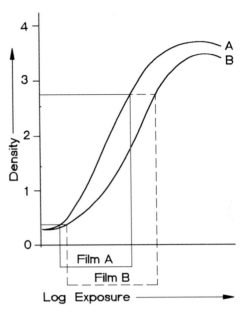

FIGURE 26-6. The effect of the D log E curve on contrast. As the slope of the curve becomes steeper, contrast is increased. Film A possesses higher contrast than film B, because Film A compresses the visible density range into a narrower exposure range.

sity range is compressed into a narrower exposure range. Film A is a high contrast, narrow latitude film. Film B is a low contrast, wide latitude film because the visible density range is expanded across a wider exposure range.

Processing
Increasing film developer time, temperature, or replenishment rate will increase the chemical fog on the film. These changes produce a decrease in the slope of the curve especially in the toe region (Figure 26–7). When any processing factor causes a change in base fog, contrast is affected. Developer temperature and immersion time, replenishment, and developer contamination are the primary processing factors that cause objectionable fog levels. Increased developer temperature, time, and replenishment rates cause increased fog and decreased contrast. As shown in Figure 21–10, film processing has an optimal range and any factor that causes processing to deviate from optimal values will decrease contrast. Developer contamination by fixer causes

increased fog and decreased contrast because the chemical ability of the developer reducing agents is seriously impaired by the pH change in the solution.

Subject Contrast
Subject contrast is the range of differences in the intensity of the x-ray beam after it has been attenuated by the subject. It is dependent on kilovoltage and the amount and type of irradiated material.

Kilovoltage
Kilovoltage peak (kVp) is the primary controller of subject contrast. As kVp increases, a wider range of photon energies is produced (Figure 7–6). The wider the range of photon energies, the greater the ability of the photons to penetrate the body tissues. This leads to a wider range of densities on the film, which results in an overall lower contrast.

As long as the kVp is adequate to penetrate the part being examined, low kVp will produce high subject contrast. When the kVp is too low, most of the photons do not reach the film because they are absorbed in the

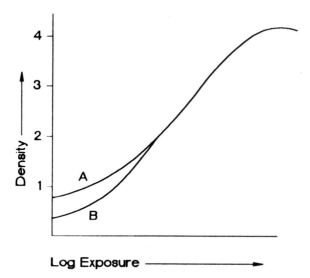

FIGURE 26-7. The effect of processing fog on contrast. In curve A, increased fog raises the toe of curve and decreases its slope, thus decreasing contrast.

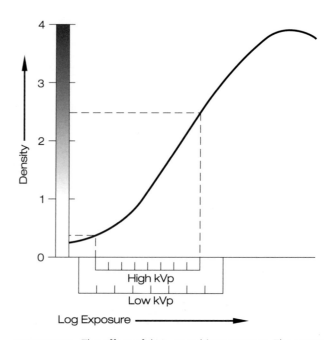

FIGURE 26-8. The effect of kVp on subject contrast. The range of transmitted photon intensities for high kVp produces a compressed range of relative exposures, which are reflected within the visible density range by the slope of the curve. The expanded range of exposures produced by low kVp is too wide for the curve to reflect within the visible density range. This causes some of the lowest and highest photon intensities not to be visible when low kVp is used.

patient. Low kVp produces higher subject contrast because most of these low energy photons are absorbed by thicker parts while more penetrate the thin part. With high kVp, subject contrast is decreased because more uniform penetration occurs between thick and thin parts.

The effect of kVp on subject contrast can be detailed by examining the D log E curve. Figure 26–8 shows the range of transmitted photon intensities forming the exposure to the film for both high and low kVp techniques for the same film type. High kVp produces a compressed range of relative exposures, which the slope of the D log E curve reflects within the visible density range. Low kVp produces an expanded range of relative exposures, which the slope of the D log E curve is unable to reflect within the visible density range. This causes some of the lowest and highest exposures to fall outside the visible density range. Increasing kVp causes density differences that were previously undetectable to become visible, resulting in an increase in the diagnostic information provided by the image.

This concept is demonstrated nicely by comparing chest radiographs to radiographs of the ribs. In chest radiography high kVps result in a wide range of radi-

ographic densities that fall within the visible range. Both the air-filled lungs and the bony structures are demonstrated within the visible range. No structures appear under or overexposed. In rib radiography low kVps are used to enhance the differences between the air-filled lungs and the overlying bony structures. The air-filled lungs demonstrate increased radiographic density, while the bony structures demonstrate decreased radiographic density compared to the chest film.

In addition to kVp, radiation fog has a significant effect on contrast. It is the result of x-ray interactions with matter, primarily Compton scatter. As kVp increases the percentage of Compton interactions increases. As a result of this increase in the amount of scatter reaching the film, contrast is decreased. Scatter raises the base plus fog (the toe) and decreases the slope of the curve (Figure 26–7). These changes cause the lightest densities to be "fogged over" so they can no longer be distinguished from one another (Figure 26–9). The resulting image no longer includes a clear or pure "white" region, and therefore has less contrast.

Fog can be caused by factors other than scatter radiation. These include subjecting film to heat, low level ionizing radiation, or chemical fumes. Developer temperature, replenishment, and developer contamination may also cause objectionable fog levels. The effect of fog on contrast must be considered during clinical radiography because it sets the acceptance limits for contrast regulation. The radiographer should remember that any factor that results in an increase in fog will decrease contrast.

Amount of Irradiated Material

The amount of irradiated material depends on the thickness of the body part and the field size. Both these factors influence the number of x-rays transmitted to the image receptor. As body part thickness increases, x-ray absorption increases. Conversely, as body part thickness decreases so does absorption. This difference in absorption between various thicknesses influences subject contrast. When the difference between adjacent thicknesses of various body parts is great, subject contrast is increased. When little difference exists in the thickness of adjacent body parts, subject contrast is decreased.

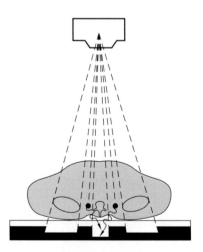

FIGURE 26-9. The effect of scatter radiation on contrast. Scatter radiation producing image densitiy (and incorrect information) in a region of high subject density (under the vertebral column). The scatter interferes with the ability of the bone to cast a light shadow on the film.

When the overall thickness of a body part increases, or when field size increases, the amount of scatter created will increase. This results in a decrease in subject contrast. A decrease in overall body part thickness or field size results in increased subject contrast.

Type of Irradiated Material

The type of irradiated material is influenced by the atomic number of the material and its density. Both these factors influence subject contrast.

Materials with a higher atomic number, such as lead and iodine, absorb a greater percentage of the x-ray beam than low atomic number materials, such as hydrogen, carbon, and calcium. This results from the presence of a greater number of electrons, which enables more interactions to occur. When the difference between the average atomic number of adjacent tissues is great, subject contrast is increased. When little difference exists between them, subject contrast is decreased. For example, bone has a higher average atomic number than soft tissue. Therefore, subject contrast between bone and soft tissue is greater than the contrast between adjacent soft tissue structures. Contrast media increase subject contrast by introducing greater differences in atomic number variations than those that exist naturally.

Tissue density describes how tightly the atoms of a given substance are packed together. When the difference between the densities of adjacent tissues is great, subject contrast is increased. When little difference exists between them, subject contrast is decreased. For example, bone tissue is a denser substance than lung tissue. Therefore subject contrast between bone and lung tissue is greater.

Evaluating Contrast

The major consideration in evaluating visible contrast is **verification that a proper range of densities are visible throughout the anatomical area of interest** on the radiograph. Proper density alone is not enough. The anatomical structures of interest are visible only when sufficient contrast between the densities exists. Of course, these densities must be well within the range of human visibility (OD 0.25–2.50).

Unlike the evaluation of density, contrast assessment requires more than just sufficient density within the visibility range. Adequate contrast must demonstrate enough distinctly different densities within the range to satisfy diagnostic quality requirements for the particular examination. Much of this ability is the result of clinical experience. It is obvious that proper contrast is not the same for all tissues. Knowledge of anatomy and physiology, both normal and abnormal, as well as pathology and technical factors, is critical for proper contrast evaluation. Only when these skills are combined with an experienced and trained professional eye, can proper contrast evaluation occur.

Because there is more information recorded on a radiograph than is seen, the diagnostic importance of contrast is a matter of how many densities are included in the visible contrast range. To some extent, it can be said that low contrast images have more information. However, the critical point is that the various densities must be discernible.

The human eye is limited in its ability to discern light and dark. This essentially establishes an OD value for the lightest and darkest visible shades of gray. When additional shades of gray are added to the visible range of contrast, they must fit between these two densities. Each additional shade of gray reduces the magnitude of the density difference, or the contrast, between the lightest and darkest grays. Eventually a point is reached where additional shades of gray do not have enough density difference to be visible (Figure 26–1A). Of course, this occurs at different points, depending on individual visual abilities. A 30 percent density difference has been used as the minimum change to cause a visible difference because this magnitude is discernible by nearly everyone. However, some professionals may be able to discern as little contrast as a 15 percent density difference, which means they are capable of seeing twice as many shades of gray as someone who can discern only a 30 percent change.

Discerning contrast can be extremely difficult for even the experienced radiographer when the image exhibits poor density. **Contrast evaluation can be made only when sufficient density exists to permit the range of contrast to be seen.** The eye tends to consider nearby densities and contrast when evaluating image quality. It is so difficult for the eye to ignore nearby factors that a contrast mask is often helpful (Figure 26–10). A contrast mask is a simple tool to help focus on the contrast in a selected area. When a contrast mask is used with an image, adjacent information is eliminated. This makes the evaluation much easier as the contrast problem becomes evident as well as easier to evaluate (Figure 26–11). Because of the difficulty in ignoring nearby density problems (either too light or dark) even the experienced radiographer will find a contrast mask useful in making some evaluations.

Selecting The Appropriate kVp

There are no established rules concerning how much contrast is desirable in all situations. Experience and knowledge enable the radiographer to determine when a change in contrast will increase the diagnostic quality of an image. Many radiologists find it desirable to have uniform contrast throughout a single examination to permit comparisons between projections. Low contrast can be achieved to some degree by utilizing a fixed kilovoltage technique system. Other radiologists prefer a higher contrast. This can be achieved to some degree by utilizing a variable kilovoltage technique system.

The radiographs in Figures 26–1 and 26–12 illustrate the effect of contrast on image quality. Notice in Figure 26–12 that the contrast varies as the kVp varies. Also notice that the contrast varies for the same kVp with different body part thickness (different subject densities). The exposure factors for these images used different mAs values to compensate for the differences in scatter radiation as the kVp was changed.

The radiographs in Figure 11–2 illustrate the effect of kVp on image density. To perceive a contrast change, density should be maintained at a uniform level. The 15 percent rule is an acceptable method of achieving uni-

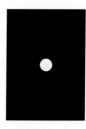

FIGURE 26-10. A contrast mask.

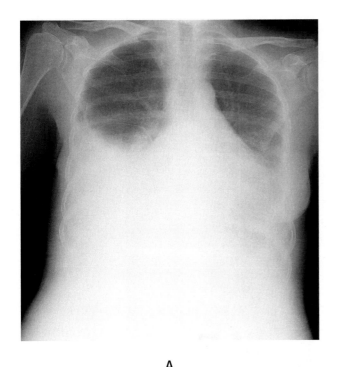
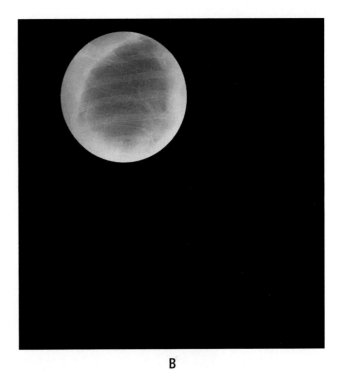

A B

FIGURE 26-11. Using a contrast mask. (A) A radiograph of a chest that appears too light, making contrast evaluation difficult. (B) The same radiograph with the contrast mask applied to the right upper lobe of the lung, making contrast evaluation easier.

form density when changing contrast. **A visible change in contrast will not be perceived until kVp is changed by 4–12 percent, depending on the kVp range** (Table 26–2). There is no reason to repeat an exposure for contrast reasons unless at least a 4–5 percent change is made, although higher kVps require even greater changes. The effects of mAs and the influencing factors on image contrast are not exact because of the wide variety of variables that are part of the imaging system. Many of the variables affect the contrast of the image as a side effect of other changes.

Both the quantity and quality of the x-ray beam will vary with changes in kilovoltage. There are too many variables to be quantified into a reliable formula. Because the 15 percent rule is used so much when maintaining density, it is convenient to use it as the minimum practical change within the diagnostic range. Remember that the 15 percent rule is a misnomer as the actual changes necessary to maintain density vary from 15–25 percent (Figure 25–4).

When a radiograph is outside acceptance limits, it needs to be repeated. All acceptance limits permit some degree of variation, at least 8–15 percent change in contrast. **The rule for contrast changes is to make adjustments in increments of 15 or 8 percent.** If the radiograph does not require an 8 percent change in kVp and contrast, it seldom requires repeating. Exceptions to this rule are fine adjustments of 8 percent that are crucial to demonstrate small structures. Radiographers may adjust

TABLE 26–2. Changes Necessary To Produce Visible Contrast Differences

Level	Change Necessary to Produce Visible Change	Change to Equal Percent Change
30–50 kVp	4–5 percent	1–3 kVp
50–90 kVp	8–9 percent	4–8 kVp
90–130 kVp	10–12 percent	9–16 kVp

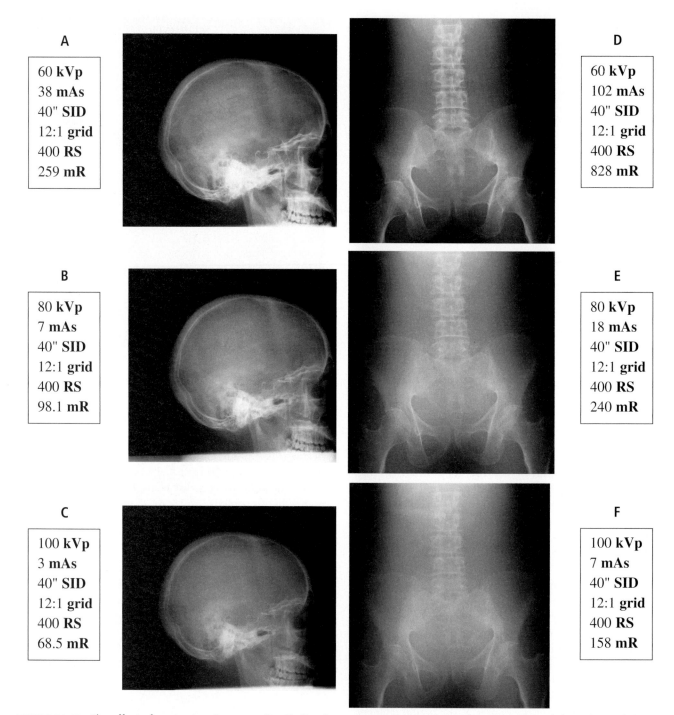

A

60 kVp
38 mAs
40" SID
12:1 grid
400 RS
259 mR

B

80 kVp
7 mAs
40" SID
12:1 grid
400 RS
98.1 mR

C

100 kVp
3 mAs
40" SID
12:1 grid
400 RS
68.5 mR

D

60 kVp
102 mAs
40" SID
12:1 grid
400 RS
828 mR

E

80 kVp
18 mAs
40" SID
12:1 grid
400 RS
240 mR

F

100 kVp
7 mAs
40" SID
12:1 grid
400 RS
158 mR

FIGURE 26-12. The effect of contrast on image quality. Skull radiographs produced at (A) 60 kVp; (B) 80 kVp; (C) 100 kVp. Abdomen radiographs produced at (D) 60 kVp; (E) 80 kVp; (F) 100 kVp. Compare these images, noting contrast changes due to anatomical part differences.

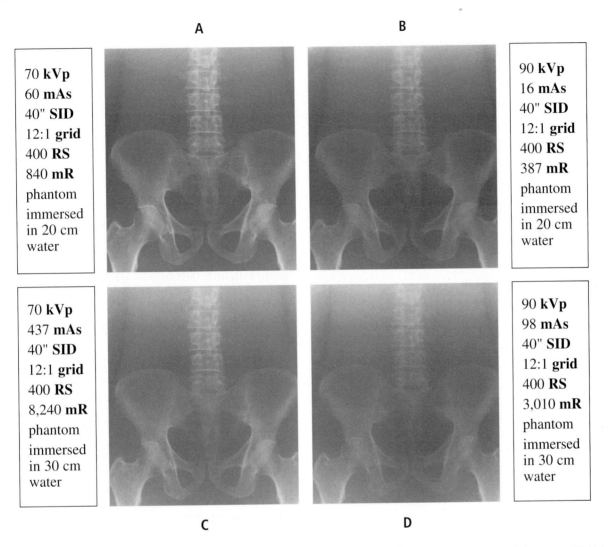

A

70 kVp
60 mAs
40" SID
12:1 grid
400 RS
840 mR
phantom
immersed
in 20 cm
water

B

90 kVp
16 mAs
40" SID
12:1 grid
400 RS
387 mR
phantom
immersed
in 20 cm
water

70 kVp
437 mAs
40" SID
12:1 grid
400 RS
8,240 mR
phantom
immersed
in 30 cm
water

90 kVp
98 mAs
40" SID
12:1 grid
400 RS
3,010 mR
phantom
immersed
in 30 cm
water

C

D

FIGURE 26-13. Increased contrast on 20 and 30 cm abdomens. (A) 20 cm abdomen at 70 kVp; (B) 20 cm abdomen at 90 kVp; (C) 30 cm abdomen at 70 kVp; (D) 30 cm abdomen at 90 kVp. All images were exposed with the same AEC and have the same overall density values. (Note the differences in mAs and mR dose.)

technique charts by an 8 percent margin, but will seldom subject the patient to a second exposure for such a minor change. As with density adjustments, contrast changes require bold action or no action at all.

In some instances it may be desirable to decrease kVp to increase contrast when mAs must be increased. A radiograph of a 20 cm abdomen produced at 90 kVp demonstrates a relatively low contrast (Figure 26–13B). When the same abdomen is radiographed at 70 kVp, a significantly higher contrast results (Figure 26–13A). The reduced kVp produced less scatter radiation, thus producing higher contrast. The natural tendency to increase kVp for thicker parts will not produce satisfactory radiographs if the effect of increased Compton scatter on contrast is not considered first.

Radiographic image contrast occurs due to the photoelectric effect's total absorption of photons in the subject. High contrast is directly related to the number of photoelectric effect interactions that occur in the subject. Because Compton interactions produce scatter, low contrast is directly related to the amount of Compton scatter that occurs in the subject. Image contrast can be controlled by adjusting kVp. The kVp controls the relationship between the number of photoelectric versus Compton interactions.

Contrast can be determined by matching the average incident photon energy with the average inner-shell binding energy of the predominant subject material, as shown in Figure 12–8. For example, when maximum contrast is desired for bone tissue, technical factors that increase the percentage of photoelectric interactions should be used. Photoelectric effect interactions increase as kVp decreases.

Factors Affecting Contrast

The controlling and influencing factors that affect contrast are shown in Figure 26–14. **The controlling factor that affects contrast has the most direct effect on the image.** When it is changed the image will change as a primary result. The influencing factors that control contrast have a **less direct effect** on the image or change other factors as well as contrast. When the influencing factors are changed the contrast is affected, but not as directly as with the controlling factor. With some of the factors this change is so small that it is essentially negligible.

Kilovoltage as the Controlling Factor

Kilovoltage peak (kVp) is the controller of contrast. As kVp increases contrast decreases. As kVp decreases contrast increases. In most instances the control of contrast rests with the radiographer by selecting an appropriate kVp setting from a technique chart developed for the particular x-ray unit in use. Other variables such as generator configuration (phase, falling load, or frequency) may also affect the final decision. A generator configuration that increases the effective kVp will result in a decrease in contrast. For example, for a given kVp a three-phase generator will produce a lower contrast than a single-phase unit.

Kilovoltage also controls the amount of scatter radiation produced. Increasing kVp increases the amount of radiation fog, thereby decreasing contrast.

The radiographer must adapt the suggested kVp setting for the individual procedure. Experience and study of various body habitus, pathologies, positioning, and equipment quickly provides the radiographer with clinical knowledge that can be used for these adjustments.

Influencing Factors

Influencing factors include milliampere-seconds (mAs), focal spot size, anode heel effect, distance, filtration, beam restriction, anatomical part, grids, film/screen combinations, and processing

Milliampere-Seconds (mAs)
Milliampere-seconds alters film density of the image and therefore affects contrast. When the change is sufficient to move density differences out of the range of human vision, either too dark or too light, the contrast is decreased (Figure 26–5).

Focal Spot Size
The possibility of the focal spot size altering contrast enough to be visible is extremely unlikely. Focal spot sizes have such a small effect on density that it is unlikely that their effect on contrast could be detected.

Anode Heel Effect
The anode heel effect alters the intensity of radiation, and therefore affects film density which can affect contrast. The intensity of radiation is greater at the cathode end of the tube. This difference would become visible only with open collimation and a small anode target angle (less than 12°). The anode heel has very little effect on contrast.

Distance
Source-to-image receptor distance (SID) alters the intensity of the beam reaching the image receptor according to the inverse square law. This affects film density and therefore contrast. Greater distance decreases density while less distance increases it. As distance alters density it can change the contrast exactly as does mAs.

Object-to-image receptor distance (OID) also has an effect on film density and contrast. An air-gap technique increases object-to-film distance and this permits scatter radiation to avoid the image receptor. This scatter radiation would normally contribute radiation fog to the density. Removing scatter from the image will increase contrast.

Filtration   Filtration increases the effect of kVp by changing the average photon energy of the beam. All types of filtration — inherent, added, and total — alter film density and contrast. Filtration affects contrast by changing the average photon energy and decreasing beam intensity. The increase in the average photon energy causes more Compton scatter production and this decreases contrast. The decreased intensity decreases density, which

decreases contrast. This change is negligible, however, because most of these low energy photons do not exit the patient to contribute to film density. The predominant effect of filtration is caused by changes in average photon energy, therefore increased filtration decreases contrast.

Beam Restriction   Restricting the beam, collimating, or reducing the primary beam field size reduces the total number of photons available. This reduces the amount of scatter radiation and therefore increases contrast.

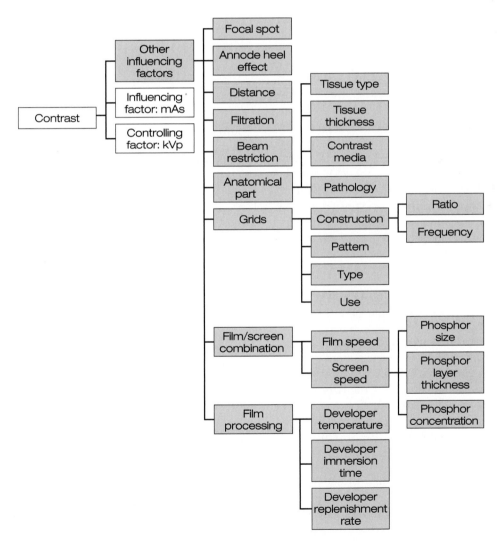

FIGURE 26 -14. Radiographic image quality: factors affecting contrast.

Anatomical Part   Because the patient is the prime attenuator of the beam, both the amount and type of tissue being examined greatly influence the density and contrast of the film. As the anatomical part size increases, the amount of scatter created by the part also increases, resulting in a decrease in contrast. As tissue density increases, the amount of scatter increases, which also results in a decrease in contrast. As average atomic number increases (i.e., using contrast media) there is more photoelectric absorption resulting in higher or increased contrast.

As with density adjustments, compensation for anatomical part changes depends on an ability to assess tissue type, thickness, pathology, etc. This ability is achieved only through clinical experience.

Grids   The primary function of a grid is contrast improvement (Figure 26–15). Grids improve contrast by removing scatter before it reaches the image. The contrast improvement factor (K) is the best measure of how well a grid accomplishes this function. The contrast improvement factor is dependent on the amount of scatter produced, which is controlled by the kVp and the amount and type of irradiated tissue. As the amount of scatter radiation increases, the lower the contrast and the lower the contrast improvement factor. The contrast improvement factor K is measured by using the average gradient (or gamma) of the straight line portion of the D log E curve:

$$K = \frac{\text{average gradient with the grid}}{\text{average gradient without the grid}}$$

If K = 1, then no improvement in contrast has occurred. Most grids have contrast improvement factors between 1.5 and 3.5 so their contrast is 1.5–3.5 times better than an identical non-grid film. The higher the K factor, the greater the contrast improvement.

Higher ratio grids remove more scatter and therefore have a greater contrast improvement factor. This results in a higher contrast image.

Film/Screen Combinations   The primary determinant of the shape of the D log E curve is the physical composition of the film emulsion. As the slope of the curve becomes steeper, contrast is increased. Intensifying screens create an inherently higher contrast image.

Contrast is always lower for a film exposed to x-rays only than it is for the same film exposed to light from intensifying screens.

Processing   Increasing film developer time, temperature, or replenishment rate from the optimal range will increase the chemical fog on the film. These changes produce a decrease in the slope of the curve, which results in a decrease in contrast. Decreasing film development time, temperature, or replenishment rate from the optimal range will decrease the film's density, which in turn will decrease contrast.

Summary

Contrast is one of the two photographic properties that comprise visibility of detail. Visibility of detail refers to the fact that the radiographic image is visible to the human eye only because sufficient contrast (and density) exists to permit structural details to be perceived. Radiographic contrast is the difference between adjacent densities. It can be mathematically evaluated as the percentage or ratio of the differences between densities. These differences can range from clear white through various shades of gray to black.

When the differences between adjacent densities that comprise contrast are great, the image is described as high contrast. The result is fewer discernible shades of gray. Conversely, when the differences are minimal the image is described as low contrast.

Short scale contrast is also called high contrast, or increased contrast, while long scale contrast is called low contrast, or decreased contrast. Physical contrast is the total range of density values recorded by the image receptor whereas visible contrast is the total range of density values that can be perceived by the human eye in a single image.

Radiographic contrast is the total amount of contrast acquired from both the anatomical part and the film. These are described as image receptor (film) contrast and subject contrast respectively. Image receptor (film) contrast is the range of densities that the image receptor is capable of recording. Film contrast depends on four factors: the use of intensifying screens, film density, the D log E curve, and processing. Subject contrast is the range

80 kVp	3.2 mAs	40" **SID**
No **grid**	400 **RS**	45.2 **mR**

80 kVp	17 mAs	40" **SID**
12:1 **grid**	400 **RS**	226 **mR**

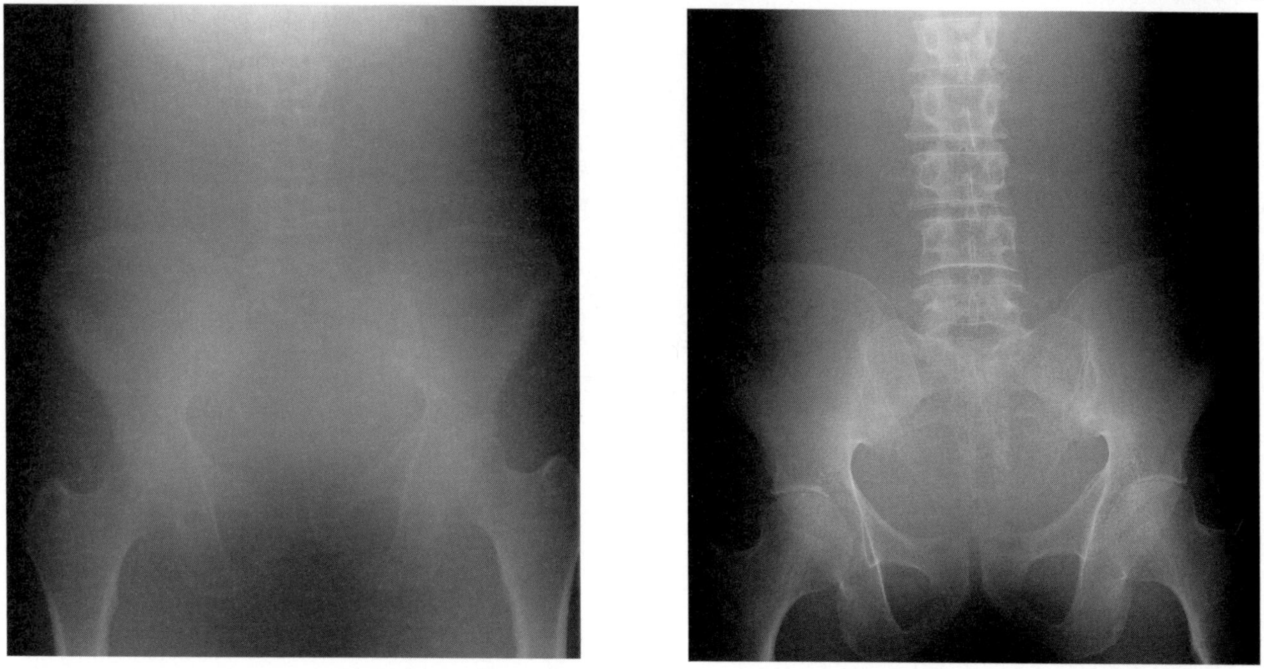

A

B

FIGURE 26-15. The effect of a grid on contrast. (A) 80 kVp without a grid; (B) 80 kVp with a grid. Both images were exposed with the same AEC and have the same overall density values. (Note the differences in mAs and mR dose.)

of differences in the intensity of the x-ray beam after it has been attenuated by the subject. It is dependent on kilovoltage and the amount and type of irradiated material.

The major consideration in evaluating visible contrast is verification that a proper range of densities are visible throughout the anatomical area of interest on the radiograph. Proper density alone is not enough. The anatomical structures of interest can be visualized only when sufficient contrast between the densities exists. To perceive a contrast change, density should be maintained at a uniform level. The 15 percent rule is an acceptable method of achieving this.

A wide variety of factors affect radiographic contrast. These factors are classified as either controlling or influencing factors. The controlling factor is kVp and it

should be used as the principle method for altering the contrast. The influencing factors include milliamperage-seconds, focal spot size, anode heel effect, distance, filtration, beam restriction, anatomical part, grids, film/screen combination, and film processing.

When the controlling factor or any of the influencing factors is altered, some change in contrast will occur, however with some of the factors the effect is often neglible. Table 26–3 illustrates the effect on contrast when the various factors are changed. For the purpose of this review, assume that compensation has been made for the changes in the radiographic density. Remember that if no compensation is made for the changes in density, and the resulting image is too light or too dark, contrast will always decrease.

TABLE 26–3. Effects of Changing Factors on Contrast

+ = increases contrast
− = decreases contrast
∅ = negligible effect

Controlling Factor
− Increasing kilovoltage
+ Decreasing kilovoltage
− Increasing number of pulses in the generator waveform
+ Decreasing number of pulses in the generator waveform

Influencing Factors
∅ Increasing milliamperage-seconds*
∅ Decreasing milliamperage-seconds*
∅ Focal-spot size changes
∅ Anode heel effect
∅ Increasing SID
∅ Decreasing SID
+ Increasing OID
− Decreasing OID
− Increasing filtration
+ Decreasing filtration
+ Increasing beam restriction/collimation
− Decreasing beam restriction/collimation
− Increasing amount of irradiated tissue
+ Decreasing amount of irradiated tissue
− Increasing atomic number or density of tissue
+ Decreasing atomic number or density of tissue
+ Using contrast media (increasing or decreasing atomic number)
− Additive pathological conditions
+ Destructive pathological conditions
+ Increasing grid ratio
− Decreasing grid ratio
∅ Increasing film/screen combination relative speed
∅ Decreasing film/screen combination relative speed
+ Use of intensifying screens
− Increasing or decreasing film processing developer time and temperature beyond optimal

*For example, changing mAs while maintaining density by SID changes.

REVIEW QUESTIONS

1. Define radiographic contrast.

2. How do high contrast images differ from low contrast images?

3. What is the difference between physical and visible contrast?

4. What factors affect image receptor (film) contrast and subject contrast?

5. How does film density affect image receptor contrast?

6. What is the controlling factor of subject contrast and how does it affect it?

7. How do variations in the anatomical part affect contrast?

8. What is the effect of a grid on contrast?

9. How does film processing affect contrast?

REFERENCES AND RECOMMENDED READING

Abildgaard, A. & Notthellen, J. A. (1992). Increasing contrast when viewing radiographic images. *Radiology. 185*(2), 475–478.

Bauer, R. G. (1970). High kilovoltage chest radiography with an air gap. *Radiologic Technology. 42*, 10–14.

Bierman, A. & Boldingh, W. H. (1951). The relation between tension and exposure times in radiography. *Acta Radiologica. 35*, 22–26.

Bloom, W. L., Hollenbach, J. L., & Morgan, J. A. (1965). *Medical radiographic technic* (3rd ed.). Springfield, IL: Charles C. Thomas Publishers.

Bryan, G. J. (1970). *Diagnostic radiography: A manual for radiologic technologists.* Baltimore: Williams & Wilkins.

Cahoon, J. B. (1961). Radiographic technique: Its origin, concept, practical application and evaluation of radiation dosage. *The X-Ray Technician. 32*, 354–364.

Carlton, R. R. & McKenna, A. (1989). Repeating radiographs: Setting imaging standards. *Postgraduate Advances in Radiologic Technology.* Berryville, VA: Forum Medicum.

Carroll, Q. B. (1993). *Evaluating radiographs.* Springfield, IL: Charles C. Thomas Publishers.

Carroll, Q. B. (1993). *Fuchs's radiographic exposure, processing, and quality control* (5th ed.). Springfield, IL: Charles C. Thomas Publishers.

Chow, M. F. (1988). The effect of a film's sensitivity to its speed, contrast, and latitude. *The Canadian Journal of Medical Radiation Technology. 19*(4), 147.

Clark, K. C. (1953). An introduction to high-voltage technique. *Radiography. 19*, 21–33.

Cullinan, A. & Cullinan, J. (1994). *Producing quality radiographs* (2nd ed.). Philadelphia: J. B. Lippincott.

Distance — technique relationship of angulated projections. (1980). *Radiologic Technology. 52*(3), 301.

DuPont Company Photosystems & Electronic Products Department. *Positioning and Exposure Guide for General Radiography*. Wilmington, DE: Publication R-53806-1.

Eastman Kodak Company. (1980). Health Sciences Markets Division. *The Fundamentals of Radiography* (12th ed.). Rochester, NY: Kodak Publication M1–18.

Eastman, T. R. (1969). Chest technique through body habitus. *Radiologic Technology. 41*, 80–84.

Eastman, T. R. *The radiographic technique guide*. Wilmington, DE: DuPont deNemours, Inc. Photo Products Department Publication A-99101.

Files, G. W. (1952). *Medical Radiographic Technique*. Springfield, IL: Charles C. Thomas Publishers.

Files, G. W. (1935). Maximum tissue differentiation. *The X-Ray Technician. 7*, 17–24+.

Fuchs, A. W. (1958). *Principles of radiographic exposure and processing*. Springfield, IL: Charles C. Thomas Publishers.

Fuchs, A. W. (1950). The rationale of radiographic exposure. *The X-Ray Technician. 22*, 62–68, 76.

Fuchs, A. W. (1948). Relationship of tissue thickness to kilovoltage. *The X-Ray Technician. 19*, 287–293.

Fuchs, A. W. (1940). Balance in the radiographic image. *The X-Ray Technician. 12*(3), 81–84, 118.

Funke, T. (1966). Pegged kilovoltage technic. *Radiologic Technology. 37*, 202–213.

General Electric Company Medical Systems Department. *How to Prepare an X-ray Technic Chart*. Milwaukee: Publication 4301A.

Gratale, P., Turner, G. W., & Burns, C. B. (1986). Using the same exposure factors for wet and dry casts. *Radiologic Technology. 57*(4), 325–328.

Hiss, S. S. (1993). *Understanding radiography* (3rd ed.). Springfield, IL: Charles C. Thomas Publishers.

Jenkins, D. (1980). *Radiographic photography and imaging processes*. Lancaster, England: MTP Press Limited.

Jerman, E. C. (1928). *Modern x-ray technic*. St. Paul: Bruce Publishing.

Kelsey, C. A. (1982). Comparison of Nodule Detection with 70 kVp and 120 kVp Chest Radiographs. *Radiology*. (June), 609.

Kodera, Y., Schmidt, R. A., Chan, H., & Doi, K. (1984). Backscatter from metal surfaces in diagnostic radiology. *Radiology*. (Jan.), 231.

Koenig, G. F. (1957). Kilovoltage as a qualitative factor. *The X-Ray Technician. 29*, 1–4, 13.

Lauer, O. G., Mayes, J. B., & Thurston, R. P. (1990). *Evaluating radiographic quality: The variables and their effects*. Mankato, MN: The Burnell Company Publishers.

Mattsson, O. (1955). Practical photographic problems in radiography. *Acta Radiologica. Supplementum*. 1201–1206.

McEnerney, P. (1960). Evaluation of radiographic contrast after uncompensated factor changes. *Radiologic Technology. 32*(1), 23.

Mitchell, F. (1991). Scattered radiation and the lateral lumbar spine part 1: Initial research. *Radiography Today. 57*(644), 18–20.

Mitchell, F., Leung, C., Ahuja, A., & Metreweli, C. (1991). Scattered radiation and the lateral lumbar spine part 2: Clinical research. *Radiography Today. 57*(645), 12–14.

Morgan, J. A. (1977). *The art and science of medical radiography* (5th ed.). St. Louis: Catholic Hospital Association.

Morgan, R. H. (1946). An analysis of the physical factors controlling the diagnostic quality of roentgen images: Part III. Contrast and the intensity distribution function of a Roentgen image. *American Journal of Roentgenology and Radiation Therapy. 55*(1), 67–89.

Morgan, R. H. (1946). An analysis of the physical factors controlling the diagnostic quality of roentgen images: Part IV. Contrast and the film contrast factor. *American Journal of Roentgenology and Radiation Therapy. 55*(5), 627–633.

Newman, H. (1933). Relation of kilovolts to thickness of part—x-ray technic. *The X-Ray Technician. 5*, 21–26.

Roderick, J. F. (1950). Photographic contrast in roentgenology. *The X-Ray Technician. 22*, 141–150, 163.

Schwarz, G. S. (1961). *Unit-step radiography.* Springfield, IL: Charles C. Thomas Publishers.

Schwarz, G. S. (1960). Kilovoltage conversion in radiography. *The X-Ray Technician. 31*, 373–379, 436.

Schwarz, G. S. (1959). Kilovoltage and radiographic effect. *Radiology. 73*, 749–760.

Seeman, H. E. (1968). *Physical and photographic principles of medical radiography.* New York: Wiley & Sons.

Spiegler, G. (1950). The story of contrast and definition. *Radiography. 41*(189), 177–182.

Thompson, M. A., Hattaway, M. P., Hall, J. D., & Dowd, S. B. (1994). *Principles of imaging science and protection.* Philadelphia: W. B. Saunders.

Tortorici, M. (1992). *Concepts in medical radiographic imaging.* Philadelphia: W. B. Saunders.

Trout, E. D., Graves, D. E., & Slauson, D. B. (1949). High kilovoltage radiography. *Radiology. 52*, 669–683.

United States War Department. (1941). *Technical manual: Roentgenographic technicians*, TM 8–240, July 3.

Wegelius, C. (1954). The diagnostic use of high voltage rays in relationship to the physical background of mass absorption. *Acta Radiologica. Supplementum 116*, 589–597.

Wilks, R. J. (1981). *Principles of radiological physics.* Edinburgh: Churchill Livingstone.

Wilsey, R. B. (1921). The intensity of scattered x-rays in radiography. *American Journal of Roentgenology. 8*, 328–338.

CHAPTER 27

Recorded Detail

One look is worth a thousand listens.

Merrill C. Sosman, *"A Radiologist's Opinion of the Stethoscope."*

OBJECTIVES

Upon completion of this chapter, the student should be able to:

▶ Define recorded detail, including synonymous terms and derived units.

▶ Explain the effect of various distances on recorded detail.

▶ Describe the factors that affect penumbra size.

▶ Describe the effect of film/screen combinations on the resolution of recorded detail.

▶ Discuss the relationship of the three intensifying screen factors to recorded detail.

▶ Describe appropriate techniques to prevent patient motion.

▶ Synthesize various geometrical factors into a clinical protocol for improving resolution.

▶ Recommend techniques for reducing motion, including immobilization devices.

Assessing Recorded Detail

Recorded detail is one of the two geometric proper-ties of radiographic image quality. Unlike the pho-tographic properties of density and contrast, which con-trol the visibility of detail, the geometric properties con-trol detail itself. **Recorded detail is the degree of geo-metric sharpness or accuracy of the structural lines actually recorded in the radiographic image.** Good detail exists even when it cannot be seen due to poor vis-ibility of detail or, in other words, when the density and/or contrast are poor. Recorded detail is one of the easiest of the prime technical factors to evaluate and adjust.

Recorded detail is also referred to as **definition, sharp-ness, resolution, or simply as detail**. When the term detail is used by itself it usually refers to the recorded detail of the radiographic image. Detail is easily quanti-fied and even has a derived unit. The term resolution is applied to quantified discussions of recorded detail. The **unit of resolution** is line pairs per millimeter (lp/mm) or cycles per mm. A radiographic resolution tool is com-posed of pairs of lines a set distance from one another (Figure 27–1). The point at which the viewer can discern the closest pair of lines from each other represents the lp/mm reading. Most human visual acuity is limited to the range of 5 lp/mm. At this level each line is 0.1 mm wide, so a structure of this size could be discerned. Unfortunately, most radiographic imaging systems do not provide this level of resolution.

All radiographic images have less recorded detail than the object itself. In other words, the radiographic image exhibits some, but never all, of the detail of the anatom-ical part. The art of radiography involves controlling the degree of **unsharpness** so that it does not interfere with image diagnosis.

The effect of poor resolution on the image is seen as a lack of sharp definition of fine detail. This is caused by unacceptable levels of penumbra as compared to the umbral shadows that are expected from the part. Evaluation of resolution is best accomplished when an image has high contrast and a diagnostic quality density.

Recorded detail is usually evaluated during quality control testing by imaging a resolution test tool. In a clinical situation, small structures are the easiest to exam-

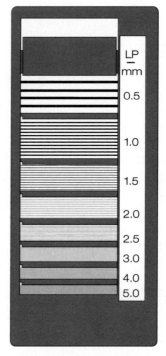

FIGURE 27-1 A resolution tool. The tool is read by discerning the point at which the finest lines are still visible as separated from one another. This point is then compared to the scale to determine the lp/mm reading. *(Courtesy of Nuclear Associates, Inc., 100 Voice Road, Carle Place, NY 11514)*

ine to evaluate recorded detail. The trabeculae of bone is an excellent guidepost to image resolution. Much of the ability to assess when the resolution is too poor to be of diagnostic quality is a matter of clinical experience (Figure 27–2).

Effects on Image Appearance

Resolution affects the image appearance by demon-strating fine detail structures, often very close to the size limits of the naked eye. When fine detail is lacking, the image will often appear blurred.

Motion unsharpness is often not perceived by the beginning student, partially because students must learn to critically examine each image in a methodical manner. Another reason is that a thorough knowledge of how var-

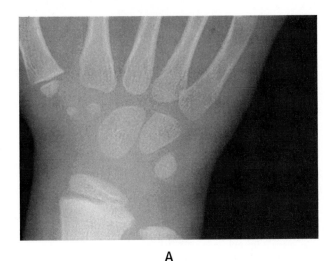

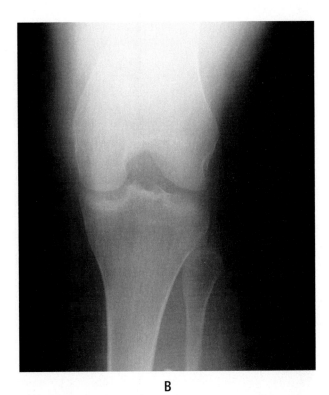

FIGURE 27-2. Assessing resolution. (A) A pediatric wrist exhibiting good resolution. (B) An adult knee exhibiting fair resolution in the tibia and poor resolution in the femur.

ious anatomical structures should appear radiographically is necessary in order to recognize when motion causes them to appear unacceptable (Figure 27–3). The assessment of motion is a matter of obtaining sufficient clinical experience. Progress in professional competence has been achieved when the beginning radiographer easily discerns motion·unsharpness.

Factors Affecting Recorded Detail

The factors that control recorded detail are shown in Figure 27–4. Close consideration of these factors will reveal that recorded detail is improved only through factors that increase the patient dose. This makes consideration of how much resolution is necessary for a particular study a patient radiation protection issue. Resolution problems should be approached in this order:

1. Eliminate **motion**;

2. Reduce **OID** (OFD);

3. Reduce **focal spot size**;

4. Reduce **intensifying screen phosphor size and concentration**; and

5. Increase **SID** (FFD).

Geometry

The geometry of the beam is the most important factor in establishing the level of resolution desired for recorded detail. Because the x-ray beam emanates from a small point (the focal spot), the further the photons move from their source, the further they diverge. In Figure 27–5 note how much more tissue is imaged and exposed at the level of the spine than at the level of the collimator light beam. This is the basis of the inverse square law and it applies to the geometry of the beam as well.

Distance The distances between the source or focal spot (S), object or part (0) and image receptor (I) are

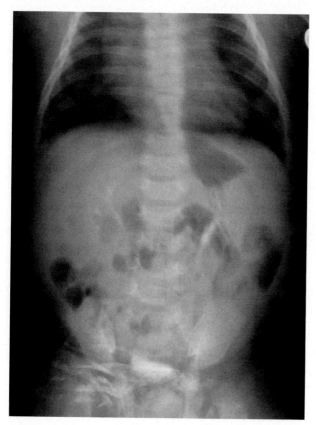

FIGURE 27-3. Motion unsharpness. The diaphragm, heart and bowel are all unsharp due to motion of this pediatric patient.

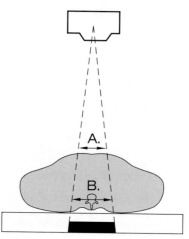

FIGURE 27-5. Divergence of the x-ray beam. More tissue is imaged and exposed at the level of the spine (point B) than at the level of the collimator light beam (point A).

critical in establishing sufficient recorded detail. These distances are referred to, as shown in Figure 27–6, so that SOD + OID = SID. **Resolution is improved when OID decreases** and degraded whenever it increases. This is why the affected side or part of interest is always positioned as close to the film as possible.

Resolution is improved when SID increases and degraded when it decreases. Increasing SID improves the

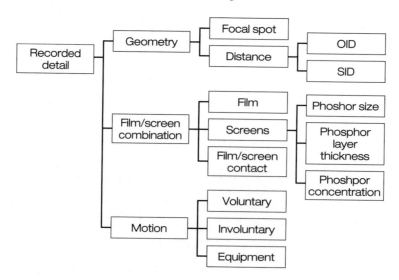

FIGURE 27-4. Radiographic image quality: factors affecting recorded detail.

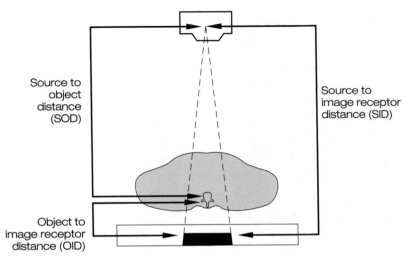

FIGURE 27-6. Critical distances in radiography.

recorded detail of the image enough that numerous leaders in radiography are currently advocating a routine 48" (120 cm) distance in place of the current 40" (100 cm) distance.

When it is necessary to make adjustments in order to improve detail, OID should be evaluated first. **The minimum OID should be used to improve detail.** The details of the positioning and the equipment in use should be carefully considered. In many instances a change in positioning will accomplish a remarkable improvement in detail. In fact, most positioning routines were established with OID as a critical factor. For example, the PA chest projection is preferred because it places the heart closer to the film than does the AP projection. The left lateral stomach, AP kidney and AP lumbar projections were all developed for the same reason.

The OID can also be minimized by considering the distance between the surface supporting the part and the film cassette. Differences between the **tabletop-to-Bucky tray distance can have a considerable influence on OID.** Of course, the minimal OID is obtained with non-Bucky procedures that place the part directly on the cassette, as is routine in extremity radiography. However, once the need for a grid supersedes the resolution that is lost by using a Bucky tray, careful consideration can still result in significant differences in detail. For example, whereas a head unit will often permit an OID of 1–2 cm, a floating top table may permit an OID of only 10

cm. The differences in image quality are significant (Figure 27–7).

Once the OID has been minimized, **resolution is improved when SID increases** and degraded when it decreases. Again, positioning routines were established to take advantage of this relationship. For example, the lateral cervical is usually performed at 72" (180 cm) instead of 40" (100 cm) because the OID cannot be reduced due to the distance between the neck and shoulder. Increased SID is the only method that can produce a lateral image comparable to the AP and oblique projections, which have a much smaller OID.

Focal Spot Size Focal spot size is controlled by the line focus principle (see Figure 6–13). A multitude of tube designs have been used over the years to minimize the effective focal spot while maximizing the actual focal spot to absorb the heat.

The umbra is the distinctly sharp area of a shadow or the region of complete shadow. **The penumbra is the imperfect, unsharp shadow surrounding the umbra.** With light, it is the region of partial illumination that surrounds the complete shadow. It is also referred to as the edge gradient. The focal spot size is a major controller of image resolution because it controls penumbra. The fact that the source of the x-ray photons is not a point source, although it is sometimes convenient to think of it as such, is what causes penumbra. Figures

80 kVp	10 mAs	40" **SID**
8:1 **grid**	400 **RS**	57.3 **mR**

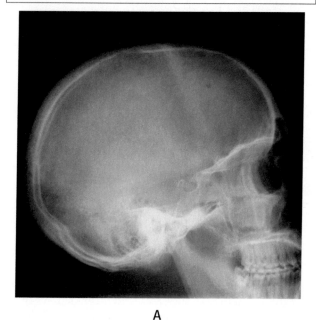

A

80 kVp	10 mAs	40" **SID**
8:1 **grid**	400 **RS**	57.3 **mR**

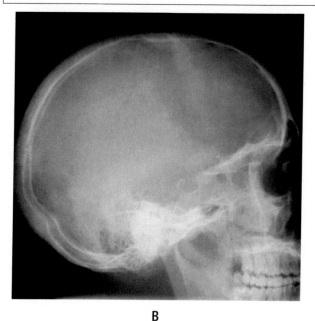

B

FIGURE 27-7. (A) 7 cm OID (OFD); (B) 14 cm OID (OFD)

27–8A and B illustrate the umbra and penumbra caused by the focal spot size and configuration. As the focal spot decreases in size, penumbra also decreases, thus increasing resolution. Focal spots are usually not capable of imaging structures smaller than the focal spots themselves.

The width of the penumbra (unsharpness) can be mathematically calculated using the following formula:

$$P = \frac{\text{Focal Spot Size} \times \text{OID}}{\text{SOD}}$$

Example: Calculate the penumbra for an image taken with a 1.0 mm focal spot, at a 40" distance and an OID of 3".

Answer:

$$P = \frac{\text{Focal Spot Size} \times \text{OID}}{\text{SOD}}$$

If the SID is 40" and the OID is 3", then the SOD = 40"– 3" = 37".

$$P = \frac{1.0 \times 3"}{37} = \frac{3}{37} = 0.08 \text{ mm}$$

Example: Calculate the penumbra for an image taken with a 2.0 mm focal spot, at a 40" distance and an OID of 3".

Answer:

$$P = \frac{\text{Focal Spot Size} \times \text{OID}}{\text{SOD}}$$

If the SID is 40" and the OID is 3", then the SOD = 40" – 3" = 37".

$$P = \frac{2.0 \times 3"}{37} = \frac{6}{37} = 0.16 \text{ mm}$$

Example: Calculate the penumbra for an image taken with a 1.0 mm focal spot, at a 40" distance and an OID of 8".

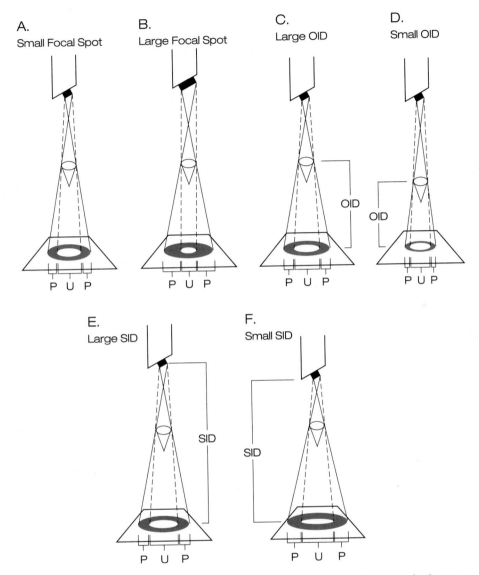

FIGURE 27-8. Umbra and penumbra. The umbral area receives essentially no photons. The penumbral area receives more photons at the outer edges with progressively fewer photons toward the umbral area, thus creating an imperfect, unsharp shadow around the umbra. (A and B) The effect of focal-spot size on resolution as focal-spot size decreases. (C and D) The effect of object-to-image receptor distance (OID) on resolution. As the OID decreases, penumbra is reduced and resolution increases. (E and F) The effect of source-to-image distance (SID) on resolution. As SID increases, penumbra is reduced and resolution increases.

Answer:

$$P = \frac{Focal\ Spot\ Size \times OID}{SOD}$$

If the SID is 40" and the OID is 8", then the SOD = 40" − 8" = 32".

$$P = \frac{1.0 \times 8"}{32} = \frac{8}{32} = 0.25\ mm$$

Example: Calculate the penumbra for an image taken with a 1.0 mm focal spot, at a 72" distance and an OID of 3".

Answer:

$$P = \frac{\text{Focal Spot Size} \times \text{OID}}{\text{SOD}}$$

If the SID is 72" and the OID is 3", then the SOD = 72" − 3" = 69".

$$P = \frac{1.0 \times 3"}{69} = \frac{3}{69} = 0.04 \text{ mm}$$

From these examples, it is evident that penumbra decreases when the focal spot decreases, when the OID decreases and when the SID increases.

Figures 27–8C and D illustrate that as OID decreases, penumbra also decreases. Figures 27–8E and F illustrate that as SID increases, penumbra decreases. When penumbra decreases, resolution is increased.

Penumbra is increased by another phenomenon known as attenuation or absorption unsharpness. Because of the divergence of the incident x-ray beam, only an object that is trapezoidal would have a perfectly sharp edge (Figure 27–9A). A trapezoidal object would have a relatively equal object thickness that would attenuate the beam, causing an equal proportion of the beam to reach the image. A square object would project an edge with a gradually increasing attenuation (Figure 27–9B). Circular objects, which predominate in the human body, have an attenuation that varies throughout the entire object, reaching a maximum at a single point (Figure 27–9C). Consequently, the attenuation of the object itself causes a continuously varying projected density, which, when added to the penumbra, causes structures in the human body to have gradual instead of sharp abrupt edges.

Film/Screen Combinations

Film/screen combinations are most commonly classified by speed. Within a single phosphor type, there is an inverse relationship between film/screen combination speed and resolution. In other words, a slow film/screen combination will demonstrate better resolution than a fast one. This is such a definite relationship that many slow film/screen combinations are labeled as detail combinations.

Once the geometrical considerations of recorded detail have been maximized, the most common source of better resolution is the film/screen combination. Most institutions utilize at least two different film/screen combinations in recognition of the better detail required by extremity examinations. This policy permits higher speed film/screens to be used to reduce patient dose for other examinations that do not require such high resolution.

Film   Although various types of film have a wide variety of resolving capabilities, in radiography the intensifying screen always has poorer resolution than the film. Radiographic film usually has resolving capabilities in the range of 100 lp/mm, far beyond the ability of any screen or human eye. As long as the film is sensitive to the light emitted by the screens, film speed and resolution are not important issues in radiographic imaging.

Although obsolete due to excessive patient dose, non-screen or direct exposure film possesses the highest resolution possible. Direct exposure film often required 20–100 times the mAs of a film/screen exposure.

Adjustment of film speed is seldom considered for resolution purposes. However, when a decision is made to use a higher resolution intensifying screen, its slower speed may be somewhat compensated for by using a higher speed film to help reduce patient dose.

Intensifying Screens   The resolving power of an intensifying screen depends on three factors: **phosphor size, phosphor layer thickness and phosphor concentration**. The relationship of these factors to recorded detail, patient dose and density are shown in Table 27–1. As phosphor size and layer thickness decrease, resolution increases along with patient dose; however, increasing phosphor concentrations will result in an intensifying screen that is better able to record details while reducing patient dose. Overall, as intensifying screen speed is decreased, there is a gain in resolution but patient dose must be increased. This creates a classical confrontation in radiography that pits recorded detail against patient dose. The decision is often left to the radiographer, who must consider all elements of both sides of the issue. Detail speed screens can resolve about 15 lp/mm, regular speed screens about 10 lp/mm, and high speed screens about 7 lp/mm. These differences in recorded detail are easily visualized (Figure 23–3).

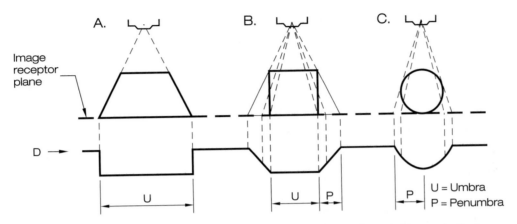

FIGURE 27-9. Attenuation unsharpness. The D line represents the amount of density that would occur in the image receptor under each object. (A) A trapezoidal object shaped congruent to the divergence of the beam. (B) A square object produces density shadings that form the penumbra. (C) A round object produces a penumbra that is incorporated into the continuously varying density of the shape itself.

Recall that because of their higher conversion efficiency, rare-earth phosphors have significantly better resolving abilities than similar speed calcium tungstate screens.

Quantum mottle is a phenomenon that may dramatically affect recorded detail when high speed intensifying screens are used with extremely low mAs. Modern intensifying screen technology is so advanced that it is now possible to obtain screens that are so sensitive that suffi-cient radiographic density can be achieved at extremely low mAs. If the total number of incident photons reaching the intensifying screen are insufficient to activate enough phosphors to emit light to cover the entire surface of the film, quantum mottle results (Figure 22–6). When using diagnostic radiographic intensifying screens, quantum mottle is corrected **only** by increasing mAs.

When resolution is unsatisfactory and the geometric solutions have been exhausted, a higher resolution film/screen combination should be used. It is important to remember that this decision includes a significant increase in patient dose. Conversely, if resolution is more than satisfactory for the examination, a lower resolution film/screen combination should be considered to reduce patient dose.

TABLE 27–1. Effects Of Intensifying Screen Factors On Resolution

Phosphor Change	Effect on Image Resolution	Effect on Patient Dose	Effect on Density
Phosphor size			
increases	decreases	decreases	increases
decreases	increases	increases	decreases
Layer thickness			
increases	decreases	decreases	increases
decreases	increases	increases	decreases
Phosphor concentration (Packing density)			
increases	increases	decreases	increases
decreases	decreases	increases	decreases

Film/Screen Contact The radiographic film and intensifying screens are sandwiched together in the cassette by pressure pads that keep them in immediate direct contact with one another. When the film/screen contact is broken, even over a small area of the cassette, the image detail is not as sharp because of increased penumbra (Figure 22–5).

The only adjustment for poor film/screen contact is repairing or discarding the cassette. The procedures for testing cassettes for film/screen contact are part of a quality control program.

Motion

Motion affects recorded detail because it fails to permit enough time for a well-defined image to form. Instead, the image is spread over a linear distance and appears as a blurred series of densities in which no fine detail can be perceived.

Voluntary Motion
Voluntary motion is that which is under the direct control of the patient. For the most part, this comprises the voluntary nervous system in cognizant adults (children and incognizant adults may be excepted in some cases). For **all** patients, including children and incognizant adults, **communication**, especially in a manner that establishes a professional and competent atmosphere, is the best method of controlling voluntary motion. There are a few examinations, such as most headwork, where immobilization greatly decreases the potential need for a repeated exposure.

For most examinations, when the radiographer effectively communicates positioning instructions, the patient is able to cooperate in reducing motion. Instructions must be given in a kindly and concerned manner. They must be in an understandable language, which includes avoiding medical terminology when appropriate, using proper pronunciation of foreign language instructions, at a proper volume and properly enunciated. Even infants and incognizant adults will respond to a kindly tone of voice and gentle handling. Never assume that your patient is unable to understand your instructions. Many young children can be amazingly cooperative when they wish to be and incognizant adults will often remember fragments of conversations when they regain full cognizance.

Involuntary Motion
Involuntary motion is not under the conscious control of the patient. For the most part, involuntary motion is controlled by the involuntary nervous system and is physiological in nature. Heartbeat and peristalsis are the most common examples. Involuntary motion can be best reduced by decreasing exposure time.

Equipment Motion
Although often overlooked, motion of equipment can also be an occasional problem. If the movement of the reciprocating grid mechanism is not dampened, it can cause vibration of the cassette in the Bucky tray. If the x-ray tube suspension system is not bal-

anced and isolated from other moving devices, especially overhead suspended units, it can vibrate or drift. This type of motion is extremely difficult to detect. It is usually suspected only when a variety of patients examined with the same x-ray unit appear to have motion problems.

Communication
The best method of reducing motion is patient communication. It is assumed that appropriate aids to positioning, such as foam pads, angle sponges and sandbags, are already in use. The radiographer should consider the instructions that are given to be sure that they are clear, concise and understandable.

Exposure Time Reduction
When the patient is unable to cooperate, the best method is a reduction in exposure time with a corresponding increase in mA to maintain sufficient mAs and density. Involuntary motion can be best reduced by a reduction in exposure time. Other methods of decreasing exposure time while maintaining density include using higher speed film and screens, decreasing SID and increasing kVp. Increasing kVp is not a preferred method because of the accompanying contrast change. Table 27–2 summarizes the pros and cons of each method.

Immobilization
When communication and exposure time reduction are not sufficient to reduce motion, partial immobilization must be considered. Immobilization devices, such as foam pads, angle sponges and sandbags, should be considered routine positioning aids. Patient motion can be expected when these aids are not provided. If students find it uncomfortable or difficult to hold radiographic positions during laboratory positioning practice, imagine how an ill patient who is in pain (most likely lying on the most acute area) must feel. The use of positioning aids is part

TABLE 27–2. Effects Of Various Methods For Reducing Exposure Time To Avoid Motion

Method	Density	Contrast	Resolution	Distortion
mA increase	maintains	maintains	maintains	maintains
kVp increase	maintains	decreases	maintains	maintains
Film/screen speed increase	maintains	maintains	decreases	maintains
SID decrease	maintains	maintains	decreases	increases

of professionalism. Even when they are in short supply, the radiographer should try to locate the proper aids for the patient.

For some examinations, especially headwork, immobilization greatly reduces the potential need for repeated exposures and should be used routinely. A wide range of immobilization devices and techniques have been developed over the years; some are available commercially while others are homemade.

Experienced radiographers often say that tape is the radiographer's best friend. Tape should certainly be carried at all times by radiographers and used freely when warranted. A strip of tape across the forehead (folded sticky side out across skin surfaces) has avoided many repeated cranial exposures.

Some devices, especially in pediatrics, are designed to immobilize the entire body. Pediatric boards, mummy wrapping techniques, Pig-O-Stats™ and compression bands are common examples. Individual parts can usually be immobilized with combinations of tape, sandbags, long-handled paddles, compression bands and sheet wrapping. As a **last** resort, human immobilizers may be used to hold the patient in position. Male relatives are the first choice, female relatives second, then nonradiology hospital personnel and nonprofessional radiology personnel. Radiographers are the last choice. Under no circumstances should anyone be expected to routinely hold patients.

Summary

Recorded detail is one of the two geometric properties of radiographic image quality. Unlike the photographic properties of density and contrast, which control the visibility of detail, the geometric properties control detail itself. Recorded detail is the degree of geometric sharpness or accuracy of the structural lines actually recorded in the radiographic image. Good detail exists even when it cannot be seen due to poor visibility of detail or, in other words, when the density and/or contrast are poor.

Recorded detail is also referred to as definition, sharpness, resolution, or simply as detail. When the term detail is used by itself, it usually refers to the recorded detail of the radiographic image. Detail is easily quantified and even has a derived unit. The term resolution is

applied to quantified discussions of recorded detail. The unit of resolution is line pairs per millimeter (lp/mm) or cycles per mm.

The factors that affect recorded detail are geometry, including SID, OID and focal spot size; film/screen combinations, including film, intensifying screens and film/screen contact; and motion.

When the factors that affect recorded detail are altered, some change in the recorded detail will occur. No effect will occur unless one of these factors is altered. Table 27–3 illustrates the effect on recorded detail when the various factors are changed.

REVIEW QUESTIONS

1. What is recorded detail?
2. How is resolution measured?
3. How do the SID and the OID affect recorded detail?
4. What is the relationship between focal spot size and recorded detail?

TABLE 27–3. Effect Of Changing Factors On Recorded Detail

+	= increases recorded detail (resolution)
−	= decreases recorded detail (resolution)

Geometry
+ Increasing SID
− Decreasing SID
− Increasing OID
+ Decreasing OID
− Increasing patient thickness
+ Decreasing patient thickness
− Increasing focal-spot size
+ Decreasing focal-spot size

Film/Screen Combination
− Increasing film/screen speed
+ Decreasing film/screen speed
+ Good film/screen contact
− Poor film/screen contact

Motion
− Increasing motion
+ Decreasing motion

5. What is the difference between umbra and penumbra?

6. What three factors affect the resolving power of intensifying screens?

7. What is the difference between voluntary and involuntary motion?

8. What are the methods which can be used to reduce the possibility of motion?

REFERENCES AND RECOMMENDED READING

American Registry of Radiologic Technologists. (1987). Use of 'penumbra' studied. *Radiologic Technology. 58*(1), 74.

Ball, J. & Price, T. (1989). *Chesneys' radiographic imaging.* Oxford: Blackwell Scientific Publishing.

Bushong, S. C. (1997). *Radiologic science for technologists: Physics, biology, and protection* (6th ed.). St. Louis: C.V. Mosby.

Cahoon, J. B. (1961). Radiographic technique: Its origin, concept, practical application and evaluation of radiation dosage. *The X-Ray Technician. 32*, 354–364.

Carroll, Q. B. (1993). *Evaluating radiographs.* Springfield, IL: Charles C. Thomas Publishers.

Carroll, Q. B. (1993). *Fuchs's radiographic exposure, processing, and quality control* (5th ed.). Springfield, IL: Charles C. Thomas Publishers.

Crooks, H. E. (1973). Some aspects of radiographic quality with special reference to image sharpness. *Radiography. 39*(468), 317–327.

Cullinan, A. & Cullinan, J. (1994). *Producing quality radiographs* (2nd ed.). Philadelphia: J. B. Lippincott.

Eastman Kodak Company. (1980). Health Sciences Markets Division. *The Fundamentals of Radiography* (12th ed.). Rochester, NY: Kodak Publication M1-18.

Eastman Kodak Company. (1977). *Image insight 1: The quality image.* Rochester, NY: Eastman Kodak Company, Publication M3-182.

Eastman Kodak Company. (1977). *Image insight 2: Geometry of image formation: Detail.* Rochester, NY: Eastman Kodak Company, Publication M3-184.

Eastman, T. R. *The radiographic technique guide.* Wilmington, DE: DuPont deNemours, Inc. Photo Products Department Publication A-99101.

Engel, T. L. (1979). Effect of kilovoltage and milliamperage on focal spot size. *Radiologic Technology. 50*(5), 559–561.

Files, G. W. (1952). *Medical radiographic technique.* Springfield, IL: Charles C. Thomas Publishers.

Files, G. W. (1935). Maximum tissue differentiation. *The X-Ray Technician. 7*, 17–24+.

Fodor, J. & Malott, J. C. (1993). *The Art and Science of Medical Radiography* (7th ed.). St. Louis: C. V. Mosby.

Fuchs, A. W. (1958). *Principles of radiographic exposure and processing.* Springfield, Illinois: Charles C. Thomas Publishers.

Fuchs, A. W. (1950). The rationale of radiographic exposure. *The X-Ray Technician. 22*, 62-68, 76.

Fuchs, A. W. (1940). Balance in the radiographic image. *The X-Ray Technician. 12*(3), 81–84, 118.

Geometrical fallacies. (1983). *Radiologic Technology. 54*(4), 297.

Godderidge, C. (1995). *Pediatric imaging.* Philadelphia: W. B. Saunders.

Hage, S. J. (1974). Modulation transfer function and film-screen combinations. *Applied Radiology.* (May/June).

Haus, A. G. (1985). Evaluation of image blur (unsharpness) in medical imaging. *Medical Radiography and Photography. 61*(1–2), 42–53.

Haus, A. G. (1980). Effects of geometric and screen-film unsharpness in conventional and 350 kVp chest radiography. *Radiology.* (Oct.), 197.

Hiss, S. S. (1993). *Understanding radiography* (3rd ed.). Springfield, IL: Charles C. Thomas Publishers.

Jenkins, D. (1980). *Radiographic photography and imaging processes.* Lancaster, England: MTP Press Limited.

Jerman, E. C. (1928). *Modern x-ray technic.* St. Paul: Bruce Publishing.

Lauer, O. G., Mayes, J. B., & Thurston, R. P. (1990). *Evaluating radiographic quality: The variables and their effects.* Mankato, MN: The Burnell Company Publishers.

Morgan, J. A. (1977). *The art and science of medical radiography* (5th ed.). St. Louis: Catholic Hospital Association.

Morgan, R. H. (1945). An analysis of the physical factors controlling the diagnostic quality of roentgen images: Part I. Introduction. *American Journal of Roentgenology and Radiation Therapy. 54*(2), 128–135.

Morgan, R. H. (1945). An analysis of the physical factors controlling the diagnostic quality of roentgen images: Part II. Maximum resolving power and resolution coefficient. *American Journal of Roentgenology and Radiation Therapy. 54*(4), 395–402.

Morgan, R. H. (1949). An analysis of the physical factors controlling the diagnostic quality of roentgen images: Part V. Unsharpness. *American Journal of Roentgenology and Radiation Therapy. 62*(6), 870–880.

Seeman, H. E. (1968). *Physical and photographic principles of medical radiography*. New York: Wiley & Sons.

Sparks, O. J. (1960). Possibilities and limitations of definition. *Radiologic Technology. 32*(2), 148.

Spiegler, G. (1950). The story of contrast and definition. *Radiography. 41*(189), 177–182.

Stears, J. G., Gray, J. E., & Frank, E. D. (1989). Radiologic exchange (resolution by focal spot size). *Radiologic Technology. 60*(5), 429–430.

Stockley, S. M. (1986). *A manual of radiographic equipment*. Edinburgh: Churchill Livingstone.

Sweeney, R. J. (1975). Some factors affecting image clarity and detail perception in the radiograph. *Radiologic Technology. 46*(6), 443.

Thompson, M. A., Hattaway, M. P., Hall, J. D., & Dowd, S. B. (1994). *Principles of imaging science and protection*. Philadelphia: W. B. Saunders.

Tortorici, M. (1992). *Concepts in medical radiographic imaging*. Philadelphia: W. B. Saunders.

United States War Department. (1941). *Technical manual: Roentgenographic technicians*, TM 8-240, July 3.

Wilks, R. J. (1981). *Principles of radiological physics*. Edinburgh: Churchill Livingstone.

CHAPTER 28

Distortion

Hans Castorp peered through the lighted window, peered into Joachim Ziemssen's empty skeleton. The breastbone and spine fell together in a single dark column. The frontal structure of the ribs was cut across by the paler structure of the back. Above, the collar-bones branched off on both sides, and the framework of the shoulder, with the joint and beginning of Joachim's arm, showed sharp and bare through the soft envelope of flesh. The thoracic cavity was light, but blood-vessels were to be seen, some dark spots, a blackish shadow.

Thomas Mann, Der Zauberberg (The Magic Mountain).

Objectives

Upon completion of this chapter, the student should be able to:

▶ Define size and shape distortion.

▶ Explain the effects of SID and OID on image distortion.

▶ Discuss various methods of minimizing distortion through variation of SID and OID.

▶ Explain why elongation and foreshortening are relational definitions.

▶ Describe the routine relationships between central ray, anatomical part and image receptor.

▶ Explain the proper terms used to describe angulation direction and degree.

▶ Differentiate distorted images from routine projections.

▶ Calculate the magnification factor when given SID and SOD.

▶ Calculate the actual size of an object when given the projected size, SID and OID.

▶ Describe adjustments of SID and OID that will minimize magnification.

▶ Describe adjustments of central ray, anatomical part and image receptor that will minimize shape distortion.

Assessing Distortion

*D*istortion is the second of the two geometric properties affecting radiographic image quality. Unlike
the photographic properties of density and contrast,
which control the visibility of detail, the geometric properties control detail itself. **Distortion is a misrepresentation of the size or shape of the structures being examined.** It creates a misrepresentation of the size and/or
shape of the anatomical part being imaged. This misrepresentation can be classified as either size or shape distortion. Distortion, like detail, exists even when it cannot be
seen due to poor visibility or, in other words, when the
density and/or contrast are poor. The evaluation and
adjustment of distortion require a thorough familiarity
with normal radiographic anatomy. Unless the normal
size and shape of a structure are known, comparison of
the size and shape cannot be accomplished. Distortion
can be difficult to determine even when normal sizes and
shapes are known. Because the objective of radiography is
to provide accurate images of structures, methods of minimizing distortion are important to diagnosis.

The factors that control distortion are shown in
Figure 28–1. Careful examination of these factors will
reveal that distortion is directly related to positioning.
Only careful attention to the distances, direction and
angulation between the anatomical part, central ray and
image receptor can minimize distortion.

Factors Affecting Size Distortion

Size distortion can be only magnification in radiography. Radiographic minification is impossible, due to the
divergent property of x-ray photons. Since it is not possible to reflect or refract x-ray photons by ordinary methods, they can only diverge from their point source. Thus,
only magnification is possible and all size distortion is
controlled by the radiographic distances, SID (FFD) and
OID (OFD). In all instances, **reduced magnification
size distortion increases the resolution of recorded
detail.** Therefore, the objective in most radiography is to
minimize magnification as much as possible.
Magnification radiography is an exception to this rule.
In this instance, the principles of magnification geometry are used to increase the size of structures that are too
small to be easily visualized. Special conditions must be
created to achieve diagnostically acceptable magnification images.

Magnification size distortion is controlled by positioning the body part and tube to maximize SID while
minimizing OID. This can be accomplished by various
procedures and by positioning. For example, an upright
oblique cervical vertebra projection can be performed at
72" (180 cm) while a supine projection is performed at
40" (100 cm). An AP chest may place the heart 6" (15
cm) from the film while a PA projection would place it
2" (5 cm) away.

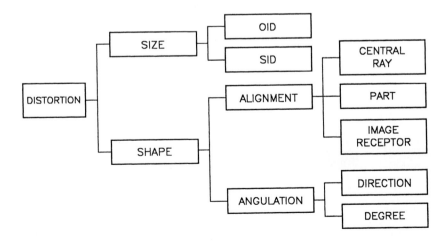

FIGURE 28-1. Radiographic image quality: factors affecting distortion.

Source-to-Image Receptor Distance

The SID has a major effect on magnification (Figure 28–2). **The greater the SID, the smaller the magnification**, because as SID increases the percentage of the total distance that makes up OID decreases. The OID is the critical distance for magnification and resolution.

Although 40" (100 cm) has developed as the current routine SID, this was not always so. The popular SID has been increasing since the advent of radiography and will probably continue to do so. The first x-ray techniques book in the U.S. is generally recognized to be the 1918 *Extract from the United States Army X-Ray Manual*, in which 20" (50 cm) is discussed as a reasonable SID. When Ed Jerman developed the first positioning and technique book, *Modern X-Ray Technic*, in 1928, he recommended distances varying from 25" (63 cm) to 36" (90 cm). Of course, in those days shorter distances were necessary because the x-ray tubes were not capable of

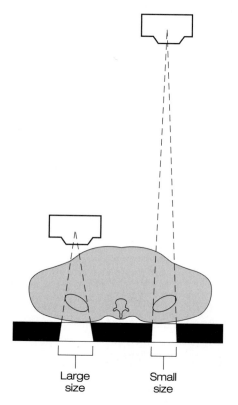

FIGURE 28-2. The effect of SID on image size magnification. Magnification size distortion is minimized by increasing SID.

Large size   Small size

handling the load required to provide sufficient density with the film and screens of the time. As generator technology advanced, the SID increased.

Glenn Files' 1945 book, *Medical Radiographic Technic*, established the 40" (100 cm) SID. For over 40 years this has remained the standard distance, but now there are institutions that use 48" (120 cm) as a routine distance and the movement appears to be growing. Although a change demands new grids as well as careful consideration of x-ray unit design so that tube-to-tabletop distances can be achieved, and low table design so that radiographers can reach the tube, the increased resolution is worth the expense and trouble.

For many, many years chest radiography has routinely been performed at 72" (180 cm) because the erect positioning arrangement permits a horizontal beam to be used and the increased SID effectively minimizes the magnification of the heart shadow. Any examination that permits a horizontal beam to be used can easily be established at an SID greater than 40" (100 cm), and in many places the lateral cervical vertebral examination is performed at 72" (180 cm) as well.

The source-to-object distance (SOD) is seldom discussed because it is included in descriptions of SID and OID, which are more critical. The SID is the distance that must be established by the radiographer when positioning.

The SID must be maximized to decrease magnification. Examinations of body parts with large inherent OID, such as the lateral cervical vertebra and the chest, use large SID whenever possible. In addition, the historical trend to increase the routine SID should be continued.

Object-to-Image Receptor Distance

The OID is also a critical distance in both magnification and resolution. Figure 28–3 illustrates two major facets of OID. First, when objects within a structure are at different levels (Figure 28–3, objects A and B) they will be projected onto the image as different sizes. This is similar to the manner in which the eye processes information for depth perception; smaller objects are perceived as more distant and larger objects as closer.

The radiographer should develop a stereoscopic perception of the radiographic image, which is difficult because radiographic perceptions are in reverse of the normal information the eye is accustomed to processing. This is because objects that are further from the image receptor will be magnified. For example, in a chest radiograph the ribs are seen as wider as they become more posterior. This effect should make them appear closer, which is the opposite of the truth for the PA projection. Nevertheless, the perception of three-dimensionality can be developed and then used to determine object-to-image receptor distance visually. When describing objects, it is important to remember that the size and distance relationship in a radiographically projected image is the opposite of that perceived visually.

A more important size relationship that is controlled by OID is shown in Figure 28–3 between objects B and C, where object C appears identical in size to object B. This is an illusion because object C is much smaller but is magnified more because of its location in the part. This illustrates that a thorough knowledge of normal radiographic anatomy is a prerequisite to making judgements about size relationships. This is also one of the reasons radiographic examinations must include two projections, as close to 90° from one another as possible.

When AP and lateral projections cannot be performed because of superimposing structures, as in an examination of the kidneys, it is important to include two oblique projections at 90° to one another. The two 90° opposing images can be used to verify the positional relationship of structures. This is also a shape distortion issue.

The OID is also important in dosimetry because it establishes the source-to-entrance skin distance that is the benchmark maximum exposure to the patient. Because OID varies with the part size and position of the patient, it accounts for the increased exposure that is part of many examinations. For example, there is a significant difference in the OID between an AP and a lateral projection (Figure 28–4). Note that the SOD changes dramatically in the figure as well. Obviously the entrance skin exposure would be greater with the lateral, even if the same exposure factors were used. Consequently, larger patients receive a greater exposure simply because their entrance skin surface is closer to the source, making their SOD much less. The increased mAs that is often used to provide sufficient density then increases the exposure even more.

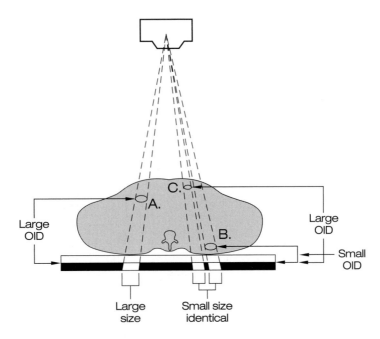

FIGURE 28-3. The effect of OID on image size magnification. Objects A and B are identical in size but their images as projected on the receptor are of significantly different sizes. Object C is significantly smaller than B, yet the image sizes are identical because of C's greater OID.

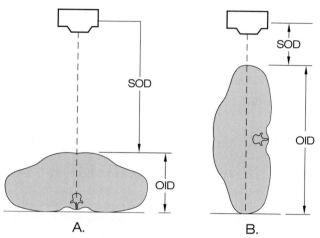

FIGURE 28-4. Variation in OID with size and projection. (A) Short OID, large SOD, low entrance skin exposure. (B) Large OID, short SOD, high entrance skin exposure.

The OID must be minimized to decrease magnification. Examinations of body parts with large inherent OID, such as the kidneys and chest, use positioning techniques to achieve as small an OID as possible.

Calculating Size Distortion

Size distortion is present in any radiographic image and can be measured very accurately by using simple geometry. **Magnification, or size distortion, can be assessed by calculation of the magnification factor.** The magnification factor is the degree of magnification and is calculated by:

$$M = \frac{SID}{SOD}$$

where M = magnification factor

The mnemonic device shown can be used (see discussion of Ohm's law in Chapter 3).

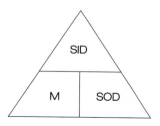

Example: If the SID is 40" (100 cm) and the SOD is 30" (75 cm), what is the magnification factor?

Answer:

$$M = \frac{SID}{SOD}$$

$$M = \frac{40"}{30"} \text{ or } M = \frac{100 \text{ cm}}{75 \text{ cm}}$$

$$M = 1.33$$

The magnification will be 33 percent or the image will be 133 percent of the object size.

Example: If the SID is 40" and the OID is 2", what is the magnification factor?

Answer: Since the SOD is not supplied, it must be found by using the formula:

$$SID = SOD + OID$$
$$40" = SOD + 2"$$
$$SOD = 40" - 2"$$
$$SOD = 38"$$

then

$$M = \frac{SID}{SOD}$$

$$M = \frac{40"}{38"}$$

$$M = 1.05$$

The magnification factor permits calculation of the actual size of an object that is projected as an image by using the formula:

$$O = \frac{I}{M}$$

where O = object size
  I = image size
  M = magnification factor

The following mnemonic device can be used.

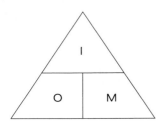

Example: If a projected image measures 5" and the magnification factor is 1.02, what is the size of the actual object?

Answer:

$$O = \frac{I}{M}$$

$$O = \frac{5"}{1.02}$$

$$O = 4.9"$$

Example: If object B in Figure 28–3 is 2" in diameter on the image and is measured to be 3" from the film (by using a lateral projection), what is its actual size if the SID is 40"?

Answer: Since the SOD is not supplied, it must be found by using the formula:

$$SID = SOD + OID$$
$$40" = SOD + 3"$$
$$SOD = 40" - 3"$$
$$SOD = 37"$$

then

$$M = \frac{SID}{SOD}$$

$$M = \frac{40"}{37"}$$

$$M = 1.08$$

then

$$O = \frac{I}{M}$$

$$O = \frac{2}{1.08}$$

$$O = 1.85"$$

If the image size and the object size are known, the percent of magnification can be determined using the following formula:

$$\frac{I - O}{O} \times 100 = \text{percent of magnification of the object}$$

Example: If an object measures 5 cm and the image measures 6 cm, what would be the percent magnification of the object?

Answer:

$$\frac{I - O}{O} \times 100 = \text{percent magnification of the object}$$

$$\frac{6 - 5}{5} \times 100 = \text{percent magnification of the object}$$

$$\frac{1}{5} \times 100 = \text{percent magnification of the object}$$

$$0.2 \times 100 = 20 \text{ percent of magnification of the object}$$

The magnification formula assumes that the focal spot is a point source. Because it is not, when the object size approaches the effective focal spot size or smaller, special problems develop from penumbral overlap (Figure 28–5). Therefore, **objects smaller than the effective focal spot cannot be demonstrated** and the magnification formula must be modified to consider the width of the focal spot.

Factors Affecting Shape Distortion

Shape distortion is the misrepresentation by unequal magnification of the actual shape of the structure being

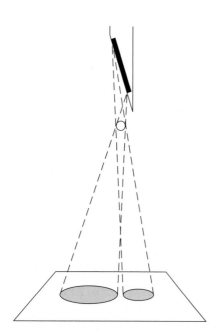

FIGURE 28-5. Objects smaller than the focal spot itself cannot be imaged due to penumbral overlap. The entire image is composed of overlapping penumbra with no umbra to define the edges.

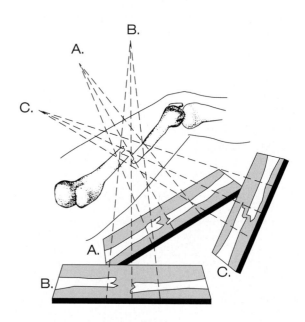

FIGURE 28-6. Shape distortion due to unequal magnification. Note how the alignment of the part appears different depending on the degree of distortion. *(Adapted with permission from Cullinan, Angeline M.,* Producing Quality Radiographs, *copyright 1987 by J. B. Lippincott, Philadelphia, PA)*

examined (Figure 28–6). Shape distortion displaces the projected image of an object from its actual position and can be described as either elongation or foreshortening. **Elongation** projects the object so it appears to be longer than it really is while **foreshortening** projects it so it appears shorter than it really is. Elongation occurs when the tube or the image receptor is improperly aligned. Foreshortening occurs only when the part is improperly aligned. Changes in the tube angle cause elongation, never foreshortening.

Shape distortion often results because structures lie normally at different levels within the body. Shape distortion also occurs because of the divergence of the x-ray beam. The projected length varies, depending on the angle between the object and the diverging beam (Figure 28–7).

Adjustment of shape distortion requires careful consideration of the beam-part-film geometry involved in the projection. This information must be combined with a knowledge of the normal projection of the structures to determine exactly how improvements can be achieved.

Alignment

Shape distortion can be caused or avoided by careful alignment of the central ray with the anatomical part and the image receptor. Proper positioning is achieved when the central ray is at right angles to the anatomical part and to the image receptor. This means the part and the image receptor must be parallel. When the position of the body part or object within the body does not permit this alignment, creative positioning must be utilized. The half-axial 30° angulation of the cranium to demonstrate the occipital bone, the 25° cephalad angulation of the pelvis to demonstrate the sigmoid colon, and the 10° caudad angulation of the coccyx, are all examples of routine procedures that were developed to minimize distortion.

Alignment adjustments involve bringing the tube central ray, the part and the film back into their correct relationship — part and film parallel to one another with the central ray perpendicular to both. Incorrect centering may occur from off-centering the tube (misalign-

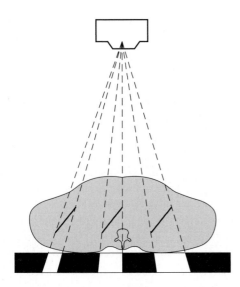

FIGURE 28-7. Shape distortion due to the angle between the object and the diverging beam. Although all three objects are at the same angle to the image receptor, the project length varies according to the angle between the object and the diverging beam.

ment of the central ray), incorrectly positioning the part or off-centering the film (Figure 28–8).

Central Ray

The central ray is the theoretical photon that exits from the exact center of the focal spot. Ideally the central ray is intended to be projected **perpendicular to both the anatomical part and the image**

receptor. Whenever the central ray is not perpendicular, some degree of shape distortion will result. This occurs in every image because only the central ray is truly perpendicular. Any structure that is not positioned at the central ray will be distorted because of the divergence of the beam—**the farther from the central ray, the greater the distortion**. This applies as distance from the central ray increases transversely as well as longitudinally. For example, an AP pelvis will have more distortion of an object near the right greater trochanter than an object near the symphysis pubis. This is why it is so important to position according to standardized central ray locations.

Long bone length studies are an example of a procedure developed to ensure accurate central ray centering. The procedure shown in Figure 28–9 uses a radiopaque ruler, positioned from above the hip joint to below the ankle joint, as a measurement control. Spot films of the critical joints — hip, knee and ankle — are then made with the central ray perpendicular to the joint space to ensure accurate measurement.

Centering away from the specified central ray entrance point is equivalent to angling the tube away from perpendicular because the entire perspective of the anatomical part is distorted. Some projections take advantage of this type of distortion. For example, a PA lumbar projection uses the divergence of the beam to open the lordotically curved intervertebral joints (Figure 28–10).

The central ray is normally positioned perpendicular to the anatomical part and to the image receptor. When

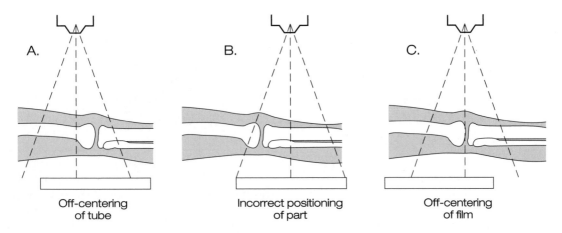

A.

Off-centering of tube

B.

Incorrect positioning of part

C.

Off-centering of film

FIGURE 28-8. Incorrect centering.

the part is superimposed over other structures, central ray angulation can be a useful tool to provide a projection that would otherwise be impossible to differentiate from overlying structures. The use of the semiaxial AP

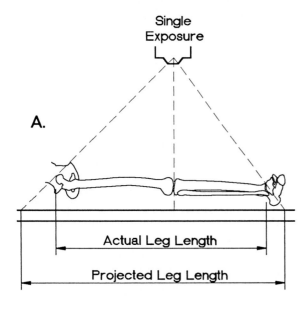

A.

Actual Leg Length

Projected Leg Length

B.

Actual Leg Length

Projected Leg Length

FIGURE 28-9. A long bone leg length study. Exact central ray location is critical to ensuring an accurate measurement of the bone lengths. (A) Inaccurate leg lengths due to beam divergence at the joints from a single exposure. (B) Accurate leg lengths with three spot exposures, each perpendicular to a joint.

projection of the skull to project the occipital region free of facial bone superimposition is an example. Failure to maintain the correct relationship between the part and the image receptor will produce a projected image that may not be comparable to norms and is therefore useless in the diagnostic process.

Anatomical Part The long axis of the anatomical part, or object, is intended to be positioned perpendicular to the central ray and parallel to the image receptor. When these positions are incorrect, distortion may occur. Elongation occurs when there is poor alignment of the tube and/or image receptor. Foreshortening occurs only when there is poor alignment of the part (Figure 28–11). Figure 28–11A shows the intended relationships of central ray, part and film. In Figure 28–11B the entire

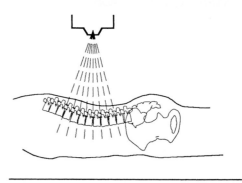

A. PA Projection

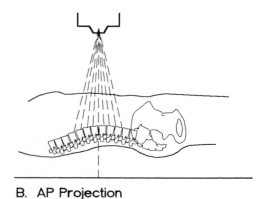

B. AP Projection

FIGURE 28-10. Divergence of the beam used to advantage. The lordotic curvature of the lumbar spine and the divergence of the beam can be used to open the intervertebral joints in a PA projection.

object is foreshortened because of the improper part-to-image receptor relationship. In addition to the entire object being foreshortened, one end is more magnified due to increased OID, which indicates that size distortion is also occurring.

In Figure 28–11C the entire object is again foreshortened with one end being more magnified due to increased OID. However, because of the differences in the actual size of the two ends, the increased size distortion of the smaller end makes both ends appear the same size.

Note especially the vast differences in the projected images of these anatomical part relationships. Figure 28–11A projects an accurate image. Figure 28–11B projects distortion of both size and shape so the entire object is foreshortened and the large end appears larger than it really is. Figure 28–11C also projects distortion of both size and shape but has distorted the relationship so both ends appear the same size.

The anatomical part is normally positioned with its long axis perpendicular to the central ray and parallel to the image receptor. As with the central ray, some routine

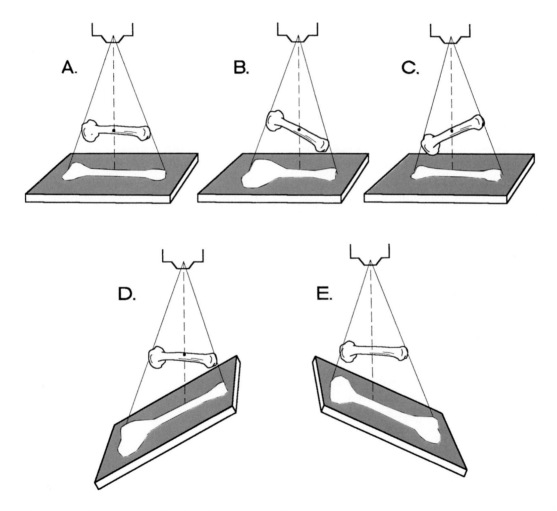

FIGURE 28-11. Foreshortening and magnification due to anatomical part and image receptor alignment. (A) Normal relationship between part and image receptor. (B and C) Foreshortening and magnification due to changes in anatomical part alignment. (D and E) Elongation and magnification due to changes in part/image receptor and central ray/image receptor alignment.

projections are designed to vary from this standard to avoid superimposition. Failure to maintain the specified relationships between the central ray and the image receptor can result in an image that is not comparable to norms and therefore of limited value in the diagnostic process.

Image Receptor   The image receptor, usually a radiographic film cassette, is intended to be positioned perpendicular to the central ray and parallel to the anatomical part. As long as the film plane is parallel to the object, the only result of off-centering of the image receptor is the clipping of a portion of the area of interest. Although this will usually result in a repeated exposure, there is no distortion of image size or shape.

However, when the film plane is not parallel to the object, or if the central ray is not centered to the part, serious shape distortion results exactly as if the object were not parallel. Figures 28–11D and E illustrate for the image receptor the same examples shown for the object in Figures 28–11B and C above.

The image receptor, or film plane, is normally positioned perpendicular to the central ray and parallel to the anatomical part. Even in routine projections designed to vary from this standard, the specified relationships must be maintained to obtain a useful diagnostic image.

Angulation

Angulation refers to the direction and degree the tube is moved from its normal position perpendicular to the image receptor. Numerous radiographic projections utilize angulation to avoid superimposition of parts. The semiaxial AP projection of the cranium, tangential os calcis and axial clavicle are all examples.

The angulation of the tube is designed to cause a controlled or expected amount of shape distortion to avoid superimposition. As long as the specified angulation is applied, the image is comparable to norms and is of diagnostic quality. Angulation of the tube also changes the SID, which, unless compensated for by a new SID, will produce a decrease in density.

Direction

The most common direction of tube angle is longitudinal. Longitudinal angulations are usually termed

cephalad when the tube is angled toward the head of the patient, and **caudad** when it is angled toward the patient's feet. Some radiographic tubes can also be angled transversely (sometimes referred to as "roll"). Transverse angulations are usually identified as right and left (in reference to the patient).

The direction of the tube angle is specified according to patient position and must be maintained as specified. When the patient position is reversed, the direction of tube angle must also be reversed to maintain the relationship. For example, 25° cephalad for an AP projection is identical to 25° caudad for a PA projection.

Degree   Degree is simply a method of describing the exact amount of angulation **and is usually stated as the angle between the central ray and the film plane from the standard reference point of perpendicularity**. Because the standard reference point is 90° from the patient's head, radiographic angles must be added or subtracted from that point. For example, 5° cephalad is 5° from perpendicular as is 5° caudad. It is important to maintain the correct degree of angle specified for a given procedure. Tube angulations also change SID, which will produce changes in magnification. Table 28–1 provides conversions for common tube angulations.

TABLE 28–1. SID Compensations For Common Tube Angulations

Tube Angulation	Overhead Scale	True SID
5°	39.8"	40"
10°	39.4"	40"
15°	38.6"	40"
20°	37.6"	40"
25°	36.2"	40"
30°	34.6"	40"
35°	32.8"	40"

From Robert J. English, *Radiologic Technology* 52:3, 304, 1980 by permission of the American Society of Radiologic Technologists.

Evaluating Shape Distortion

Shape distortion is a more subjective evaluation than size. It is much more difficult to assess because there is no effect that can be calculated, as in the magnification factor for size distortion. Instead, the entire assessment relies on the radiographer's knowledge of normal anatomy and the normal projected images for each position.

Effect on Image Appearance

Size

Size distortion is simply a matter of magnification (Figure 28–12). All magnification involves a degree of loss of resolution, even when special systems are designed to minimize the loss.

Shape

Shape distortion involves both elongation and foreshortening and is a serious alteration in the projected image (Figure 28–13). There are situations where shape distortion can be used to advantage, as in a tangential os calcis.

Summary

Distortion is the second of the two geometric properties affecting radiographic image quality. Unlike the photographic properties of density and contrast, which control the visibility of detail, the geometric properties control detail itself. Distortion is the difference between the structures being examined and the recorded image. It creates a misrepresentation of the size and/or shape of

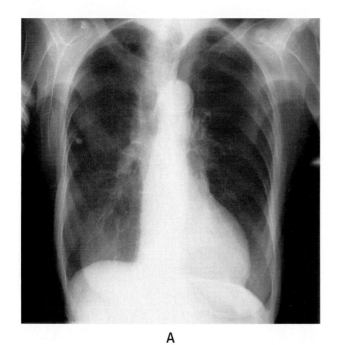

A

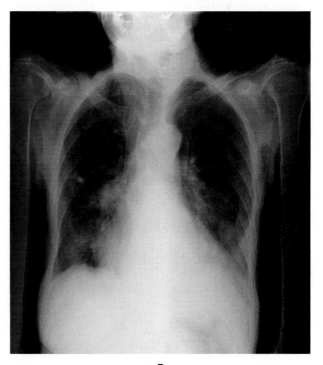

B

FIGURE 28-12. Magnification size distortion. (A) Minimal heart size magnification in a PA chest. (B) An AP projection of the same patient demonstrating greater heart size magnification. *(Courtesy of Tracy Thegze, RT(R), Community Hospital, Munster, IN)*

60 kVp	15 mAs	72" SID
No grid	100 RS	11.9 mR

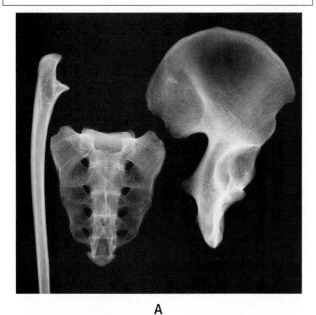

A

60 kVp	15 mAs	72" SID
No grid	100 RS	11.9 mR

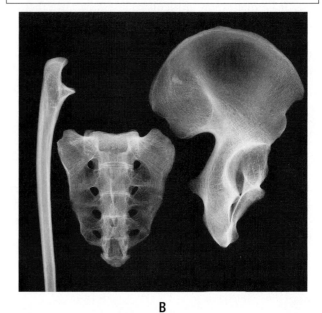

B

FIGURE 28-13. Shape distortion. (A) This radiograph was taken with the central ray perpendicular and centered to the center of the film. (B) This radiograph was taken with the central ray perpendicular but off center to the left (away from the pelvis). The effect on distortion is not significant; however, changes in the image appearance are evident, particularly when studying the pelvis, which was furthest from the central ray. (C) This radiograph was taken with a central ray angle of 25 degrees and centered to the center of the film. Notice the significant distortion created by angling the central ray.

60 kVp	15 mAs	72" SID
No grid	100 RS	11.9 mR

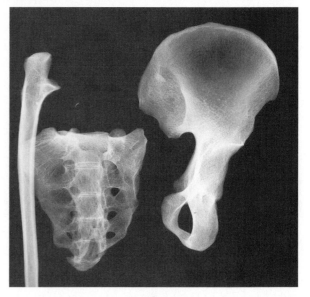

C

the anatomical part being imaged. This misrepresentation can be classified as either size or shape distortion. Distortion, like detail, exists even when it cannot be seen due to poor visibility or, in other words, when the density and/or contrast are poor. The evaluation and adjustment of distortion require a thorough familiarity with normal radiographic anatomy. Unless the normal size and shape of a structure are known, comparisons of size and shape cannot be accomplished.

When the factors that affect size and shape distortion are altered, some change in distortion will occur. No change will occur unless one of these factors is altered. Table 28–2 illustrates the effect on distortion when the various factors are changed.

REVIEW QUESTIONS

1. What is distortion?

2. What is the difference between size and shape distortion?

3. How do the SID and the OID affect size distortion?

4. What is the magnification factor formula?

5. What is the difference between elongation and foreshortening?

6. How does the alignment of the anatomical part affect shape distortion?

7. How do the direction and degree of angulation affect shape distortion?

8. How can shape distortion be used to advantage?

REFERENCES AND RECOMMENDED READING

Ball, J. & Price, T. (1989). *Chesneys' radiographic imaging.* Oxford: Blackwell Scientific Publishing.

Bushong, S. C. (1997). *Radiologic science for technologists: Physics, biology, and protection* (6th ed.). St. Louis: C. V. Mosby.

Cahoon, J. B. (1961). Radiographic technique: Its origin, concept, practical application and evaluation of radiation dosage. *The X-Ray Technician. 32,* 354–364.

TABLE 28–2. Effect of Changing Factors on Distortion

+	= increases distortion
−	= decreases distortion

Size Distortion
− Increasing SID
+ Decreasing SID
+ Increasing OID
− Decreasing OID
+ Increasing patient thickness
− Decreasing patient thickness

Shape Distortion
+ Improper central ray alignment
+ Improper anatomical part alignment
+ Improper image receptor alignment
+ Improper direction of central ray angle
+ Improper degree of central ray angle

Carroll, Q. B. (1993). *Evaluating radiographs.* Springfield, IL: Charles C. Thomas Publishers.

Carroll, Q. B. (1993). *Fuchs's radiographic exposure, processing, and quality control* (5th ed.). Springfield, IL: Charles C. Thomas Publishers.

Cullinan, A. & Cullinan, J. (1994). *Producing quality radiographs* (2nd ed.). Philadelphia: J. B. Lippincott.

Distance — technique relationship of angulated projections. (1980). *Radiologic Technology. 52*(3), 301.

Distortion in imaging. (1989). *Radiography Today. 55*(628), 31.

Eastman Kodak Company. (1977). *Image insight 2: Geometry of image formation: Detail.* Rochester, NY: Eastman Kodak Company, Publication M3-184.

English, R. J. (1980). Distance-technique relationship of angulated projections. *Radiologic Technology. 52*(3), 301–304.

Files, G. W. (1952). *Medical radiographic technique.* Springfield, IL: Charles C. Thomas Publishers.

Haus, A. G. (1985). Evaluation of image blur (unsharpness) in medical imaging. *Medical Radiography and Photography. 61*(1–2), 42–53.

Haus, A. G. (1980). Effects of geometric and screen-film unsharpness in conventional and 350 kVp chest radiography. *Radiology.* (Oct.), 197.

Hiss, S. S. (1993). *Understanding radiography* (3rd ed.). Springfield, IL: Charles C. Thomas Publishers.

Jenkins, D. (1980). *Radiographic photography and imaging processes.* Lancaster, England: MTP Press Limited.

Jerman, E. C. (1928). *Modern x-ray technic.* St. Paul: Bruce Publishing.

Lauer, O. G., Mayes, J. B., & Thurston, R. P. (1990). *Evaluating radiographic quality: The variables and their effects.* Mankato, MN: The Burnell Company Publishers.

Morgan, J. A. (1977). *The art and science of medical radiography* (5th ed.). St. Louis: Catholic Hospital Association.

Morgan, R. H. (1945). An analysis of the physical factors controlling the diagnostic quality of roentgen images: Part I. Introduction. *American Journal of Roentgenology and Radiation Therapy. 54*(2), 128–135.

Morgan, R. H. (1945). An analysis of the physical factors controlling the diagnostic quality of roentgen images: Part II. Maximum resolving power and resolution coefficient. *American Journal of Roentgenology and Radiation Therapy. 54*(4), 395–402.

Morgan, R. H. (1949). An analysis of the physical factors controlling the diagnostic quality of roentgen images: Part V. Unsharpness. *American Journal of Roentgenology and Radiation Therapy. 62*(6), 870–880.

Pearson, G. R. (1951). Radiographic projection studies. *Radiologic Technology. 23*(1), 1.

Petersen, T. D. & Rohr, W. (1987). Improved assessment of lower extremity alignment using new roentgenographic techniques. *Clinical Orthopaedics. 219*, 112–119.

Riles, G. W. (1943). *Medical roentgenographic technique.* Springfield, IL: Charles C. Thomas Publishers.

Seeman, H. E. (1968). *Physical and photographic principles of medical radiography.* New York: Wiley & Sons.

Stockley, S. M. (1986). *A manual of radiographic equipment.* Edinburgh: Churchill Livingstone.

Tarrant, R. M. (1952). Maintaining desired anode-film distance and alignment after angling the x-ray tube. *Radiologic Technology. 23*(5), 349.

Thompson, M. A., Hattaway, M. P., Hall, J. D., & Dowd, S. B. (1994). *Principles of imaging science and protection.* Philadelphia: W. B. Saunders.

Tortorici, M. (1992). *Concepts in medical radiographic imaging.* Philadelphia: W. B. Saunders.

United States War Department. (1941). *Technical manual: Roentgenographic technicians,* TM 8–240, July 3.

Wilks, R. J. (1981). *Principles of radiological physics.* Edinburgh: Churchill Livingstone.

CHAPTER 29

The Art of Film Critique

If all the factors involved in the making of a . . . radiograph are known, it then becomes a simple matter, by means of . . . (a) method of analysis, to decide what may be done to improve the quality of that radiograph.

Ed. C. Jerman, The Father of Radiologic Technology.

OBJECTIVES

Upon completion of this chapter, the student should be able to:

▶ Discuss the elements of a diagnostic image as they relate to the art of film critique.

▶ Identify the steps of the decision making process.

▶ Describe an effective film critique method, incorporating critical problem solving skills.

▶ Use an effective film critique method.

▶ Explain the differences between technical factor problems, procedural factor problems and equipment malfunctions.

▶ Apply an effective film critique method to a wide range of problems specific to clinical situations beyond those presented in this chapter.

Implementing Imaging Standards

Radiographers are required to make critical decisions every day about the quality of their radiographic images. Critiquing an image is a very complex process which requires a thorough knowledge of all aspects of radiography. Deciding if an image is acceptable or unacceptable should be approached in a logical, organized manner. Film critique is an analytical process that involves many of the steps of diagnostic decision making, including critical problem solving.

The Diagnostic Image

The art of film critique revolves around the concept of deciding exactly where in the diagnostic quality spectrum a particular radiographic image lies. A practical technical definition of a diagnostic quality image has never been established because the artistic elements involved to produce the required medical information vary so much from one situation to another. The exponential number of variables involved make radiography as much an art as a science.

The production of a diagnostic image involves an overwhelming number of variables, including such elements as patient anatomy, pathological conditions, radiographic positioning, patient preparation, radiation protection, x-ray equipment, prime technical factor selections, collimation, film/screen combinations, film processing, density and contrast perceptions, detail and distortion. In other words, nearly all of the elements of anatomy, positioning, physics and principles of exposure are involved. **The art of film critique is the application of scientific knowledge to an analysis of the image.**

The Analytical Process

It is important to remember that not even radiologists are trained in the finer points of creating and analyzing the quality of a radiographic image. The radiographer is the expert and has the responsibility of proceeding with image analysis. Only with an acceptable image can a radiologist make an accurate diagnosis. It is the radiographer's professional responsibility to create the best possible image given each individual circumstance.

To determine whether an image is of diagnostic quality, the steps of an analytical decision making process must be followed.

The process begins with a review of the entire image. This is essential to avoid premature narrowing. During the review the radiographer watches for anything that is different from a diagnostic quality image. When differences are noticed, a pattern is sought, especially when there is more than one cue. Cues and patterns focus attention on a suspicious area, thus narrowing the search. Cues and patterns are then used to seek hypotheses. An effort is made to formulate a hypothesis that will explain all the cues. Cues that do not fit the hypothesis are held in reserve. The hypothesis is then tested by guided information seeking, with general questioning to produce more cue information. The last step is an evaluation of the final hypothesis. The hypothesis attempts to resolve the greatest number of cues and patterns.

There are myriad factors that can affect the quality of a radiographic image and these factors can act upon each other to create an astronomical number of possible imaging problems. A film critique system uses the diagnostic problem solving process to critically think through the problem and help resolve the situation.

Identifying An Imaging Problem

The identification of an imaging problem requires the use of a full range of radiographic expertise. The radiographer must first recall that the purpose of the radiographic image is to provide information about the medical condition of the patient. The information needed may vary greatly, depending on the suspected medical problem and the anatomical region to be examined. For example, alignment of a nail during a hip-pinning operation requires a type of information different from that needed for detection of a small blood vessel constriction during cerebral angiography.

The meaning of the expression "diagnostic quality image" is quite different in these two cases. The hip pinning requires two images at right angles to one another as fast as possible with a major consideration being patient dose. The cerebral angiograph requires maximum visibility of detail and resolution from a high speed exposure with less consideration of patient dose. Any definition of a diagnostic quality image must consider the clinical situation while providing a good balance between visibility of detail (density and contrast) and the geometry of the image (recorded detail or distortion).

The primary problem encountered by radiographers in successfully critiquing images is the tendency to glance at radiographs instead of critically evaluating them for image quality. The professional approaches each image as a window in the diagnostic process.

In her introductory text for radiologists, *Fundamentals of Radiology,* Dr. Lucy Frank Squire emphasizes to aspiring radiologists that, "While the single-glance approach has its value, it is full of danger to the patient, because the presence of a very obvious abnormality tends to suppress psychologically your search for more subtle changes." She suggests that students utilize a systematic approach to evaluating radiographs, primarily by looking at various structures in a deliberate order, concentrating on each structure while excluding the superimposed shadows of other structures. Radiographers should adopt an identical process by looking at each technical and procedural factor in a systematic fashion before jumping to any "glancing" conclusions.

An Effective Film Critique Method

An effective film critique method is a three-step process involving:

1. **the classification of the image,**

2. **the determination of the cause of the problem and**

3. **the recommendation of corrective action** (Figure 29–1).

This approach is designed to provide the radiographer with an organized and systematic protocol for critiquing a radiograph. When consistently used, the system will be found to be a thorough and dependable method for establishing and maintaining professional skills at the very highest level of competence. The form in Figure 29–2 illustrates the application of this film critique method.

Classification of the Image

The first step in classifying the image is to evaluate it to determine if it is within the diagnostic acceptance limits. If the image is within the acceptance limits it should be critically examined to determine if it is of **optimal** diagnostic quality. If it is satisfactory in every respect, the pride of professional competence is the radiographer's reward. If the image is within acceptance limits but not of optimal diagnostic quality, the radiographer should continue the critique to refine his or her technical skills. Although the radiograph may be submitted for diagnosis, a continued critique provides an opportunity to improve the quality of care for future patients.

If the film is outside the acceptance limits, a continued critique is mandatory prior to attempting to repeat the exposure. Failure to continue the critique is ethically unacceptable for a radiographer because it subjects the patient to additional radiation exposure without ascertaining how to produce an acceptable image.

Determination of the Cause of the Problem

The actual diagnostic problem solving begins with determination of the cause of the unacceptable or suboptimal image. In most instances there is more than one cause and this can complicate the problem solving process immensely. Searching for cues or patterns is primarily a matter of clinical experience. It is best to slowly narrow the search process by first trying to classify the problem into one of three major categories:

1. **a technical factor problem,**

2. **a procedural factor problem or**

3. **an equipment malfunction problem.**

All of these categories are then further subdivided in an effort to determine the exact cause of the problem.

Technical Factor Problems
Technical factor problems can be arranged into two categories: **a photographic problem with visibility of detail or a geometric problem with detail.** (Of course, some images will have problems with both visibility of detail and detail.) The photographic problems concern maintaining sufficient density and contrast to make the detail of the image vis-

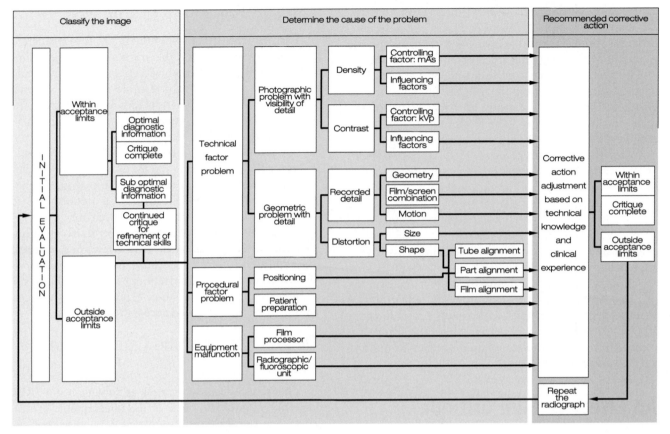

FIGURE 29-1. An effective film critique method.

ible. Even with good detail present, anatomical structures cannot be visualized unless appropriate density and contrast are also present. An image that appears totally black may still possess good detail; it is simply beyond the ability of the human eye to discern it. Geometric problems directly concern the production of detail (also called definition, sharpness and resolution). (See Unit IV, Radiographic Image Quality Flow Chart, p. 358.)

Photographic problems with visibility of detail are further classified as **density** or **contrast** problems. Density problems may be the result of the mAs selection and/or a variety of other influencing factors, including the film/screen combination, the selected kVp level, distance, grid selection, beam restriction, a pathology problem, etc. Contrast problems are the result of the kVp selection and/or a variety of influencing factors, including field size, patient thickness, grid selection, etc.

Geometric problems with detail are further classified as **recorded detail** or **distortion** problems. Recorded detail problems are the result of the geometry of the beam (focal spot size, SID or OID), the film/screen combination, and/or patient motion. Distortion is further classified as size distortion (magnification) or shape distortion. Size distortion problems are the result of SID or OID. Shape distortion problems are the result of improper tube, part and/or film alignment.

Procedural Factor Problems

A procedural factor problem can be classified as one that involves **patient positioning** or **patient preparation** for the x-ray examination. Proper patient positioning results when the part, the film and the tube (central ray) are correctly aligned with one another. The result is an image which demonstrates the anatomical structures of interest from the

FILM CRITIQUE FORM

I. CLASSIFY THE RADIOGRAPHIC IMAGE AS:
☐ **WITHIN ACCEPTANCE LIMITS**
    ☐ Optimal diagnostic information (critique is complete)
    <u>(all checkmarks below this line require completion of section II and III)</u>
    ☐ Suboptimal diagnostic information
☐ **OUTSIDE ACCEPTANCE LIMITS**

II. DETERMINE THE CAUSE OF THE PROBLEM AS:
☐   **A:**   **Technical Factors**
    ☐ Photographic problem with visibility of detail
        ☐ Density
            ☐ mAs_____
            ☐ Influencing factor (specify) _____
        ☐ Contrast
            ☐ kVp _____
            ☐ Influencing factor (specify) _____
    ☐ Geometric problem with detail
        ☐ Recorded detail
            ☐ Geometry (specify) _____
            ☐ Film/Screen combination (specify) _____
            ☐ Motion _____
        ☐ Distortion
            ☐ Size (Magnification) (specify) _____
            ☐ Shape (Part/Film/Tube Alignment) (specify) _____
☐   **B:**   **Procedural Factors**
    ☐ Patient Positioning
        ☐ Tube Alignment _____
        ☐ Part Alignment _____
        ☐ Film Alignment _____
    ☐ Patient Preparation (specify) _____
☐   **C:**   **Equipment Malfunction**
    ☐ Processing Equipment (specify) _____
    ☐ Radiographic/Fluoroscopic Equipment (specify) _____

III. RECOMMENDED CORRECTIVE ACTION For each cause specified above:
_____
_____
_____

FIGURE 29-2. Form used for film critique.

proper perspective. Of course, a thorough knowledge of the anatomy being visualized for a given radiographic procedure is essential to determine if the positioning is accurate. When studying an image for accuracy in positioning, three alignment factors should be reviewed separately:

1. the tube alignment,
2. the part alignment and
3. the film alignment.

The second procedural factor problem involves preparation of the patient for the examination. Proper patient preparation includes removing radiopaque objects from the area of interest (i.e., jewelry, safety pins, etc.), proper bowel cleansing for a gastrointestinal study, recording a thorough history, communicating clear instructions to the patient, etc.

Equipment Malfunction

The last major category in the classification of the causes of an imaging problem is equipment malfunction. While the technical and procedural factors may have been correctly determined, a problem can still result when the equipment being used for the examination does not function properly. Problems normally occur with the processing equipment or with the radiographic/fluoroscopic equipment. These problems can be kept to a minimum through an effective quality control program.

Recommendation of Corrective Action

Each identified cause requires an appropriate corrective action that will resolve the problem. Corrective action adjustments are based on knowledge and clinical experience. Clinical experience is gained through careful attention to problems and successes. Remember that clinical knowledge is gained by critiquing acceptable but suboptimal images, analyzing repeated images and recording successful results.

It is recommended that radiographers purchase or make a personal technique system booklet that can be easily carried while performing clinical examinations. This booklet should record appropriate technical factors, including the specific tube used (by room number or location), kVp, mAs, distance, grid, the relative speed of the film/screen combination, anatomical projection, part

thickness and any other variable factors (adjustable filtration, focal spot size, etc.). By using a personal technique system booklet, the radiographer has a quick reference for establishing the technical and procedural factors for a specific examination. Additionally, this guide can be useful for determining accurate adjustments in order to correct a problem.

Applying The Film Critique Method

Figure 29–3 illustrates how to use the film critique method that has been outlined. The radiograph in Figure 29–3A is classified as an image which is outside the acceptance limits of image quality. To determine the cause of this problem, the entire image should be studied for technical and procedural accuracy as well as for potential equipment malfunction problems.

From this review, it is determined that the image exhibits a technical factor problem and a procedural problem, but no apparent equipment problem. Further searching narrows the technical factor problem to a photographic problem of visibility of detail and the procedural problem to patient positioning. This narrowing is based on observations that the image is too dark and that not all of the anatomical structures of interest are demonstrated on the film. These two cues narrow the search by eliminating geometric problems of detail, patient preparation and equipment malfunction as probable causes. Once suspected problem areas are defined, the cues and patterns should be used to form a hypothesis about the probable cause of the problem.

The photographic problem of visibility of detail can be further narrowed to a density problem. The possible causes of excessive density are then reviewed to determine the most likely cause. Although too much mAs is the most common cause, a number of secondary factors, such as the film/screen combination, the grid selection and the kVp level, need to be considered and checked to test the hypothesis. This is a necessary part of evaluating the hypothesis.

Next, the procedural problem should be reviewed to determine the most likely cause. The problem is first narrowed to a patient positioning problem and then to an alignment problem.

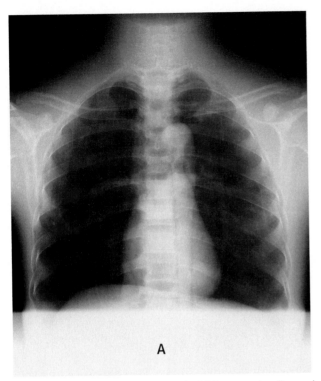
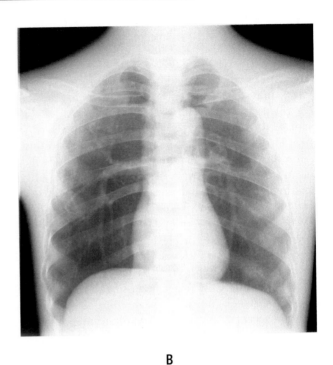

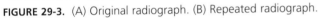
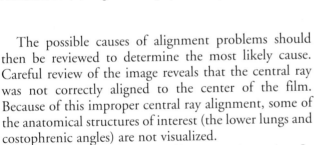

FIGURE 29-3. (A) Original radiograph. (B) Repeated radiograph.

The possible causes of alignment problems should then be reviewed to determine the most likely cause. Careful review of the image reveals that the central ray was not correctly aligned to the center of the film. Because of this improper central ray alignment, some of the anatomical structures of interest (the lower lungs and costophrenic angles) are not visualized.

The final step is recommending corrective action. In the example, the corrective action involves changes in technical factor selection and patient positioning. The mAs is reduced by one-half the original amount to correct the density problem and the central ray is properly aligned to the midline of the film. Figure 29–3B illustrates the result after these adjustments were made.

A thorough understanding of the concepts involved in producing an acceptable diagnostic quality image is important. Because of the large number of variables in the imaging process, acceptable images will not always result from the initial exposure. Even the best of radiographers will be required to repeat radiographs because of the vast number of variables. By applying a systematic film critique method, radiographers are practicing one of the most complex skills of the profession. This analytical and effective film critique method will help to ensure the best possible patient care by minimizing the need to repeat an exposure.

Summary

Critiquing an image is a very complex process which requires a thorough knowledge of all aspects of radiography. Deciding if an image is acceptable or unacceptable should be approached in a logical, organized manner. Film critiquing is an analytical process that involves many of the steps involved in diagnostic decision making, including critical problem solving.

To determine whether an image is of diagnostic quality, the steps of an analytical decision making process must be followed.

The process begins with a review of the entire image to avoid premature narrowing. When differences are noticed, a pattern is sought, especially when there is more than one cue. Cues and patterns focus attention on a suspicious area, thus narrowing the search. Cues and patterns are then used to seek hypotheses. An effort is made to formulate a hypothesis that will explain all the cues. The hypothesis is then tested by guided information seeking, with general questioning to produce more cue information. The last step is an evaluation of the final hypothesis. The hypothesis attempts to resolve the greatest number of cues and patterns.

An effective film critique method is a three-step process involving: 1) the classification of the image, 2) the determination of the cause of the problem and 3) the recommendation of corrective action.

In the first step, the image is classified to determine if it is within the diagnostic acceptance limits. If the image is within acceptance limits but not of optimal diagnostic quality, the radiographer should continue the critique to refine his or her technical skills. If the film is outside the acceptance limits, a continued critique is mandatory prior to attempting to repeat the exposure.

The actual diagnostic problem solving begins with determination of the cause of the unacceptable or sub-optimal image. Searching for cues or patterns is primarily a matter of clinical experience. It is best to slowly narrow the search process by first trying to classify the problem into one of three major categories: 1) a technical factor problem, 2) a procedural factor problem or 3) an equipment malfunction problem.

Each identified cause requires an appropriate corrective action that will resolve the problem. Corrective action adjustments are based on knowledge and clinical experience. Clinical experience is gained through careful attention to problems and successes.

Even the best of radiographers will be required to repeat radiographs. Using an effective film critique method will help to assure the best possible patient care by minimizing the need to repeat an exposure.

REVIEW QUESTIONS

1. What is the purpose of film critique?

2. During the analytical process of critiquing a radiograph, how are cues and patterns used?

3. What are the three steps in an effective film critique method?

4. What are the three classifications of imaging problems?

5. What are the two categories of technical factor problems?

6. A necklace is seen on a chest radiograph. What type of imaging problem would this be?

7. A film is jammed in the processor and destroyed. What type of imaging problem would this be?

8. How does a radiographer determine the appropriate corrective action for an imaging problem?

REFERENCES AND RECOMMENDED READING

Adler, A. M. & Carlton, R. R. (1990). Perceiving the radiographic image. *Postgraduate Advances in Radiologic Technology*. Berryville, VA: Forum Medicum.

Adler, A. M. & Carlton, R. R. (1989). Repeating radiographs: Critiquing the image. *Postgraduate Advances in Radiologic Technology*. Berryville, VA: Forum Medicum.

Carlton, R. R. (1992). Another dimension of quality assurance in radiology. *Introduction to Radiologic Technology* (3rd ed.). Editors: Gurley, L. T. & Callaway, W. J. St. Louis: C. V. Mosby, 149–166.

Carlton, R. R. & McKenna, A. (1989). Repeating radiographs: Setting imaging standards. *Postgraduate Advances in Radiologic Technology*. Berryville, VA: Forum Medicum.

Carnevali, D. L., Mitchell, P. H., Woods, N. F., & Tanner, C. A. (1984). *Diagnostic reasoning in nursing*. Philadelphia: J. B. Lippincott.

Carroll, Q. B. (1993). *Evaluating radiographs*. Springfield, IL: Charles C. Thomas Publishers.

Cullinan, A. & Cullinan, J. (1994). *Producing quality radiographs* (2nd ed.). Philadelphia: J. B. Lippincott.

Cullinan, J. E. (1981). A 'perfect' chest radiograph — or a compromise? *Radiologic Technology. 53*(2), 121.

Dowd, S. B. (1995). *Encyclopedia of radiographic positioning.* Philadelphia: W. B. Saunders.

Goldman, L. W. (1977). Effects of film processing variability on patient dose and image quality. *Second Image Receptor Conference: Radiographic Film Processing: Proceedings of a Conference held in Washington, D.C., March 31 - April 2, 1977.* Rockville, MD: U.S. Department of Health, Education, and Welfare, Public Health Service, Food and Drug Administration, Bureau of Radiological Health, HEW Publication (FDA) 77-8036, 55–63.

Hiss, S. S. (1993). *Understanding radiography* (3rd ed.). Springfield, IL: Charles C. Thomas Publishers.

Jerman, E. C. (1926). An analysis of the end-result: The radiograph. *Radiology. 6*, 59–62.

Lauer, O. G., Mayes, J. B., & Thurston, R. P. (1990). *Evaluating radiographic quality: The variables and their effects.* Mankato, MN: The Burnell Company Publishers.

Singer, B. H. (1971). The aesthetic method in radiographic exposure. *Radiologic Technology. 42*(6), 411.

Squire, L. F. & Novelline, R. A. (1988). *Fundamentals of radiology* (4th ed.). Cambridge: Harvard University Press.

CHAPTER 30

Quality Management

. . . a quality assurance program maximizes the likelihood that the images will consistently provide adequate diagnostic information for the least possible radiation exposure and cost to the patient.

William R. Hendee and Raymond P. Rossi,
Quality Assurance for Radiographic X-Ray Units and Associated Equipment.

OBJECTIVES

Upon completion of this chapter, the student should be able to:

▶ Define quality assurance and control and discuss their relationship to excellence in radiography.

▶ Describe the process of identifying imaging requirements, developing equipment specifications, selecting equipment, installing and testing equipment, and training the technical staff.

▶ Describe the objectives and responsibilities of monitoring equipment performance.

▶ Discuss primary automatic film processor quality control monitoring and maintenance procedures.

▶ Discuss primary quality control tests for external radiation beam monitoring of diagnostic radiographic systems, fluoroscopic systems, tomographic systems and automatic exposure controls.

▶ List primary quality control tests for miscellaneous ancillary equipment, including cassettes and view boxes.

▶ Explain the rationale behind the data collection process and the basic analysis of a radiographic repeat-rate study.

▶ Describe a basic troubleshooting procedure.

Quality Assurance and Quality Control

Regulation and Accreditation

*I*n the United States, the federal government initiated radiologic and imaging sciences quality management regulations after the Radiation Control and Safety Act of 1968. The 1981 Consumer-Patient Radiation Health and Safety Act added considerably to the scope of this effort as did the 1990 Safe Medical Devices Act (SMDA) and the 1992 Mammography Quality Standards Act (MQSA). Today these acts and others relating to radiologic and imaging sciences are developed and enforced by the Center for Devices and Radiological Health (CDRH), which is part of the Food and Drug Administration (FDA) under the Department of Health and Human Services (HHS).

Of the acts currently in place, the SMDA and MQSA have had the greatest impact on the practice of the radiologic and imaging sciences. SMDA mandates that any serious injury or death due to a medical device be reported. MQSA requires mammography facilities to be approved by the FDA.

There are also voluntary accreditation procedures available and they are used by the vast majority of hospitals in the United States. The largest hospital accreditation agency is the Joint Commission on the Accreditation of Healthcare Organizations (JCAHO). Their approval is linked to many medical activities, most importantly to reimbursement by the federal and state governments and many insurance companies. Accreditation agencies establish quality standards, assess them, and provide certification that individual institutions have met the agency's standards.

Although there are numerous quality measurement consultants, books, and process methods, one is worthy of remembering in all medical settings. The Hospital Corporation of America's FOCUS-PDCA method has gained great acceptance. It functions as shown in Table 30–1.

Quality management consists of a coherent system designed to monitor equipment performance through a variety of quality assurance and quality control standards or benchmarks.

TABLE 30–1. FOCUS-PDCA Method

Find and define a problem.
Organize a team to work on improvement.
Clarify the problem with current knowledge.
Understand the problem and its causes.
Select a method to improve the process.
Plan implementation.
Do the implementation and measure change.
Check the results.
Act to continue improvements.

Quality Assurance

Quality assurance consists of activities that provide adequate confidence that a radiology service will render consistently high quality images and services. It is an evolutionary process that assesses everything that affects patient care. It may be medically, technically or managerially oriented. Quality assurance includes evaluating activities such as interpretation of examinations, maintenance of equipment, performance of procedures, filing systems, staff development, scheduling of examinations and supply lines.

The quality assurance process operates by identifying problems or potential problem areas, monitoring the problem and then resolving it. Monitoring problems involves several steps, including establishing criteria, performing monitoring, and collecting, analyzing and evaluating data. It is these steps of the monitoring process that are of greatest concern to the quality assurance radiographer.

Quality Control

Quality control is the aspect of quality assurance that monitors technical equipment to maintain quality standards. The concept of quality control is rooted in the need to stabilize the various equipment components of the radiographic imaging chain. From incoming line current through x-ray production to the processing of the radiograph, erratic equipment performance causes repeat radiographs and unnecessary patient exposure to radiation. The term quality control is sometimes used to describe the evaluation of individual radiographs according to acceptance limits standards. It is probably better to think of this image evaluation process as film critiquing or quality checking rather than quality control, although the quality control process is certainly a critical part of the critique evaluation.

Technical expertise will not ensure success in radiography unless the equipment is reliable. Because radiographic equipment changes as it ages, there are often great differences between the results obtained on one unit and those obtained on another. The same unit cannot be counted on to produce exactly the same beam for the radiographer to control and analyze unless it is properly checked on a regular basis. The system of checks to accomplish a measure of consistency in beam output is the quality control.

Ensuring the quality of the radiographic image is a prime responsibility of the radiologic technologist. Every patient expects to receive the highest possible quality, or excellence, of service, from a medical facility. No one wants to be exposed to ionizing radiation by a radiographer incapable of producing excellent images.

It is important that quality control be seen as a method of controlling the radiographic image from start to finish. To do this requires a series of procedures (Figure 30–1). Unfortunately, some quality control begins with the last step instead of the first. An effective program cannot be achieved simply by monitoring equipment performance, although this is unquestionably the most involved step. The thought process preceding equipment purchase is critical.

Purchasing Equipment

Identification of Imaging Requirements

It is not always apparent exactly what type of equipment is needed when new purchases are being considered. Historically, this decision was made by the chief radiologist or administrative technologist. Rarely are the actual operators of the equipment, the radiographers, consulted. The result has been that nearly every x-ray department owns a radiological monstrosity that is avoided by radiographers and radiologists alike. These units are often inconvenient, overly sophisticated, or unable to produce quality images. Careful identification of imaging requirements can prevent these problems.

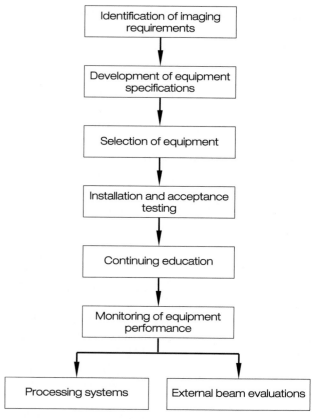

FIGURE 30-1. A total quality control system. *(Adapted from William R. Hendee and Raymond P. Rossi,* Quality Assurance for Radiographic X-Ray Units and Associated Equipment. *Rockville, MD: U.S. DHEW, PHS, FDA, Bureau of Radiological Health, HEW Publication FDA 79-8094, 1979)*

It is not necessary to be an expert in imaging physics and technology in order to be capable of contributing to the process of identifying the imaging requirements. Each member of the radiological team can contribute his or her expertise. The person who will make the final decision should interview the radiologists, administrators, supervisors and staff technologists who will use the equipment. In many instances the needs of the radiologist will determine the basic parameters for the purchase. Administrators must often impose financial and space restraints, although they can also create new funds and space when necessary. Supervisors are often able to provide important information on patient flow and staffing needs. After the radiologists, the radiographers are the most important persons to have input because their experiences with equipment provide a wealth of information.

Development of Equipment Specifications

Generic equipment specifications should be developed from the interview information. It is important that the person formulating the specifications have the technical background to state exactly what is needed to meet the imaging requirements. An imaging physicist should be involved at this point. The best specifications include detailed statements of what the equipment should be capable of doing. For example, "Maintain mA linearity within ±10 percent to produce equal film density when mAs is maintained but mA is varied." This must include a change from highest to lowest setting. When the specifications are complete they are sent to vendors for bidding.

Selection of Equipment

The actual selection of equipment becomes simple if the investigation into the first two steps has been thorough. When the bids arrive they can be compared for meeting specifications, cost and service. The actual decision is then academic. A pitfall in the process can occur when radiologists in the institution show a preference to a particular vendor, thus weakening the bargaining position of the department administrator. In many institutions this pitfall should be expanded to include interference by administrative officers unfamiliar with imaging equipment.

Installation and Acceptance Testing of Equipment

Installation and acceptance testing of equipment is the responsibility of the vendor and/or manufacturer. The quality control technologist must verify that the equipment specifications have been met. Normally this includes supervising the testing procedures and results. It is suggested that the exact methods for acceptance testing be included in the original specifications. The data from these tests will form the standard for all future quality control monitoring.

Continuing Education

It is normally the responsibility of the vendor to familiarize the users of the equipment with its proper operation. With simple equipment, such as ancillary devices, the equipment manual may be sufficient for use in inservice training. More complex equipment should be demonstrated and explained by the vendor **to at least two persons** as part of the purchase contract. Continuing education **must** be an ongoing procedure. It is advisable to include both the quality control and inservice education coordinators in the initial training demonstrations. A good inservice program will include an orientation procedure as well as periodic updates on all complex equipment.

Monitoring Equipment Performance

The final procedure of a total program is commonly considered to be the whole of quality control. Monitoring equipment performance includes routine checks of all radiographic equipment. Although they are interdependent, monitoring can be divided into two parts: (1) **film processing systems** and (2) **external beam evaluation**. Objectives for a performance monitoring system are to:

1. monitor the quality of the film processing systems,

2. measure the quality of the external radiation beams and

3. specify faults within these systems to allow corrective measures to be taken.

Evidence shows that a properly working quality control system will reduce equipment down-time and the number of repeated exposures. This will also reduce patient dose, patient waiting time, and supply costs, as well as increase confidence in diagnostic consultation and boost departmental morale.

Responsibility

Professional service personnel or medical physicists are not required to perform routine quality control procedures. Many procedures must be done daily, and to use these experts would be too costly. Radiographers, who are more available and knowledgeable about potential problems, should do the equipment monitoring. An initial cost outlay for testing equipment is required. To maintain a program, staff technologists must be given time to perform the procedures and to evaluate them.

Processor Monitoring

Processor monitoring is designed to permit an automatic film processor to fluctuate within set limits. These tests may be performed by anyone who has been oriented to the use of the equipment involved. Only a radiographer or processor maintenance person should perform the corrective actions.

Action must be taken to correct problems whenever the limits are exceeded. A quality control program that is not backed up by a commitment to shut down processors that are outside limits is of little value. Manufacturers' suggestions should be followed for the start-up and for the regular maintenance of the processor.

There are also several monitoring tests that should be done on a daily basis. These include a darkroom fog test, also known as a safelight test, and processor sensitometry to monitor speed, contrast and base fog of film. See Chapters 19, 20, and 21 for details.

External Beam Evaluation

The second part of performance monitoring involves the evaluation of the external primary radiation beam. These tests must be performed by a radiographer who has a knowledge of the physical operation of the equipment and all related accessories. Corrective action should be taken only by an authorized service person.

Some monitoring equipment can be made very inexpensively; other equipment must be purchased. A dosimeter is an essential piece of equipment and reasonable quality control cannot be performed without one. Computerized dosimeters are available that permit readouts and printouts of many quality control parameters from a single exposure. Figure 30–2 illustrates common quality control equipment. A room log should be kept to record test results, maintenance, and repairs performed on each x-ray tube and other system in each room.

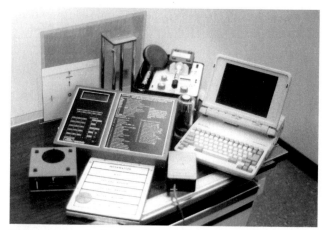

FIGURE 30-2. Radiographic quality control equipment. Clockwise from upper left: wire mesh film/screen contact tool, collimator accuracy tool, pinhole focal spot camera, digital dosimeter with computer, synchronous spinning top and penetrometer tool, and kVp test cassette with star pattern focal spot tool. In center: noninvasive beam evaluator (NERO™ computerized unit with ionization chamber) and resolution pattern focal spot test tool.

Diagnostic Radiographic Systems The tests that should be performed on diagnostic radiographic systems should be done on a **semi-annual** schedule. The tests for x-ray tubes should include:

Focal spot size estimation. An estimate of focal spot size is important so that it is kept within acceptable limits to ensure proper image detail. There are three types of focal spot test tools: line pair resolution tools, star test patterns, and pinhole cameras. Both line pair resolution tools and star test patterns function by imaging a resolution pattern on a film. The image can then be analyzed to estimate the focal spot size. A pinhole camera permits measurement of the focal spot by creating an image of the effective focal spot on a film (Figure 30–3).

The National Electrical Manufacturers Association (NEMA) specifies that focal spots of 0.3 mm and smaller may be measured with a star test pattern. Focal spots larger than 0.3 mm should be measured with a pinhole camera. In clinical quality control assurance testing a pinhole camera is avoided because it is difficult to use accurately and requires massive tube loading. A star test pattern will satisfactorily monitor focal spot size growth in most instances. When the focal spot grows to an unacceptable size, the x-ray tube must be replaced. NEMA

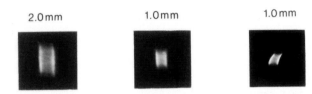

2.0 mm   1.0 mm   1.0 mm

FIGURE 30-3. Focal spot images produced on dental x-ray film with a pinhole camera. *(Courtesy of J. E. Gray and M. Trefler, Pinhole cameras: Artifacts, modifications, and recording of pinhole images on screen film systems.* Radiologic Technology *52:3, 277-282, 1980 by permission of the American Society of Radiologic Technologists from* Quality Control in Diagnostic Imaging, *Aspen Publishers, Inc., Rockville, MD, 1983 by permission of the Mayo Foundation)*

specifies that focal spots smaller than 0.8 mm may be 50 percent larger than the stated nominal size. Focal spots between 0.8 mm and 1.5 mm may be 40 percent larger than nominal and focal spots larger than 1.5 mm may be 30 percent larger than nominal. For example, a 0.5 mm focal spot may actually be 0.75 mm and still be considered acceptable.

Half-value layer. The amount of total filtration in the primary beam is important for both radiation protection and image quality. Radiation protection is assured by eliminating low-energy photons that are incapable of reaching the image receptor. Image quality is ensured by making appropriate contrast adjustments. Half-value layers are measured by using dosimetry equipment to detect the quality of aluminum filtration that will reduce the beam intensity to half the original value. Computerized quality control dosimeters provide a digital readout of the half-value layer. Half-value layer recommendations or requirements vary depending on the kVp. If insufficient filtration is present, the tube housing must be modified to supply additional aluminum filtration.

Collimator, central ray, and Bucky tray accuracy. The congruence of the projected centering light field and the central ray with the actual collimated primary x-ray beam and Bucky tray is of critical importance for radiation protection. Radiation protection is ensured by avoiding repeated radiographs due to over-collimation errors and by avoiding irradiation of tissue unless it will be imaged. A collimator test tool is simply a lead marker for each corner of the light beam plus cross-hairs or a

lead marker, placed several centimeters above the cassette surface, for the central ray. A 2 percent SID error is allowed between the primary-beam image and the light field size (this is a U.S. federal standard). The centering mark should be within 1 percent of the light field central ray. The positive beam limitation (PBL) mechanism should not permit the primary beam to be larger than the cassette in the Bucky tray unless the override lock is activated. When these margins of error are exceeded, the collimator light or PBL mechanism must be adjusted.

Distance and centering indicators' accuracy. Many older x-ray units have inaccurate distance indicators located on tube support stands or overhead readouts. In addition, both distance and centering locks, stops and detents may not be accurate. Assurance that distance and centering are accurate avoids the need for repeated exposures due to the inverse square law, misalignment of the central ray and primary beam collimation. Distance indicators should be checked with a tape measure (point zero should be measured from the focal spot, which is approximately 1 cm from the bottom of the tube housing end cap). Centering indicators can be checked by visual inspection of the collimator light beam (assuming a collimator and central ray accuracy test has been done). Distance indicators should be ±10 percent and centering indicators should be ±2 percent. If the indicators are not within these limits they should be adjusted.

Angulator or protractor accuracy. X-ray tables, Bucky units and tubes with angulators or protractors must provide accurate readings for positioning baselines. They can be evaluated by using a large protractor for angle measurements and a level to verify that locks, stops and detents are set to establish horizontal and perpendicular surfaces. Angles should be ±1 percent, with adjustments made when necessary.

The tests for x-ray generators should include:

Kilovoltage accuracy. Kilovoltage settings tend to drift over time, primarily as a result of tube aging. Their accuracy is essential in maintaining image quality. The scale of contrast and density cannot be predicted unless the kVp is accurate. Verification and calibration of the kVp ensure that technique exposure charts will produce diagnostic quality images. Computerized dosimeters provide digital readouts or printouts of average and single-pulse kVp. If the settings drift beyond the ±5 kVp of the labeled setting, the generator must be recalibrated.

Timer accuracy. Exposure time settings also tend to drift over time. Their accuracy is essential in maintaining image quality because image density cannot be predicted unless the time is accurate. Verification and calibration of the timer ensure that technique exposure charts will produce diagnostic quality images. Computerized dosimeters provide digital readouts or printouts of the exposure time, or a spinning top may be used to measure 1ϕ generators and a motorized synchronous top may be used for 3ϕ units. The tops are less accurate, more time-consuming and difficult to use. Exposure time settings should be maintained within ±5 percent of the label. If the settings drift beyond this limit the timing circuit or mechanism must be recalibrated.

mR/mAs and milliamperage linearity. Milliamperage settings also tend to drift over time, primarily as a result of tube aging. Their accuracy is essential to maintaining image quality because density cannot be predicted unless the mA is accurate. Assurance is needed that technique exposure charts will accurately produce diagnostic quality images. Milliamperage cannot be measured by noninvasive quality control methods. Consequently, mA station accuracy must be inferred by comparing mR/mAs measurements after both time and kVp accuracy have been verified. Comparative measurements are made for the same mAs at different mA and time settings to evaluate the linearity of the mA stations. Computerized dosimeters provide digital readouts or printouts of mR/mAs. Milliamperage stations should be maintained within ±10 percent of each other but some sources recommend maintaining the entire generator within ±10 percent. If the settings drift beyond the established limit the generator must be recalibrated.

Exposure reproduceability. Generators must be capable of repeating exposures accurately. This is ensured by measuring the mR/mAs of several different exposures with the same technical factors. Computerized dosimeters provide digital readouts or printouts of mR/mAs. Reproduceability should be maintained within ±5 percent. If the readings are beyond this limit the entire series of tube and generator tests should be analyzed to attempt to isolate the problem.

Specialized radiographic systems, such as fluoroscopy, tomography and automatic exposure controls, require additional tests.

Fluoroscopic Systems
The tests for fluoroscopic systems should include:

Exposure reproduceability. Fluoroscopic spot film devices use automatic exposure controls (AECs) and they should be evaluated according to the AEC tests below.

Exposure rate. Fluoroscopic exposure rates are measured by a dosimeter exactly as diagnostic mR/mAs. The exposure rate should not exceed 5 R/min. If the rate exceeds this limit the automatic brightness control or other systems may require calibration or repair.

Field size accuracy and beam alignment. As with collimation accuracy in diagnostic radiography, fluoroscopic units should not be capable of irradiating tissue outside the image receptor area. In addition to the evaluation performed for a diagnostic unit, fluoroscopic units should display everything within 1 cm of the edges of the image intensifier tube, and the primary beam should be aligned to the center of the image intensifier. Correction of the tube collimation, image intensification system or video display system may be required (further testing by a service engineer is necessary).

Source-to-skin distance limits. Fluoroscopic units should not be capable of placing the tube target closer than 15" (38 cm) (or 12" [30 cm] for a mobile fluoroscopy unit) to the patient's skin surface (this is a U.S. federal requirement). Without making any exposure, the source-to-image receptor distance should be verified. If it is not within limits, the unit should not be used until a mechanical device is fitted to set a minimum source-to-skin distance.

Intensifier viewing system resolution. Because fluoroscopic resolution is much poorer than radiographic resolution, periodic assurance that it has not deteriorated is critical in maintaining confidence in diagnosis. A fluoroscopic mesh test tool or a resolution pattern test tool can be imaged to permit visualization of the maximum resolving ability of the system. If the resolution appears to be deteriorating, a service engineer should be consulted.

Intensifier viewing system contrast. Because fluoroscopic contrast is much higher than radiographic contrast, it is important to periodically determine approximately how low contrast a structure may be imaged. Special low contrast fluoroscopic test tools are available that consist of two plates of aluminum with holes of 1–7 mm drilled in one of the plates. When the plates are sandwiched together and imaged on a fluoroscopy system, low contrast evaluation can be made based on the smallest visible hole.

TV monitors and recorders. The vast majority of modern fluoroscopic systems use video systems for image display because of the reduction in patient dose. Although a video signal generator is the test tool of choice, its expense and limited application in radiography usually prohibit its use for routine testing. A fluoroscopic mesh test tool or a resolution test tool and a piece of wire mesh are more commonly used. The resolution test tool can be imaged on the fluoroscopy unit to permit visual measurement of the system resolution. The wire mesh can be imaged to permit visualization of distortion (Figure 30–4). When degradation in resolution or distortion is observed, a service engineer should be consulted.

Automatic brightness control. Although there are a number of types of automatic brightness controls, the term is used here in a generic sense. These controls are designed to function like an AEC in that variations in subject density are automatically compensated for,

resulting in a relatively uniform image density. A computerized dosimeter can be used to measure exposure after the beam passes through a phantom. When the phantom thickness is decreased by half, the exposure should be similarly reduced. If there is a great discrepancy between phantom thickness and exposure reduction, a service engineer should be consulted.

Tomographic Systems The tests for tomographic systems should include:

Uniformity and completeness of motion. Tomography relies on the motion of the tube during exposure to produce a sectional image of the subject. Assurance of the uniformity and completeness of tube motion are basic tests. The test tool is simply a lead mask with a pinhole that is positioned several centimeters above the tomographic fulcrum. If the pinhole is centered to the film and then imaged with a full tomographic motion, images similar to Figure 30–5 may be obtained. Erratic tube motion is demonstrated by the uneven densities. If the motion were incomplete there would not be a full length of the tracing. If the motion is erratic or incomplete, the mechanisms involved in the

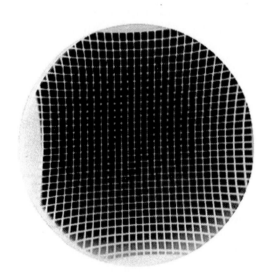

FIGURE 30-4. Normal distortion of a wire mesh test tool imaged with a conventional fluoroscopy system. *(Reprinted from Joel E. Gray, Norlin T. Winkler, John Stears, and Eugene D. Frank,* Quality Control in Diagnostic Imaging. *Rockville, MD: Aspen Publishers, Inc., 1983 by permission of Mayo Foundation)*

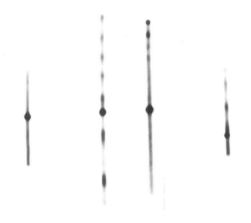

FIGURE 30-5. Tomographic uniformity and completeness of motion test with a pinhole trace image. Both exposures were erratic, as demonstrated by the uneven densities along the entire pinhole exposure. *(Reprinted from Joel E. Gray, Norlin T. Winkler, John Stears, and Eugene D. Frank,* Quality Control in Diagnostic Imaging. *Rockville, MD: Aspen Publishers, Inc., 1983 by permission of Mayo Foundation)*

tomographic motion should be cleaned (rails, guide-wheels, etc.) and the test repeated. If the problem continues, a service engineer should be consulted.

Section depth indicator accuracy. Tomographic units are designed to provide an image that is sharp (possessing good detail) only at the fulcrum level. Assurance that the fulcrum indicator is accurate is essential in diagnosing the location of structures within the subject. Commercial test tools are available or a penetrometer with lead numbered steps can be used. When a tomographic image is made of the test tool, the number that was at the level of the fulcrum should appear sharp. If it doesn't, the fulcrum indicator should be adjusted to the appropriate level. Additional testing may be required to ascertain the proper adjustment.

Section thickness accuracy. The sharp section of a tomograph should be of a known thickness, depending on the total arc of the tomographic motion (exact section thickness per arc is usually stated in the equipment manual). Commercial test tools are available or an angled wire mesh can be used. When the angled resolution mesh is imaged, the section thickness can be determined by measuring the region of sharpness on the image. If the section thickness is inaccurate, the pinhole trace should be consulted. If it appears unacceptable, a service engineer should be consulted.

Resolution. Tomographic resolution is determined by imaging a resolution test pattern at the fulcrum level. The resulting image can be visually inspected to determine the resolving capability of the system. When resolution deteriorates, standard diagnostic quality control measures should be consulted first, then a service engineer.

Automatic Exposure Controls

The tests for automatic exposure controls (AECs) should include:

Exposure reproduceability. The same reproduceability standards for diagnostic radiography systems are applied to AECs. Using the same procedure, with the addition of a subject phantom, densitometer readings of images produced with the AEC should be within OD ±0.1 in the same areas. Reproduceability cannot be achieved on an AEC with dosimeter mR/mAs readings. Radiographs must be produced and measured with a densitometer. If the readings are not within limits, the generator AEC circuits must be calibrated.

Ion chamber sensitivity. Most AECs utilize three ion chambers and permit activation of various combinations during exposures. It is important to ensure that each ion chamber is equally sensitive by comparing the reproduceability of each chamber individually. Exact chamber locations should be verified by producing an image of the ion chambers by using the AEC without a subject at extremely low kVp. After this step is completed, the test is done by using a lead brick to block all chambers but the one to be tested. The AEC reproduceability test is then performed for the unblocked chamber. If all chambers do not respond within ±10 percent, a service engineer should be consulted to recalibrate the generator AEC circuitry.

Density variation control accuracy. Nearly all AEC units provide controls to decrease and increase density by changing the sensitivity of the ion chamber. These controls vary tremendously from one unit to another. Consultation of equipment manuals will provide the percentage of change each control is designed to produce. A computerized dosimeter can then be employed to obtain mR/mAs measurements to verify the intensity differences for each control. If the controls are not accurate, the generator AEC circuits must be calibrated.

Response capability. Each AEC has a minimum response capability (which varies with manufacturer and model). If the AEC cannot respond at the minimum time, there is no assurance that diagnostic quality images can be produced. Response capability is best evaluated by using a computerized dosimeter readout or printout to determine exposure time for AEC exposures made with a small lucite phantom. As the phantom thickness is reduced, the AEC should produce exposures within ±10 percent mR/mAs of one another until a time below the minimum exposure time is used. If the minimum response time is greater than specified, the AEC should not be used until the problem is corrected.

Back-up timer verification. Occasionally even the best radiographers will forget to activate the proper tube or AEC. When this occurs, patient radiation protection requires that AEC back-up timers be functioning to terminate exposures and protect both patient and tube. When a lead plate is placed over the AEC ionization chamber and an exposure is made, the back-up timer should terminate the exposure and a visual and an audible warning should occur. If the back-up timer or signals fail, the AEC should not be used until the problem is corrected.

Ancillary Equipment

Ancillary equipment must also be monitored on a regular basis. This includes cassette cleaning, film/screen contact tests and view box reproduceability.

Cassette Cleaning and Inspection

During normal use, radiographic intensifying screens are exposed to dust and other foreign particles as cassettes are opened during loading and unloading of film. Periodic cleaning of the screens with a specially formulated antistatic solution removes these artifacts and eliminates the potential for misdiagnosis. At the time they are cleaned, cassettes should also be inspected for wear at corners, edges and especially at hinges. When excessive wear is observed, the cassette should be tested to see if it is lightproof. All cassettes should have a leaded identification number to assist in locating the source of artifacts during use.

Film/Screen Contact

Cassette backs and fronts may warp due to improper storage or traumatic handling. This can lead to loss of contact between the film and the intensifying screen. When poor film-to-screen contact exists, the diverging light photons from the screen cause loss of detail and contrast. A wire mesh test tool should be imaged and the radiograph examined for areas of poor detail. Although rescreening cassettes will replace the pressure pads and sometimes resolve the problem, many institutions prefer to replace the entire cassette.

View Box Uniformity

View boxes, or illuminators, should emit a uniform intensity of light. One of the greatest sources of misunderstanding between radiographers and radiologists is the difference in light intensity of different view boxes because it directly affects the perceived radiographic density. When radiographs consistently exhibit different densities on different view boxes, they become difficult to evaluate. View boxes should be monitored with a light meter periodically to alleviate this problem. View boxes are measured in NITs, the unit of luminance (1 NIT = 1 candela/m^2). Normal view boxes emit around 1700 NIT, while mammography view boxes should be in the 3500 NIT range. When inconsistencies are discovered, they should be brought to the attention of all professional staff.

Correction of the problem, when many view boxes are involved, can be expensive because most institutions have collected view boxes of different models and manufacturers over many years. The thickness and translucency of the plastic surface must be identical for all view boxes. Differences in the plastic are the most common cause of illumination problems. Old view boxes may require painting of their reflectors so the exact tone and reflecting ability of the paint matches newer models. Finally, the bulbs of all view boxes must not only be of the same manufacture and model but should be from the same production run. Attempts to solve view box problems should be carried out in the above order.

Repeat Film Studies

The careful analysis of repeated radiographs has proven a valuable aid in diagnosing the radiographic process. Repeated radiographs are also referred to as reject, retake, or double-dose studies. Even excellent repeat film studies need take little time or effort to pinpoint conditions that may be easily corrected. Significant reductions in patient dose, radiographer time and effort and supply costs can be achieved with properly executed repeat film studies.

Obtaining Data

A repeat film study involves retaining all repeated radiographs, regardless of cause, for analysis. Any image outside the acceptance limits and scrap film should be included. Boxes labeled as to cause of repeat should be provided near each film processor and the room and tube used should be noted on each film before it is discarded. Typical causes of repeats are shown in Table 30–2.

The most important rule when analyzing repeated images is to not discipline radiographers based on the

TABLE 30–2. Causes Of Repeated Radiographs

Total exposure	55 percent
Light	34 percent
Dark	21 percent
Positioning	30 percent
Motion	3 percent

information obtained. The analysis must be used in a constructive manner to improve working conditions and to point out areas where further technical training may be helpful. Radiographers must be informed of the intent of the study and asked to cooperate in a positive manner to improve both patient care and working conditions. Most radiographers are aware of numerous items they believe contribute to repeat radiographs and welcome an opportunity to find justification for their change. Incompetent radiographers should be disciplined through normal administrative procedures based on actual performance, not as a finding of a repeat film study. Failure by management to follow this suggestion may result in inaccurate repeat-study data when films are not submitted for analysis.

Analysis of Data

The analysis of collected data begins with the classification and counting of images by cause of repeat, room, tube and radiographer. Data should also be separated according to time (weekly is most common). The compiled data should be examined for obvious problems. For example, a large number of images from a single room with an artifact in the same location might indicate a barium or iodine stain on a grid or table. Once obvious problems are addressed, the data should be examined for unequal distribution of repeats. Tables 30–3 and 30–4 illustrate how distributions can be diagnosed.

The **total repeat rate** is a valuable figure to monitor over long periods of time. It is calculated as a percentage of the total number of images produced during the period of the study. The total image figure can be extracted from institutional data in some cases or can be estimated by multiplying the number of examinations by the average number of images produced per examination. For example, a chest unit that produced 600 examina-

TABLE 30–3. Retake Percentage By Room

REASON	ROOM # 1	2	3	4	5
Dark	29	37	36	33	33
Light	(45)	31	32	32	37
Positioning	20	18	18	19	17
Centering	10	11	(20)	9	9
Motion	6	7	6	5	5
Other	8	6	7	7	6
Total:	118	110	119	105	107

Technique exposure chart error?

Collimator misaligned?

Retake percentage by room. (Adapted from Lee W. Goldman and Scott Beech, *Analysis of Retakes: Understanding, Managing and Using an Analysis of Retakes Program for Quality Assurance.* Rockville, MD: U.S. DHEW, PHS, FDA, Bureau of Radiological Health, HEW Publication FDA 79 – 8097, 1979.)

TABLE 30–4. Retake Percentage By Technologist

REASON	TECHNOLOGIST # 1	2	3	4	5
Dark	35	31	32	30	43
Light	32	31	31	34	30
Positioning	20	18	18	(30)	17
Centering	13	12	11	12	11
Motion	5	(11)	4	4	4
Error	(10)	4	5	3	3
Other	5	7	6	6	7
Total:	120	112	107	119	115

Needs to be more careful?

Using long exposure times?

Has difficulty with some exams?

Retake percentage by radiographer. (Adapted from Lee W. Goldman and Scott Beech, *Analysis of Retakes: Understanding, Managing and Using an Analysis of Retakes Program for Quality Assurance.* Rockville, MD: U.S. DHEW, PHS, FDA, Bureau of Radiological Health, HEW Publication FDA 79 – 8097, 1979.)

tions in a week could be calculated to have produced 1,200 images (PA + lateral × 600). Repeat rates may suffer from a start-up effect where data may not be reliable for the first three weeks due to unfamiliarity with the requirements of the study or various psychological phenomena from stress to hypermotivation. Data indicates that radiographer repeat rates should be between 3 and 10 percent, with the average at 8 percent. One study demonstrated the student reject rates average to be slightly above 9 percent. Data also appear to indicate that when the rate drops below 3 percent there is a problem in data collection or an extremely wide acceptance limit in effect. It is important to realize that repeat rates are not only affected by film processing equipment, x-ray equipment, patient condition and radiographer competence, but also by the acceptance limits of the radiologists. In some instances a high repeat rate may indicate extremely high quality standards in the institution while the same rate may also indicate poor quality radiographers. Caution in interpretation is essential, and all aspects of the analysis should be carefully studied before conclusions are drawn.

Troubleshooting

Troubleshooting (locating problems when equipment malfunctions) is a diagnostic process. The same reasoning process that a physician uses to diagnose a disease can be applied to radiographic equipment. Beginning with the symptoms, the radiographer can work step-by-step through a problem solving procedure to eliminate possible problems until the source of trouble is isolated.

Although radiographers are not qualified to perform invasive procedures on electronic equipment, they can often pinpoint the general source of the problem. For example, an increase in density could be caused by nearly all equipment in the radiographic imaging chain. However, a problem solving approach may discover that all radiographs have increased density, not just the radiographs from a single unit. This would focus attention on the film processor. If the developer temperature is checked and found to be within normal limits, the radiographer might then check the replenishment tank only to discover that it is empty. To solve the problem, the

radiographer might fill the tank, remove air locks from the replenishment lines and restock the developer tank solution. A complete troubleshooting guide is provided in Appendix B.

Summary

Quality assurance consists of activities that provide adequate confidence that a radiology service will render consistently high quality images and services. Quality assurance includes evaluating activities such as interpretation of examinations, maintenance of equipment, performance of procedures, filing systems, staff development, scheduling of examinations and supply lines. The quality assurance process operates by identifying problems or potential problem areas, monitoring the problem and then resolving it.

Quality control is the aspect of quality assurance that monitors technical equipment to maintain quality standards. The concept of quality control is rooted in the need to stabilize the various equipment components of the radiographic imaging chain. From incoming line current through x-ray production to the processing of the radiograph, erratic equipment performance causes repeat radiographs and unnecessary patient exposure to radiation.

Equipment purchasing decisions should involve each member of the radiological team. Specific imaging requirements should be identified and equipment specifications should be developed. Once the equipment is selected it is then installed and tested.

Monitoring equipment performance is an integral part of quality assurance. It involves the film processing systems as well as the external radiation beams. Ancillary equipment should also be checked.

Monitoring the quality of the film processing systems includes routine processor sensitometry and darkroom safelight testing. External beam evaluations involve monitoring the diagnostic radiographic systems, fluoroscopic systems, tomographic systems and automated exposure controls. A wide variety of tests on each of the systems are performed to assure equipment accuracy. Ancillary equipment, such as cassettes and view boxes, are also monitored.

A careful analysis of repeat radiographs is also a valuable aid in diagnosing the radiographic process. Significant reductions in patient dose, radiographer time and effort and supply costs can be achieved with properly executed repeat-film studies.

REVIEW QUESTIONS

1. Why are quality assurance and control so important?

2. What factors should be considered when making equipment purchasing decisions?

3. How should film processing systems be monitored?

4. How often should tests be performed on diagnostic radiographic systems?

5. What tests should be performed routinely on the x-ray generator?

6. What tests should be performed routinely on automatic exposure controls?

7. Why are repeat film studies a valuable part of quality assurance?

REFERENCES AND RECOMMENDED READING

Adams, M. J., Barsotti, J. B., Kohler, T. D., & Reel, L. A. (1994). Film processor quality assurance: Increasing reliability while decreasing costs. *American Journal of Roentgenology. 163*, 709–710.

Adler, A. M. & Carlton, R. R. (1989). Repeating radiographs: Critiquing the image. *Postgraduate Advances in Radiologic Technology*. Berryville, VA: Forum Medicum.

Adler, A. M., Carlton, R. R., & Wold, B. (1992). An analysis of radiographic repeat rate data. *Radiologic Technology. 63*(5), 308–314.

Adler, A. M., Carlton, R. R., & Wold, B. (1992). A comparison of student radiographic reject rates. *Radiologic Technology. 64*(1), 26–32.

American Association of Physicists in Medicine. (1978). *Diagnostic radiology committee task force on quality assurance protocol: Basic quality control in diagnostic radiology*. AAPM Report No. 4, Chicago: AAPM.

American College of Radiology. (1981). *Quality Assurance in Diagnostic Radiology and Nuclear Medicine — The Obvious Decision*. Rockville, MD: U.S. Department of Health, Education, and Welfare, Public Health Service, Food and Drug Administration, Bureau of Radiological Health, HEW Publication (FDA) 81–8141.

Ardran, G. M. & Crooks, H. E. (1968). Checking diagnostic x-ray beam quality. *British Journal of Radiology. 41*, 193.

Ardran, G. M., Crooks, H. E., & James, V. (1969). Testing x-ray cassettes for film-intensifying screen contact. *Radiography. 35*(414), 143.

Barber, T. C. & Thomas, M. (1983). *Radiologic quality control manual*. Reston, VA: Reston Publishing.

Basart, J. A. (1974). Developer pH: Its significance in quality control. *Radiographic Technology. 45*(6), 413.

Berry, G. C., Starchman, D. E., & Howland, W. J. (1980). Objective equipment selection and performance evaluation. *Radiology Management. 2*(5), 14.

Bowers, J., Lin, P., & Rogers, L. (1978). Impact of equipment specifications on purchases, *Workshop in Purchase Specifications and Performance Evaluation of Radiologic Imaging Equipment Proceedings*. Chicago: Midwest Chapter American Association of Physicists in Medicine, Northwestern University Medical School and Northwestern Memorial Hospital, May 12–13.

Brookstein, J. J. & Steck, W. (1971). Effective focal spot size. *Radiology. 98*, 31–33.

Burkhart, R. L. (1983). *A basic quality assurance program for small diagnostic radiology facilities*. Rockville, MD: U.S. Department of Health and Human Services, Public Health Service, Food and Drug Administration, National Center for Devices and Radiological Health, HHS Publication FDA 83–8218.

Carlton, R. (1980). Establishing a total quality assurance program in diagnostic radiology. *Radiologic Technology. 52*, 23–38.

Carlton, R. R. (1992). Another dimension of quality assurance in radiology. *Introduction to Radiologic Technology* (3rd ed.). Editors: Gurley, L. T. & Callaway, W. J. St. Louis: C. V. Mosby, 149-166.

Carlton, R. R. & McKenna, A. (1989). Repeating radiographs: Setting imaging standards. *Postgraduate Advances in Radiologic Technology.* Berryville, VA: Forum Medicum.

Carroll, Q. B. (1993). *Fuchs's radiographic exposure, processing, and quality control* (5th ed.). Springfield, IL: Charles C. Thomas Publishers.

Chu, W. K., Ferguson, S., Wunder, B., Smith, R., & Vanhoutte, J. J. (1979). A two-year reject/retake profile analysis in pediatric radiology. *Health Physics.* 42(1), 53–59.

Corr, B. (1985). Quality control in radiology: An administrative overview. *The Canadian Journal of Medical Radiation Technology.* 16(1), 4.

Corr, B. (1978). A basic quality control system — Part 1. *The Canadian Journal of Medical Radiation Technology.* 9(3), 129.

Crooks, H. E. (1980). A device for checking the speeds and quality of x-ray films and efficiency of film processors. *Radiography.* 46(545), 128.

Crooks, H. E. (1975). Control of image quality, voltage, and filtration. *Radiography.* 41(481), 3.

Cullinan, A. & Cullinan, J. (1994). *Producing quality radiographs* (2nd ed.). Philadelphia: J. B. Lippincott.

Cullinan, J. E. (1981). A 'perfect' chest radiograph — or a compromise? *Radiologic Technology.* 53(2), 121.

David, G. & Price, S. C. (1991). Improved calibrations using personal computers. *Radiologic Technology.* 63(1), 32–39.

Dodd, B. C. (1983). Repeat analysis in radiology: A method of quality control. *The Canadian Journal of Medical Radiation Technology.* 14(2), 37.

Dowd, S. B. (1995). *Encyclopedia of radiographic positioning.* Philadelphia: W. B. Saunders.

Duffey, R. M. (1984). Quality assurance/department audits — new buzzwords in health care. *The Canadian Journal of Medical Radiation Technology.* 15(4), 134.

Eastman, T. R. (1993). Technique charts are vital to quality. *Radiologic Technology.* 65(1), 19.

Eisenberg, R. L., Akin, J. R., & Hedgcock, M. W. (1980). Optimal use of portable and stat examination. *American Journal of Roentgenology.* (March), 523–524.

Engel, T. L. (1979). Effect of kilovoltage and milliamperage on focal spot size. *Radiologic Technology.* 50(5), 559.

Everson, J. D. & Gray, J. E. (1987). Focal-spot measurement: Comparison of slit, pinhole, and star resolution pattern techniques. *Radiology.* 165(1), 261–264.

Fairbanks, R. & Doust, C. (1979). Methods for studying the focal spot size and resolution of diagnostic x-ray tubes. *Radiography.* 45(533), 89.

Finney, W. (1999). Introduction to radiographic quality assurance. In Ballinger, P. W. *Merrill's Atlas of Radiographic Positions and Radiologic Procedures* (7th ed.). St. Louis: C. V. Mosby, 305–320.

Gildenhorn, H. L., Rehman, I., Pape, L., & Baker, S. (1960). Standardization of physical factors in radiographic exposures. *Radiology.* 75, 262–267.

Gilbert, M. & Carlton, W. (1978). Performance evaluations for diagnostic x-ray equipment. *Radiologic Technology.* 50, 243–248.

Goldman, L. W. & Beech, S. (1979). *Analysis of retakes: Understanding, managing, and using an analysis of retakes program for quality assurance.* Rockville, MD: U.S. Department of Health, Education, and Welfare, Public Health Service, Food and Drug Administration, Bureau of Radiological Health, HEW Publication (FDA) 79–8097.

Gray, J. E. & Trefler, M. (1980). Pinhole cameras: artifacts, modifications, and recording of pinhole images on screen film systems. *Radiologic Technology.* 52(3), 277.

Gray, J. E., Winkler, N. T., Stears, J. G., & Frank, E. D. (1983). *Quality control in diagnostic imaging: A quality control cookbook.* Baltimore: University Park Press.

Guglielmo, J. (1980). Processor quality control science. *Radiology Management.* 2(4), 2.

Hall, C. L. (1977). Economic analysis from a quality control program. *Proceedings of the Society of Photo-optical Instrumentation Engineers.* 127, 271–275.

Haus, A. G. (1993). *Film processing in medical imaging.* Madison, WI: Medical Physics Publishing.

Hendee, W. R. & Ritenour, R. (1993). *Medical imaging physics* (3rd ed.). St. Louis: C. V. Mosby.

Hendee, W. R. & Rossi, R. P. (1980). *Quality assurance for conventional tomographic x-ray units.* Rockville, MD: U.S. Department of Health, Education, and Welfare, Public Health Service, Food and Drug Administration, Bureau of Radiological Health, HEW Publication (FDA) 80–8096.

Hendee, W. R. & Rossi, R. P. (1979). *Quality assurance for radiographic x-ray units and associated equipment.* Rockville, MD: U.S. Department of Health, Education, and Welfare, Public Health Service, Food and Drug Administration, Bureau of Radiological Health, HEW Publication (FDA) 79–8094.

High and Normal Speed Rotors: Effect on Focal Spot Size, Resolution and Density. (1981). *Radiologic Technology.* 53(1).

Hill, C. (1991). Introducing a radiographic quality control system at Crawley District General Hospital. *Radiography Today.* 57(649), 16–21.

Irfan, A. Y., Pugh, V. I., & Jeffery, C. D. (1985). Some practical aspects of peak kilovoltage measurements. *Radiography.* 51(599), 251–254.

Joint Commission on Accreditation of Healthcare Organizations. (1994). *Accreditation Manual for Hospitals.* Chicago: Joint Commission on Accreditation of Healthcare Organizations, Diagnostic Radiology Services.

Kalivoda, F. J. (1979). Ancillary audits in the radiology services: Improving patient care. *Radiology Management.* (Fall), 2–10.

Kebart, R. C. & James, C. D. (1991). Benefits of increasing focal film distance. *Radiologic Technology.* 62(6), 434–441.

Lam, R. W. & Price, S. C. (1989). The influence of film-screen color sensitivity and type of measurement device on kVp measurements. *Radiologic Technology.* 60(4), 319–321.

Lowthian, J. & McFadden, B. (1989). Quality control for chest radiography. *Canadian Journal of Medical Radiation Technology.* 18(2), 93–97.

MacLean, B. (1984). Quality Control Report 1981–82: 9 months of operations. *The Canadian Journal of Medical Radiation Technology.* 15(1), 4.

McFadden, B. (1989). Half value layer calibration. *Canadian Journal of Medical Radiation Technology.* 20(2), 67–74.

McKinney, W. E. J. (1993). Another look at film processor quality. *Radiologic Technology.* 64(4), 211–212.

McKinney, W. (1988). *Radiographic processing and quality control.* Philadelphia: J. B. Lippincott.

McLemore, J. M. (1981). *Quality assurance in diagnostic radiology.* Chicago: Yearbook Medical Publishers.

Moores, B. M., Henshaw, E. T., Watkinson, S. A. A., & Pearcy, B. J. (1987). *Practical guide to quality assurance in medical imaging.* New York: Wiley.

National Electrical Manufacturers Association. (1985). Measurements of dimensions and properties of focal spots of diagnostic x-ray tubes. NEMA Standards Publication No. XR-5-1984.

Nelson, M. T. (1994). Continuous quality improvement (CQI) in radiology: An overview. *Applied Radiology.* 23(7), 11–16.

Nelson, R. E., Barnes, G. T., & Witten, D. M. (1977). Economic analysis of a comprehensive quality assurance program. *Radiologic Technology.* 49, 129–134.

Paleen, R., Skundberg, P. A., & Schwartz, H. (1989). How much is quality assurance costing your department? *Radiology Management.* 11(1), 24.

Pirtle, O. L. (1994). X-ray machine calibration: A study of failure rates. *Radiologic Technology.* 65(5), 291–298.

Potsaid, M. S., Rhea, J. T., Llewellyn, H. J. (1978). Quality assessment and assurance in diagnostic imaging. *Radiology* (June), 583–588.

Price, R. (1981). The continuous assessment of x-ray tubes and generators. *Radiography.* 47(553), 2.

Pugin, M. (1986). Teaching quality control in radiological imaging. *The Canadian Journal of Medical Radiation Technology.* 17(4), 14.

Rhatigan, L. & Montague, E. (1987). Computerized quality assurance. *Radiologic Technology.* 58(6), 523.

Rogers, K. D., Matthews, I. P., & Roberts, C. J. (1987). Variation in repeat rates between 18 radiology departments. *The British Journal of Radiology.* 60, 463–468.

Rouse, S. & Cowen, A. R. (1983). Quality assurance of fluorographic camera systems. *Radiography.* 49(587), 251.

Rowley, R. (1985). The practical use of test films for x-ray film processor quality control. *The Canadian Journal of Medical Radiation Technology.* *16*(3), 123.

Rozenfeld, M. & Jette, D. (1984). Quality assurance of radiation dosage: Usefulness of redundancy. *Radiology.* (Jan.), 241.

Stears, J. G., Gray, J. E., Webbles, W. E., & Frank, E. D. (1989). Radiologic exchange (kVp measurements). *Radiologic Technology.* *60*(3), 233–236.

Stears, J. G., Gray, J. E., Webbles, W. E., & Frank, E. D. (1985). X-ray waveform monitoring for radiographic quality control. *Radiologic Technology.* *57*(1), 9–15.

Sweeney, R. J. (1983). *Radiographic artifacts: Their cause and control.* Philadelphia: J. B. Lippincott.

Thompson, M. A., Hattaway, M. P., Hall, J. D., & Dowd, S. B. (1994). *Principles of imaging science and protection.* Philadelphia: W. B. Saunders.

Thornhill, P. J. (1987). Quality assurance in diagnostic radiography: Are we using it correctly and what is its future? *Radiography.* *53*(610), 161–163.

Tortorici, M. (1992). *Concepts in medical radiographic imaging.* Philadelphia: W. B. Saunders.

Watkinson, S. & Moores, B. M. (1984). Reject analysis: Its role in quality assurance. *Radiography.* *50*(593), 189–194.

Watkinson, S., Shaw, M., Moores, B. M., & Eddleston, E. (1983). Quality assurance: A practical programme. *Radiography.* *49*(578), 27.

Watkinson, S. A. (1985). Economic aspects of quality assurance. *Radiography.* *51*(597), 133.

Wheeler, W. N. (1980). Equipment specifications and performance standards for equipment pertaining to the nuclear medicine department. *Radiology Management.* *2*(5), 43.

World Health Organization. (1982). *Quality assurance in diagnostic radiology.* Geneva: World Health Organization.

Zimmer, E. A. (1960). *Artifacts and handling and processing faults on x-ray films.* New York: Grune & Stratton.

UNIT V

Comparing Exposure Systems

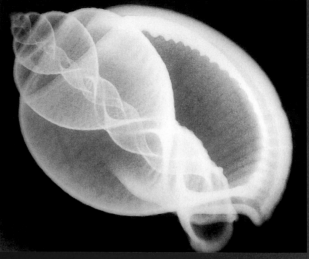

Once a thorough background knowledge has been acquired, the radiographer must then analyze the clinical conditions and synthesize the information into a workable exposure system. The objective is to provide a method of producing consistent image quality. Consistency facilitates the diagnostic process by permitting more valid comparisons between examinations and confidence in the amount of information presented in the image. A balance must exist between image quality, patient situation, and dose.

This unit presents various exposure systems that have been developed and assists in evaluating which system is most appropriate for particular clinical situations. All radiographers must have a thorough understanding of how an exposure system functions if it is to be used successfully. The practice of radiography involves so many nonroutine situations, unusual conditions and unique patients that simply following guidelines established by someone else does not permit the radiographer with the necessary skills to provide the patient with the best quality of care.

It is even more important to establish appropriate exposure factors when using computed or digital radiography systems and automatic exposure control (AEC) devices (phototimers). These automated systems cannot function unless the incoming photons are at the correct intensity and proper attenuation ranges to permit the computer or mechanical system to provide an appropriate range of input data for the processing of the image.

Because of the tremendous number of variables in the radiographic imaging chain, the most successful exposure systems maintain them all except a single variable for a given range of conditions. For example, a variable kVp system maintains all factors except kVp, which is varied to obtain appropriate image density for different subject densities and contrasts. This unit begins with a technical discussion on **developing exposure charts** as a guide to establishing functional systems for clinical practice. This is followed by specific details in the development of **fixed kVp systems** and **variable kVp systems,** the most popular exposure systems. **Other exposure sys-** tems that are more complicated in nature are then explained, followed by **automatic exposure controls** that are used for more exposures than any other system. A full chapter of **exposure conversion problems** provides methods for solving complex problems similar to the nonroutine situations that arise in practice.

CHAPTER 31

Developing Exposure Charts

[The radiograph] is not an anatomical snapshot taken at random.

Arthur W. Fuchs, Preface to the first edition of Principles of Radiographic Exposure and Processing.

Objectives

Upon completion of this chapter, the student should be able to:

▶ Compare various exposure systems.

▶ Describe the advantages and disadvantages of fixed and variable kVp systems.

▶ Discuss other exposure systems that have influenced radiographic technique.

▶ Explain why measurement of part thickness is critical to the accurate use of technique charts.

▶ Describe the function of the radiographer when using automatic exposure control systems.

▶ Describe how programmed exposure control systems function.

▶ State the steps necessary to establish a technique chart.

▶ Explain a basic phantom testing procedure.

▶ Describe the process of selecting an optimal image range.

▶ Extrapolate a technique chart from a limited number of phantom test images.

▶ Describe the clinical trial and fine tuning processes.

System Selection

*T*he foundations of the principles of radiographic exposure technique were laid in the 1920s by Ed. C. Jerman, known as the father of radiologic technology in the United States, and were developed into a scientific system in the 1940s by Arthur W. Fuchs.

Because radiographic exposure is such a complex process, technique systems function best when the large number of variables can be held constant while a single factor is permitted to vary. The goal of any radiographic exposure system is to provide a method of consistency in the quality of image production. Each type of exposure system functions in a different way to accomplish this goal, but all require the routine use of technique charts. Radiographers should consult a technique chart prior to making each exposure. Failure to follow this practice results in a higher personal repeat rate and excessive, unwarranted, patient dose.

A radiography department can expect to produce consistent results only when accurate technique charts are provided for each x-ray unit. Monitoring and revising these charts is part of the quality control function. Institutions that develop and enforce policies requiring radiographers to utilize posted technique charts experience lower repeat rates. Radiographers are advised to follow posted technique charts and to bring inaccuracies to the attention of quality control personnel immediately to avoid continued poor-quality images and excessive patient dose.

Comparing Exposure Systems

Each exposure system has its advantages and disadvantages and professionals quickly develop a rationale for their favorite system. The student must study each system in detail to learn its advantages and disadvantages before forming a personal professional judgment. It is important to recognize that any exposure system is designed to provide consistency in image quality and requires that all users of equipment in a single institution adhere to the same technique charts. Although personal philosophy may differ from institutional procedures and policies, the professional must let personal preference become secondary to the primary goal of widespread consistency in image quality. The following information

outlines the various exposure systems that are explained in detail in this unit.

Fixed Kilovoltage Systems

Fixed kVp systems were developed by Fuchs in 1943 during World War II. They have strong theoretical support in the literature and among many radiographers because they tend to decrease patient dose, provide more information on the image, increase the consistency of image density and contrast, lengthen exposure latitude, reduce x-ray tube wear, decrease time settings and therefore patient motion, and are easier to remember. However, these systems produce more scatter radiation, which tends to provide a lower contrast than a variable kilovoltage system. Low contrast is usually perceived as less pleasing to the eye and for this reason many institutions have not adopted the fixed kVp system.

Variable Kilovoltage Systems

Variable kVp systems were the first methodical approach to radiographic technique. They were proposed by Jerman in 1925 and predominated until x-ray generators became powerful enough to support fixed kVp techniques in the 1940s. They permit small incremental changes in exposure to compensate for variation in body part thickness. Most x-ray generators permit finer adjustment of kVp stations than of time or mA settings. Variable kVp systems produce higher contrast images, which enhance the visibility of fine detail and increase the perception of resolution. Institutions that have not adopted a variable kVp system cite the overwhelming advantages of fixed kVp to patient dose, image information, tube wear, etc.

Other Exposure Systems

Over the years since the work of Jerman and Fuchs there have been many attempts to refine exposure systems. During the 1950s and 1960s attempts were made to use mathematical formulas to quantify the relationship between the primary factors, especially kVp and mAs. A number of these formulas have been proven invalid. Only the systems based on $\log_{10}$ have survived, although there is some support for body habitus and proportional anatomy systems. However, several exposure systems have been developed that have either had a major effect on thinking about radiographic technique or have proven to be accurate in clinical situations.

Bit System   The Bit System was called the Du Pont Bit System because it was developed, by computer analysis, by Robert Trinkle of E. I. Du Pont de Nemours and Company, Inc. (now Sterling Diagnostics). Du Pont published the system in the 1970s and has supported it through numerous editions. The Bit System is a log-based system that utilizes points to quantify a vast number of radiographic variables, such as film density and contrast, distance, anatomical thickness, kVp, mAs, pathology, grids, development time, etc. The concept was simply that each projection required an established number of bits. Any balanced combination of variables that equaled the required bits would produce a diagnostic-quality image. The Bit System even permits calculation of approximate entrance skin exposure.

XVS System   The X-Ray Value Scale (XVS) system was designed by Gerhart Schwarz in 1960. It was patterned after the photographic Exposure Value Scale (EVS) system, but with the addition of research into the effect of part thickness on kVp's effect on image density. The system was the first used to quantify the primary radiographic variables. It permitted variance of exposure factors, much as with the Bit System. The basis of the system was a caliper that measured part thickness in XVS numbers. Any total of XVS numbers that equaled the caliper measurement could be obtained from special markings on the x-ray machine's distance, mA, time and kVp indicators. The lack of standardization of all but a single factor resulted in too many variables for consistent diagnostic confidence. In addition, when manufacturers began to build units with XVS numbers replacing technical controls, radiographers experienced difficulty in adapting to specific clinical situations.

Siemens Point System   The Siemens Point System was designed as a parallel system to the XVS system. It predated the Bit System, and although it was not as sophisticated, it permitted the radiographer to control the exposure variables much better than with the XVS system.

Supertech™ Calculator   In 1973 a log-based, slide rule technique calculator was developed by Brice Kratzer, patented, trademarked, and marketed as the Supertech™ Calculator by Supertech, Inc. Circular and slide rule calculators had been presented in the radiographic literature by C. W. Reed in 1939 and 1949 and William A. Williams had developed a circular calculator technique system in 1960. Several of these calculators were distributed by commercial film companies, but only the Supertech™ Calculator has survived to the present and is updated continually. The most recent version includes an acrylic penetrometer with a calibration master film for elementary quality control testing of machine output. After a short testing procedure, each machine can be assigned a correction factor that takes into account such variations as kVp, mA, time, part thickness, patient age, projection, distance, grid, pathology, etc. In addition, the slide rule style calculator provides positioning instructions, principles of exposure and anatomy review and even serves as an angulator and basic quality control tool. A computer disk provides a technique data reference to accompany the slide rule system. The Supertech™ Calculator remains a viable technique system, especially in low volume clinics, physician's offices and in ancillary radiographic service situations, such as chiropractics and podiatry.

Proportional Anatomy Systems   A body habitus system for chest radiography was proposed by Terry Eastman in 1969. Proportional anatomy systems were presented by Quinn Carroll in 1985 and by Eugene Frank and Norlin T. Winkler in 1987. These systems classify body parts and habitus into groups of similar subject density and contrast. The body habitus system determined technical factors for the chest from patient height and weight. The proportional anatomy systems use ratios or conversion factors to extrapolate a technique chart for the entire body from a control exposure.

Measurement of Part Thickness

Nearly all variables in exposure systems are changed according to the thickness of the anatomical part being radiographed and no exposure system can be expected to function accurately unless the radiographer measures part thickness. Part thicknesses for various regions in the average adult were detailed by Arthur Fuchs (Table 31–1).

Failure to measure consistently will cause unnecessary repeated exposures, resulting in excessive patient dose.

TABLE 31–1. Average Adult Part Thickness By Region

Region		Average Thickness Adult—CMS			Percent Frequency
		AP	PA	Lat	
Thumb, Fingers		1.5–4			99
Hand		3–5			99
				7–10	93
Wrist		3–6			99
				5–8	98
Forearm		6–8			94
				7–9	92
Elbow		6–8			96
				7–9	87
Arm		7–10			95
				7–10	94
Shoulder		12–16			79
Clavicle			13–17		82
Foot		6–8			92
				7–9	91
Ankle		8–10			86
				6–9	96
Leg		10–12			85
				9–11	89
Knee		10–13			92
				9–12	92
Thigh		14–17			77
				13–16	76
Hip		17–21			76
Cervical Vertebrae	C1–3	12–14			77
	C4–7	11–14			98
	C1–7			10–13	90
Thoracic Vertebrae		20–24			76
				28–32	81
Lumbar Vertebrae		18–22			69
				27–32	77
Pelvis		19–23			78
Skull			18–21		96
				14–17	88
Sinuses	Frontal		18–21		97
	Max.		18–22		88
Mandible				13–17	96
				10–12	82
Chest			20–25		82
				27–32	84

Reprinted with permission of the American Society of Radiologic Technologists from Arthur W. Fuchs's Relationship of tissue thickness to kilovoltage. *The X-ray Technician* [now *Radiologic Technology*] 19:6, 287 – 293, 1948.

The device used to measure a part thickness is a **caliper**. Improper use of a caliper will result in improper technical factors and a repeated exposure. Caliper measurements are made either by central ray entrance and exit or by thickest part. It is critical that all radiographers using a particular technique chart measure by the same method and in exactly the same manner.

Central ray measurements should be made from the point of central ray entrance to exit. For example, in Figure 31–1, the chest should be measured at point B, not point A or C. Thickest part measurements should be made at the thickest part of the area of interest. If another special measurement point or method has been established, it must be followed by all users of the chart.

Phototiming (AEC) Systems

When automatic exposure control (AEC) systems are used, the selection of exposure time factors, and thereby mAs selection, are eliminated. The radiographer must still exercise professional judgment to determine all other factors, including mA (which can be used to influence the time), kVp, distance, etc. Part of the art of phototiming is learning when to use AECs and when to avoid them.

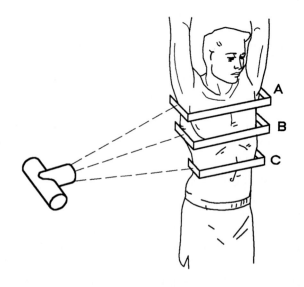

FIGURE 31-1. Proper caliper measurement of part thickness by using the central ray entrance-to-exit method as shown in B.

Anatomically Programmed Radiography

The most exciting developments are currently in computerized exposure control systems. These systems are simply computerized technique charts utilizing existing exposure systems but storing the data in a memory bank that is an inherent part of the x-ray control console. Many of these units have anatomically based programming (Figure 31–2). For example, when the radiographer pushes a button to indicate a lumbar spine, a screen may provide a choice of projections. When the lateral projection is indicated, a suggested series of technical factors may be set on the x-ray console. If the exposure is begun, the computerized factors will be used. However, if the radiographer determines that nonroutine conditions exist, the technical factors can be modified prior to exposure. The computerized control can be programmed to display any desired exposure system and then be fine tuned to meet existing needs. If the programmed console or consoles are monitored and maintained to display accurate techniques, they can be consulted for techniques for an entire department. Only an mAs correction factor would be needed for each room to make the chart accurate.

Establishing A Technique Chart

The process of establishing a technique chart begins with collecting exposure data. The first step is to make a single exposure that produces an optimal diagnostic quality radiograph. This original image must be at the optimal center of the acceptance limits curve. Although any projection can be used as a starting point in collecting data, it is preferred that the first data be from a subject part size and kVp in the middle of the diagnostic range. Ideal part sizes are 10–25 cm and ideal kilovoltage is in the 60–80 range.

Figure 31–3 illustrates the steps in setting up a radiographic technique chart for any exposure system.

Initial Phantom Images

Initially, a series of test exposures is made to determine the optimal quality image. This is accomplished by using an appropriate phantom to produce radiographs at a variety of technical factor combinations both above and below the average level. It is essential that the density remain the same at a control point to avoid misperception of the contrast range. It is preferred that the images be produced using an AEC to control the density. If an AEC is not available, or cannot be used due to other circumstances, a density reference control point must be established and measured with a densitometer. For example, the exact center of the body of L4 could be measured on each film. It would be necessary to adjust milliampere-second values until all images exhibited control point densities within OD 0.3 of one another.

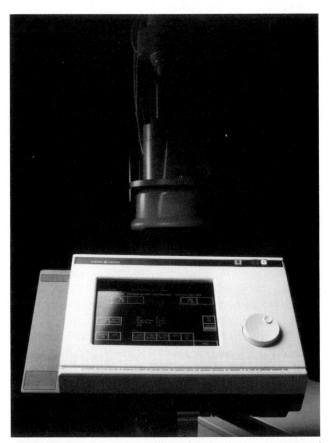

FIGURE 31-2 A programmed, computerized exposure control console. *(Courtesy of GE Medical Systems)*

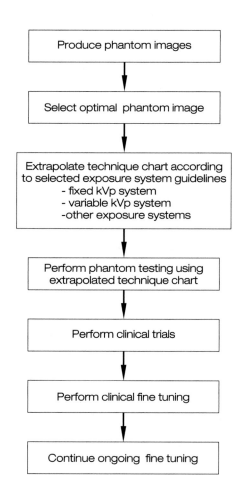

FIGURE 31-3. A systematic approach to establishing a technique chart.

Select Optimal Phantom Image

Once the series of phantom test images has been produced, it must be shown to all radiologists, who will be asked to diagnose the images, and to the supervisory radiographers, who will be responsible for image quality control checking. These professionals should not be asked to select the best image but to select those images they believe to be outside acceptance limits, because when any group of professionals is asked to select the best image there will be differences of opinion, leaving no consensus as to which is the best image. Conversely,

elimination of those images that are not acceptable will often result in a series of images that are acceptable to all, although "perfect" to only a few.

Extrapolate Technique Chart

Next, a series of preliminary clinical trials should be performed by preparing a technique chart that adjusts current technical factors to those that are newly established as optimal. This is normally done by using the 15 percent rule and other guides for part thickness adjustments for particular exposure systems. Particular attention should be given to projections that have a narrow range of part thicknesses or few choices of technical factors. For example, the variations in a wrist or PA chest chart both require careful calculation, the wrist because the normal thickness range encompasses only about 3 cm and the PA chest because the extremely high kVp with a normal thickness range of only about 5 cm amplifies minute changes in mAs.

Phantom Testing

The new chart is then tested with a phantom to verify its effectiveness. Minimum phantom testing should include a median, small and large part thickness. At this point the chart is completed for all part thicknesses for each projection.

Clinical Trials

Finally, a limited series of clinical trial examinations should be performed using the new chart. Each examination should be recorded and all repeated images should be saved for analysis. The series of clinical examinations should then be shown to each person who participated in the determination of the original standards. If the new image quality is accepted, a new exposure technique chart should be designed and implemented. If the new image quality experiences limited acceptance, adjustments should be made to satisfy deficiencies and all of the phantom testing and clinical trial steps should be repeated. Under no circumstance should clinical trials be performed until phantom testing and the other preliminary steps have been properly completed. Whenever new equipment is added to the imaging chain, especially a new x-ray tube, intensifying screens, type of processing chemistry, or film, the phantom testing and/or clinical trial steps should be repeated until confidence in the chart is re-established.

Clinical Fine Tuning

Clinical fine tuning requires that the technical factors for each exposure be recorded, regardless of whether the image is within acceptance limits. Each image is then used to fine tune the chart. Excellent quality images permit technical factors for the part thicknesses to be verified, while all other images permit adjustments of the technical factors for their respective part sizes.

Ongoing Fine Tuning

It is important that a system of ongoing fine tuning be established as a quality control monitoring method. The quality control radiographer should be consulted whenever a technique chart produces an unacceptable image and the cause is not evident. A series of unexplained rejected images may signify a change in one of the system's components that can be determined by quality control testing. The problem can often be fixed by a service engineer, although aging processes (such as filament wear, focal spot deterioration and tube gas) may require adjustments of the technique chart.

Summary

The goal of any radiographic exposure system is to provide a method of consistency in the quality of image production. Each type of exposure system functions in a different way to accomplish this goal, but all require the routine use of technique charts. Radiographers should consult a technique chart prior to making each exposure. Failure to follow this practice results in a higher personal repeat rate and excessive, unwarranted patient dose.

A radiography department can expect to produce consistent results only when accurate technique charts are provided for each x-ray unit. Monitoring and revising these charts is part of the quality control program. Institutions that develop and enforce policies requiring radiographers to utilize posted technique charts experience lower repeat rates.

Each exposure system has its advantages and disadvantages and professionals quickly develop a rationale for their favorite system. It is important to recognize that any exposure system is designed to provide consistency in image quality and this requires that all users of equipment in a single institution adhere to the same technique charts. The two most popular exposure systems are the fixed kVp system and the variable kVp system. Other exposure systems include the Du Pont Bit System, the XVS System, the Siemens Point System, the Supertech™ Calculator, and various proportional anatomy systems.

A systematic process for establishing a technique chart involves producing initial phantom images, selecting the optimal phantom image, extrapolating a technique chart for a given exposure system, performing phantom testing using the extrapolated technique chart data, performing clinical trials, clinical fine tuning and, finally, establishing a system of ongoing fine tuning.

REVIEW QUESTIONS

1. What is the principle goal of a radiographic exposure system?

2. Why is it important for radiographers to utilize technique charts?

3. What are some of the advantages of the fixed kVp system?

4. What are some of the advantages of the variable kVp system?

5. What are the two methods used for taking caliper measurements?

6. What are the steps involved in establishing a technique chart?

7. What should be done when a technique chart produces an unacceptable image and the cause is not evident?

REFERENCES AND RECOMMENDED READING

Cahoon, J. B. (1961). Radiographic technique: Its origin, concept, practical application and evaluation of radiation dosage. *The X-Ray Technician. 32*, 354–364.

Carroll, Q. B. (1993). *Fuchs's radiographic exposure, processing, and quality control.* (5th ed.). Springfield, IL: Charles C. Thomas Publishers.

Compton, S. (1987). Bit conversion of technical factors in vascular procedures. *Radiologic Technology. 58*(5), 413.

Cullinan, A. & Cullinan, J. (1994). *Producing quality radiographs.* (2nd ed.). Philadelphia: J. B. Lippincott.

Du Pont Company Photosystems & Electronic Products Department. *Positioning and exposure guide for general radiography.* Wilmington, DE: Publication R-53806-1.

Dyke, W. P. (1975). Depth resolution: A mechanism by which high kilovoltage improves visibility in chest films. *Radiology. 117*, 159–164.

Eastman Kodak Company. (1980). Health Sciences Markets Division. *The Fundamentals of Radiography* (12th ed.). Rochester, NY: Kodak Publication M1-18.

Eastman, T. R. (1994). Technique charts improve x-ray quality. *Radiologic Technology. 65*(3), 183–186.

Eastman, T. R. (1979). *Radiographic fundamentals and technique guide.* St. Louis: C. V. Mosby.

Eastman, T. R. (1978). A history of radiographic technique. *Applied Radiology.* (July/August), 97–100.

Eastman, T. R. (1975). Technique charts: The key to radiographic quality. *Radiologic Technology. 46*, 365–368.

Eastman, T. R. (1973). Measurement: The key to exposure with manual techniques. *Radiologic Technology. 45*, 75–78.

Eastman, T. R. (1971). Automated exposures in contemporary radiography. *Radiologic Technology. 43*(2), 80–83.

Eastman, T. R. (1969). Chest technique through body habitus. *Radiologic Technology. 41*, 80–84.

Eastman, T. R. *The radiographic technique guide.* Wilmington, DE: Du Pont deNemours Inc. Photo Products Department Publication A-99101.

Files, G. W. (1952). *Medical radiographic technique.* Springfield, IL: Charles C. Thomas Publishers.

Fodor, J. & Malott, J. C. (1993). *The art and science of medical radiography.* (7th ed.). St. Louis: C. V. Mosby.

Fuchs, A. W. (1950). The rationale of radiographic exposure. *The X-Ray Technician. 22*, 62–68, 76.

Fuchs, A. W. (1949). Control of radiographic density. *The X-Ray Technician. 20*, 271–273, 291.

Fuchs, A. W. (1948). Relationship of tissue thickness to kilovoltage. *The X-Ray Technician. 19*, 287–293.

Fuchs, A. W. (1934). Radiography of entire body employing one film and a single exposure. *Radiography and Clinical Photography. 10*, 9–14.

Funke, T. (1966). Pegged kilovoltage technic. *Radiologic Technology. 37*, 202–213.

General Electric Company Medical Systems Department. *How to prepare an x-ray technic chart.* Milwaukee: Publication 4301A.

Gyss, E. E. (1957). A medical radiographic technique chart based on constants. *Radiologic Technology. 29*(2), 76.

Hiss, S. S. (1993). *Understanding radiography* (3rd ed.). Springfield, IL: Charles C. Thomas Publishers.

Hiss, S. S. (1975). Technique management. *Radiologic Technology. 46*(5), 369.

Hochschild, T. J. & Cremin, B. J. (1975). Technique in infant chest radiography. *Radiography. 41*(481), 21.

Jenkins, D. (1980). *Radiographic photography and imaging processes.* Lancaster, England: MTP Press Limited.

Jerman, E. C. (1928). *Modern x-ray technic.* St. Paul: Bruce Publishing.

Jerman, E. C. (1926). Extremity technic. *Radiology. 6*, 252–254.

Jerman, E. C. (1926). Potter-Bucky diaphragm technic. *Radiology. 6*, 336–338.

Lauer, O. G., Mayes, J. B., & Thurston, R. P. (1990). *Evaluating radiographic quality: The variables and their effects.* Mankato, MN: The Burnell Company Publishers.

Lex, J. K. (1957). The x-ray exposure chart. *The X-Ray Technician. 28*(4), 250.

Mattsson, O. (1955). Practical photographic problems in radiography. *Acta Radiologica. Supplementum 120*, 1–206.

McFadden, B. (1985). Principles of radiographic exposure: A new approach. *The Canadian Journal of Radiography, Radiotherapy, and Nuclear Medicine. 16*(2), 45–54.

Morgan, J. A. (1977). *The art and science of medical radiography* (5th ed.). St. Louis: Catholic Hospital Association.

Nemet, A., Cox, W. F., & Hills, T. H. (1953). The contrast problem in high kilovoltage radiography. *British Journal of Radiology. 26*, 185–192.

Revesz, G., Shea, F. J., & Kundel, H. L. (1982). The effects of kilovoltage on diagnostic accuracy in chest radiography. *Radiology. 142*, 615–618.

Schwarz, G. S. (1961). *Unit-Step Radiography*. Springfield, IL: Charles C. Thomas Publishers.

Schwarz, G. S. (1960). Kilovoltage conversion in radiography. *The X-Ray Technician. 31*, 373–379, 436.

Schwarz, G. S. (1959). Extended range radiography. *Radiology, 69*. 419–423, 1957.

Schwarz, G. S. (1959). Kilovoltage and radiographic effect. *Radiology. 73*, 749–760.

Schwarz G. S. (1958). A simple universal unit system of radiographic exposures suited to departmental, national, and international standardization. *Radiology. 71*, 573-574.

Seeman, H. E. (1968). *Physical and photographic principles of medical radiography*. New York: Wiley & Sons.

Thomas, J. B. (1959). High kilovoltage equipment and technique. *The X-Ray Technician. 30*(6), 500.

Thompson, M. A., Hattaway, M. P., Hall, J. D., & Dowd, S. B. (1994). *Principles of imaging science and protection*. Philadelphia: W. B. Saunders.

Tortorici, M. (1992). *Concepts in medical radiographic imaging*. Philadelphia: W. B. Saunders.

United States Army. (1955). *Principles of radiographic exposure*. TM 8-282, March.

United States War Department. (1941). *Technical manual: Roentgenographic technicians*, TM 8-240, July 3.

Williams, W. A. (1960). Standardization of x-ray technique. *The X-Ray Technician. 32*(2), 137.

CHAPTER **32**

Fixed Kilovoltage Systems

The future trend is toward the use of optimum and higher kilovoltage values and a more widespread knowledge regarding the photographic function of each exposure factor.

John B. Cahoon, Jr., from the 15th Jerman Memorial Lecture
at the 1961 Annual Meeting of the American Society of X-Ray Technicians.

OBJECTIVES

Upon completion of this chapter, the student should be able to:

▶ Describe the principles of fixed kVp technique theory.

▶ Discuss the primary advantages and disadvantages of fixed kVp technique systems.

▶ Define optimal kilovoltage.

▶ Explain how to establish fixed kVp for various subject parts.

▶ Describe the steps in establishing a fixed kVp technique chart.

▶ Synthesize a fixed kVp technique chart from control radiographs.

Principles of Fixed Kilovoltage Exposure Systems

*B*ecause radiographic exposure is such a complex process, technique systems function best when the large number of variables can be held constant while a single factor is permitted to vary. **In a fixed kilovoltage system, the kVp is held constant for a given range of subject densities and contrasts while the mAs is varied to achieve an appropriate image density.** The kVp has a profound effect on many radiographic factors, such as contrast, type of interaction, production of scatter radiation and average photon energy. In addition, it varies depending on generator phase, filtration, machine calibration, intensifying screen phosphor conversion efficiency, subject inner shell binding energy range, etc. Consequently, a technique chart that makes kVp a constant eliminates the effects of these variables on the exposure system. The basis of a fixed kilovoltage exposure system therefore becomes the concept of the optimal kilovoltage peak.

In keeping with the goal of any radiographic exposure system to provide consistency in the quality of image production, a fixed kilovoltage system provides a relatively uniform contrast and an easily remembered series of kilovoltages to which mAs values can be added to produce images within established acceptance limits. The uniform contrast contributes to radiologists' confidence in the information in the image as they do not have to contend with a variable gray scale.

Advantages and Disadvantages

There are a number of advantages to the fixed kilovoltage technique systems. These systems tend to decrease patient dose, as the kilovoltage is always at the maximum possible level, and this permits decreased mAs in compensation. The decreased mAs contributes to decreased patient dose. In addition, the consistency in kVp levels results in uniform radiographic contrast, permitting the radiologist to compare radiographs of a given projection or patient, and provides more confidence in the diagnostic process. The higher average kVps that the optimal kVp concept produces lengthen exposure latitude. It also decreases mAs, thereby decreasing the aver-

age mA, which lowers x-ray tube heating and extends tube life, and/or decreasing time, which reduces the possibility of patient motion.

There are also disadvantages to a fixed kilovoltage technique system. These systems tend to provide a lower overall contrast than do variable kilovoltage systems and this is usually perceived by radiologists as less pleasing to the eye. Without question, the lower contrast produces much more scattered radiation and films that are less artistically beautiful. Additionally, small incremental changes in exposure for variations in body part thickness may not be possible with systems that fix kVp and vary mAs, due to less variety in mA stations and exposure times as compared to the kVp settings.

Optimal Kilovoltage Peak

The optimal kVp is the maximum kVp level that will produce images with appropriate contrast that are consistently within acceptance limits. This kVp level must ensure sufficient penetration of the subject as well as provide acceptable radiographic contrast. Insufficient penetration of the area of interest, especially in contrast media studies, limits the diagnostic region to the edges of the contrast media. Sufficient penetration permits visualization through the contrast media and increases the diagnostic information available.

The use of the maximum kVp as optimal causes a corresponding decrease in the mAs required to produce acceptable image density. The mAs reduction contributes to both reduced mA and time. Reduced mA decreases x-ray tube heating and prolongs filament and anode life. Reduced time minimizes the possibility of patient motion. **The optimal kVp produces lower contrast and the minimum patient dose.** The fixed kVp system takes advantage of the only situation in radiography where image quality can be increased (low contrast and therefore more diagnostic shades of gray) and patient dose decreased (less mAs and therefore less mR/mAs).

Establishing Optimal Kilovoltage Peak

A number of optimal kVps are established for a fixed kVp system; each is specific for a range of subject densities and contrasts. In other words, the so-called "fixed kVp" is fixed only for a specific range of part thicknesses for a particular procedure. For example, where 80 kVp may be selected as the optimal kVp for noncontrast media abdominal examinations, 50 kVp may be determined to be the maximum for contrast that is acceptable for imaging the trabeculae of the smaller extremities. The optimal kVp should not be changed unless the conditions under which it was set have changed, or the acceptance limits are changed.

Establishing A Fixed Kilovoltage Peak Technique Chart

The specific steps to setting up a fixed kVp technique chart follow the basic outline provided in Chapter 31.

Initial Phantom Images

Setting up a fixed kVp system requires that a series of test exposures be obtained to determine the optimal kVp. This is accomplished by using an abdomen or pelvis phantom to produce radiographs at a variety of kVps above and below the average level. It is essential that the density remain the same at a control point to avoid misperception of the contrast range (Figure 32–1). It is preferred that the images be exposed using an AEC, although a density reference control point can be used.

Select Optimal Phantom Image

Once the series of phantom test images has been produced, the optimal phantom image must be selected. The objective of optimal kVp is to determine the **highest** kVp and **lowest** contrast that is within acceptance limits, not the best image. The optimal kVp is the highest of the acceptable images. Remember that this process is one of elimination, not of selection. In other words, radiologists and quality control radiographers should be asked to eliminate unacceptable images, not to choose the single best quality image.

Careful consideration must be given to the variety of subject densities and contrasts in the human body before establishing the optimal kVps for other procedures. Table 32–1 illustrates common optimal kVp ranges for the major body regions, but individual requirements often vary.

Extrapolate Technique Chart

Once the optimal kVp has been determined, an extrapolated technique chart should be obtained by adjusting current technical factors to the newly established optimal kVp. This is normally done by using the 15 percent rule to modify existing technical factors until the desired kVp has been achieved.

Milliampere-seconds is designed to be the primary variable for a fixed kVp exposure system. The mAs values for the technique chart must be set at minimum increments of 30 percent because values less than 30 percent are not visibly significant.

Because there is no linearity of the film/screen combination and other variables, no accurate formula can be given for extrapolating mAs values. However, most systems have been found to operate in the range of doubling or halving the mAs for every 5 cm of subject thickness. For example, if 80 mAs produces a diagnostic quality image of a 20 cm part, a 15 cm part will require about 40 mAs, while a 25 cm part will require about 160 mAs. This is often applied to variable kVp technique charts as a "2 kVp/cm rule," which is fairly consistent with the 15 percent rule and ensures sufficient penetration.

Phantom Testing

Phantom testing is recommended prior to performing patient examinations. As a minimum, phantom testing should be done for a medium, small and large part size.

TABLE 32–1. Common Optimal kVp Ranges For The Major Body Regions

Region	Optimal kVp Range
Small extremities	50–60
Iodine-based contrast media studies	68
Large extremities	70
Skull	80
Abdomen and ribs	80
AP vertebral column	80
Lateral vertebral column	90
Chest	120
Barium-based contrast media studies	120

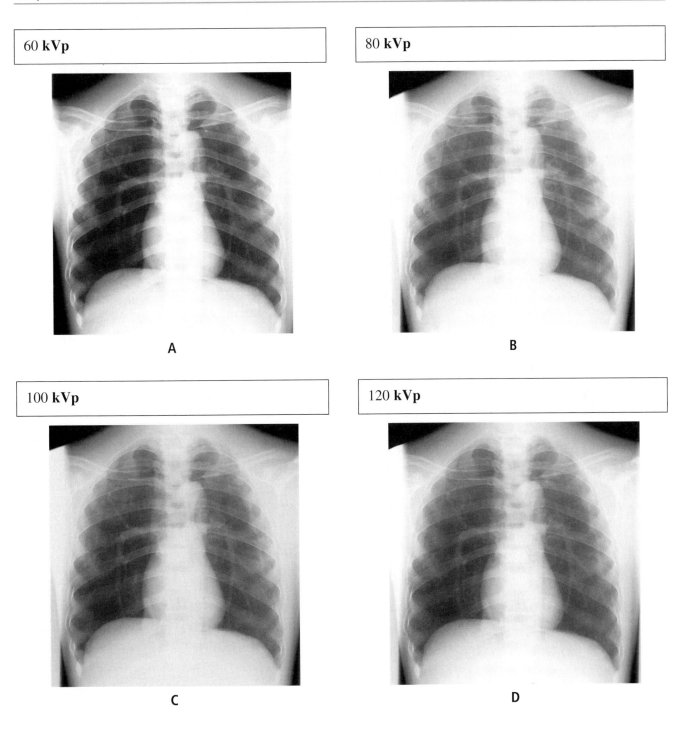

60 kVp

A

80 kVp

B

100 kVp

C

120 kVp

D

FIGURE 32-1. A series of chest radiographs produced at 60, 80, 100, and 120 kVp to determine the optimal kVp. While 60 kVp may be selected as optimal for ribs, 120 kVp may be determined to be optimal for the chest.

Because of the nonlinearity of the exposure systems and the inadequacy of the 15 percent rule, phantom testing should always be employed when the part size is less than 10 cm or the kVp is outside the median diagnostic range of 60–80.

Phantom testing also serves as a fine tuning mechanism for the extrapolated chart prior to clinical use. Once several mAs values have been set, extrapolation of the mAs for subject thickness can be done accurately. For example, if 68 kVp is set as the optimal fixed kVp for iodine-based contrast media abdominal work, a technique chart might

be established from a base diagnostic quality 20 cm phantom image at 50 mAs (Table 32–2). Step 1 illustrates a blank chart with the phantom technique. Using the 15 percent rule, several additional mAs values can be extrapolated for phantom testing, as shown in Step 2. Upon phantom testing, the extrapolated mAs values may require fine tuning, as shown in Step 3. Once phantom fine tuning is accomplished, the extrapolation of the final mAs values can be completed, as shown in Step 4. At this point the chart has been proven within acceptance limits by phantom testing and is ready for clinical trials.

TABLE 32–2. Fixed kVp Technique Chart

Blank Chart with Phantom Technique			Extrapolation of Additional mAs Values	Fine Tuning of Extrapolated mAs Values	Extrapolation of Final mAs V
		Step 1	Step 2	Step 3	Step 4
cm	*kVp*	*mAs*			
16	68				30
17	68				35
18	68				40
19	68				45
20	68	50	50	50	50
21	68				60
22	68				70
23	68				80
24	68				90
25	68		100	100	100
26	68				115
27	68				130
28	68				145
29	68				160
30	68		200	180	180
31	68				215
32	68				250
33	68				285
34	68				320
35	68		400	360	360

Clinical Trials

Limited clinical trials are permissible with the new chart. All images should be recorded, with repeated images saved for analysis. When clinical trials are proceeding without excess repeated exposures, the new technique chart can move into the clinical fine tuning stage.

Clinical Fine Tuning

The clinical fine tuning process will adjust and finally validate the entire chart. At this point the new technique chart can be adopted. However, ongoing fine tuning then begins as a permanent process.

Ongoing Fine Tuning

Ongoing fine tuning is the process that maintains the accuracy of the entire exposure system and gives radiographers and radiologists confidence in the exposure and diagnostic processes.

Summary

Technique systems function best when the large number of variables can be held constant while a single factor is permitted to vary. In a fixed kilovoltage system the kVp is held constant for a given range of subject densities and contrasts, while the mAs is varied to achieve an appropriate image density.

Fixed kilovoltage technique systems tend to decrease patient dose because the kilovoltage is always at the maximum possible level. In addition, the consistency in kVp levels results in a uniform radiographic contrast and a lengthened exposure latitude. There are also disadvantages to a fixed kilovoltage technique system. These systems tend to provide a lower overall contrast than do variable kilovoltage systems and this is usually perceived by radiologists as less pleasing to the eye. Additionally, small incremental changes in exposure for variations in body part thickness may not be possible with systems that fix kVp and vary mAs, due to less variety in mA stations and exposure times as compared to the kVp settings.

The optimal kVp is the maximum kVp level that will produce images with appropriate contrast that are consistently within acceptance limits. This kVp level must ensure sufficient penetration of the subject as well as provide acceptable radiographic contrast. A number of optimal kVps are established for a fixed kVp system and are specific for a range of subject densities and contrasts. In other words, the so-called "fixed kVp" is fixed only for a specific range of part thicknesses for a particular procedure.

Establishing a fixed kVp technique chart involves producing phantom images, selecting the optimal phantom image, extrapolating a technique chart, and performing phantom testing, clinical trials, clinical fine tuning and ongoing fine tuning.

REVIEW QUESTIONS

1. What is the principle of a fixed kVp exposure system?

2. What are the basic advantages of a fixed kVp exposure system?

3. What are the basic disadvantages of a fixed kVp exposure system?

4. Define optimal kVp.

5. How is the optimal kVp established?

6. What should be the minimal mAs increments used for variations in part thickness when using a fixed kVp exposure system?

REFERENCES AND RECOMMENDED READING

Bryan, G. J. (1970). *Diagnostic radiography: A manual for radiologic technologists.* Baltimore: Williams & Wilkins.

Cahoon, J. B. (1961). Radiographic technique: Its origin, concept, practical application and evaluation of radiation dosage. *The X-Ray Technician. 32,* 354–364.

Carlstein, C. J. (1971). Radiography of compressed air workers using optimum kilovoltage. *Radiologic Technology.* 43(1), 10–14.

Carroll, Q. B. (1993). *Fuchs's radiographic exposure, processing, and quality control* (5th ed.). Springfield, IL: Charles C. Thomas Publishers.

Clark, K. C. (1953). An introduction to high-voltage technique. *Radiography. 19*, 21–33.

Compton, S. (1987). Bit conversion of technical factors in vascular procedures. *Radiologic Technology. 58*(5), 413.

Cullinan, A. & Cullinan, J. (1994). *Producing quality radiographs* (2nd ed.). Philadelphia: J. B. Lippincott.

Du Pont Company Photosystems & Electronic Products Department. *Positioning and exposure guide for general radiography.* Wilmington, DE: Publication R-53806-1.

Du Pont, E. I. de Nemours & Co. Medical Products Department, Customer Technology Center. *Bit system of technique conversion.* Wilmington, DE.

Dyke, W. P. (1975). Depth resolution: A mechanism by which high kilovoltage improves visibility in chest films. *Radiology. 117*, 159–164.

Eastman Kodak Company. (1980). Health Sciences Markets Division. *The fundamentals of radiography* (12th ed.). Rochester, NY: Kodak Publication M1-18.

Eastman, T. R. (1979). *Radiographic fundamentals and technique guide.* St. Louis: C. V. Mosby.

Eastman, T. R. (1978). A history of radiographic technique. *Applied Radiology.* (July/August), 97–100.

Eastman, T. R. (1975). Technique charts: The key to radiographic quality. *Radiologic Technology. 46*, 365–368.

Eastman, T. R. (1973). Measurement: The key to exposure with manual techniques. *Radiologic Technology. 45*, 75–78.

Eastman, T. R. (1971). Automated exposures in contemporary radiography. *Radiologic Technology. 43*(2), 80–83.

Eastman, T. R. (1969). Chest technique through body habitus. *Radiologic Technology. 41*, 80-84.

Eastman, T. R. *The Radiographic Technique Guide.* Wilmington, DE: DuPont deNemours, Inc. Photo Products Department Publication A-99101.

Files, G. W. (1952). *Medical radiographic technique.* Springfield, IL: Charles C. Thomas Publishers.

Fodor, J. & Malott, J. C. (1993). *The art and science of medical radiography* (7th ed.). St. Louis: C. V. Mosby.

Fodor, J., Malott, J. C., Ross, J. A., & Porter, M. (1985). Indications for the use of high kVp in the plain film examination of the abdomen. *Radiologic Technology. 57*(2), 159–161.

Fuchs, A. W. (1958). *Principles of radiographic exposure and processing* (2nd ed.). Springfield, IL: Charles C. Thomas Publishers.

Fuchs, A. W. (1950). The rationale of radiographic exposure. *The X-Ray Technician. 22*, 62–68, 76.

Fuchs, A. W. (1949). Control of radiographic density. *The X-Ray Technician. 20*, 271–273, 291.

Fuchs, A. W. (1948). Relationship of tissue thickness to kilovoltage. *The X-Ray Technician. 19*, 287–293.

Fuchs, A. W. (1945). Military photoroentgen technique employing optimum kilovolt (peak) principles. *The American Journal of Roentgenology. 53*, 587–596.

Fuchs, A. W. (1943). The optimum kilovoltage technique in military roentgenography. *American Journal of Roentgenology. 50*, 358–365.

Fuchs, A. W. (1938). Higher kilovoltage technic with high-definition screens. *Radiography and Clinical Photography. 14*(3), 2–8.

Fuchs, A. W. (1934). Radiography of entire body employing one film and a single exposure. *Radiography and Clinical Photography. 10*, 9–14.

Funke, T. (1966). Pegged kilovoltage technic. *Radiologic Technology. 37*, 202–213.

General Electric Company Medical Systems Department. *How to prepare an x-ray technic chart.* Milwaukee: Publication 4301A.

Gratale, P., Turner, G. W., & Burns, C. B. (1986). Using the same exposure factors for wet and dry casts. *Radiologic Technology. 57*(4), 325–328.

Hiss, S. S. (1993). *Understanding radiography* (3rd ed.). Springfield, IL: Charles C. Thomas Publishers.

Hiss, S. S. (1975). Technique management. *Radiologic Technology. 46*(5), 369.

Hopper, B. S. (1957). Radiography above 100 peak kilovolts. *The X-Ray Technician. 29*(1), 9.

Jenkins, D. (1980). *Radiographic photography and imaging processes.* Lancaster, England: MTP Press Limited.

Jerman, E. C. (1928). *Modern x-ray technic.* St. Paul: Bruce Publishing.

Jerman, E. C. (1926). Extremity technic. *Radiology. 6,* 252–254.

Jerman, E. C. (1926). Potter-Bucky diaphragm technic. *Radiology. 6,* 336–338.

Koenig, G. F. (1966). Potential. *Radiologic Technology. 37*(4), 184–198.

Koenig, G. F. (1957). Kilovoltage as a Qualitative Factor. *The X-Ray Technician. 29,* 1–4, 13.

Kratzer, B. (1973). A technique computer: Scientific approach to radiologic technology. *Radiologic Technology. 42*(4), 142–150.

Lyon, N. J. (1962). Optimum kilovoltage techniques. *The X-Ray Technician. 33,* 398–401.

McDaniel, C. T. (1965). Tissue absorption theory applied to formulation of radiographic technique resulting in time as the variable factor. *Radiologic Technology. 37*(2), 51–55.

Mahoney, G. J. (1959). A slide rule for kVp-mAs adjustments facilitating the use of high kilovoltage. *The X-Ray Technician. 31,* 35–38.

Merrill, H. F. (1960). High kilovoltage radiography. *The X-Ray Technician. 32*(3), 259.

Morgan, J. A. (1977). *The art and science of medical radiography* (5th ed.). St. Louis: Catholic Hospital Association.

Morgan, R. H. (1961). Physics of diagnostic radiology. *Physical Foundations of Radiology* (3rd ed.). New York: Paul Hoeber/Harper & Row.

Morgan, R. H. An analysis of the physical factors controlling the diagnostic quality of roentgen images. American *Journal of Roentgenology and Radiation Therapy. 54,* 128. *54,* 395. *55,* 67. *55,* 627.

Ott, T. T. (1963). Extending the range of medical radiography to 150 kilovolts. *The X-Ray Technician. 34*(6), 335–343.

Reed, C. W. (1939). *The X-Ray Technician. 11*(1).

Revesz, G., Shea, F. J., & Kundel, H. L. (1982). The effects of kilovoltage on diagnostic accuracy in chest radiography. *Radiology. 142,* 615–618.

Roderick, J. F. (1952). Latitude in roentgenology. *The X-Ray Technician. 24,* 187–196, 220.

Roderick, J. F. (1950). Photographic contrast in roentgenology. *The X-Ray Technician. 22,* 141–150, 163.

Sante, L. R. (1942). *Manual of Roentgenological technique* (9th ed.). Ann Arbor, MI: Edwards Brothers.

Schwarz, G. S. (1961). *Unit-step radiography.* Springfield, IL: Charles C. Thomas Publishers.

Schwarz, G. S. (1960). Kilovoltage conversion in radiography. *The X-Ray Technician. 31,* 373–379, 436.

Schwarz, G. S. (1959). Extended range radiography, *Radiology, 69*: 419–423, 1957.

Schwarz, G. S. (1959). Kilovoltage and radiographic effect. *Radiology. 73,* 749–760.

Schwarz, G. S. (1958). A simple universal unit system of radiographic exposures suited to departmental, national, and international standardization. *Radiology. 71,* 573–574.

Seeman, H. E. (1968). *Physical and photographic principles of medical radiography.* New York: Wiley & Sons.

Thomas, J. B. (1959). High kilovoltage equipment and technique. *The X-Ray Technician. 30*(6), 500.

Trout, E. D., Graves, D. E., & Slauson, D. B. (1949). High kilovoltage radiography. *Radiology. 52,* 669–683.

Tuddenham, W. J., Hale, J., & Pendergrass, E. P. (1953). Supervoltage diagnostic roentgenography. *American Journal of Roentgenology. 70*(5), 759–765.

United States Army. (1955). *Principles of radiographic exposure.* TM 8-282, March.

United States War Department. (1941). *Technical manual: Roentgenographic technicians,* TM 8-240, July 3.

van Dijk, D. (1955). Some factors influencing the results in radiography. *Medicamundi. 1,* 27–32.

Williams, W. A. (1960). Standardization of x-ray technique. *The X-Ray Technician. 32*(2), 137.

Wilsey, R. B. (1921). The intensity of scatter x-rays in radi-ography. *American Journal of Roentgenology. 8*, 328–338.

Wynroe, R. F. (1955). Some observations on kilovoltage vari-ations. *Radiography. 21*(251), 242–243.

Yurcessen, E. H. (1954). Trend for higher kilovoltage for adequate penetration. *The X-Ray Technician. 26*(2), 96.

The Case of the Last Dinner

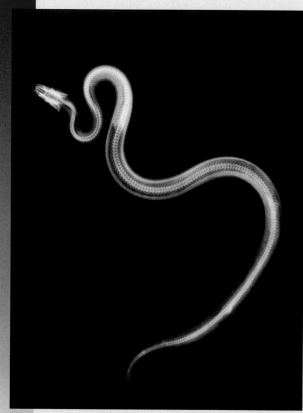

Of course this is a snake, but can you tell if the last dinner is still within the GI tract?

Answers to the case studies can be found in Appendix E.

(Reprinted by permission of the International Society of Radiographers and Radiological Technicians from the K. C. Clark Archives, Middlesex Hospital, London, England)

CHAPTER 33

Variable Kilovoltage Systems

The [radiographer] who does his work by the "hunch method" can never successfully compete with one who having mastered the fundamentals is enabled to develop a proper procedure and put into the film any quality that may be desired.

Ed. C. Jerman, the Father of Radiography in the United States.

Objectives

Upon completion of this chapter, the student should be able to:

▶ Describe a variable kilovoltage technique system.

▶ Discuss the primary advantages and disadvantages of variable kVp technique systems.

▶ State the 2 kVp rule.

▶ Explain why more than a single kilovoltage scale is required.

▶ Calculate new exposure factors from a single satisfactory exposure when mAs ratios are provided.

▶ Synthesize a stepped variable kVp technique chart from control radiographs.

Principles of a Variable Kilovoltage Peak Exposure System

A variable kilovoltage x-ray exposure technique system is one in which the kilovoltage to be used for a particular projection is varied depending on measured body part thickness. The thicker the body part, the higher the value of kilovoltage assigned. A milliampere-second value is specified for each body part to be examined. Its value depends on image receptor speed and other parameters.

In use, the radiographer sets the mAs specified for the part and measured part thickness. The value of kVp corresponding to that thickness is found on the chart. For example, in Table 33–1, a 12 cm-thick part will require 54 kVp (i.e., an average shoulder).

Advantages and Disadvantages

Technique systems that use variable kilovoltage offer the advantage of permitting small incremental changes in exposure to compensate for variation in body part thickness. These changes in exposure may not be possible with systems that fix kilovoltage and vary milliampere-seconds because of an insufficient number of settings on the exposure timers of many x-ray generators.

A potential disadvantage of the variable kilovoltage technique arises when one considers the complexity of the effect of changing kilovoltage on the way the subject is imaged on the radiograph. Increasing kilovoltage reduces radiographic contrast. Reducing contrast may be helpful if the initial kilovoltage is too low to provide adequate penetration of the part (Figure 33–1A). The reduction in contrast that occurs when kilovoltage is too high can reduce the radiologist's ability to see fine detail in the image (Figure 33–1C). A useful variable kilovoltage system must use values of kilovoltage that provide adequate penetration of the part and result in a level of contrast that is acceptable to the radiologist (Figure 33–1B).

The radiation exposure to the patient is strongly dependent upon the kilovoltage used for the projection. In general, the higher the kilovoltage, the lower the patient dose. When kilovoltage is at an appropriate level for the body part examined, patient dose considerations are less of a factor when deciding whether to establish an exposure system using fixed or variable kVp.

Historical Development

In the early days of radiography it was common practice to use a change of 2 kVp for every one centimeter of tissue thickness. A kilovoltage progression could be readily computed by taking two times the centimeter measurement. To this value a constant, such as 30 kVp, was added to achieve a kVp value high enough to penetrate the part. This produces a basic variable kVp formula:

$$(2 \text{ kVp} \times \text{part cm}) + 30 \text{ kVp} = \text{new kVp}$$

Example: What is the proper kilovoltage for a 20 cm part thickness?

Answer:

$$(2 \text{ kVp} \times \text{part cm}) + 30 \text{ kVp} = \text{new kVp}$$
$$(2 \text{ kVp} \times 20 \text{ cm}) + 30 \text{ kVp} = \text{new kVp}$$
$$(40 \text{ kVp/cm}) + 30 \text{ kVp} = 70 \text{ kVp}$$

It was found that multiple kilovoltage scales were needed because the values selected from the progression could be too low to provide adequate penetration of body parts, such as the shoulder or cervical spine, which contain dense bone with little soft tissue (Table 33–2A). Higher kilovoltage scales were created by increasing the base kilovoltage added. For example, if kilovoltage were computed using 40 kVp instead of 30 kVp, the formula would be:

$$(2 \text{ kVp} \times \text{part cm}) + 40 \text{ kVp} = \text{new kVp}$$

Example: What is the proper kilovoltage for the same 20 cm part thickness, using the new formula?

Answer:

$$(2 \text{ kVp} \times \text{part cm}) + 40 \text{ kVp} = \text{new kVp}$$

TABLE 33–1. 2 kVp Per cm Chart

cm	10	11	12	13	14
kVp	50	52	54	56	58

52 kVp	1200 mAs	42" **SID**
16:1 **grid**	300 **RS**	1550 **mR**

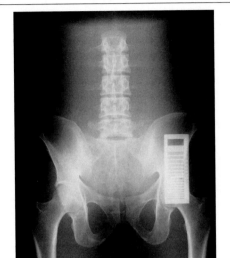

A

$$(2 \text{ kVp} \times 20 \text{ cm}) + 40 \text{ kVp} = \text{new kVp}$$
$$(40 \text{ kVp/cm}) + 40 \text{ kVp} = 80 \text{ kVp}$$

All values would be correspondingly higher with the new formula. For example, the values of shoulder and cervical spine views measuring 12 cm would be 64 kVp instead of the 54 kVp previously obtained. By increasing or decreasing the value of kVp added as a constant, it is possible to create an array of kilovoltage scales. The scales shown in Tables 33–2A–C were computed using 30, 40 and 50 kVp as the constant:

$$(2 \text{ kVp} \times \text{part cm}) + 30 \text{ kVp} = \text{new kVp}$$
$$(2 \text{ kVp} \times \text{part cm}) + 40 \text{ kVp} = \text{new kVp}$$
$$(2 \text{ kVp} \times \text{part cm}) + 50 \text{ kVp} = \text{new kVp}$$

Note that the kilovoltage values for a 20 cm-thick body part are shown as 70 kVp, 80 kVp and 90 kVp, depending on the scale selected.

Changes of 10 kVp in the base number added were used in the belief that a change of ±10 kVp would compensate for doubling and halving mAs. In practice 30, 40 or 50 can be easily added to centimeters doubled by the radiographer mentally and the assigned value of kVp can thus be readily determined when charts are not available. Milliampere-second values were found by trial and error but, once determined, were listed for a particular body

70 kVp	160 mAs	42" **SID**
16:1 **grid**	300 **RS**	580 **mR**

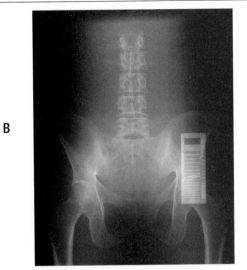

B

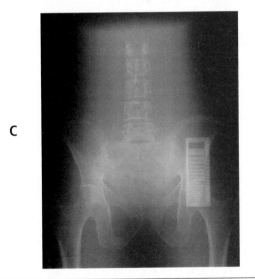

C

115 kVp	10 mAs	42" **SID**
16:1 **grid**	400 **RS**	106 **mR**

FIGURE 33-1. Comparison of contrast produced at three kilovoltage ranges: (A) high contrast at low (52) kilovoltage, (B) ideal contrast produced at approximate (70) kilovoltage, and (C) low contrast produced at high (115) kilovoltage.

TABLE 33–2. Variable Kilovoltage Scales

A		B		C	
2 kVp/cm + 30		**2 kVp/cm + 40**		**2 kVp/cm + 50**	
cm	kVp	cm	kVp	cm	kVp
2	34	2	44	2	54
3	36	3	46	3	56
4	38	4	48	4	58
5	40	5	50	5	60
6	42	6	52	6	62
7	44	7	54	7	64
8	46	8	56	8	66
9	48	9	58	9	68
10	50	10	60	10	70
11	52	11	62	11	72
12	54	12	64	12	74
13	56	13	66	13	76
14	58	14	68	14	78
15	60	15	70	15	80
16	62	16	72	16	82
17	64	17	74	17	84
18	66	18	76	18	86
19	68	19	78	19	88
20	70	20	80	20	90
21	72	21	82	21	92
22	74	22	84	22	94
23	76	23	86	23	96
24	78	24	88	24	98
25	80	25	90	25	100
26	82	26	92	26	102
27	84	27	94	27	104
28	86	28	96	28	106
29	88	29	98	29	108
30	90	30	100	30	110
31	92	31	102	31	112
32	94	32	104	32	114
33	96	33	106	33	116
34	98	34	108	34	118
35	100	35	110	35	120
36	102	36	112	36	122

part and kilovoltage selected by measuring the part. A useful technique chart was thus created.

It was found in practice that 80 kVp for a 20 cm abdomen using equipment and image receptors of the time was nearly ideal. In 1948, Fuchs suggested that kVp be fixed at 80 for the abdomen, with mAs varied to compensate for the size difference of patients. Fixed kilovoltage techniques, sometimes called optimum techniques, are described in Chapter 32. They are mentioned here to point out that similar results may be obtained regardless of the system employed in order to handle the variables of kVp, mA, and time.

Although the kilovoltage scales shown in Tables 33–2A, B, and C were useful in practical patient radiography, and in fact would still be useful, two assumptions used in their computation were found to be false. The notion that a ±10 kVp change will balance a change of double or half mAs has largely given way to the so-called 15 percent rule. This rule suggests decreasing kVp by 15 percent to reduce exposure by half and increasing kVp by 15 percent to double exposure. Although the 15 percent rule better reflects the exponentially nonlinear changes that occur when kilovoltage is altered, it is not totally accurate either. These relationships are among the most complex in radiography and remain difficult to quantify.

When the 15 percent rule is applied, it can be readily seen that a 7.5 kVp change is required at 50 kVp (15 percent × 50 kVp) to balance a 50 percent reduction in mAs, while at 100 kVp, a 15 kVp change (15 percent × 100 kVp) is required. This reflects the fact that at low kilovoltage a small change in kVp can have a large effect on film exposure, while at higher kilovoltage a larger change will be required to produce the same effect. A uniform change of 2 kVp per centimeter in tissue thickness will not function satisfactorily over a wide range of tissue thicknesses. At a fixed value of mAs and proper exposure of an average patient, radiographs of thicker patients will become increasingly underexposed as patient size increases.

Early users of variable kilovoltage techniques computed kVp scales using 2 kVp per centimeter plus a constant and ±10 kVp between the scales. They were able to use such charts successfully chiefly because the range of variation in adult body part thicknesses is small (Table 31–1). Thus, kilovoltage values used for a particular body part are within a relatively narrow range. Since mAs values were found by trial and error using kilovoltage from the scales according to patient measurement, problems due to the use of ±10 kVp change between the scales were minimized, if not entirely eliminated. In addition, a patient whose body habitus varies from the norm is easily recognized by an experienced radiographer, and it was common practice then, as now, to increase or decrease the mAs according to the radiographer's professional judgment in compensation for body habitus and known pathological conditions.

Establishing a Stepped Variable kVp System

The variable kilovoltage technique systems used today have evolved from the earlier systems. A modern stepped kVp system can be developed in a manner similar to the "pegged kilovoltage technic" system published by Funke in 1966. These systems are based on the concept that straight variable kilovoltage charts are inadequate (such as those shown in Tables 33–2A, B, and C). They all recommend kVp settings for extremely small parts that may not provide adequate penetration. These charts also recommend kVp settings for extremely large parts that may produce excessive scatter fog. In other words, unsatisfactory contrast is produced for both small and large part sizes with a straight variable kilovoltage chart.

The kVp Scale

This problem is remedied by establishing a limited variable kilovoltage scale that meets three criteria:

1. All film contrast is acceptable to the radiologists.
2. Small part size kVp recommendations provide adequate penetration.
3. Large part size kVp recommendations avoid excessive scatter fog.

Initial Phantom Images

The limited variable kilovoltage scale is determined by producing a series of radiographs according to a straight variable kilovoltage charts such as those shown in Tables 33–2A, B, and C. A phantom in a variable depth water bath is used to simulate the various part thicknesses. A variable depth water bath is made by placing a radiographic phantom in a watertight Plexiglas box and then filling it with water to the desired centimeter thickness. A much less complicated, although suboptimal simulation of this procedure, is to simply radiograph a phantom at various kVp levels without changing the part thickness. Both procedures will produce a series of phantom images ranging from very high (or even inadequate penetration) contrast to very low contrast with excessive scatter fog.

Select Optimal Phantom Image

If the resulting radiograph is too light or dark, a repeat radiograph with an appropriate mAs adjustment is made. This process is continued on subsequent patients until ideal diagnostic quality radiographs are obtained. The kVp should not be altered from the value shown for part thickness in Table 33–3.

The use of a patient equivalent phantom can reduce or eliminate the need for patient exposures. The American National Standards Institute (ANSI) patient equivalent phantom (PEP) is recommended for this purpose. Technical factors required to produce a film density of OD 1.4 with the PEP are suited for use on a 21 cm AP lumbar spine patient. Use the kVp for a 21 cm patient from the chart and find the mAs required by trial exposures. If an ANSI phantom is not available, a smooth bottom plastic wastebasket filled with tap water to a depth of 17 cm has been used successfully for technique development. Use kVp from the chart for a 21 cm AP lumbar spine, and by trial exposure find the mAs required to produce OD 1.4.

The series of images that are produced will demonstrate a wide range of contrast. They are evaluated by **all** radiologists and those other physicians deemed critical to the image quality process. Each physician indicates those images they are not willing to accept for diagnosis. When this evaluation is complete, the variable kilovoltage scale is reduced to only those kVp levels that are within the acceptable diagnostic range for the physicians who will be diagnosing from the images. This reduction will eliminate some of the part sizes from the chart (Table 33–3, Step 1).

Extrapolate Technique Chart

Once the range of acceptable diagnostic radiographs has been established, a complete technique chart can be computed. The elimination of suboptimal images leaves only the kVp ranges acceptable to the physicians and forms a limited "step" of acceptable kilovoltage. Steps should be formed in groups of 4–5 cm increments as this makes mAs adjustments much simpler.

The mAs Scale

Establishing the kVp steps in increments of 4–5 cm permits simple doubling or halving of mAs to maintain image density. Changes of 4–5 cm in tissue thickness require doubling or halving of mAs to maintain approximately the same image density (see Chapter 25). The chart is revised to eliminate the rejected kVp ranges by establishing extrapolated kVp steps for the entire chart (Table 33–3, Step 2). At this point in the development of the chart it should be obvious that there are a number of inappropriate kVp ranges. For example, a 14 cm part should not be radiographed at 84 kVp, nor should a 31 cm part be radiographed at 70 kVp. Therefore it is necessary to fine tune the extrapolated kVp steps to bring these kVp values within appropriate ranges for penetration and scatter control (Table 33–3, Step 3). This is accomplished by applying the 4–5 cm rule and/or the 15 percent rule to modify the kVp to an appropriate value while maintaining an acceptable density. Note that in Table 33–3, Step 3, the kVp steps follow an even 4 cm, doubling or halving of mAs pattern with only the 20 mAs values utilizing the entire accepted range of 70–84 kVp. This is because the fine tuning process determined that the upper kVp range (78–84 kVp) produced overpenetration of the small part sizes while the lower kVp range (70 –78 kVp) did not adequately penetrate the larger part sizes.

Phantom Testing

Phantom testing is recommended prior to performing patient examinations. At the minimum, phantom testing should be done for a median, small, and large part size as a fine tuning mechanism for the extrapolated chart prior to clinical use.

TABLE 33–3. Stepped Variable kVp Technique Chart

2 kVp/cm + 40

Establishing a Limited Variable kVp Scale Step 1				Extrapolating kVp Steps Step 2		Fine Tuning of Extrapolated kVp Values Step 3	
cm	kVp	mAs	evaluation	kVp	mAs	kVp	mAs
4	54	20	reject	70	5	70	5
6	56	20	reject	72	5	72	5
8	58	20	reject	74	5	74	5
10	60	20	reject	76	5	76	5
11	62	20	reject	78	5	70	10
12	64	20	reject	80	5	72	10
13	66	20	reject	82	5	74	10
14	68	20	reject	84	5	76	10
15	70	20	acceptable	70	20	70	20
16	72	20	acceptable	72	20	72	20
17	74	20	acceptable	74	20	74	20
18	76	20	acceptable	76	20	76	20
19	78	20	acceptable	78	20	78	20
20	80	20	acceptable	80	20	80	20
21	82	20	acceptable	82	20	82	20
22	84	20	acceptable	84	20	84	20
23	86	20	reject	70	80	78	40
24	88	20	reject	72	80	80	40
25	90	20	reject	74	80	82	40
26	92	20	reject	76	80	84	40
27	94	20	reject	78	80	78	80
28	96	20	reject	80	80	80	80
29	98	20	reject	82	80	82	80
30	100	20	reject	84	80	84	80
31	102	20	reject	70	320	78	160
32	104	20	reject	72	320	80	160
33	106	20	reject	74	320	82	160
34	108	20	reject	76	320	84	160
35	110	20	reject	78	320	78	320
36	112	20	reject	80	320	80	320
37	114	20	reject	82	320	82	320
38	118	20	reject	84	320	84	320

Clinical Trials

Limited clinical trials are then permissible with the new chart. All images should be recorded with repeated images saved for analysis. When clinical trials are proceeding without excess repeated exposures, the new technique chart can move into the clinical fine tuning stage.

Clinical Fine Tuning

The clinical fine tuning process is designed to adjust and validate the entire chart. At this point the new technique chart can be adapted. However, ongoing fine tuning then begins as a permanent process.

Ongoing Fine Tuning

Ongoing fine tuning is the process that maintains the accuracy of the entire exposure system and is crucial to both radiographers and radiologists developing a confidence in the exposure and diagnostic processes. It is performed by maintaining an accurate record of modifications to existing techniques for review by the person responsible for quality control.

The Mayo Clinic Variable kVp System

A modern version of a variable kilovoltage chart currently in use in the Mayo Clinic Department of Diagnostic Radiology is shown in Table 33–4. A precursor to this chart was originally established by Raymond Runge of Mayo Clinic about 1925. As was common practice, the first versions were constructed using kilovoltage corresponding to two times the centimeter measurement plus a constant. Runge recognized the deficiencies of this approach and made revisions in his later experiments by using a water phantom, which greatly improved the results. Modifications were made by Winkler to further refine the kilovoltage progressions and, most recently, by Stears and Frank with the introduction of rare-earth intensifying screens.

The kVp Scale

The kilovoltage versus measured centimeter thickness chart shown in Table 33–4 has the kilovoltage values arranged in seven columns plus one column corresponding to centimeter thickness of the part examined. For a given centimeter thickness there are up to seven kVp values that may be selected. For a 21 cm patient thickness these values are 52, 58, 63, 72, 80, 95 and 115 kVp. Note that the kilovoltage columns are labeled Scale 8, Scale 4, Scale 2, Scale 1, 1/2 Scale, 1/4 Scale and 1/8 Scale. The kilovoltage change from one scale to the next at any given centimeter thickness is that amount that will be equal to reducing mAs by half or doubling it. For example, using kilovoltage values from Scale 1 as a base at the 21 cm level (72 kVp), a shift to 1/2 Scale (80 kVp) will permit reducing mAs by 1/2. A change from Scale 1 to 1/4 Scale allows mAs to be reduced to 1/4 the value for kVp Scale 1, while kVp from the 1/8 Scale would allow use of 1/8 the mAs. Use of the lower kVp values obtained from Scale 2, Scale 4 and Scale 8 would require the use of two times, four times or eight times the mAs used with the kVp from Scale 1.

Radiographs obtained are similarly exposed but, because of the extreme range of kilovoltage used (52–115), vary widely from too high to too low contrast (Figure 33–1). In practice, the column from which kilovoltage is selected is specified to produce a level of contrast preferred by radiologists. For a patient 21 cm in thickness, the 1/2 Scale value, 80 kVp, is used if the generator is single phase. Lower kVp from Scale 1 (72 kVp) is chosen to maintain similar radiographic contrast if a three-phase generator is used. Arrangement of the kilovoltage columns such that the kVp changes by moving from any column to its neighbor permits halving or doubling mAs while allowing great flexibility in the use of the scales. This also permits selection of a kVp value to provide adequate penetration of any examined part, and thus produces optimum radiographic contrast.

The kilovoltage change necessary between the scales to balance doubling or halving mAs was initially derived from water phantom experiments. Kilovoltage progression (the increase in kilovoltage needed for each increase of one centimeter of tissue thickness) was obtained by using a doubling increase in kilovoltage for each 5 cm increase in part thickness. For example, in Table 33–4, the kVp value for a 21 cm measurement shown in 1/2 Scale (80 kVp) is listed in Scale 1 for a 26 cm measurement and the 1/2 Scale value for 26 cm (95 kVp) is listed in Scale 1 corresponding to 31 cm. All scales have

TABLE 33–4. Kilovoltage vs. Measured Centimeter Thickness Chart

SCALE 8	SCALE 4	SCALE 2	SCALE 1	CM	1/2 SCALE	1/4 SCALE	1/8 SCALE
		47	52	6	58	63	72
		48	53	7	59	64	73
		49	54	8	60	66	74
		50	55	9	61	68	76
	SCALE 4	51	56	10	62	70	78
	47	52	58	11	63	72	80
	48	53	59	12	64	73	82
	49	54	60	13	66	74	84
	50	55	61	14	68	76	87
SCALE 8	51	56	62	15	70	78	91
47	52	58	63	16	72	80	95
48	53	59	64	17	73	82	98
49	54	60	66	18	74	84	101
50	55	61	68	19	76	87	105
51	56	62	70	20	78	91	110
52	58	63	72	21	80	95	115
53	59	64	73	22	82	98	120
54	60	66	74	23	84	101	125
55	61	68	76	24	87	105	130
56	62	70	78	25	91	110	135
58	63	72	80	26	95	115	140
59	64	73	82	27	98	120	
60	66	74	84	28	101	125	
61	68	76	87	29	105		
62	70	78	91	30	110		
63	72	80	95	31	115		
64	73	82	98	32	120		
66	74	84	101	33	125		
68	76	87	105	34	130		
70	78	91	110	35	135		
72	80	95	115	36	140		
73	82	98	120	37			
74	84	101	125	38			
76	87	105	130	39			
78	91	110	135	40			
80	95	115	140	41			

EXTREMITY CASSETTE

CM	kVp
1	45
2	47
3	49
4	52
5	55
6	58
7	61
8	64
9	67
10	70

continues

TABLE 33–4. Kilovoltage vs. Measured Centimeter Thickness Chart (continued)

Extremity—Non-Bucky	TIME	mA	kVp			TFD	CASSETTE
REGULAR CASSETTE						45" (ALL)	
Ankle/Elbow	.016	200	1/4			48"	24 × 30 cm
Tibia-Fibula	.016	200	1/4			48"	14 × 17 in
Calcaneous	.016	200	1/2			48"	8 × 10 in
Wrist-Carpal Tunnel	.033	200	65 kVp			48"	8 × 10 in
Cast - Plaster	.033	200	1/4			48"	
Cast - Fiberglass	.016	200	1/4			48"	
EXTREMITY CASSETTE			SM	MED	LG		
Hand/Wrist PA/OBL	.025	200	58	60	62	48"	24 × 30 cm
Hand/Wrist LAT	.025	200	63	65	67	48"	8 × 10 in
Forearm	.025	200	Extremity Scale			48"	7 × 17 in
Toes	.025	200	58	60	62	48"	24 × 30 cm
Foot	.025	200	63	65	67	48"	24 ×
Lateral Calcaneous	.025	200	63	65	67	45"	8 × 10 in

©1988 Mayo Clinic (Reprinted by permission of the Mayo Clinic, Rochester, MN)

been constructed using a double technique kVp value for each 5 centimeter change in thickness. Values for centimeters between the technique doubling points are chosen to provide a smooth progression but rounded off to the nearest whole kVp.

Determination of kilovoltage, though important, gives only one of the primary exposure factors. In a variable kVp technique system, kilovoltage selection is made by first measuring the examined part and then selecting a value from the kVp tables, as previously described. Values of distance, milliamperage and time must also be determined in any useful technique system.

Source-to-Image Receptor Distance

The inverse square relationship between SID (FFD) and radiation intensity at the film permits a small difference in SID to translate into a large difference in exposure of the radiograph. For this reason, the SID should be specified for each examination.

As a practical matter, and to avoid off focal distance grid cut-off of primary radiation, the focal distance of the x-ray table Bucky should be used. Because some table grids are difficult to examine without dismantling the x-ray table, it may be helpful to know that most equip-

ment manufacturers provide 40" focal distance grids for most x-ray tables. For this reason, a 40" SID is often the best choice, unless the particular Bucky grid employed is known to have been manufactured for use at another focal range.

A useful SID selection for most routine radiography would be 40" (100 cm) for flat Bucky work and extremities, with 72" (180 cm) used for upright chest work. It is important that whatever SID is selected, the value be noted on the technique chart, and that all users of the chart recognize that an alteration in technique must be made if the specified SID is not used for a particular examination.

mAs A useful technique system requires determination of the value of mAs that will provide proper exposure to the film when used in combination with the kilovoltage chosen. During phantom testing, milliamperage-seconds are increased or decreased in doubling or halving increments for sequential radiographs until proper exposure is achieved. The mAs value that has been determined is then recorded in terms of mAs or mA and time use on the technique chart. This method of determining mAs by trial and error was thoroughly described by Fuchs. Kratzer's Supertech™, Trinkle's Du Pont Bit

System, the Siemens Point System, and Schwartz's XVS system are examples of other systems and devices that have been designed to assist in the process of x-ray technique development (see Chapter 34). Although the number of trial and error exposures that must be made can be dramatically reduced with the use of any of the systems mentioned above, the development of an effective x-ray technique system for an individual x-ray department can be successfully accomplished only by that department.

mAs Ratios

In the late 1980s Frank and Winkler presented a method of computing an x-ray exposure technique with the use of mAs ratios. The system of mAs ratios was devised by Winkler, who set up mathematical relationships from trial and error exposure determinations for various body parts that had been made by Runge. Reference to the kilovoltage scales in Table 33–4 is made to select values of kVp for use with mAs values for the examined part, which are computed using the mAs ratios after a base exposure is found. The advantage of the system lies in the radiographer's ability to compute mAs values for all body parts once the mAs value for only one body part has been found by trial and error. The need to examine large numbers of patients with multiple trials is eliminated. Minor changes in computed mAs values found for some views may be desirable following a period of use.

The resulting technique system of mAs ratios combined with kilovoltage varied with part thickness may be categorized as **variable kVp within an optimal range**. For example, the average thickness for an adult shoulder ranges from 12–16 cm. Kilovoltage for these extremes will be 64–72 kVp (from 1/2 Scale, shown in Table 33–4). Thus, the actual kilovoltage range typically used is narrow for any given body part. The best features of variable kVp techniques (small incremental changes) and fixed kVp techniques (optimal contrast) are obtained.

As previously described, the thickness of the examined part is measured where specified or along the path of the central ray. The value of the kVp corresponding to the thickness of the part is selected from the kVp chart. For example, for a shoulder measuring 14 cm, 1/2 Scale is specified with a three-phase generator and a value of 68 kVp is found, while the mAs is fixed.

The mAs ratios used in technique computation are shown in Table 33–5. Computed mAs values are used with kilovoltage corresponding to part thickness from the chart in Table 33–4. In this system, the AP projection of the lumbar spine is assigned a value of 1.0. Existing exposure techniques, which had been established by Runge using trial and error exposure for each body part, were used in computing the ratios by the following formula:

$$\frac{\text{mAs for body part}}{\text{mAs for AP lumbar}} = \text{mAs ratio for body part}$$

Establishing a Mayo Clinic Variable kVp Chart

Initial Phantom Images

When a new technique chart is computed using the mAs ratios, mAs for the AP lumbar spine is first found by patient examination. In the process, the patient's thickness is measured, kVp is selected from the kilovoltage chart found in Table 33–4 and the required mAs is estimated based on previous experience. Only those patients referred for a lumbar spine examination should be involved in the process.

Select Optimal Phantom Image

If the resulting radiograph is too light or dark, a repeat radiograph with an appropriate mAs adjustment is made. This process is continued on subsequent patients until ideal diagnostic quality radiographs are obtained. The kVp should not be altered from the value shown for part thickness in Table 33–4.

The use of a patient equivalent phantom can reduce or eliminate the need for patient exposures. The American National Standards Institute (ANSI) patient equivalent phantom (PEP) is recommended for this purpose. Technical factors required to produce a film density of OD 1.4 with the PEP are suited for use on a 21 cm AP lumbar spine patient. Use the kVp for a 21 cm patient from the chart and find the mAs required by trial exposures.

TABLE 33–5. mAs Ratios
Body Parts

Examination	mAs Ratios	kVp 3–Phase	kVp 1–Phase
Skull AP & LAT Adult	.45	1/2 scale	1/4 scale
Cervical AP	.60	1/2	1/4
Lateral (Cross Table)	.15	1/2	1/4
OBL (Tabletop)	.20	1/2	1/4
Swimmers	.75	1	1/2
Odontoid (30")	.25	1/2	1/4
Pillar	1.00	1/4	1/8
Thoracic AP (Filter)	1.50	1	1/2
(without Filter)	.75	1	1/2
Thoracic LAT (Filter)	3.04	2	1
(without Filter)	.50	2	1
Thoracic Lower LAT (No Filter)	.60	2	1
Lumbar AP and Abdomen (19–23 cm)	1.00	1	1/2
Lumbar OBL (19–23 cm)	1.50	1	1/2
Lumbar LAT	1.50	1	1/2
Lumbar LOC LAT	1.50	1	1/2
Lumbar Graft LAT (L5–S1)	3.04	2	1
Lumbar Flexion/Extension	3.04	2	1
Pelvis & Hip/OBL	1.50	1	1/2
Hips LAT	1.50	1	1/2
Sacrum AP	1.50	1	1/2
Coccyx AP	1.50	1	1/2
Sacrum, Coccyx LAT	3.00	2	1
S-I Joints	1.50	1	1/2
Shoulder AP	.30	1/2	1/4
Y or Neer View	.30	1/2	1/4
Transthoracic Lateral	.13	1/2	1/4
Axillary (Grid)	.30	1/2	1/4
Scapula AP & LAT OBL	.39	1/2	1/4
Clavicle	.30	1/2	1/4
Humerus	.30	1/2	1/4
Femur	.60	1/2	1/4
LAT & OBL for Vessels	.40	1/2	1/4
Knee	.19	1/4	1/8
Intercondylar Notch	.075	1/2	1/4
Patella (Merchants)	.075	1/4	1/8
Chest, AP Supine, All	.025	1/2	1/4
Bucky Chest	.17	1/2	1/4
Chest, Lateral Supine (Bucky)	.25	1	1/2
Chest, Lateral Decubitus (Grid)	.13	1/2	1/4
Lateral Sternum	1.50	1	1/2
Ribs Above Diaphragm	.25	1	1/2
Ribs Below Diaphragm (19–23 cm)	1.00	1	1/2

continues

**TABLE 33–5. mAs Ratios (continued)
Extremities[1]**

Examination	mAs Ratios Extremities[1]	kVp 3–Phase	kVp 1–Phase
Regular cassette: Non-Bucky			
Ankle/Elbow	.075	$1/2$ scale	$1/4$ scale
Tibia-Fibula	.075	$1/2$	$1/4$
Calcaneous	.075	$1/4$	$1/8$
Wrist-Carpal Tunnel	.075	65 kVp	73 kVp (no caliper)
Cast-Plaster	.15	$1/2$	$1/4$
Cast-Fiberglass	.10	$1/2$	$1/4$
Extremity cassette: Non-Bucky			
Hand/Wrist-PA/OBL	.25	58 60 62	
Hand/Wrist-LAT	.25	63 65 67	
Forearm	.25	EXT Scale (use caliper)	
Toes	.25	58 60 62	
Foot	.25	63 65 67	

—mAs ratios are based on: Lumbar AP, 21 cm technique and a film density of 1.4 (± 0.10) from the standard phantom. [2] Always use this *base technique* for the calculations.

—All values are for bucky/grid unless specified.

—All values are for adult techniques.

—All values are for 48" unless specified.

—The following examinations each have three exposure time and kVp values. The mAs ratio is for the *middle measurement* (19–23 cm): Lumbar AP and Abdomen; Lumbar Oblique; Ribs below diaphragm.

[1] May vary depending upon tabletop attenuation and speed of system.

[2] Gray, Winkler, Stears, Frank. *Quality Control in Diagnostic Radiology.* Aspen Publishers Incorporated, Rockville, 1983.

© 1988 Mayo Clinic (Reprinted by permission of Mayo Clinic, Rochester, MN)

Extrapolate Technique Chart

Once the mAs value that produces an optimal diagnostic quality image for the AP lumbar spine has been established, a complete technique chart is computed from that value as follows:

1. Values are substituted in the mAs ratio formula. For example, if 66 mAs was found to be a good value for the AP lumbar, it becomes the constant for all further calculations.

2. The mAs ratio for the body part is found in Table 33–5 and the formula is used to calculate the new mAs for the body part.

Example: The shoulder has an mAs ratio of 0.30. What is the appropriate mAs value that should be used for a system that produces a satisfactory AP lumbar at 66 mAs?

Answer:

$$\frac{\text{mAs for body part}}{\text{mAs for AP lumbar}} = \text{mAs ratio for body part}$$

$$\frac{\text{mAs for body part}}{66 \text{ mAs}} = 0.30$$

mAs for body part = 66 mAs x 0.30

mAs for body part = 19.8 $\approx$ 20 mAs

The kilovoltage is selected from 1/2 Scale (Table 33–4), which yields 64 kVp for a shoulder measuring 12 centimeters. Technical factors for the shoulder are 20 mAs, 64 kVp. An appropriate mA and time selection for 20 mAs might be 200 mA at 0.10 second.

Computed techniques should be entered in a technique chart that is prominently posted in the x-ray control booth for ready reference by the radiographers (Table 33–6).

It is usually most advantageous to list values of mA and time rather than mAs unless only mAs is shown on the control. This approach frees the radiographer from being required to calculate appropriate mA and time values and reduces the likelihood of errors that could cause repeats. Additionally, the use of a single mA setting eliminates the potential for exposure problems caused by variations in x-ray output that may exist between the mA stations available on a generator, and calculations of technical factors are simplified.

Example: Assume that 66 mAs was found to be appropriate for the AP lumbar spine and the 200 mA station at 0.33 seconds was used. If the 200 mA station is chosen as a constant, only the exposure time for the AP lumbar needs to be used with the mAs ratio to compute the exposure time for other body parts. What exposure time should be used for a pelvis, when the pelvis ratio is 1.5?

Answer:

$$\frac{\text{mAs for body part}}{\text{mAs for AP lumbar}} = \text{mAs ratio for body part}$$

When the mA station is a constant, only the exposure time needs to be calculated:

$$\frac{\text{sec for body part}}{0.33 \text{ sec}} = 1.5$$

$$\text{sec for body part} = 0.33 \text{ sec} \times 1.5$$
$$\text{sec for body part} = 0.495 \approx 0.5 \text{ sec}$$

In this example, the technique for the pelvis is found to be 0.5 second at 200 mA, with the kVp measured from kVp Scale 1. Time values for other body parts are computed in the same way and entered in the technique chart. When an exact match between the time value computed cannot be made because of the limited number of time selections available on the x-ray control, the next greater time value should be used.

mA Station Selection The speed of image receptors currently used, in combination with thermal load capacities of x-ray tubes usually supplied with x-ray equipment, will generally allow the use of the small focal spot at 100 mA single phase and 200 mA three phase for nearly all common procedures. However, reference must be made to the single exposure rating chart for the tube to assure that exposures computed are indeed within the capacity of the small focal spot. For example, the single-phase tube rating chart that was previously shown in Figure 6–24 would permit a maximum of 0.2 second at 200 mA and 80 kVp. Thus the exposure computed for the pelvis in the preceding example (0.5 sec, 200 mA and kVp as measured) would not be allowed with a single-phase generator and this x-ray tube on the small focal spot. Use of the large focal spot would be necessary. However, for a 150 mA small focal spot, a maximum exposure of 4 sec at 80 kVp is permitted. Thus the 150 mA station could be used at the small focal spot. It is important to check the tube's single exposure rating chart and to be certain that the correct chart for the focal spot size, generator type, and rotor speed is used as the tube's ratings are strongly dependent on these factors.

Measurement of Part Thickness

Effective use of a variable kVp technique chart requires precise measurement of part thickness. This is accomplished with a measuring caliper. As a rule, measurement of part thickness along the path of the central x-ray beam is used. For accuracy in measurement, the measuring caliper should be angled if the x-ray beam is angled. However, if the technique chart was constructed by someone using different measuring standards, the same rules used for the chart must be followed by everyone who uses it.

There are two exceptions to this general rule of measuring along the path of the central x-ray beam when the mAs ratio system in Table 33–5 is used. These are the AP projection of the lumbar spine and/or abdomen and the lateral lumbar spine. The AP lumbar or abdomen should be measured just below the tip of the sternum. The lateral lumbar spine should be measured at L2.

TABLE 33–6. Variable Kilovoltage Technique Chart

EXAMINATION	TIME	mA	kVp	mAs	TFD	CASSETTE
SKULL					45" (ALL)	
SKULL, AP, LAT Adult	.20	200	$1/4$	40	48"	24 × 30 cm
CERBRAL SPINE						
Cevical AP 10° ↑	.15	200	$1/4$	30	48"	8 × 10 in
Lateral (Cross-Table) (NON-GRID)	.05	200	$1/4$	10.2	48"	24 × 30 cm
OBL (Table Top)	.066	200	$1/4$	13.2	48"	24 × 30 cm
Swimmer's	.40	200	$1/2$	80	48"	24 × 30 cm
Odontoid	.20	200	$1/4$	40	30"	8 × 10 in
Piller 30° ↓	.30	200	$1/8$	60	48"	24 × 30 cm
THORACIC SPINE						
Thoracic AP (Filter)	.40	200	$1/2$	80	48"	24 × 30 cm
Thoracic LAT (Filter)	.60	↓	1	120	48"	24 × 30 cm
THIN 100 mAs AVERAGE 150 mAs PORTLY 200 mAs						
Thoracic Lower LAT (Filter)	.30	200	1	60	48"	24 × 30 cm
LUMBAR SPINE/ABDOMEN						
Lumbar AP 5° ↑ and Abdomen						
−18 cm	.15	200	$1/4$	30	48"	24 × 30 cm
19−23 cm	.30	200	$1/2$	60	48"	24 × 30 cm
24 cm -	.60	200	1	120	48"	24 × 30 cm
Lumbar OBL 42° 5° ↑						
−18 cm	.10	200	$1/8$	20	48"	24 × 30 cm
19−23 cm	.20	200	$1/4$	40	48"	24 × 30 cm
24 cm -	.50	200	$1/2$	100	48"	24 × 30 cm
Lumbar LAT Meas L−2	.40	200	$1/2$	80	48"	30 × 35 cm
Lumbar Loc LAT Meas L−5	.40	200	$1/2$	80	48"	8 × 10 in
Lumbar Graft LAT	.40	200	$1/2$	80	48"	24 × 30 cm
Lumbar Flexion & Extension	.40	200	$1/2$	80	48"	30 × 35 cm

continues

TABLE 33–6. Variable Kilovoltage Technique Chart (continued)

EXAMINATION	TIME	mA	kVp	mAs	TFD	CASSETTE
PELVIC REGION						
Pelvis & Hips AP / OBL 5° ↓	.40	200	$1/2$	80	48"	35 × 43 cm
Hips LAT	.80	200	$1/2$	160	48"	24 × 30 cm
Sacrum AP 5° ↑	.40	200	$1/2$	80	48"	24 × 30 cm
Coccyx AP 10° ↓	.40	200	$1/2$	80	48"	24 × 30 cm
Sacrum, Coccyx LAT	.80	200	1	160	48"	24 × 30 cm
S–I Joints (R & LPO 20°)	.40	200	$1/2$	80	48"	24 × 30 cm
SHOULDER						
Shoulder AP	.10	200	$1/4$	20	48"	24 × 30 cm
Neer View	.10	200	$1/4$	20	48"	24 × 30 cm
Transthoracic Lateral	.10	200	$1/2$	20	48"	35 × 43 cm
Axillary Grid	.10	200	$1/4$	20	48"	24 × 30 cm
Scapula AP & LAT OBL	.10	200	$1/4$	20	30"	24 × 30 cm
Clavicle	.10	200	$1/4$	20	48"	24 × 30 cm
Humerus	.10	200	$1/4$	20	48"	35 × 43 cm
Westpoint View (non-grid)	.033	200	$1/4$	6.6		
FEMUR, KNEE						
Femur	.10	200	$1/4$	20	48"	35 × 43 cm
LAT & OBL for Vessels	.10	200	$1/4$	20	48"	35 × 43 cm
Knee	.05	200	$1/8$	10	48"	24 × 30 cm
Intercondylar Notch	.025	200	$1/4$	5	48"	Non-Bucky
Patella (Merchants)	.033	200	$1/8$	6.6	48"	Non-Bucky
Ingrowth knee	.066	200	$1/8$	13.2	45"	35 × 43 cm
CHEST						
AP Supine, All (non-grid)	.10	200	$1/4$	20	48"	Non-Bucky
Bucky Chest	.05	200	$1/4$	10	45"	
Lateral Supine (Bucky)	.066	200	$1/2$	13.2	48"	35 × 43 cm
Lateral Decubitus (Grid)	.05	200	$1/4$	10	48"	35 × 43 cm
Lateral Sternum	.40	200	$1/2$	80	48"	30 × 35 cm
RAO AP-Sternum	.20	200	1	40	45"	24 × 30 cm
RIBS						
Ribs Above Diaphragm	.10	↓	$1/2$	varies	48"	24 × 30 cm
	THIN 150 mA	AVERAGE 200 mA		PORTLY 300 mA		
Ribs Below Diaphragm						
−18 cm	.15	200	$1/4$	30	48"	24 × 30 cm
19–23 cm	.30	200	$1/2$	60	48"	24 × 30 cm
24 cm -	.60	200	1	120	48"	24 × 30 cm

Technique charts of the type used at the Mayo Clinic, Rochester, Minnesota. Computed for a single-phase generator using mAs ratios in Table 33 – 5. © 1988 Mayo Clinic. (Reprinted by permission of Mayo Clinic, Rochester, MN.)

Special Considerations

The range of part thickness found in patients is relatively narrow for most body parts, such as the skull, knee or shoulder (see Table 31–1). For this reason, the use of a single kVp progression can be specified for these examinations without the kVp becoming so low on the thinner patients as to result in underpenetration and such high contrast or so high on the thicker patients as to produce radiographs with insufficient contrast. However, in abdominal examinations patient thickness in the AP dimension varies over an extremely wide range. Though most patients will fall into the range of 19–23 cm, patients who measure as little as 17 cm or as much as 34 cm will frequently be found. Although the kilovoltage range used with a 1φ generator for most patients (19–23 cm) will be relatively narrow, 76 to 84 kVp (Table 33–4, 1/2 Scale), extended use of the same variable kVp scale for the 17 cm thick patient would show 73 kVp and for the 34 cm patient 130 kVp. Body part penetration and the resultant radiographic contrast are strongly influenced by kVp level. Should these values be used, it will quickly be noted that 73 kVp is too low and 130 kVp too high for the best results. To avoid this problem in practice, the mAs should be reduced to half and the kVp value increased for the small patients. The mAs should be doubled and the kVp value decreased for the larger patients, resulting in the following modification to the AP lumbar technique chart:

Part thickness	Chart scale to be used with 1φ generator	Chart scale to be used with 3φ or high frequency generator
18 cm and below	1/4 Scale	1/2 Scale
19–23 cm	1/2 Scale	Scale 1
24	Scale 1	Scale 2

In practice, this maintains kVp within the range of 76–84 kVp for a 1φ unit, and image contrast problems attendant with the use of too low or too high kVp are avoided.

Phantom Testing

Phantom testing is recommended prior to performing patient examinations. As a minimum, phantom testing should be done for a small, medium and large part size

as a fine tuning mechanism for the extrapolated chart prior to clinical use.

Clinical Trials

Limited clinical trials are permissible with the new chart. All images should be recorded, with repeated images saved for analysis. When clinical trials are proceeding without excess repeated exposures, the new technique chart can move into the clinical fine tuning stage.

Clinical Fine Tuning

The clinical fine tuning process will adjust and finally validate the entire chart. At this point the new technique chart can be adopted. However, ongoing fine tuning then begins as a permanent process.

Ongoing Fine Tuning

Ongoing fine tuning is the process that maintains the accuracy of the entire exposure system and gives radiographers and radiologists confidence in the exposure and diagnostic processes.

Summary

A variable kilovoltage x-ray exposure technique system is one in which the kilovoltage to be used for a particular projection is varied depending on measured body part thickness. A milliampere-second value is specified for each body part to be examined.

Technique systems that use variable kilovoltage offer the advantage of permitting small incremental changes in exposure to compensate for variation in body part thickness. A potential disadvantage of the variable kilovoltage technique arises when one considers that the effect of changing kilovoltage on the way the subject is imaged on the radiograph is complex. Increasing kilovoltage reduces radiographic contrast. Reducing contrast may be helpful if the initial kilovoltage is too low to provide adequate penetration of the part. A reduction in contrast that occurs when kilovoltage is too high can reduce the radiologist's ability to see fine detail in the image. A useful variable kilovoltage system must use values of kilovoltage that provide adequate penetration of the part and result in a level of contrast that is acceptable to the radiologist.

Initially, variable kVp systems were established using a 2 kVp change for each centimeter of tissue thickness. A constant was added to this value, such as 30, 40 or 50 kVp, to get the kVp level up to a value that would provide adequate penetration. Application of the 15 percent rule shows that a uniform increase of 2 kVp for each centimeter change will not work satisfactorily over a wide range of tissue thicknesses.

Based on a number of years of field testing, a variable kVp system was established which reflects the need to adjust the kVp level based on the examination being performed. Seven scales were developed with the kVp change from one scale to the next at any given centimeter of thickness being the amount that will balance cutting the mAs in half or doubling it. Once the selected kVp scale is determined, the mAs values are computed using mAs ratios after a base exposure is found. The AP lumbar projection is used for the base exposure. This eliminates the need for multiple trial and error exposures.

The effective use of a variable kVp system requires precise measurement with the use of calipers.

REVIEW QUESTIONS

1. Which exposure factor(s) become constant(s) in a variable kilovoltage technique system?

2. What are the primary advantages and disadvantages of variable kVp technique systems?

3. What is the 2 kVp rule?

4. Why is more than a single kilovoltage scale required?

5. What is a stepped variable kVp chart?

6. What is the formula that is used to calculate new exposure factors from a single satisfactory exposure when mAs ratios are provided?

REFERENCES AND RECOMMENDED READING

Cahoon, J. B. (1961). Radiographic technique: Its origin, concept, practical application and evaluation of radiation dosage. *The X-Ray Technician. 32*, 354–364.

Carroll, Q. B. (1993). *Fuchs's radiographic exposure, processing, and quality control* (5th ed.). Springfield, IL: Charles C. Thomas Publishers.

Cullinan, A. & Cullinan, J. (1994). *Producing quality radiographs* (2nd ed.). Philadelphia: J. B. Lippincott.

Du Pont Company Photosystems & Electronic Products Department. *Positioning and exposure guide for general radiography*. Wilmington, DE: Publication R-53806-1.

Du Pont, E.I. de Nemours & Co. Medical Products Department, Customer Technology Center. *Bit system of technique conversion*. Wilmington, DE.

Eastman Kodak Company. (1980). Health Sciences Markets Division. *The fundamentals of radiography* (12th ed.). Rochester, NY: Kodak Publication M1-18.

Eastman, T. R. (1979). *Radiographic fundamentals and technique guide*. St. Louis: C. V. Mosby.

Eastman, T. R. (1978). A history of radiographic technique. *Applied Radiology*. (July/August), 97–100.

Eastman, T. R. (1975). Technique charts: The key to radiographic quality. *Radiologic Technology. 46*, 365–368.

Eastman, T. R. (1973). Measurement: The key to exposure with manual techniques. *Radiologic Technology. 45*, 75–78.

Eastman, T. R. (1969). Chest technique through body habitus. *Radiologic Technology. 41*, 80–84.

Eastman, T. R. *The radiographic technique guide*. Wilmington, DE: Du Pont deNemours Inc. Photo Products Department Publication A-99101.

Files, G. W. (1952). *Medical radiographic technique*. Springfield, IL: Charles C. Thomas Publishers.

Fodor, J. & Malott, J. C. (1993). *The art and science of medical radiography* (7th ed.). St. Louis: C. V. Mosby.

Fodor, J., Malott, J. C., Ross, J. A., & Porter, M. (1985). Indications for the use of high kVp in the plain film examination of the abdomen. *Radiologic Technology. 57*(2), 159–161.

Fuchs, A. W. (1958). *Principles of radiographic exposure and processing* (2nd ed.). Springfield, IL: Charles C. Thomas Publishers.

Fuchs, A. W. (1950). The rationale of radiographic exposure. *The X-Ray Technician.* 22, 62–68, 76.

Fuchs, A. W. (1949). Control of radiographic density. *The X-Ray Technician.* 20, 271–273, 291.

Fuchs, A. W. (1948). Relationship of tissue thickness to kilovoltage. *The X-Ray Technician.* 19, 287–293.

Fuchs, A. W. (1934). Radiography of entire body employing one film and a single exposure. *Radiography and Clinical Photography.* 10, 9–14.

Funke, T. (1966). Pegged kilovoltage technic. *Radiologic Technology.* 37, 202–213.

General Electric Company Medical Systems Department. *How to Prepare an X-ray Technic Chart.* Milwaukee: Publication 4301A.

Gratale, P., Turner, G. W., & Burns, C. B. (1986). Using the same exposure factors for wet and dry casts. *Radiologic Technology.* 57(4), 325–328.

Hiss, S. S. (1993). *Understanding radiography.* (3rd ed.). Springfield, IL: Charles C. Thomas Publishers.

Hiss, S. S. (1975). Technique management. *Radiologic Technology.* 46(5), 369.

Hopper, B. S. (1957). Radiography above 100 peak kilovolts. *The X-Ray Technician.* 29(1), 9.

Jenkins, D. (1980). *Radiographic photography and imaging processes.* Lancaster, England: MTP Press Limited.

Jerman, E. C. (1928). *Modern x-ray technic.* St. Paul: Bruce Publishing.

Jerman, E. C. (1926). Extremity technic. *Radiology.* 6, 252–254.

Jerman, E. C. (1926). Potter-Bucky diaphragm technic. *Radiology.* 6, 336–338.

Koenig, G. F. (1966). Potential. *Radiologic Technology.* 37(4), 184–198.

Koenig, G. F. (1957). Kilovoltage as a qualitative factor. *The X-Ray Technician.* 29, 1–4, 13.

Kratzer, B. (1973). A technique computer: Scientific approach to radiologic technology. *Radiologic Technology.* 42(4), 142–150.

Mahoney, G. J. (1959). A slide rule for kVp-mAs adjustments facilitating the use of high kilovoltage. *The X-Ray Technician.* 31, 35–38.

McDaniel, C. T. (1965). Tissue absorption theory applied to formulation of radiographic technique resulting in time as the variable factor. *Radiologic Technology.* 37(2), 51–55.

Morgan, J. A. (1977). *The art and science of medical radiography.* (5th ed.). St. Louis: Catholic Hospital Association.

Morgan, R. H. (1961). Physics of diagnostic radiology. *Physical Foundations of Radiology.* (3rd ed.). New York: Paul Hoeber/Harper & Row.

Morgan, R. H. An analysis of the physical factors controlling the diagnostic quality of roentgen images. *American Journal of Roentgenology and Radiation Therapy.* 54, 128. 54, 395. 55, 67. 55, 627.

Ott, T. T. (1963). Extending the range of medical radiography to 150 kilovolts. *The X-Ray Technician.* 34(6), 335–343.

Reed, C. W. (1939). *The X-ray Technician.* 11(1).

Revesz, G., Shea, F. J., & Kundel, H. L. (1982). The effects of kilovoltage on diagnostic accuracy in chest radiography. *Radiology.* 142, 615–618.

Roderick, J. F. (1952). Latitude in roentgenology. *The X-Ray Technician.* 24, 187–196, 220.

Roderick, J. F. (1950). Photographic contrast in roentgenology. *The X-Ray Technician.* 22, 141–150, 163.

Sante, L. R. (1942). *Manual of roentgenological technique.* (9th ed.). Ann Arbor, MI: Edwards Brothers.

Schwarz, G. S. (1961). *Unit-step radiography.* Springfield, IL: Charles C. Thomas Publishers.

Schwarz, G. S. (1960). Kilovoltage conversion in radiography. *The X-Ray Technician.* 31, 373–379, 436.

Schwarz, G. S. (1959). Kilovoltage and radiographic effect. *Radiology.* 73, 749–760.

Schwarz, G. S. (1959). Extended range radiography, *Radiology,* 69: 419–423, 1957.

Schwarz, G. S. (1958). A simple universal unit system of radiographic exposures suited to departmental, national, and international standardization. *Radiology.* 71, 573–574.

Seeman, H. E. (1968). *Physical and photographic principles of medical radiography.* New York: Wiley & Sons.

United States Army. (1955). *Principles of radiographic exposure.* TM 8-282, March.

United States War Department. (1941). *Technical manual: Roentgenographic technicians*, TM 8-240, July 3.

van Dijk, D. (1955). Some factors influencing the results in radiography. *Medicamundi. 1*, 27–32.

Williams, W. A. (1960). Standardization of x-ray technique. *The X-Ray Technician. 32*(2), 137.

Wilsey, R. B. (1921). The intensity of scatter x-rays in radiography. *American Journal of Roentgenology. 8*, 328–338.

Wynroe, R. F. (1955). Some observations on kilovoltage variations. *Radiography. 21*(251), 242–243.

CHAPTER 34

Other Exposure Systems

Pride in one's profession is demanded . . . a vital feeling of belonging to a favored profession, which gives many rights but also requires many duties. All our ambitions should be directed toward a faithful fulfillment of duties toward others as well as toward ourselves. . . .

W. C. Röntgen, upon assuming the position of Rector of the University of Wurzburg.

Objectives

Upon completion of this chapter, the student should be able to:

▶ Describe the concept of a log-based point system for technique chart conversion and development.

▶ Discuss the value of exposure systems other than fixed or variable kVp when developing technique charts.

▶ Validate a fixed or variable kVp system by using another exposure system.

▶ Explain the concept of proportional anatomy exposure systems, including extrapolation of a technique chart from control images via constants or ratios.

*A*lthough fixed and variable kVp exposure systems are the most popular systems in use, there are situations where other exposure systems are easier to use or more accurate. Each of the following exposure systems has advantages and disadvantages. Students can test their knowledge of the principles of radiographic exposure and increase their understanding of the relationships between technical factors by careful study of each of these systems.

Each system was developed by a radiographer, except for the XVS unit step system, which was developed by a radiologist. Except for the proportional anatomy systems, they are all based on logarithmic scales. Each was subjected to extensive study and experimentation and was designed to provide consistency in image quality while quantifying variables into a useful format. These systems have either had a major effect on thinking about radiographic technique or have proven to be accurate in clinical situations and are still in use.

XVS Unit Step System

Considerable attention was given to the quantification of radiographic exposure factors during the 1950s. Many authors, notably Reed (in 1939) and Williams (in 1956, 1958 and 1960) attempted to prove a radiographic effect (RE) formula as a corollary to the photographic effect (PE) formula that had gained acceptance for measuring photographic image density. The problems these researchers encountered stemmed from their failure to recognize the full effect of subject density and contrast, primarily through part thickness, on the production of scatter radiation. In 1959, Gerhart Schwarz published a study of these effects and from this work continued his research to develop the X-Ray Value Scale (XVS) system, which was published as a book entitled Unit-Step Radiography in 1960.

The XVS system was patterned after the photographic Exposure Value Scale (EVS) system but with the addition of Schwarz's research into the effect of subject thickness on kVp's effect on image density. The system was not strictly log-based, although the basis of this type of system was present. The XVS system was the first to quantify the primary radiographic variables. It permitted variance of kVp, mA, time and filtration, as the Bit

System would later, but did not address other variables.

The system functioned by using a caliper to measure subject part thickness in XVS numbers instead of centimeters. Any total of XVS numbers that equaled the caliper measurement could be obtained from special markings on the x-ray machine's mA, time and kVp indicators. Schwarz proposed mechanical systems that would automatically set the x-ray control after measuring patient thickness with photocells. One major manufacturer even built a control console that gave XVS numbers instead of radiographic exposure factors. In later years this concept was adopted in a revised form and marketed by another major manufacturer. Of course, radiographers are crippled by these types of systems because they effectively blindfold the operator by requiring him or her to guess at technical factors. One of the greatest triumphs of the professionalism of radiographers occurred when this type of equipment labeling was rejected by purchasers because it limited the skills of the operators.

An interesting note in Schwarz's book is that he had to impose rigid requirements on radiographers during the original clinical trials of the XVS system because it became an easy game to discover which XVS numbers were hiding which exposure factors on the control consoles. The radiographers then proceeded to improve image quality by ignoring the XVS units when necessary. Schwarz conceded that the radiographer must retain the right to exercise his or her professional judgment by deviating from average values.

Although Schwarz proposed several modifications of the system, the lack of standardization of all but a single factor, plus the ignorance of the many other variables, resulted in the eventual demise of the system. However, the theory of the interrelationships between the variables is a basic concept in understanding radiographic exposure factors and remains worthy of study.

Equipment with variations of unit step labeling is available for use in regions of the world where it is not possible to adequately train x-ray operators. For a time, the benefit of providing basic radiographic services far outweighs the risk of inadequate training. The Basic Radiological System (BRS), which operates on this principle, is supported by the International Society of Radiographers and Radiological Technicians (ISRRT) and the World Health Organization (WHO).

Bit System

The Bit System was developed by Robert J. Trinkle of E. I. Du Pont de Nemours and Company, Inc. (now Sterling Diagnostic), in 1957. The system is similar to the Polaroid light value exposure (LVS) system, the XVS unit step system of Schwarz described above, and the Siemens Point System described below. Trinkle used a computer to analyze vast quantities of exposure system data, and named the system after the computer processing bit to emphasize the use of computerized data. The Du Pont company publishes a pocket guide to the system and routinely revises it. The system uses log-base$_2$ points to quantify variables with the objective of maintaining image density within acceptance limits. Each point, or bit, either doubles or halves the exposure.

The Bit System is designed as a technique conversion system, although an experienced radiographer can make valid extrapolations using guide totals for the major subject density and contrast regions of the body. The 10th edition of the Bit System, with step-by-step instructions on its use, is provided in Appendix C.

The system is used as the basis for the computerized Du Pont technique charts that are available to customers. As with any other system, following the steps to establish a technique chart will produce a functional system. Each projection must be rated for an established number of bits. Any balanced combination of variables that equal the established bits will produce a diagnostic quality image. The key is to maintain a balanced combination of variables. Conversion of a technique by more than a full bit (doubling or halving) is not recommended. The Bit System also permits calculation of approximate entrance skin exposure by applying distance, mAs and converted kVp bits to an exposure table.

Siemens Point System

The Siemens Point System, developed in 1950 by the Siemens Corporation, was based on work by F. Claassen. Siemens publishes and revises the system, which is more commonly used in Europe than elsewhere. The system uses log-base$_{10}$ points to quantify variables, with the objective of maintaining image density within acceptance limits. Technically, each point increases exposure by 25.9 percent, although for all practical purposes it is easier to consider a one-point increase as increasing exposure by 25 percent and a one-point decrease as decreasing exposure by 20 percent. Even simpler is to remember that the system requires three points to double or halve the exposure.

The Siemens Point System is designed to serve as a complete technique chart system. It must be calibrated by determining an initial exposure value point for each anatomical area. If the suggested initial exposure values do not produce an optimal image, correcting points must be established for all subsequent exposures. The chart provided by Siemens is usually modified by the correcting points to establish normal exposure value points. The normal exposure value points provide an accurate exposure system. Each anatomical area is listed on the chart as an average part thickness. Compensation for part size variations is one point per centimeter except for chest radiography, where the compensation is one point per 1.5 cm. The ancillary charts must be consulted to estimate appropriate technical factor changes when correction points must be added or subtracted. The system can be easily used for technique conversions in the same manner as the Du Pont Bit System. A current version of the system is provided in Appendix D.

Supertech™ Calculator

Brice Kratzer published an article in 1973 reporting on research experience with a log-based slide rule technique calculator. It was later developed, patented, trademarked and marketed as the Supertech™ Calculator by Supertech, Inc. Slide rule-style calculators, both circular and linear, had been developed by Reed in 1939 and 1949 and Williams had developed a circular calculator technique system in 1960. These calculators were limited to the relationship between 1–2 factors, for example the relationship between kVp and mAs. Two commercial film companies in the United States published and distributed the calculators for many years. The Supertech™ Calculator is the only one that has survived to the present and is revised regularly.

Supertech™ includes elements of quality control testing, positioning guidelines, principles of exposure and anatomy review, and can serve as an angulator. It is sold as a kit with an acrylic penetrometer and calibration master film for elementary quality control testing of machine output (Figure 34–1). After a short testing procedure, each machine can be assigned a correction factor that takes into account over a dozen different variables. Supertech™ remains a viable technique system and has found acceptance in low volume clinical sites, and in situations where radiography is an ancillary service, such as physicians' offices, chiropractics and podiatry.

Proportional Anatomy Systems

Proportional Anatomy Systems are based on the concept that the body can be classified into regions of similar subject densities and contrasts and that these similarities can be correlated to exposure factors.

Terry Eastman reported on a body habitus technique system for chest radiography in 1969. The system was based on observations that chest density and contrast were closely related to various body habitus factors, especially height and weight. Eastman collected data on adult averages and then codified an effective technique chart that correlated exposure factors with the patient's height and weight. Although limited to chest radiography, the system remains in use in some institutions where a high volume of essentially normal chest radiography is performed.

To date, two true Proportional Anatomy Systems have been presented, one by Quinn Carroll in 1985 and the other by Norlin T. Winkler and Eugene Frank in 1987. Carroll's system is presented in his revision of *Fuchs's Principles of Radiographic Exposure, Processing and Quality Control.* Winkler and Frank have presented their data at the annual meetings of the American Society of Radiologic Technologists. Their data are the cumulation of research begun by Raymond Runge and encompass experiences at the Mayo Clinic in Rochester, Minnesota, since 1925. Both of these systems classify body parts, habitus and projections into groups of similar subject density and contrast. Carroll uses conversion factors while Winkler and Frank use mAs ratios to extrapolate a technique chart for the entire body from a control exposure. Winkler presents the Mayo Clinic system as the current state of the art for variable kVp systems (see Table 33–5).

Summary

Although fixed and variable kVp systems are the most popular systems in use, there are situations where other systems are easier to use or more accurate. These other systems include the XVS Unit Step System, the Du Pont Bit System, the Siemens Point System, the Supertech™ Calculator and Proportional Anatomy Systems.

The XVS system was patterned after the photographic Exposure Value Scale (EVS) system but with the addition of Schwarz's research into the effect of subject thickness on kVp's effect on image density. The XVS system was the first to quantify the primary radiographic variables. The system functioned by using a caliper to measure subject part thickness in XVS numbers instead of centimeters. Any total of XVS numbers that equaled the caliper measurement could be obtained from special markings on the x-ray machine's mA, time and kVp indicators.

The Du Pont Bit System was developed using a computer to analyze vast quantities of exposure system data, and it was named after the computer processing bit to emphasize the use of computerized data. The system uses

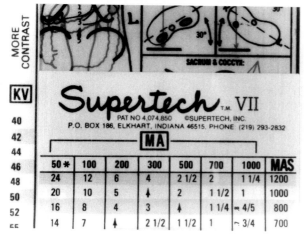

FIGURE 34-1. The Supertech™ Calculator. *(Courtesy of Supertech, Inc.)*

log-base$_2$ points to quantify variables with the objective of maintaining image density within acceptance limits. Each point, or bit, either doubles or halves the exposure. Each projection is rated for an established number of bits. Any balanced combination of variables that equal the established bits will produce a diagnostic quality image.

The Siemens Point System uses log-base$_{10}$ points to quantify variables with the objective of maintaining image density within acceptance limits. The system requires three points to double or halve the exposure. Each anatomical area is listed with an average part thickness. Compensation for part size variations is one point per centimeter except for chest radiography, where the compensation is one point per 1.5 cm.

The Supertech™ Calculator is a log-based slide rule technique system. After a short testing period, each machine can be assigned a correction factor that takes into account over a dozen different variables.

Proportional Anatomy Systems are based on the concept that the body can be classified into regions of similar subject densities and contrasts and that these similarities can be correlated to exposure factors. Two true Proportional Anatomy Systems (Carroll and Frank/Winkler) classify body parts, habitus and projections into groups of similar subject density and contrast. Carroll uses conversion factors while Winkler and Frank use mAs ratios to extrapolate a technique chart for the entire body from a control exposure.

REVIEW QUESTIONS

1. What do all of the various exposure systems have in common?

2. What four primary radiographic variables were quantified in the XVS System?

3. Why was the Du Pont Bit System so named?

4. What is the relationship between a bit and radiographic density?

5. What is the Supertech™ Calculator?

6. On what concept are Proportional Anatomy Systems based?

REFERENCES AND RECOMMENDED READING

Bierman, A. & Boldingh, W. H. (1951). The relation between tension and exposure times in radiography. *Acta Radiologica. 35*, 22–26.

Bryan, G. J. (1970). *Diagnostic radiography: A manual for radiologic technologists.* Baltimore: Williams & Wilkins.

Cahoon, J. B. (1961). Radiographic technique: Its origin, concept, practical application and evaluation of radiation dosage. *The X-Ray Technician. 32*, 354–364.

Carroll, Q. B. (1993). *Fuchs's radiographic exposure, processing, and quality control.* (5th ed.). Springfield, IL: Charles C. Thomas Publishers.

Compton, S. (1987). Bit conversion of technical factors in vascular procedures. *Radiologic Technology. 58*(5), 413.

Cullinan, A. & Cullinan, J. (1994). *Producing quality radiographs.* (2nd ed.). Philadelphia: J. B. Lippincott.

Du Pont Company Photosystems & Electronic Products Department. *Positioning and exposure guide for general radiography.* Wilmington, DE: Publication R-53806-1.

Du Pont, E.I. de Nemours & Co. Medical Products Department, Customer Technology Center. *Bit system of technique conversion.* Wilmington, DE.

Eastman, T. R. (1979). *Radiographic fundamentals and technique guide.* St. Louis: C. V. Mosby.

Eastman, T. R. (1978). A history of radiographic technique. *Applied Radiology.* (July/August), 97–100.

Eastman, T. R. (1975). Technique charts: The key to radiographic quality. *Radiologic Technology. 46*, 365–368.

Eastman, T. R. (1973). Measurement: The key to exposure with manual techniques. *Radiologic Technology. 45*, 75–78.

Eastman, T. R. (1971). Automated exposures in contemporary radiography. *Radiologic Technology. 43*(2), 80–83.

Eastman, T. R. (1969). Chest technique through body habitus. *Radiologic Technology. 41*, 80–84.

Eastman, T. R. *The radiographic technique guide.* Wilmington, DE: Du Pont deNemours Inc. Photo Products Department Publication A-99101.

Files, G. W. (1952). *Medical radiographic technique.* Springfield, IL: Charles C. Thomas Publishers.

Files, G. W. (1935). Maximum tissue differentiation. *The X-Ray Technician. 7*, 17–24+.

Fodor, J. & Malott, J. C. (1993). *The art and science of medical radiography.* (7th ed.). St. Louis: C. V. Mosby.

Frank, E. D. & Winkler, N. T. (1988). Preparing an accurate x-ray exposure technique chart. Rochester, MN: Mayo Foundation (Postgraduate course from American Society of Radiologic Technologists annual meeting).

Fuchs, A. W. (1958). *Principles of radiographic exposure and processing.* (2nd ed.). Springfield, IL: Charles C. Thomas Publishers.

Fuchs, A. W. (1950). The rationale of radiographic exposure. *The X-Ray Technician. 22*, 62–68, 76.

Fuchs, A. W. (1949). Control of radiographic density. *The X-Ray Technician. 20*, 271–273, 291.

Fuchs, A. W. (1948). Relationship of tissue thickness to kilovoltage. *The X-Ray Technician. 19*, 287–293.

Fuchs, A. W. (1945). Military photoroentgen technique employing optimum kilovolt (peak) principles. *The American Journal of Roentgenology. 53*, 587–596.

Fuchs, A. W. (1943). The optimum kilovoltage technique in military roentgenography. *American Journal of Roentgenology. 50*, 358–365.

Fuchs, A. W. (1938). Higher kilovoltage technic with high-definition screens. *Radiography and Clinical Photography. 14*(3), 2–8.

Funke, T. (1966). Pegged kilovoltage technic. *Radiologic Technology. 37*, 202–213.

General Electric Company Medical Systems Department. *How to prepare an x-ray technic chart.* Milwaukee: Publication 4301A.

Hiss, S. S. (1993). *Understanding radiography.* (3rd ed.). Springfield, IL: Charles C. Thomas Publishers.

Hiss, S. S. (1975). Technique management. *Radiologic Technology. 46*(5), 369.

Horsington, G. (1974). A radiographic exposure calculator. *Radiography. 40*(472), 77–83.

Jenkins, D. (1980). *Radiographic photography and imaging processes.* Lancaster, England: MTP Press Limited.

Jerman, E. C. (1928). *Modern X-Ray Technic.* St. Paul: Bruce Publishing.

Jerman, E. C. (1926). Extremity technic. *Radiology. 6*, 252–254.

Jerman, E. C. (1926). Potter-Bucky diaphragm technic. *Radiology. 6*, 336–338.

Jerman, E. C. (1925). X-ray technic: From the old to the new. *Radiology. 5*(September), 6.

Kratzer, B. (1973). A technique computer: Scientific approach to radiologic technology. *Radiologic Technology. 42*(4), 142–150.

Lyon, N. J. (1962). Optimum kilovoltage techniques. *The X-Ray Technician. 33*, 398–401.

Mahoney, G. J. (1959). A slide rule for kVp-mAs adjustments facilitating the use of high kilovoltage. *The X-Ray Technician. 31*, 35–38.

Morgan, J. A. (1977). *The art and science of medical radiography.* (5th ed.). St. Louis: Catholic Hospital Association.

Palmer, P. E. S. (1985). The World Health Organization: Basic radiological system. *Radiography. 51*(597), 169–178.

Reed, C. W. (1939). *The X-ray Technician. 11*(1).

Sante, L. R. (1942). *Manual of roentgenological technique.* (9th ed.). Ann Arbor, MI: Edwards Brothers.

Schwarz, G. S. (1961). *Unit-step radiography.* Springfield, IL: Charles C. Thomas Publishers.

Schwarz, G. S. (1960). Kilovoltage conversion in radiography. *The X-Ray Technician. 31*, 373–379, 436.

Schwarz, G. S. (1959). Kilovoltage and radiographic effect. *Radiology. 73*, 749–760.

Schwarz, G. S. (1959). Extended range radiography, *Radiology, 69*: 419–423, 1957.

Schwarz, G. S. (1958). A simple universal unit system of radiographic exposures suited to departmental, national, and international standardization. *Radiology. 71*, 573–574.

Seeman, H. E. (1968). *Physical and photographic principles of medical radiography*. New York: Wiley & Sons.

Stopford, J. E. (1979). Log$_{10}$ technique charts. *Radiologic Technology. 51*(3), 331–333.

Trinkle, R. J. (1966). The bit system of technic conversion. Unpublished paper presented at American Society of Radiologic Technologists annual meeting, Boston (June).

Trout, E. D., Graves, D. E., & Slauson, D. B. (1949). High kilovoltage radiography. *Radiology. 52*, 669–683.

United States Army. (1955). *Principles of radiographic exposure*. TM 8-282, March.

United States War Department. (1941). *Technical manual: Roentgenographic technicians*. TM 8-240, July 3.

Williams, W. A. (1960). Standardization of x-ray technique. *The X-Ray Technician. 32*(2), 137.

Williams, W. A. (1956). Radiographic effect formula: Its practical application. *The X-Ray Technician. 28*, 1–6, 67.

World Health Organization. (1985). *Manual of radiographic technique*. Geneva: World Health Organization Publications.

The Case of the Very Dense Object

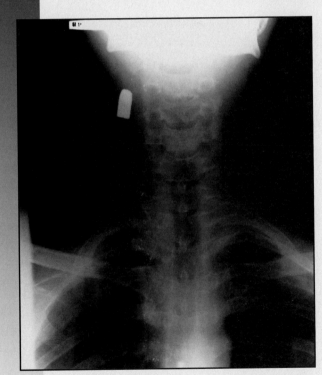

What could be causing the image of the very dense object on the right side of the fourth cervical vertebra?

Answers to the case studies can be found in Appendix E.

CHAPTER 35

Automatic Exposure Controls

The art of using AECs is the art of positioning.

Objectives

Upon completion of this chapter, the student should be able to:

▶ Explain why the art of phototiming is the art of positioning.

▶ Accurately identify configuration size, shape and position for various brands of ionization chambers.

▶ Describe how to modify density, contrast and time when using an automatic exposure control.

▶ Describe various common subject density and subject contrast problems when using AECs.

▶ Explain the effect of collimation on AEC image quality.

▶ Provide solutions to minimum response time and back-up time problems.

▶ Explain how to modify the suggested technical factors on an anatomically programmed control unit.

▶ Discuss the advisability of the creative use of AECs.

The operation of ionization chamber automatic exposure controls (AECs) was discussed in Chapter 5, X-Ray Equipment. It is important to remember that although the term phototiming may be used in clinical practice, the generic terms automatic exposure control (AEC) and automatic exposure device (AED) refer to both antique phototiming devices and the ionization chambers currently in use. Although referred to as phototiming, the term actually refers to the use of ionization chambers. In nearly all instances the principles are applicable to phototimers as well as ionization chambers.

AECs have been popular since their introduction by Russell H. Morgan in 1942. He designed the first phototimer for use with mass chest screening photofluorographic units. It was designed to react to the dominant area of the radiograph that is proportional to the general appearance of the entire image.

The ionization chamber is designed for a single purpose, best illustrated by the proper term for the device — **automatic exposure control**. The single function of an AEC is to eliminate the need for the radiographer to set an exposure **time**. The radiographer loses control over time, and as a result **mAs**, when using an AEC. All other factors, **especially mA and kVp**, must still be set manually.

Radiographers can fall into the habit of depending on AECs to produce diagnostic radiographs in situations for which they were never designed. When using an AEC it is critical that the **location** of the ionization chamber be determined and the precise **positioning** of tissue over that location be achieved. These factors can be remembered by thinking of the use of AECs as another of the radiographic **arts** based on professional expertise and a sound technical understanding.

Ionization Chambers

The most critical element in using AECs is the exact position of the ionization chambers because positions differ for various brands and models of equipment (Figure 35–1). **Automatic exposure devices provide a diagnostic quality density only for structures positioned directly above the ionization chambers.** Therefore the most important fact to remember when using automatic exposure devices is that **the art of using AECs is the art of positioning**. Experienced radiographers become extremely adept, often to the point of being artistic, in carefully positioning exactly the right amount of tissue over the chambers.

Ionization chamber AECs are usually used in a three chamber configuration. The most common relationship of the three chambers is with the center chamber at the center of the image receptor with right and left chambers slightly higher. This configuration places the center chamber below the duodenum and transverse colon for most abdominal examinations, thus eliminating problems with gastric and bowel gas being placed over the chamber. This configuration also places the right and left chambers away from the mediastinum and completely within the lobes of the lungs during chest radiography. As long as the exact chamber locations are known, this configuration will not affect phototiming ability during other examinations.

Determining Configurations

Determining the location of the AEC chambers can be a difficult task. Some manufacturers provide plastic inserts for collimators that project an image of the chamber location, size and shape with the positioning light beam (Figure 35–2). These inserts are accurate for only the specified SID (usually printed in a corner of the insert.) When projection inserts are not provided, the radiographer must be capable of determining the location, size and shape. This can be accomplished by producing a radiograph without a body part as the subject, exposed at very low kVp for maximum contrast (Figure 35–1).

Controlling Configurations

AEC consoles permit various combinations of the ionization chambers to be activated in order to control the exposure. Most units permit any single cell or all three cells to be activated. Some units permit other combinations to be utilized, for example, right and left chambers together or all three at once. In these situations, often termed "averaging," the signals from the cells are sent to a special operational amplifier which sums the voltages received from each cell and divides by the number of cells that have been activated. When the appropriate voltage for a diagnostic quality density is reached, the exposure is terminated by the operational amplifier.

| 52 kVp | 4 mAs | 72" SID |
| 16:1 grid | 200 RS | 3.12 mR |

| 40 kVp | 5.1 mAs | 40" SID |
| 10:1 grid | 200 RS | 9.66 mR |

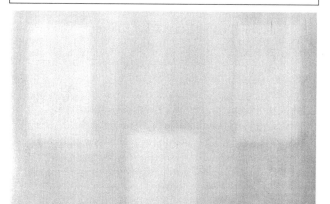

A

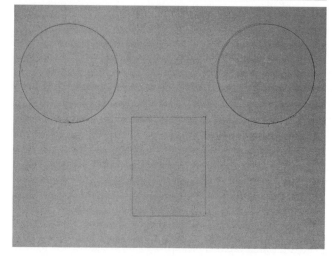

B

FIGURE 35-1. Automatic exposure control ionization chamber configurations. (A) A radiograph of a configuration with square ionization chambers. The middle cell is centered to the image receptor while the outside cells are placed high. (B) A radiograph of a configuration with both square and circular chambers (outlined in pencil). The middle cell is square and centered to the image receptor while the outside cells are round and high. (C) Actual square ionization chamber configuration. The middle cell is centered to the image receptor while the outside cells are high. Note the wire leads to each ionization chamber. *(Photograph courtesy of Eugene Frank, Mayo Clinic)*

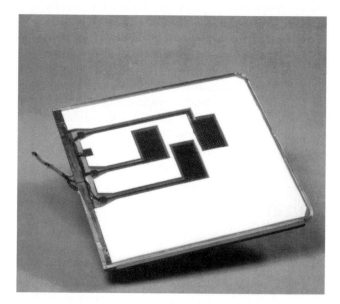

C

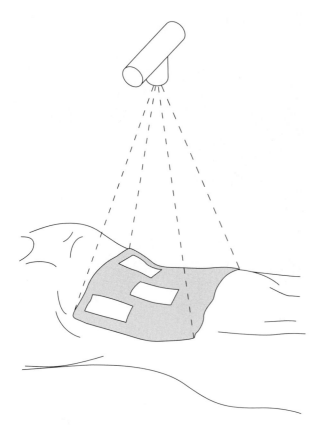

FIGURE 35-2. Projection of AEC locations from collimator positioning light.

Density Controls

All AEC systems permit the adjustment of the amount of radiation necessary to send the exposure termination signal. These controls regulate the image density but often have different labels, depending on the manufacturer. Typical AEC density control labels are –3, –2, –1, 0, 1, 2, 3, or 1/4, 1/2, N, 1 1/4, 1 1/2. Most labels use the center control as the normal density (0 and N in the two examples) and permit both increases and decreases. Some units use a single density control while others use a major and a minor control. Major controls operate large density changes while minor controls operate fine adjustment.

The density controls should not be used to compensate for patient part thickness or kVp changes. The AEC system is designed to calculate this compensation automatically. Proper use of the density controls is accomplished when the configuration of the ionization chamber cells cannot be adapted to the necessary positioning, for example, when an image is produced that is slightly too dark for the lung fields and a decrease in density is desired even though the patient and ionization chambers are properly positioned.

Exposure Technique Charts

Automatic exposure controls require the use of exposure technique charts that specify the technical parameters to be used. The only difference from non-AEC charts is that cell locations are given while time settings are eliminated, as the AEC fulfills that function automatically.

Positioning Skills

The AEC will produce a diagnostic density for whatever tissue is placed directly over the chamber. When the radiographer possesses good positioning skills, the vast majority of AEC exposures will produce diagnostic quality results. Poor positioning skills result in an increased repeat rate when using AECs. There are numerous instances when variables in tissue density and contrast may complicate the precise location of the tissue of interest over the ionization chamber. Knowledge of when these instances are likely to occur and the experience to

When more than one cell is activated, the cell receiving the most radiation will contribute the greatest electrical signal and therefore have the most influence on density. For example, if three cells are activated and an abdomen is positioned so that barium is over one cell and normal tissue over the other two cells, the resultant image will be slightly overexposed because the operational amplifier was dividing the incoming voltage by all three cells but only two cells were contributing to the signal. If the cell under the barium was the only one activated, the image would be greatly overexposed, probably to the back-up time limit, because insufficient radiation was received to terminate the exposure. Cell selection is therefore determined by the radiographer based on knowledge of anatomy and positioning.

adequately compensate for them are important. When not enough of the structure of interest is positioned over the activated ionization chamber, the AEC cell will attempt to produce a diagnostic quality density for whatever is over it (Figures 35–3 and 35–4).

The skilled radiographer detects the majority of these conditions through careful observation of the patient and consideration of the patient's history. A proper clinical history can reduce the number of repeated radiographs and produce excellent images.

Subject Density and Contrast Problems

AEC problems with subject density and contrast occur whenever an unexpected density is present or when an expected density is lacking. For example, fluid in the lungs causes increased subject density and contrast, for which the AEC would remain on longer, making an aerated lung much too dark for diagnosis. A case of emphysema would produce the opposite result.

Collimation

Collimation of the primary beam is another important consideration when using AECs. Attempts to tight-

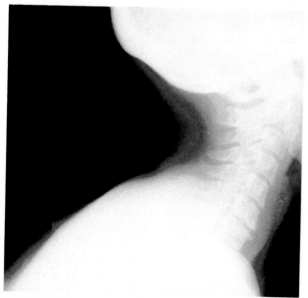

FIGURE 35-3. Improper positioning over AEC cell. Although this lateral cervical spine is too light, note that the region at the center of the film, where the AEC cell was activated, is nearly perfect density.

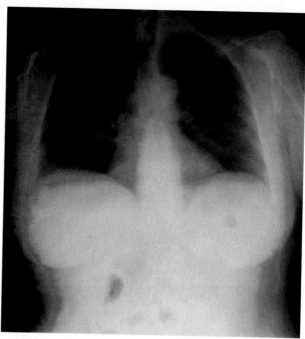

FIGURE 35-4. Improper AEC cell selection. Although this PA chest is too dark, note that the region at the center of the film, where the AEC cell was activated is of perfect density for the thoracic spine.

ly collimate should be avoided near ionization chamber locations. If the primary beam is collimated from an activated chamber, the chamber operates as if the tissue is extremely dense. The resulting long exposure will create a dark radiograph.

The use of wider collimation can also create problems because the full primary beam will produce scatter radiation that may undercut the patient (Figure 35–5). This undercutting scatter will cause the AEC to terminate the exposure while some areas of the image are still too light.

Timing Problems

Minimum response time and the proper use of a back-up time are important considerations when using AECs. The minimum response time is the length of time necessary for the AEC to respond to the ionization and send a signal to terminate the exposure. Modern AECs have a minimum response time in the region of 0.001 second. However, the use of extremely high speed intensifying screens for smaller part sizes can cause problems when AECs need less than 0.001 second to produce a diagnostic quality density. In these instances, mA should be decreased to permit longer AEC time.

The back-up time should be set at 150 percent of the anticipated manual exposure time, although U.S. public law requires that generators automatically terminate AEC exposures at 600 mAs or 60 kilowatt seconds (kWs) (kVp × mA × time) above 50 kVp, and 2,000 mAs below 50 kVp. When the back-up time is too short, it will terminate the exposure before the AEC signal, thus producing a light image. In these instances, the back-up time should be increased to a level where the AEC is terminating the exposure at the proper time.

Anatomically Programmed Radiography

Anatomically programmed radiography (APR) units combine an AEC system with a technique chart that is computerized to correspond to anatomical procedures. The control console permits the choice of an anatomical region (for example, the chest) and the projection (for example, PA). This choice results in the computer entering the suggested average technique (for example, 120 kVp, 600 mA, with the right and left ionization chambers activated). The radiographer may override the suggested technique when patient condition, pathology or other factors make it desirable to do so.

Creative Positioning

The experienced radiographer often becomes extremely adept at positioning exactly the right amount of tissue over the chambers. Experienced radiographers should remember that **a manual technique will always provide a precisely repeatable exposure** whereas an AEC exposure leaves the radiographer guessing.

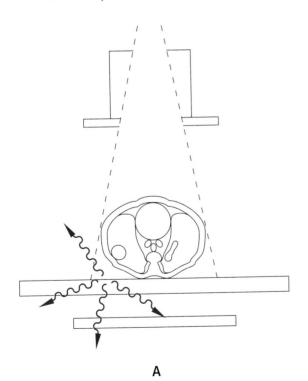

A

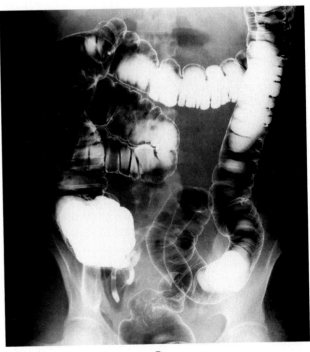

B

FIGURE 35-5. Undercutting scatter. (A) The uncollimated primary beam produces scatter that undercuts the patient and causes the AEC to prematurely terminate the exposure. (B) An image that is too dark in the upper right quadrant due to undercutting. *(Reprinted from Automatic exposure control: A primer, [1988].* Radiologic Technology, *Vol. 59, No. 5, 1988, p. 425. Radiograph courtesy of Seymour Sterling.)*

Care must be taken when AEC cells are not completely covered by tissue. The most common compensation in this circumstance is to deactivate the uncovered cell. However, if no cell is covered by normal tissue for the area of interest, deactivation is not the answer. In these instances, creative techniques must be used. For example, if a cell is covered by an appropriate percentage of tissue, it may react with an appropriate density. These techniques require much experience and should not be attempted by inexperienced radiographers.

Summary

The ionization chamber is designed for a single purpose, best illustrated by the proper term for the device — automatic exposure control. The single function of an AEC is to eliminate the need for the radiographer to set an exposure time. The radiographer loses control over time, and as a result mAs, when using an AEC. All other factors, especially mA and kVp, must still be set manually.

When using an AEC, it is critical that the location of the ionization chamber be determined and that the precise positioning of tissue over that location be achieved. AEC locations differ for various brands and models of equipment. Automatic exposure devices provide a diagnostic quality density only for structures positioned directly above the ionization chambers. AECs are usually used in a three chamber configuration. The most common relationship of the three chambers is with the center chamber at the center of the image receptor with right and left chambers slightly higher.

AEC consoles permit various combinations of the ionization chambers to be activated in order to control the exposure. When more than one cell is used, the signals from the cells are sent to a special operational amplifier which sums the voltages received from each cell, divides by the number of cells that have been activated, and then terminates the exposure.

All AEC systems permit the adjustment of the amount of radiation necessary to send the exposure termination signal. These controls regulate the density but often have different labels, depending on the manufacturer. Typical AEC density control labels are –3, –2, –1, 0, 1, 2, 3, or 1/4, 1/2, N, 1 1/4, 1 1/2. Some units use a single density control while others use a major and a minor control.

Problems can result with the use of AEC devices when variations occur in subject density or contrast. Collimation must also be used consistently to assure proper results. The AEC's minimum response time can also cause exposure problems when very fast film/screen combinations are used. Back-up times should be set at 150 percent of the expected manual technique time.

REVIEW QUESTIONS

1. What is the principle function of the automatic exposure control?

2. What are the typical number and configuration of the ionization chambers?

3. What is the purpose of an operational amplifier?

4. When should the density controls be used?

5. How can changes in subject density result in AEC problems?

6. How can collimation affect AEC image quality?

7. Define minimum response time.

REFERENCES AND RECOMMENDED READING

Bruce, G. (1976). Automatic exposure control: A few notes. *Radiography. 42*(503), 235.

Bushberg, J. T., Seibert, J. A., Leidholdt, E. M., & Boone, J. M. (1994). *The essential physics of medical imaging.* Baltimore: Williams & Wilkins.

Bushong, S. C. (1997). *Radiologic science for technologists: Physics, biology, and protection* (6th ed.). St. Louis: C. V. Mosby.

Croft, M. J. (1986). Filtration, the answer to the automatic exposure control response problem. *Radiologic Technology. 57*(5), 447.

Cullinan, A. & Cullinan, J. (1994). *Producing quality radiographs.* (2nd ed.). Philadelphia: J. B. Lippincott.

Curry, T. S., Dowdey, J. E., & Murry, R. C. (1990). *Christensen's introduction to the physics of diagnostic radiology.* (4th ed.). Philadelphia: Lea and Febiger.

Eastman, T. R. (1971). Automated exposures in contemporary radiography. *Radiologic Technology. 43*(2), 80–83.

Fodor, J. & Malott, J. C. (1993). *The art and science of medical radiography.* (7th ed.). St. Louis: C. V. Mosby.

Hiss, S. S. (1993). *Understanding radiography.* (3rd ed.). Springfield, IL: Charles C. Thomas Publishers.

Jenkins, D. (1980). *Radiographic photography and imaging processes.* Lancaster, England: MTP Press Limited.

Karila, K. T. K. (1989). Manual or automatic exposure controller imaging in mammography. *Radiography Today. 54*(618), 35.

Morel, J. M. (1957). Phototiming. *Radiologic Technology. 29*(3), 165.

Morgan, R. H. (1943). The automatic control of exposure in photofluorography. *Public Health Reports. 58*, 1,533–1,541.

Morgan, R. H. (1943). The control of diagnostic quality in roentgenograms of the chest. *American Journal of Roentgenography and Radium Therapy. 50*, 149–161.

Morgan, R. H. (1942). A photoelectric timing mechanism for the automatic control of roentgenographic exposure. *American Journal of Roentgenography and Radium Therapy. 48*, 220–228.

Olson, A. & High, M. (1981). Performance of automatic exposure controls when used with rare-earth intensifying screens. *Radiology.* p. 491.

Seeram, E. (1985). *X-ray imaging equipment: An introduction.* Springfield: Charles C. Thomas.

Sprawls, P. (1990). *Principles of radiography for technologists.* Rockville, MD: Aspen Publishers.

Sprawls, P. (1987). *Physical principles of medical imaging.* Rockville, MD: Aspen Publishers.

Stears, J. G., Gray, J. E., & Frank, E. D. (1988). Radiologic exchange (automatic exposure control function). *Radiologic Technology. 59*(6), 521–522.

Sterling, S. (1988). Automatic exposure control: A primer. *Radiologic Technology. 59*(5), 421–427.

Thompson, T. T. (1985). *A practical approach to modern imaging equipment.* (2nd ed.). Boston: Little, Brown, & Co.

CHAPTER 36

Exposure Conversion Problems

Never lose your courage.

Professor Wilhelm Röntgen.

Objectives

Upon completion of this chapter, the student should be able to:

▶ Discuss the limitations of standard conversion tables.

▶ Explain the concept of direct and inverse relationships versus proportions.

▶ Calculate appropriate new exposure factors for multiple changes in exposure factor variables.

Standard Conversion Relationships and Tables

*A*primary concern when using conversion tables is their tendency to oversimplify complex exposure problems. It is safer to think of radiographic exposure factors as relationships to one another rather than as direct conversions. The radiographer uses conversion tables as guidelines, with the realization that the great number of variables in any imaging system make all conversion factors variables, not constants. Conversion tables are designed to assist in producing an image within acceptance limits. Production of an image of optimal diagnostic quality usually requires fine tuning. Conversion tables, like all other factors, require fine tuning before being integrated into an exposure system.

Most conversion tables are designed to provide a method of maintaining radiographic density. It is important to understand the interrelationship between variables and their effects on the four image quality factors: density, contrast, recorded detail and distortion.

The effect of a particular variable is best described as either a direct relationship, in which an increase in the variable causes an increase in the effect, or an inverse relationship, in which an increase in the variable causes a decrease in the effect, and vice versa. The description of a relationship as direct or inverse does not necessarily indicate that the relationship is **proportionally** direct or inverse. In other words, a proportionally direct relationship would indicate that a linear relationship exists between the variable and the effect, whereas a direct relationship would simply indicate that as the variable changes, the effect changes in the same direction, not necessarily in a linear manner.

Table 36–1 is a master table indicating the relationship of most radiographic image variables on density, contrast, recorded detail and distortion. Conversion tables are provided for the factors that are commonly considered when converting from one exposure factor or system to another, especially regarding maintaining density. (Tables 36–2 through 36–10).

TABLE 36–1. Effects Of Radiographic Exposure Variables On The Primary Factors

D = direct relationship (when the variable changes, the effect changes in the same direction).

I = inverse relationship (when the variable changes, the effect changes in the opposite direction).

X = decreases if variable is greater or less than optimal.

0 = no effect

NOTE: Many effects are not linearly proportional.

Variable	Density	Contrast	Recorded Detail	Distortion
EQUIPMENT				
Generator Phase	D	X	0	0
Kilovoltage	D	X	0	0
Milliamperage-seconds	D	0	0	0
SID	I	0	D	I
OID	I	X	I	D
TUBE				
Focal Spot Size	0	0	I	0
Filtration	I	I	0	0
Beam Restriction	I	D	0	0
SUBJECT				
Part Thickness	I	X	I	D
Tissue Type	I	X	0	0
Additive Pathology	I	X	0	0
Destructive Pathology	D	X	0	0
IMAGE RECEPTOR				
Grid Ratio	I	D	0	0
Film/Screen Relative Speed	D	0	I	0
Film Processing				
Developer Time	D	I	0	0
Developer Temperature	D	I	0	0
Developer Replenishment	D	I	0	0

Effect On

TABLE 36–2. Density Rules

All these rules help **maintain the same density**.

• 2KVP/CM RULE

Variable kVp Theory
Maintains density by changing kVp for different part sizes.
Changes by 2 kVp for every cm of part size.
    EXAMPLE: 60 kVp for 10 cm = 64 kVp for 12 cm

• 4-5 CM RULE

Fixed kVp Theory
Maintains density by changing mAs for different part sizes.
Double or halve mAs for every 4-5 cm part size.
    EXAMPLE: 10 mAs for 20 cm = 20 mAs for 24 cm

• 15% RULE

Variable and Fixed kVp Theory
Maintains density when kVp is changed.
Increase kVp 15% AND Decrease mAs to half
    EXAMPLE: 60 kVp and 10 mAs = 69 kVp and 5 mAs
Decrease kVp 15% AND Increase mAs double
    EXAMPLE: 60 kVp and 10 mAs = 51 kVp and 20 mAs

Disclaimer: The above rules are not "Laws of Exposure" by any means. They are simply rules of thumb that have proven useful for generations of radiographers. The actual physical processes that determine exact exposure rates and image quality factors are extremely complex and vary not only from one radiographic unit to another, but over time with the same unit. **These rules may be considered useful with a range of 1-2 densities for part sizes from 10-20 cm and kVp ranges of 60-80.** However, they are often close enough to produce diagnostically useful images throughout the diagnostic radiography range of body part sizes and kVp levels.

TABLE 36–3. Conversion Factors: Effect Of Generator Phase On Radiographic Density

When Converting Generator Phase		To Maintain Radiographic Density, Multiply mAs by a
From:	**To:**	**Conversion Factor of:**
$1\phi2p$	$3\phi6p$	0.6
$1\phi2p$	$3\phi12p$/HF	0.5
$3\phi6p$	$1\phi2p$	1.6
$3\phi6p$	$3\phi12p$/HF	0.8
$3\phi12p$/HF	$1\phi2p$	2.0
$3\phi12p$/HF	$3\phi6p$	1.2

TABLE 36–4. The Fifteen Percent Rule

To maintain radiographic density when increasing kVp:
increase kVp 15 percent and reduce mAs to half.

To maintain radiographic density when decreasing kVp:
decrease kVp 15 percent and double mAs.

TABLE 36–5. The mAs Formula

$$mA \times seconds = mAs$$

TABLE 36–6. The Density Maintenance Formula

$$\frac{mAs_1}{mAs_2} = \frac{D_1^2}{D_2^2}$$

where
$$mAs_1 = \text{original mAs}$$
$$mAs_2 = \text{new mAs}$$
$$D_1 = \text{original distance}$$
$$D_2 = \text{new distance}$$

The same formula can be expressed as:

$$mAs_2 = \frac{mAs_1 \times D_2^2}{D_1^2}$$

TABLE 36–7. Recommended Compensation For Subject Part Thickness

$$mAs = 2X \text{ or } 0.5X \text{ mAs per } 5 \text{ cm} =$$
$$15\% - 20\% \text{ mAs per cm}$$
$$kVp = 2 \text{ kVp per cm}$$

NOTE: Because scatter production varies with total part thickness, these figures are based on 60 – 80 kVp for a 20 cm part. The recommendations for changes are less accurate further from this average range.

TABLE 36–8. Grid Ratio Conversion Forumla

$$\frac{mAs_1}{mAs_2} = \frac{GCF_1}{GCF_2}$$

TABLE 36–9. Grid Ratio Conversions

(Approximate values based on clinical tests of pelvis and skull.)

Grid Ratio	60 kVp	85 kVp	110 kVp
No grid	1	1	1
5:1	3	3	3
8:1	3.75	4	4.25
12:1	4.75	5.5	6.25
16:1	5.75	6.75	8

Adapted with permission from *Characteristics and Applications of X-Ray Grids*, Liebel-Flarsheim division of Sybron Corporation, Cincinnati, Ohio.

TABLE 36–10. Relative Speed Formula

$$\frac{mAs_1}{mAs_2} = \frac{RS_2}{RS_1}$$

Solving Complex Exposure Problems

The most difficult part of developing technique exposure factor skills is learning how to use the information in actual clinical situations. The difficulty lies in the fact that clinical problems usually present complex situations with more than one variable. Now that each variable has been explored in detail, it is necessary to learn how to solve complex exposure problems with many variables.

Methodology

A very simple method can be used to assess a complex exposure problem. Although the analytical decision making process can be used, it is simpler to work through the variables. If the same variables are considered for each problem, it is less likely that a factor will be missed.

Radiographic variables that should be considered when solving a clinical exposure problem can be classified into four major areas: equipment, tube, patient and image receptor. Each of these four areas has its variables, as shown in Table 36–1. The variables are easier to remember than it first appears. Equipment is composed of phase plus the four primary factors (kVp, mA, time and distance). The tube is focal spot, filtration and field size. The subject consists of part density and contrast. The image receptor includes grid and film/screen variables.

Mistakes in solving complex exposure problems are invariably caused by failure to consider one of these variables. Even when the solution to a problem appears self-evident, a moment taken to consider all the variables may reveal a hidden factor that would have been missed otherwise.

The following problems demonstrate this methodology.

Example: A satisfactory radiograph is produced as follows:

1ϕ2p, 80 kVp, 40 mAs, 40" SID, 8:1 grid, 250 RS.

If a new radiograph is to be produced with the following changes—3ϕ6p, 12:1 grid, 400 RS—what changes should be made to maintain the original density?

Answer: The following variables must be considered:

Equipment: generator phase from $1\phi2p$ to $3\phi6p$.

Image receptor: grid from 8:1 to 12:1.

Image receptor: film/screen combination from 250 RS to 400 RS.

Each variable must be converted for the new exposure:

Equipment: generator phase from $1\phi2p$ to $3\phi6p$.

The conversion factor for $1\phi2$ to $3\phi6$ = mAs $\times$ 0.6.

$$40 \text{ mAs} \times 0.6 = 24 \text{ mAs}.$$

Image receptor: grid from 8:1 to 12:1.

The conversion factor formula for grid changes is

$$\frac{mAs_1}{mAs_2} = \frac{GCF_1}{GCF_2}$$

The conversion factor for an 8:1 grid = 4

The conversion factor for a 12:1 grid = 5.5, so

$$\frac{24 \text{ mAs}}{mAs_2} = \frac{4}{5.5}$$

$$mAs_2 \times 4 = 24 \text{ mAs} \times 5.5$$

$$mAs_2 \times 4 = 132 \text{ mAs}$$

$$mAs_2 = \frac{132 \text{ mAs}}{4}$$

$$mAs_2 = 33 \text{ mAs}$$

Image receptor: film/screen combination from 250 RS to 400 RS.

The conversion formula for RS changes is

$$\frac{mAs_1}{mAs_2} = \frac{RS_2}{RS_1}$$

The RS change is from 250 RS to 400 RS, so

$$\frac{33 \text{ mAs}}{mAs_2} = \frac{400}{250}$$

$$mAs_2 \times 400 = 33 \text{ mAs} \times 250$$

$$mAs_2 \times 400 = 8,250 \text{ mAs}$$

$$mAs_2 = \frac{8,250 \text{ mAs}}{400}$$

$$mAs_2 = 20.63 \text{ mAs}$$

So the new exposure factor conditions require a change to 20.63 mAs to duplicate the density of the original exposure factors.

Example: A satisfactory radiograph is produced as follows:

$3\phi6p$, 80 kVp, 20 mAs, 72" SID, 12:1 grid, 400 RS.

If a new radiograph is to be produced with the following changes — $3\phi12p$, 68 kVp, 100 mA, 10:1 grid, 200 RS — what changes should be made to maintain the original density?

Answer: The following variables must be considered:

Equipment: generator phase from $3\phi6p$ to $3\phi12p$.

Equipment: kVp from 80 to 68.

Equipment: mAs = time $\times$ 100 mA

Image receptor: grid from 12:1 to 10:1.

Image receptor: film/screen combination from 400 RS to 200 RS.

Each variable must be converted for the new exposure:

Equipment: generator phase from $3\phi6p$ to $3\phi12p$.

The conversion factor for $3\phi6p$ to $3\phi12p$ = mAs $\times$ 0.8.

$$20 \text{ mAs} \times 0.8 = 16 \text{ mAs}$$

Equipment: kVp from 80 to 68.

The conversion when decreasing kVp by 15 percent is doubling the mAs.

$$80 \text{ kVp} \times 15\% = 12 \text{ kVp}$$

$$80 \text{ kVp} - 12 \text{ kVp} = 68 \text{ kVp}$$

so, 16 mAs $\times$ 2 = 32 mAs

Image receptor: grid from 12:1 to 10:1.

The conversion factor formula for grid changes is

$$\frac{mAs_1}{mAs_2} = \frac{GCF_1}{GCF_2}$$

The conversion factor for an 8:1 grid = 3.75.

The conversion factor for a 12:1 grid = 4.75, so

$$\frac{32 \text{ mAs}}{mAs_2} = \frac{4.75}{3.75}$$

$$mAs_2 \times 4.75 = 32 \text{ mAs} \times 3.75$$

$$mAs_2 \times 4.75 = 120 \text{ mAs}$$

$$mAs_2 = \frac{120 \text{ mAs}}{4.75}$$

$$mAs_2 = 25.3 \text{ mAs}$$

Image receptor: film/screen combination from 400 RS to 200 RS.

The conversion formula for RS changes is

$$\frac{mAs_1}{mAs_2} = \frac{RS_2}{RS_1}$$

The RS change is from 400 RS to 200 RS, so

$$\frac{25.3 \text{ mAs}}{mAs_2} = \frac{200}{400}$$

$$mAs_2 \times 200 = 25.3 \text{ mAs} \times 400$$

$$mAs_2 \times 200 = 10,120 \text{ mAs}$$

$$mAs_2 = \frac{10,120 \text{ mAs}}{200}$$

$$mAs_2 = 50.6 \text{ mAs}$$

Equipment: mAs = time × 100 mA

$$\frac{50.6 \text{ mAs}}{100 \text{ mA}} = \text{time}$$

$$0.51 = \text{time}$$

So the new exposure factor conditions require a change to 50.6 mAs to duplicate the density of the original exposure factors. Using 100 mA, the exposure time would be set at 0.51 seconds.

Summary

A primary concern when using conversion tables is their tendency to oversimplify complex exposure problems. It is safer to think of radiographic exposure factors as relationships to one another rather than as direct conversions. Conversion tables are designed to assist in producing an image within acceptance limits. Most conversion tables are designed to provide a method of maintaining density. It is important to understand the interrelationships between variables and their effects on the four image quality factors: density, contrast, recorded detail and distortion.

The effect of a particular variable is best described as either a direct relationship, in which an increase in the variable causes an increase in the effect, or an inverse relationship, in which an increase in the variable causes a decrease in the effect, and vice versa. A proportionally direct relationship would indicate that a linear relationship exists between the variables.

The most difficult part of developing technique exposure factor skills is learning how to use the information in actual clinical situations. It is necessary to learn how to solve complex exposure problems with many variables. A very simple method can be used to assess a complex exposure problem. If the same variables are considered for each problem, it is less likely that a factor will be missed.

Radiographic variables that should be considered when solving a clinical exposure problem can be classified into four major areas: equipment, tube, patient and image receptor. Mistakes in solving complex exposure problems are invariably caused by failure to consider one of the variables. Even when the solution to a problem appears self-evident, a moment taken to consider all of the variables may reveal a hidden factor that would otherwise have been missed.

REVIEW QUESTIONS

1. What is the primary purpose of conversion tables?

2. When making exposure factor conversions, it is important to consider the effect on which of the image quality factors?

3. What is the meaning of a direct relationship?

4. What is the difference between a relationship and a proportion?

5. When solving complex exposure problems, the variables can be classified into what four major areas?

REFERENCES AND RECOMMENDED READING

Cullinan, A. & Cullinan, J. (1994). *Producing quality radiographs.* (2nd ed.). Philadelphia: J. B. Lippincott.

Du Pont Company Photosystems & Electronic Products Department. *Positioning and exposure guide for general radiography.* Wilmington, DE: Publication R-53806-1.

Du Pont, E. I. de Nemours & Co. Medical Products Department, Customer Technology Center. *Bit System of Technique Conversion.* Wilmington, DE.

Eastman Kodak Company. (1980). Health Sciences Markets Division. *The fundamentals of radiography.* (12th ed.). Rochester, NY: Kodak Publication M1-18.

Eastman, T. R. (1979). *Radiographic fundamentals and technique guide.* St. Louis: C. V. Mosby.

Eastman, T. R. *The radiographic technique guide.* Wilmington, DE: Du Pont deNemours Inc. Photo Products Department Publication A-99101.

Files, G. W. (1952). *Medical radiographic technique.* Springfield, IL: Charles C. Thomas Publishers.

Fodor, J. & Malott, J. C. (1993). *The art and science of medical radiography.* (7th ed.). St. Louis: C. V. Mosby.

General Electric Company Medical Systems Department. *How to prepare an x-ray technic chart.* Milwaukee: Publication 4301A.

Gratale, P., Turner, G. W., & Burns, C. B. (1986). Using the same exposure factors for wet and dry casts. *Radiologic Technology.* 57(4), 325–328.

Hiss, S. S. (1993). *Understanding radiography.* (3rd ed.). Springfield, IL: Charles C. Thomas Publishers.

Jenkins, D. (1980). *Radiographic photography and imaging processes.* Lancaster, England: MTP Press Limited.

Jerman, E. C. (1928). *Modern x-ray technic.* St. Paul: Bruce Publishing.

Kratzer, B. (1973). A technique computer: Scientific approach to radiologic technology. *Radiologic Technology.* 42(4), 142–150.

Lauer, O. G., Mayes, J. B., & Thurston, R. P. (1990). *Evaluating radiographic quality: The variables and their effects.* Mankato, MN: The Burnell Company Publishers.

Morgan, J. A. (1977). *The art and science of medical radiography.* (5th ed.). St. Louis: Catholic Hospital Association.

Sante, L. R. (1942). *Manual of roentgenological technique.* (9th ed.). Ann Arbor, MI: Edwards Brothers.

Schwarz, G. S. (1961). *Unit-step radiography.* Springfield, IL: Charles C. Thomas Publishers.

The Case of the Dripping Film

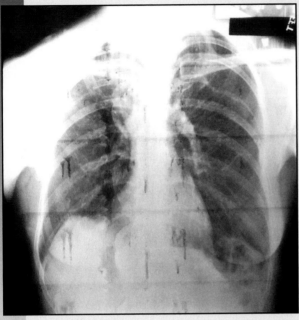

What caused the horizontal lines and dripping marks on this radiograph?

(Images courtesy of E.D. Frank and J.G. Stears, Mayo Clinic/Foundation)

Answers to the case studies can be found in Appendix E.

UNIT VI

Special Imaging Systems

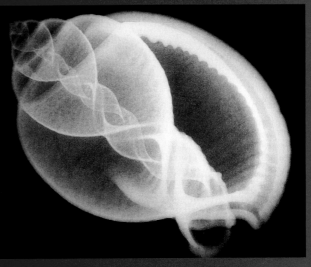

Several special imaging systems deserve consideration to complete a basic foundation in the principles of radiographic imaging. These include the use of specialized diagnostic equipment for **mobile radiography, fluoroscopy,** the oldest and most common dynamic radiographic modality, and conventional **tomography.**

The specialized systems utilized in the **technical aspects of mammography** and **vascular imaging equipment** are explored as well as the unique design requirements of these fields of radiologic science. Most modern imaging modalities utilize computers to accomplish digital image processing. Those that rely completely on digital processing include **digital radiography, computed tomography (CT),** and **magnetic resonance imaging (MRI),** which although recognized as specialty areas within radiologic technology, continue to serve as extensions of the radiographer's knowledge.

Although within the scope of departments of radiology, the specialty areas of ultrasound (diagnostic medical sonography), nuclear medicine, and radiation therapy (oncology) are not addressed in this text because they are recognized as separate established professional disciplines with their own accreditation and certification processes. Proper study of these professions generally requires a recognized educational program of one or more years in length encompassing the study of entire subjects beyond the realm of this text.

A thorough study of the six units of this text: **Creating the Beam, Protecting Patients and Personnel, Creating the Image, Analyzing the Image, Comparing Exposure Systems** and **Special Imaging Systems** provides the thorough physical basis required of the radiographer. Basic physical knowledge must be combined with an equally thorough and correlated knowledge in the anatomical sciences of anatomy, positioning, physiology, and pathology to form the complete basis of radiography knowledge. Only when this basis is added to an elementary understanding of human interactions and combined with clinical experience does the true professional radiographer emerge.

CHAPTER 37

Mobile Radiography

Come, come, and sit you down. You shall not budge!
You go not till I set you up a glass
Where you may see the inmost part of you.

Shakespeare, Hamlet, III, iv, 18.

OBJECTIVES

Upon completion of this chapter, the student should be able to:

▶ Determine factors that contribute to the difficulty of mobile radiography.

▶ Explain appropriate communications methods for mobile examinations.

▶ Describe items that must be considered when arranging a patient room for a mobile examination.

▶ Recommend methods for accomplishing acceptable variations of standard radiographic projections, especially chest examinations for air-fluid levels.

▶ Assess the radiation protection rules for mobile radiography.

▶ Differentiate light duty portable x-ray units from full power mobile units.

▶ Evaluate the advantages of capacitor discharge and battery powered mobile units.

▶ Explain why technical factor selection is more difficult during mobile radiography.

▶ Describe the effect of various generator waveforms on kVp.

▶ Identify advantages of standardizing mobile SID to one of 40″ (100 cm), 56″ (140 cm) or 72″ (180 cm).

▶ Determine appropriate grids for mobile examinations.

▶ Appraise various film/screen combinations for mobile applications.

*T*he mobile radiographic examination is often the ultimate test of the radiographer's competence and skill. Accomplishing an optimal quality image without stationary equipment on the most difficult patients is a prime achievement. An understanding of the special considerations involved in mobile examinations is important for the radiographer.

Special Patient Considerations

Mobile examinations are more difficult to accomplish because there are so many additional variables — variables that would be constants with a stationary unit — when manipulating and positioning both patient and equipment. In many instances the reason an examination is requested at the bedside is to avoid transporting the patient because of his physical condition. Special adaptations of routine projections, imaginative equipment manipulation and innovative technical factor considerations are often required.

In surgery or the emergency unit, the stress of performing in a high tension environment may be added to the patient problems. These situations often include limitations due to aseptic conditions and the presence of additional critical equipment (e.g., ventilators, multiple intravenous solutions, cardiac lines, etc.).

Communication

Although good communication with the patient is not a special consideration during mobile examinations, it is advisable for the radiographer to park the mobile unit outside a patient's room before entering to establish the proper rapport. The patient's permission must be obtained before proceeding with the examination, an explanation of the procedure should be given, and some rearrangement of equipment and room furnishings must usually be accomplished before bringing the mobile unit into the room.

The unconscious or incognizant patient requires the same explanation that a cognizant patient would receive. In many instances conscious but incognizant patients will be more cooperative if they hear a kindly voice of explanation prior to being touched. In surgery, the attending physician or operating room nurse must be consulted before entering, and this procedure should be followed even in an emergency suite.

Manipulating Equipment

Extreme care must be taken when manipulating equipment in a high technology environment such as intensive care, surgery or the emergency unit. The importance of other equipment must be considered, especially when it must be moved to make room for the x-ray unit. Care must be exercised to ensure that power supplies, oxygen tubes, catheters, intravenous lines, etc., have enough slack to permit movement. Finally, the radiographer must take care not to bump the bed or other equipment when moving the mobile unit out of the way or when driving it into position. Although this seems to be an obvious consideration, it is easily overlooked when one's mind is on the examination. Wall suspended television units are especially hazardous to both the x-ray tube and the radiographer's head. Neither the radiographer nor the patient can afford to be in a hurry when preparing for a mobile examination. It is the radiographer's duty to return all items to their original locations prior to leaving the area.

Positioning and Pathology

Patients requiring examinations with mobile equipment are often unable to assume standardized positions. Clinical experience and a thorough knowledge of acceptable positioning variants are required for this problem. For example, the inability of the patient to sit on the side of a bed requires an AP projection of the chest instead of the preferred PA projection. A patient in orthopedic traction may not be able to straighten the knee. Thus, a distal knee joint, mid-shaft and proximal hip exposure will be required to avoid gross distortion and to satisfactorily demonstrate the entire femur from a single projection. However, routine positioning practices should still be carried out to the extent possible. For example, during chest radiography most cognizant patients are capable of moving the scapula from the lung fields by rolling their shoulders forward, as they would if the examination were performed on stationary equipment.

Even with difficult or uncooperative patients, chest radiography should be performed with the patient in a semi-erect position in the vast majority of instances.

Patients who have been confined to a bed, especially when pathology is present, are prone to disease processes that cause collections of fluid. Even elevating the thorax to the level of a pillow (perhaps only 10° from supine) may provide an opportunity to demonstrate a fluid level. Ideally, air-fluid level demonstration is best accomplished with the patient in a completely erect position, utilizing a horizontal beam (Figure 37–1). Demonstration of air-fluid levels when a patient is unable to assume an erect position causes gross distortion of anatomical structures (Figure 37–2). This distortion may be great enough to render the image useless for normal chest diagnosis. **When it is determined that air-fluid demonstration is a priority, two projections may be required: one for air-fluid levels and the other for a normal projection of the chest.**

The radiographer must not assume that an apparently well patient is able to be transported to stationary equipment. For example, an ambulatory patient on whom a mobile chest examination is requested, may in fact be under observation for myocardial infarct and may be susceptible to the sudden onset of potentially serious symptoms.

The radiographer must also not assume that every mobile examination will result in a poorer image quality than examinations performed in the radiology department. The same myocardial infarct patient may be capable of providing a detailed history that makes delineation of the heart shadow the primary image quality goal, of assuming an erect position on the edge of a bed, and of holding a cassette to permit a 72" (180 cm) PA projection essentially identical in quality to an image produced with a stationary unit.

Because the mobile examination is performed at the patient's bedside, there is an increased possibility of artifacts, such as personal items (e.g., dropped hair pins, jewelry, etc.), layers of coverings (e.g., insulated blankets, several sheets, etc.), and medical equipment (e.g., nasogastric tubes, intravenous lines, catheters, electrocardiographic leads, clamps, etc.). A careful and tactful examination of the area of interest should be performed prior to exposure to locate and remove as many of these artifacts as possible. It is usually possible to carry out this examination during positioning, which also presents an opportunity to check for a necklace, bra, brace, etc. Clamps holding various tubes and lines should be moved as far from the area of interest as possible. For example, intensive care unit chest radiography often requires movement of intravenous, respiratory and cardiac lines from over the lung fields. **A nursing staff member or physician should be consulted before moving any lines, especially venous and arterial.** It is desirable to limit coverings to a single smoothed layer of gown or sheet.

Special Radiation Protection Considerations

During a mobile examination the radiographer is bringing a radiation hazard into an area not designed for radiation protection. Professional responsibility for ensuring radiation protection becomes a fundamental operating procedure during all mobile radiography. This is a prime opportunity for radiographers to educate the public, health professionals, physicians and other patients concerning proper radiation protection practices. A duty exists to protect the patient, health workers, the public and oneself. The rules shown in Table 37–1 should never be violated. The mobile unit should not be used as a portable shield. When standing behind a mobile unit, a lead apron is required to ensure sufficient

**TABLE 37–1. Radiation Protection Rules
For Mobile Radiography**

1. Recognize a duty to protect your patient, health professionals, physicians, the public and yourself.
2. Request the public, health professionals, physicians and other patients to leave the immediate area prior to exposure.   (Always inform these persons that you will be finished in a moment, request them to remain nearby, and inform them promptly when you are finished.)
3. Announce in a loud voice your intent to make each exposure and permit sufficient time for others to leave.
4. Carry at least two lead aprons: one for yourself, the other for your patient. If you have an assistant, he too must have an apron.
5. Never place your hand or any other body part within the primary beam.
6. Provide gonadal protection for your patient.
7. Achieve maximum distance from the patient (not the tube) immediately prior to exposure, in accordance with rules requiring the use of a 6' cord on mobile units.
8. Label and handle each cassette carefully to avoid repeats.

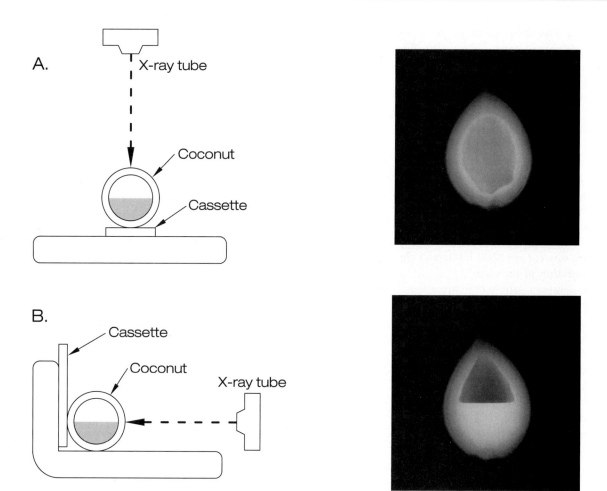

FIGURE 37-1A AND B. Demonstration of air-fluid levels. A coconut was used to demonstrate the effect of various positions and tube angles on air-fluid levels. (A) Recumbent AP projection with beam perpendicular to the air-fluid level. (B) Upright AP projection with beam parallel to the air-fluid level.

protection. Radiographers should also move to a maximum distance from the mobile unit by extending the exposure control cord prior to making the exposure.

Types of Equipment

X-ray units are available in a wide array of sizes and capabilities, many of which can be classified as mobile. Although often described as portable units (the truly portable unit can be hand carried), the proper description is mobile. The need for mobile x-ray equipment has

been apparent from the earliest days of radiography; one unit was designed to fit in a suitcase. During World War I, the Picker Corporation developed a mobile unit that has remained popular for bedside radiography in hospitals. Today there are two major classifications of mobile equipment: portable light duty units and full power institutional units (Figure 37–3).

Power Supplies

Light duty mobile units and some full power units obtain power from wall outlets. Although some older units required 220 volts, modern units are usually

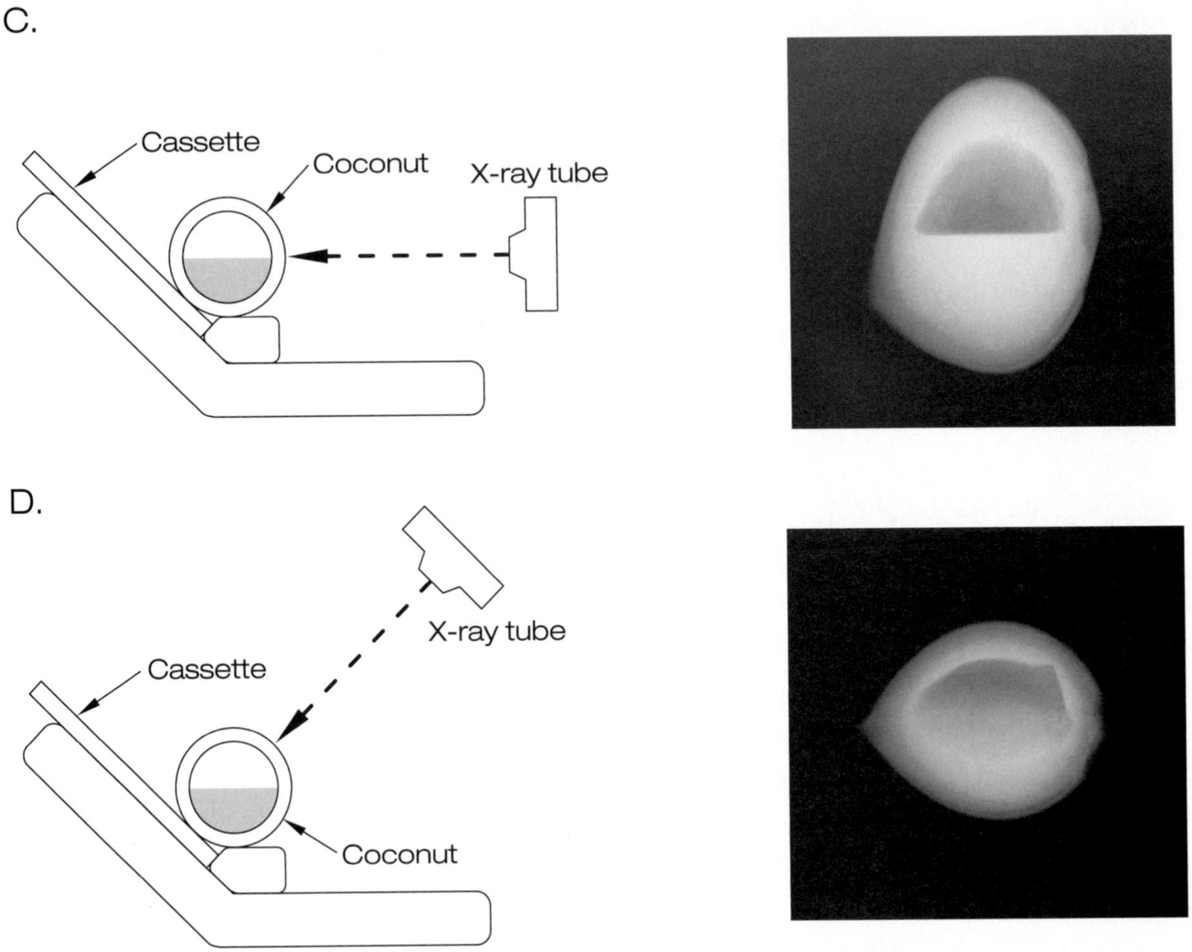

C.

D.

FIGURE 37-1C AND D. (C) The film was at a 45° angle to the plane of the floor with the beam parallel to the air-fluid level and therefore parallel to the floor. (D) The film was at a 45° angle to the plane of the floor and therefore at a 45° angle to the air-fluid level, with the beam perpendicular to the film. Note that the central ray must be parallel to the floor to demonstrate distinct air-fluid levels.

designed to use 110 volts. The more advanced full power units use batteries for a power supply and are capable of greater voltages. Units that are not battery-equipped may be susceptible to line voltage fluctuations due to other resistances operating from the same circuit.

When using a mobile unit that is drawing power from a wall outlet, the voltage compensator must be accurately adjusted immediately prior to exposure. Battery units are usually equipped with circuitry to monitor battery strength, and normal maintenance procedures include periodic replacement of old batteries. However, battery cell failure is a potential cause of erratic exposures.

Generators

Specialized generators have been developed specifically for mobile equipment. Capacitor discharge units and battery powered units are the most common. Capacitor discharge units produce a constant potential output while battery operated units produce output that is essentially 3ϕ (Figure 37–4).

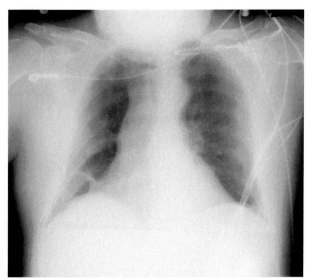

FIGURE 37-2. A chest radiograph demonstrating distortion due to improper source-to-image receptor alignment during a mobile examination. The central ray and film were not perpendicular to one another.

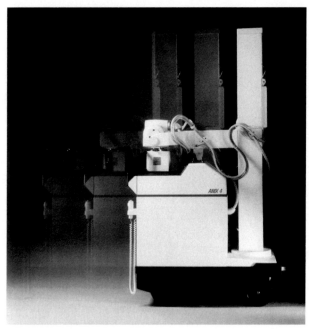

FIGURE 37-3. A typical full-powered mobile radiographic unit. *(Courtesy of GE Medical Systems)*

Power Drive

An additional advantage of a battery powered unit is that power is available to drive the unit itself. In large institutions, power driven units quickly become the radiographer's best friend. The drive switch on a mobile unit should be of the dead-man type so that its release immediately disengages the power drive. The size and weight of a battery powered mobile x-ray unit are considerable and extreme care must be observed when piloting it. Patients and staff could be seriously injured by careless driving. Radiographers must be cautious in looking ahead, especially at corners and intersections, just as when driving a car.

Automatic Exposure Control

Automatic exposure control (AEC, AED or photo-timing) is available for most mobile units in the form of a paddle ionization chamber, the Mobil-AID® Automatic Exposure Control (a registered trademark of Advanced Instrument Development, Inc.) (Figure

37–5). This unit functions exactly as an ionization chamber AEC in a stationary unit except that the chamber is contained within a paddle that can be positioned behind the cassette. The critical element in the use of the Mobil-AID® AEC is the accuracy of the positioning of the ionization chamber. All the elements of positioning used with stationary AECs must be applied to the positioning of the paddle and the positioning of the patient.

Special Technical Factor Selection Considerations

Establishing technical factors for mobile units almost always involves conversion of multiple variables (i.e., generator phase, filtration, grid, etc.) from stationary equipment technique systems. Because multiple conversions increase the risk of error, it is advisable to establish individual technique charts for each mobile unit. There are numerous special considerations when establishing these charts.

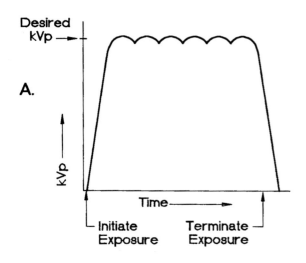

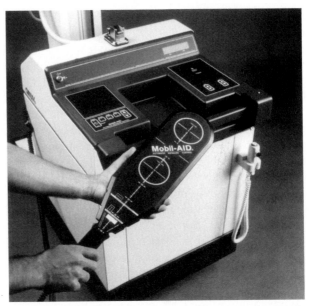

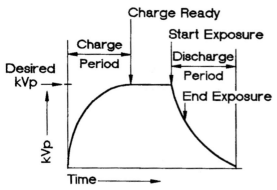

FIGURE 37-4. Mobile unit generator waveforms. (A) A battery-powered unit. (B) A capacitor discharge unit.

FIGURE 37-5. Mobil-AID® Automatic Exposure Control for mobile procedures. *(Courtesy of Advanced Instrument Development, Inc.)*

Kilovoltage

Most mobile units produce an x-ray beam with an average photon energy that is quite different from that of stationary equipment. Full power rotary 3φ units that are battery powered produce a waveform, as shown in Figure 37–4A. Because this waveform has essentially no ripple, it is actually more efficient and will produce a higher average photon emission than a 3φ, 12 pulse unit.

Capacitor discharge units have serious kilovoltage limitations. Careful examination of the waveform in Figure 37–4B illustrates the difference from pulse generators. With a capacitor discharge unit, voltage drops approximately 1 kV/mAs. Therefore voltage is about 0.5

kV/mAs less than initial kVp. The total voltage drop may be as much as 30 percent. (For example, an exposure at 80 kVp and 40 mAs would end at 56 kVp and average only 68 kV.) The mAs used with a capacitor unit should not exceed 30 percent of the kVp. For example, not more than 24 mAs should be used at 80 kVp.

Milliampere-Seconds

Low power units may not be capable of the high mAs required for grid radiography and may even require the use of kVp instead of mAs to obtain sufficient density for some examinations. When these problems are present, a motion problem will invariably develop because longer exposure times are used. For a relatively healthy and cooperative patient, a double or even triple exposure may be considered in order to overcome this problem. However, the radiographer must be **extremely** cautious not to overload the tube in this situation.

Distance

A primary cause of repeated mobile exposures is failure to measure distance. **Every mobile procedure must**

have SID measured. Radiographers who estimate SID must be within 15 percent to avoid producing a visible density difference. A 72" (180 cm) chest radiograph must be exposed between 61" (153 cm) and 83" (208 cm) to produce an optimal image from 72" (180 cm) factors.

Figure 37–6 illustrates common problems encountered in mobile chest radiography. The size of the room and the location of the bed and ancillary equipment may not permit a mobile unit to be manipulated into a position from which a standard 40" (100 cm) or 72" (180 cm) projection can be obtained. Position A may be unobtainable because of tube height limitations. Position B is usually obtainable but does not optimize information because at an SID of 40" (100 cm) it magnifies the heart and, when the patient cannot sit erect, does not provide the geometry to demonstrate air-fluid levels. Positions C and D may be obtainable when air-fluid levels are required, but position C causes magnification.

The most reliable method of eliminating density fluctuations due to distance is to use only the two standardized distances, 40" (100 cm) and 72" (180 cm), with the addition of 56" (140 cm) for mobile radiography. The 56" (140 cm) distance should be employed only when 40" (100 cm) is undesirable because of magnification, yet 72" (180 cm) is not possible due to room and/or equipment limitations. As seen earlier in Table 25–3, mAs conversions are provided to maintain density at these distances according to the rule of doubling or halving mAs with each distance change (i.e., 40" [100 cm] to 56" [140 cm] to 72" [180 cm]).

Grids

Proper alignment to a grid is difficult when the patient is supine but the grid is on a soft bedding surface, which easily permits the grid to tilt, unless the patient's weight is almost exactly distributed around the center of the grid. Proper alignment is even more difficult when the film is at an angle other than parallel or perpendicular.

Figure 37–7 illustrates the problems created by this common situation. The radiographer must attempt to align the central ray and the cassette perpendicular to one another. Although this is a relatively simple task when the relationships are as shown in Figure 37–7A, it becomes very difficult when the reference points are not parallel or perpendicular.

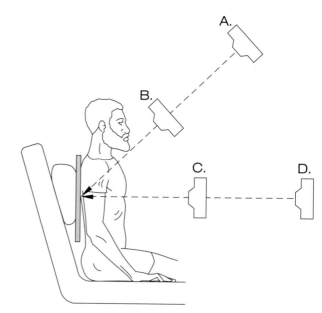

FIGURE 37-6. Common distance problems during mobile chest radiography.

Most people can draw a simple angle, such as 45°, quite accurately, but accuracy becomes more difficult when the baseline is at an angle. Figure 37–8 demonstrates this difficulty. Angling off-center to a focused grid by as little as 5° can result in sufficient grid cut-off to visibly reduce image density.

Grids that permit wide exposure and centering latitude assist in these problems. **Low-ratio grids (5:1 and 6:1) are often preferred for mobile radiography.** Use of a parallel instead of a focused grid also increases latitude.

Film/Screen Combinations

Because there are more variables with mobile radiography, it is appropriate to permit a wider latitude film and intensifying screen combination to be used. Wider latitude films usually exhibit slower speed, greater resolution and lower contrast. It is also appropriate to take the opposite position and utilize a high speed film/screen combination to reduce patient dose and overcome the limitations of lower power equipment. However, when rotary 3ϕ battery powered units are available, their output capabilities remove equipment limitation rationales.

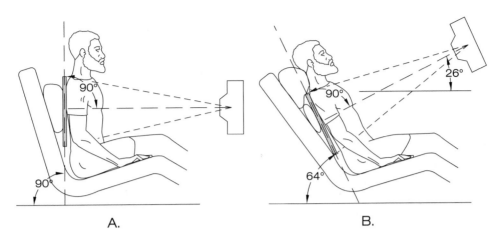

FIGURE 37-7. Alignment problems during mobile chest radiography. (A) A simple alignment problem correctly resolved. (B) A difficult alignment problem correctly resolved.

Other Factors

Other technical factors are not significantly different between mobile and stationary equipment, although the exact specifications for equipment will vary. For example, mobile equipment seldom requires fractional focal spots.

Summary

Mobile examinations are more difficult because there are so many additional variables — variables that would be constants with a stationary unit — when manipulating and positioning both patient and equipment. In many instances the reason an examination is requested at the bedside is to avoid transporting the patient because of his physical condition. Special adaptations of routine projections, imaginative equipment manipulation and innovative technical factor considerations are often required. Good communication with the patient is a necessary part of all radiographic procedures. The unconscious or incognizant patient requires the same explanation that a cognizant patient would receive.

Extreme care must be taken when manipulating equipment in a high technology environment such as intensive care, surgery or the emergency unit. Care must be exercised to ensure that power supplies, oxygen tubes,

catheters, intravenous lines, etc., have enough slack to permit movement.

Patients requiring examinations with mobile equipment are often unable to assume standardized positions. Clinical experience and a thorough knowledge of acceptable positioning variants are required for this problem. Because the mobile examination is performed at the patient's bedside, there is an increased possibility of artifacts, such as personal items, layers of coverings and medical equipment.

During a mobile examination the radiographer is bringing a radiation hazard into an area not designed for radiation protection. A duty exists to protect the patient, health workers, the public and oneself.

X-ray units are available in a wide array of sizes and capabilities, many of which can be classified as mobile. There are two major classifications of mobile equipment: portable light duty units and full power institutional units. Light duty mobile units and some full power units obtain power from wall outlets. The more advanced full power units use batteries for a power supply and are capable of greater voltages. Specialized generators have been developed specifically for mobile equipment. Capacitor discharge units and battery-powered units are the most common. Capacitor discharge units produce a constant potential output while battery operated units produce output that is essentially 3ϕ.

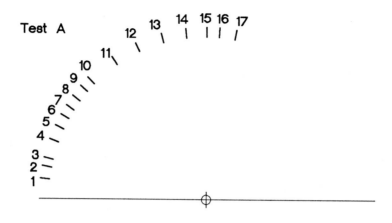

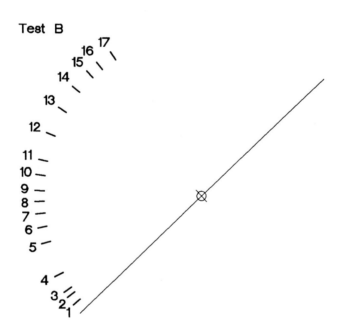

FIGURE 37-8. Difficulty of angle estimation with an angled baseline. If a line is drawn from one of the numbers to the dot, which number would create a 90° angle? A 15° angle? A 37° angle? Record your answers for both tests A and B, and then look on page 532 for the correct answers. Do not tilt your head or the book when completing Test B.

Establishing technical factors for mobile units almost always involves conversion of multiple variables (i.e., generator phase, filtration, grid, etc.) from stationary equipment technique systems. Because multiple conversions increase the risk of error, it is advisable to establish individual technique charts for each mobile unit. A number of factors should be considered when establishing mobile technique charts, including kilovoltage, milliamperage, distance, grids and film/screen combinations.

REVIEW QUESTIONS

1. Why are mobile procedures often more difficult than those performed using stationary units?

2. What should the radiographer do before bringing mobile equipment into a patient's room?

3. What must be considered when manipulating mobile equipment in a high technology environment?

4. What must a radiographer do to adequately visualize air-fluid levels on a chest radiograph?

5. What are the two most common generators used for mobile equipment?

6. What type of generator waveform is produced with a full powered battery operated mobile unit?

7. Why is it important to measure distance (SID) for all mobile procedures?

8. What type of grids are preferred for mobile procedures?

REFERENCES AND RECOMMENDED READING

Adler, A. & Carlton, R. R. (1994). *Introduction to radiography and patient care*. Philadelphia: W. B. Saunders.

Ball, J. & Price, T. (1989). *Chesneys' radiographic imaging*. Oxford: Blackwell Scientific Publishing.

Barnhard, H. J. (1978). The bedside examination: A time for analysis and appropriate action. *Radiology. 129*, 539–540.

Benbow, M. (1994). The selection of kVp during mobile radiography on the special care baby unit. *Radiography Today. 60*(686), 19–20.

Bushberg, J. T., Seibert, J. A., Leidholdt, E. M., & Boone, J. M. (1994). *The essential physics of medical imaging*. Baltimore: Williams & Wilkins.

Bushong, S. C. (1997). *Radiologic science for technologists: Physics, biology, and protection* (6th ed.). St. Louis: C. V. Mosby.

Cantwell, K. G., Press, H. C., & Anderson, J. E. (1978). Bedside radiographic examinations: Indications and contraindications. *Radiology. 129*, 383–384.

Cullinan, A. & Cullinan, J. (1994). *Producing quality radiographs*. (2nd ed.). Philadelphia: J. B. Lippincott.

A device for improving the quality of bedside decubitus exams. (1979). *Radiologic Technology. 51*(1), 88.

Dowd, S. B. (1995). *Encyclopedia of radiographic positioning*. Philadelphia: W. B. Saunders.

Drafke, M. W. (1990). *Trauma and mobile radiography*. Philadelphia: F. A. Davis.

Eisenberg, R. L., Akin, J. R., & Hedgcock, M. W. (1980). Optimal use of portable and stat examination. *The American Journal of Roentgenology. 134*, 523–524.

Evans, S. A., Harris, L., Lawinski, C. P., & Hendra, I. R. F. (1985). Mobile x-ray generators: A review. *Radiography. 51*(595), 89–107.

Floyd, C., Baker, A., Lo, J., & Ravin, C. (1992). Measurement of scatter fractions in clinical bedside radiography. *Radiology. 183*(3), 857–861.

Fry, O. E. & Gianturco, C. (1960). Bedside radiography reduction of patient exposure and orientation of grid cassettes. *Radiologic Technology. 31*(4), 387.

Hasse, R. A. (1991). New trends in portable x-ray batteries and technology. *Radiology Management. 13*(3), 42–44.

MacMahon, H., Yasillo, N., & Carlin, M. (1992). Laser alignment system for high-quality portable radiography. *RadioGraphics. 12*, 111–120.

Marlowe, J. E. (1983). *Surgical radiography*. Baltimore: University Park Press.

O'Donovan, P., Skipper, G., Litchney, J., Salupo, A., & Bortnick, J. (1992). Device for facilitating precise alignment in bedside radiography. *Radiology. 184*(1), 284.

Osborn, R. R. (1960). Improved portable radiographs of the trunk without the use of grids or Bucky. *Radiologic Technology. 32*(2), 145.

Rossi, R., Harnisch, B. D., & Hendee, W. R. (1982). Evaluation of an automatic exposure control device for mobile radiography. *Radiology.* (Dec), 823.

Schaefer, C. (1989). Improved control of image optical density with low-dose digital and conventional radiography in bedside imaging. *Radiology.* (Dec), 713.

Seeram, E. (1985). *X-ray imaging equipment: An introduction.* Springfield: Charles C. Thomas.

Thompson, M. A., Hattaway, M. P., Hall, J. D., & Dowd, S. B. (1994). *Principles of imaging science and protection.* Philadelphia: W. B. Saunders.

Tortorici, M. (1992). *Concepts in medical radiographic imaging.* Philadelphia: W. B. Saunders.

Trew, D. J. (1970). The 'cordless' mobile x-ray machine. *Radiography. 36*(427), 159–164.

Weaver, K. E., Barone, G. J., & Fewell, T. R. (1978). Selection of technique factors for mobile capacitor energy storage x-ray equipment. *Radiology. 128*, 223–228.

Wolbarst, A. B. (1993). *Physics of radiology.* Norwalk, CT: Appleton & Lange.

Answers to Figure 37–8

Test A	Test B
$90° = 15$	$90° = 15$
$15° = 3$	$15° = 4$
$37° = 8$	$37° = 7$

CHAPTER 38

Fluoroscopy

. . . in February, 1896, fantastic, vague, and startling reports emanated from the foreign press regarding a wonderful device "invented" by Professor Salvioni of Perugia, Italy, called the cryptoscope, that permitted instantaneous visualization of human, living, and moving bones. . . . At about the same time Professor McGie of Princeton University also developed a . . . skiascope. Edison also constructed a similar device about which extensive publicity soon developed. He named it the fluoroscope.

Arthur W. Fuchs, "Edison and Roentgenology."

Objectives

Upon completion of this chapter, the student should be able to:

▶ Differentiate fluoroscopic examinations from static diagnostic radiographic examinations.

▶ Describe a typical basic fluoroscopic image chain.

▶ Explain the difference between the operation of a fluoroscopic and a diagnostic x-ray tube.

▶ Describe the advantages of image intensified fluoroscopy over conventional screen fluoroscopy.

▶ Explain the functions and operation of the image intensification tube input screen, photocathode, electrostatic focusing lenses and anode and output screen.

▶ Explain the operation of a multifield magnification image intensification tube.

▶ Discuss the effects of minification and flux gain on total brightness gain.

▶ Explain the basic function of a fluoroscopic automatic brightness control.

▶ Discuss the factors that affect fluoroscopic image contrast, resolution, distortion and quantum mottle.

▶ Explain the operation of an optical mirror viewer system, video camera CCD, video camera tube and video monitor.

▶ Evaluate the three basic types of fluoroscopic viewing systems.

▶ Explain the uses of dynamic and static fluoroscopic recording systems.

▶ Evaluate various types of fluoroscopic recording systems for various clinical situations.

▶ Explain the operation of a cineradiographic camera, a spot film recording system, 105 mm chip film and 70 mm roll film recording systems and magnetic and laser video disc recorders.

▶ Discuss the resolving ability of various videotape recording equipment.

▶ Relate problems with mobile radiographic equipment to mobile fluoroscopic equipment.

▶ Discuss various methods of reducing dose to the patient, the radiographer and the radiologist during a fluoroscopic examination.

Historical Development

*F*luoroscopy (fluoro) is a dynamic radiographic examination, compared to diagnostic radiography, which is static in character. Fluoroscopy involves active diagnosis during an examination. For this reason, fluoroscopy is primarily the domain of the radiologist. The radiographer's role becomes that of an assistant during the examination, although routine post-fluoroscopic radiography is the responsibility of the radiographer. **Radiographers should perform fluoroscopy only for static examinations** where diagnosis is not involved, such as spot filming the terminal ilium.

The invention of the fluoroscope is credited to Thomas A. Edison in 1896, the year after Röntgen's discovery of x-rays. However, technically speaking, Röntgen discovered x-rays fluoroscopically when he noticed their ability to demonstrate skeletal anatomy as he brought a lead disc into the beam and observed the dynamic movement of his own fingers projected onto a fluorescent screen. Fluoroscopic procedures have, therefore, been a part of diagnostic radiography since its inception.

A fluoroscopic imaging chain consists of a specialized x-ray tube with an image receptor, called the **fluoroscopic screen**, that can be viewed during an x-ray exposure. The first fluoroscopes were held by hand in front of the patient and x-ray tube and included a viewing hood to eliminate extraneous light. Later units attached the fluoro screen to the x-ray table. In both systems, the radiologist's face and eyes received the full primary beam. A great number of the pioneers in radiology became martyrs of the science because of the design of early fluoro units. Once the biological hazards of radiation became apparent, the design of the fluoroscope was changed to permit viewing by an arrangement of mirrors. This arrangement shielded the primary beam in a leaded enclosure while the mirrors transmitted the optical image to the viewer. **Image intensification tubes** were developed in 1948 and they resulted in video camera and monitor systems (see Figure 5–1) which began to replace mirror viewers. However, there is still a significant loss of detail with a video system, a fact that cannot be appreciated unless an opportunity to view a fluorescent screen through a mirror system arises.

Fluoroscopic Uses

Although the fluoroscopic image was preferred originally, the need to document findings, coupled with immense improvements in the resolution capabilities of diagnostic radiography, not to mention reductions in the dose to the patient, caused fluoroscopy to become less popular. It is currently used only for studies that require observation of dynamic physiological functions, e.g., the flow of barium through the gastrointestinal tract, swallowing, the injection of a contrast medium into the heart, etc.

Fluoroscopic Positioning Previewing

Fluoroscopy is not intended to be used as a preview to positioning. Radiographers spend two years or more learning how to position the patient properly. There should be no reason for a radiographer to use fluoroscopy as a positioning guide. This procedure would cause unnecessary patient exposure to ionizing radiation. Radiographers should obtain a satisfactory image 95 percent of the time, and this degree of expertise entails not just positioning but technical factors and equipment variations as well.

Types of Equipment

The fluoroscopic x-ray tube and image receptor are mounted on a C-arm to maintain their alignment at all times (Figure 38–1). In the United States, federal regulations prohibit the use of a fluoroscopic x-ray tube when the entire primary beam is not resulting in an image. The C-arm permits the image receptor to be raised and lowered to vary the beam geometry for maximum resolution while the x-ray tube remains in position. It also permits scanning the length and width of the x-ray table. There are two types of C-arm arrangements, both described by the location of the x-ray tube. Under-table units have the x-ray tube under the table while over-table units suspend the tube over the patient.

The arm that supports the equipment suspended over the table is called the **carriage**. It typically includes an image intensification tube (on an under-table unit) or the x-ray tube (on an over-table unit), controls for power drive to the carriage, brightness (which regulates the tube mA), spot film selection, tube shutters, spot filming and/or cine camera, video input tube and other controls. Although it can be disengaged and pushed away from the table to gain access to the patient, exposure cannot commence until the carriage is returned to a full beam intercept position.

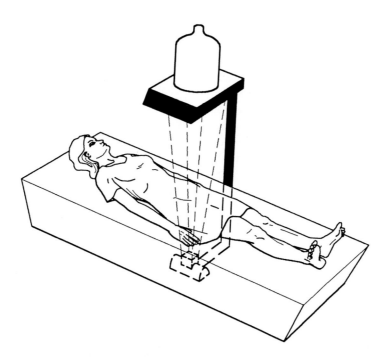

FIGURE 38-1. C-arm alignment of fluoroscopic x-ray tube and image receptor.

Fluoroscopic X-Ray Tubes

Fluoroscopic x-ray tubes are very similar to diagnostic tubes except that they are designed to operate for longer periods of time at much lower mA. Where a typical diagnostic tube operates at 50 –1,200 mA, **the fluoroscopic mA range is 0.5–5.0 mA**. The tube target must be fixed to prevent an SOD of less than 15" (38 cm). The fluoroscopic tube is operated by a foot switch, which permits the fluoroscopist to have both hands free to operate the carriage and position and palpate the patient. Care must be taken to not accidentally activate the foot switch when the unit is in operating mode before or after examinations. Fluoroscopic tubes are equipped with electrically controlled shutters that permit maintenance of close collimation from the fluoro carriage during both fluoroscopy and spot filming.

Image Intensification Tubes

Early fluoroscopic screens were very dim. Dark adaptation, a procedure in which light levels are reduced for a period of at least 10–15 minutes to permit the rods of the eye to become activated, was a time-consuming and irritating part of the radiologist's work routine. The exclusive use of the rod cells constituted a serious threat to diagnostic accuracy because visual acuity is controlled by the cones, which require daylight (photopic) levels of light in order to function. Photopic visual acuity is about 10 times greater than scotopic acuity. The brightness of the fluoro image was not raised to daylight levels until image intensification technology was developed in 1948.

An image intensification tube is designed to electronically amplify the brightness of an image. Modern image intensifiers are capable of increasing image brightness 500–8,000 times. Photopic visual acuity becomes active when the brightness is about 1,000 times that of a fluoroscopic screen. Their primary use is in fluoroscopy equipment, although variations of the design are used in other modalities.

A typical image intensifier is shown in Figure 38–2. The primary x-ray beam exits the patient and strikes the input screen of the image intensifier tube, which is a vacuum tube with a cathode and an anode. The fluorescent screen is built into the image intensifier as its input screen. **The fluorescent screen absorbs the x-ray photons and emits light photons**, which immediately encounter the photocathode (the cathode of the tube) that is in contact with the input screen to prevent divergence of the light beam. **The photocathode absorbs the light photons and emits electrons.** The electrons are then accelerated from the cathode toward the anode and the output screen by the potential difference that exists between the cathode and anode. At the same time the electron beam is focused onto the output screen, which is much smaller than the input screen. **Electrostatic lenses are used to accelerate and focus the electrons. The primary brightness gain occurs from the acceleration and focusing of the electron beam.** The acceleration of the electron beam increases its energy and its ability to emit light at the output screen. The focusing of the electron beam intensifies the image into a smaller area. **The output screen absorbs the electrons and emits light photons**, which are then available for viewing or further electronic processing by a video system. Note the changes in the quantity of photons and electrons in the image at each stage of the intensification process.

The entire image intensification tube is encased in a lead lined housing that effectively absorbs the primary beam while permitting the intensified light photon image to be transmitted to the viewer. An ion pump device called a getter is used to remove ions produced during operation and to maintain the vacuum within the tube.

Input Screen and Photocathode

The input fluorescent screen consists of a 0.1 –0.2 mm layer of sodium-activated cesium iodide (CsI) phosphors coated onto the concave surface of the image intensification tube. This surface may be made of glass, titanium, steel or aluminum and ranges from 6" (15 cm) to 23" (58 cm) in diameter, depending on the manufacturer and use. The screen is concave to maintain the same distance between each point on the input screen and its corresponding location on the output screen. Failure to maintain this distance would result in distortion of the image because points farther from the center would be more magnified. The CsI phosphors are packed together very tightly so they absorb about 66 percent of the incident beam, producing a good conversion

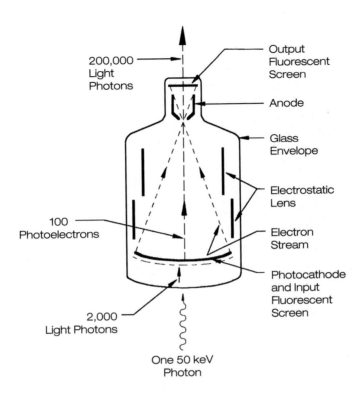

FIGURE 38-2. An image intensification tube. The quantity of photons and electrons in the image changes at each stage of the intensification process, with the output significantly greater than the input.

efficiency, or quantum yield. The phosphors then emit light photons vertically, in proportion to the absorption, thus reducing the lateral spread of light photons that would reduce the image detail. As an example, a single 25 keV incident photon would typically produce over 1,500 light photons. This conversion efficiency permits the fluoro system to function with minimal activation of the phosphors.

An extremely thin protective coating is applied to the input screen to prevent a chemical interaction with the photocathode. The photocathode material is composed of photoemissive metals, usually cesium and antimony compounds, which are applied to the protective coating. The two materials appear to be a single coating when examined. The photoemissive materials absorb the light photons and emit electrons in a process called photoemission. The process is similar to thermionic emission except that the stimulation is light instead of heat.

Electrostatic Lenses

The electrostatic lenses are a series of charged electrodes located inside the glass envelope of the tube. Because the electrons are negative, the charge of the lenses accelerates and focuses the electron stream, which carries the fluoroscopic image. As with an optically focused image, the focal point reverses the image so the output screen image is reversed from the input screen image (right becomes left and superior becomes inferior). The concave input screen reduces distortion by maintaining the same distance between all points on the input screen and their corresponding locations on the output screen, regardless of the position of the focal point.

Magnification Tubes
The greater the voltage supplied to the electrostatic lenses the greater the acceleration, and the closer the focal point moves toward the

input screen. Image intensification tubes can be designed to magnify the image electronically by changing the voltage on the electrostatic lenses. They are often called multifield, dual-field, triple-field or quad-field intensifiers.

Increased voltage focuses the electrons at a point closer to the input screen and this causes the image to be magnified when it reaches the output screen (Figure 38–3). Magnification image intensifiers are capable of 1.5–4× magnification, which is usually controlled at the fluoro carriage. Some tubes are capable of up to four different magnifications. Resolution can be increased from ≈4 lp/mm to ≈6 lp/mm when the magnification mode is used. The tubes are described according to the diameter of the area of the input screen that will be imaged. For example, a 23/15 dual-focus tube has a 9" (23 cm) input screen when operating normally and uses a 6" (15 cm) area when magnifying. The magnification factor is calculated as:

$$\text{magnification} = \frac{\text{input screen diameter}}{\begin{array}{c}\text{diameter of input screen}\\\text{used during magnification}\end{array}}$$

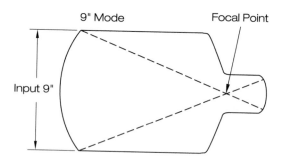

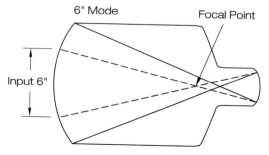

FIGURE 38-3. A magnification image intensification tube. Changes in the focal point produce the magnification.

Example: What is the magnification for an image viewed with an image intensification tube with an input screen diameter of 9" (23 cm) that is using a 5" (13 cm) diameter area during magnification?

Answer:

$$\text{magnification} = \frac{\text{input screen diameter}}{\begin{array}{c}\text{diameter of input screen}\\\text{used during magnification}\end{array}}$$

$$\text{magnification} = \frac{9"}{5"}$$

$$\text{magnification} = 1.8$$

The excess edges of the image are not transmitted by the output screen; therefore the primary beam field should be collimated to the viewing field when these tubes are operated in magnification mode. Minimal magnification is used for most studies because it reduces contrast problems due to minification and flux gain and permits viewing of the entire primary beam field.

Anode and Output Screen

The anode is positively charged and is normally supplied with about 25 kV. This charge causes a tremendous attraction of the negative electrons from the photocathode. The anode is positioned inside the glass envelope, immediately in front of the output screen. It has a hole in its center that permits the accelerated electrons to pass through the anode field and onto the output screen.

The output screen is also a glass fluorescent screen. It is a silver-activated zinc-cadmium sulfide phosphor (ZnS-CdS:Ag) that was also used as the input phosphor in early tubes. The electrons that strike the screen are converted into light photons that exit the tube. Because all phosphors emit light isotropically, an opaque filter is used under the output phosphor layer to prevent most of the light emitted in that direction from returning to the input screen, where it would degrade the image. Some newer intensifiers use a fiber optic disc in place of the glass output screen. Fiber optics eliminate the isotropic emission problem and are capable of transmitting the image some distance without loss of resolution.

Total Brightness Gain

Total brightness gain is a measurement of the increase in image intensity achieved by an image intensification tube. It is determined by two factors: minification gain and flux gain.

Minification Gain   Minification gain occurs as a result of the same number of electrons that were produced at the large input screen being compressed into the area of the small output screen. Most image intensification tubes have input screens of 6" (15 cm) or 9" (23 cm), although 12" (30 cm) and larger tubes have been available for special applications. The typical output screen has a diameter of 1" (2.5 cm). The minification gain is calculated as the ratio between the area of the input and output screens.

$$\text{minification gain} = \frac{\text{input screen diameter}^2}{\text{output screen diameter}^2}$$

Example: What is the minification gain for an image intensification tube with an input screen diameter of 6" (15 cm) and an output diameter of 1" (2.5 cm)?

Answer:

$$\text{minification gain} = \frac{\text{input screen diameter}^2}{\text{output screen diameter}^2}$$

$$\text{minification gain} = \frac{6^2}{1^2}$$

$$\text{minification gain} = \frac{36}{1}$$

$$\text{minification gain} = 36$$

Minification gain is simply an increase in brightness or intensity, not an improvement in the quality or number of photons making up the image.

Flux Gain   Flux gain is a measurement of the increase in light photons due to the conversion efficiency of the output screen. For example, if the output phosphor produces 50 light photons for each electron that strikes it, the flux gain would be 50. Flux gain does not take into account the conversion efficiency of the input screen. It deals only with the gain accomplished by the electron to light conversion at the output screen. Flux gain causes a decrease in image quality exactly as intensifying screens decrease resolution in diagnostic images as a result of the penumbral effect of individual phosphor crystals.

Total Brightness Gain   Total brightness gain can be calculated by several methods. As a function of minification and flux gain, the formula is:

$$\text{brightness gain} = \text{minification gain} \times \text{flux gain}$$

Example: What is the total brightness gain for an image intensification tube with a minification gain of 36 and a flux gain of 60?

Answer:

$$\text{brightness gain} = \text{minification gain} \times \text{flux gain}$$
$$\text{brightness gain} = 36 \times 60$$
$$\text{brightness gain} = 2,160$$

However, the original formula was:

$$\text{brightness gain} = \frac{\text{intensity of output prosphor}}{\text{intensity of Patterson B–2 fluoroscopic screen}}$$

A Patterson B–2 fluoro screen was chosen as the reference point because it was in common use at the time. This formula has lost acceptance because the Patterson B–2 screens would vary from one batch to another and their deterioration was not linear.

Because the Patterson B–2 screen is no longer available, this standard is now obsolete. Although it appears that the term brightness gain will continue in use, its measure is a conversion factor that is the ratio of the intensity of the output phosphor to the input exposure rate.

$$\text{conversion factor} = \frac{\text{intensity of output phosphor}}{\text{mR/sec}}$$

Output phosphor intensity is measured in candelas (cd), the unit of luminous intensity.

$$\text{conversion factor} = \frac{\text{cd/m}^2}{\text{mR/sec}}$$

Typical values for modern image intensifier systems are

$$80-250 \ \frac{cd/m^2}{mR/sec}$$

This represents a gain of 8,000–25,000 times.

Brightness gain deteriorates as much as 10 percent per year because, just as with intensifying screen phosphors, the input and output screen phosphors age. Although difficult to measure, brightness gain can be evaluated by monitoring the radiation dose required to obtain a diagnostic image from a standard phantom, such as an abdomen or pelvis.

Fluoroscopic Generators

The generators used for static radiography are also used for fluoroscopy. Usually the operator's console includes a control that activates the fluoroscopic system and bypasses the static radiography system.

Brightness Control

A wide variety of systems with different names are used to automatically maintain satisfactory fluoroscopic image density and contrast. Automatic brightness control (ABC) is the most common term although automatic dose control (ADC) and automatic brightness stabilization (ABS) accomplish the same result. They maintain the brightness of the image by automatically adjusting the exposure factors as necessary according to subject density and contrast. Most ABC systems monitor the current flowing between the cathode and anode of the image intensification tube or the intensity of the output screen. In all systems, the primary beam is changed when current and intensity fall below established levels. Regulation of the primary beam can be accomplished by varying kVp, mA and pulse time. Most ABCs use combinations of these methods in a manner similar to a stepped variable kVp technique system. For example, kVp is gradually increased to the maximum acceptable contrast level, then mA is doubled while kVp is stepped down to the lowest acceptable contrast level and the procedure is started over again. All ABCs have a relatively slow response time, which is noticeable during routine fluoroscopic scanning because the image density adjustment lags a moment behind rapid changes in tissue density. Automatic gain control (AGC) is part of the video camera control system. It responds very quickly but does not change the x-ray exposure factors.

Image Quality

Because the imaging chain of a fluoroscopic system is so complex, there are more factors that affect each of the quality elements of the image than in static radiography. In addition to contrast, resolution and distortion, quantum mottle must also be considered.

Contrast

Contrast is controlled by increasing the amplitude of the video signal, although it is affected by other factors. Image intensified fluoroscopic contrast is not only affected by scattered ionizing radiation but is also affected by penumbral light scatter in the input and output screens, and light scatter within the image intensification tube itself. Scattered ionizing radiation not only produces scatter photons arriving at the input phosphor but also produces some background fog from incident photons that are transmitted through the tube to the output screen or that backscatter from the output to the input screen. Light photons also scatter as they are reflected and refracted within the tube. Since light is emitted isotropically from the output phosphor, some of it will strike the input screen, causing a backscatter effect. All these effects combine to produce a background fog that raises the base density of the image. This affects image contrast exactly as film processing base plus fog affects film contrast. By raising the lowest density value, it decreases the total visible contrast. The overall effect is of reduced contrast. There is also a decrease in image contrast near the edges of the images.

Resolution

The primary limitation on most fluoroscopic resolution is the 525-line raster pattern of the video monitor. For nonvideo recording, such as spot filming or direct optical viewing, the ability to resolve recorded detail in a fluoroscopic system will vary depending on the geometrical factors, just as in static radiography. However, the geometrical factors are different, including minification gain, electrostatic focal point, input and output screen diameter and viewing system resolution (especially television system resolution), as well as OID and phosphor size and thickness. CsI image intensifiers are capable of ≈4 lp/mm. Optical mirror systems that permit indirect viewing of the fluoro screen are capable of ≈3 lp/mm. Magnification or multifield image intensifiers are capable of up to ≈6 lp/mm in the magnification mode.

Distortion

Size distortion is caused by the same factors that affect static radiographic magnification, primarily OID. Magnification image intensifiers that produce a magnified image by changing the electrostatic focal point within the tube do not significantly affect actual size distortion. Although a magnified image often appears to have more distortion, the distortion is also present in the minified image. It is simply easier to detect when enlarged.

Shape distortion is caused primarily by geometric problems in the shape of the image intensification tube. Although the input screen is concave, it does not completely eliminate edge distortion at the output screen. Electrons at the outer edges of the image tend to flare outward as they are electrostatically focused. Part of this problem is caused by the repulsion of electrons from one another due to their like charges. Figure 30–4 illustrates the edge distortion problem in image intensification tubes. This effect is called vignetting or pincushion distortion and may comprise 8–10 percent of the image area. Some of the vignetting effect is also caused by the effect of the divergence of the primary beam from the x-ray tube focal spot. Vignetting also causes image intensity to be greater at the center of the image and less at the edges. Consequently, distortion is minimized and contrast is improved at the center of the fluoro image.

Quantum Mottle

Quantum mottle is a blotchy or grainy appearance caused by insufficient radiation to create a uniform image. Since the quantity of photons is controlled by the mA and time settings, with static radiography any mA and time combination can be used to accumulate sufficient radiation to create a uniform image. With fluoroscopy, the time factor is controlled by the length of time the eye can integrate, or accumulate, light photons from the fluoro imaging chain. Because this period is 0.2 second, fluoroscopy must provide sufficient photons, through mA, to avoid mottle. Quantum mottle is also a large part of video noise and is a special problem during fluoroscopy because the units operate with the minimum number of photons possible to activate the fluoro screen. The factors that influence mottle are those that affect the total number of photons arriving at the retina of the eye. This includes radiation output, beam attenuation by the subject, the conversion efficiency of the input screen, minification gain, flux gain, total brightness gain, viewing system and the distance of the eye from the viewing system. Increasing the efficiency of any of these factors can assist in reducing quantum mottle, but the most common solution is to increase the fluoro tube mA.

Viewing Systems

A number of viewing systems have been developed to deliver the image from the output screen to the viewer. These include video, cine and spot film systems. Some of these systems permit dynamic real-time viewing while others are for static images. The viewing time, resolution and processing time vary. Table 38–1 illustrates the characteristics of each system.

Video Viewing System

The most commonly used fluoroscopic viewing system is video. Closed circuit video is used with all transmission through cables to avoid broadcast interference. A system includes a video camera attached to the image intensification tube output phosphor and a display monitor for viewing. Fluoroscopic video cameras use a vidicon or Plumbicon™ tube or a charge-coupled device (CCD).

Video Camera Tubes

The vidicon and Plumbicon™ tubes are similar in operation, differing mainly in their target layers. A

TABLE 38–1. Comparison Of Various Image Intensification Viewing Systems

System	Dynamic/Static	Real-time/Delayed	Resolution	Processing Time
Video				
Real-time	dynamic	real-time	7th highest	short
Videotape	dynamic or static	delayed	lowest	short
Cine film				
16 mm	dynamic or static	delayed	6th highest	highest
35 mm	dynamic or static	delayed	5th highest	highest
Spot film				
Cassette	static	delayed	2nd highest	high
105 mm chip	static	delayed	3rd highest	high
70 mm roll	static	delayed	4th highest	high

Plumbicon™ tube has a faster response time than a vidicon tube. The tube consists of a cathode with a control grid, a series of electromagnetic focusing and electrostatic deflecting coils, and an anode with face plate, signal plate and target (Figure 38–4).

Cathode

The cathode consists of a heating assembly that forms an electron gun by thermionically emitting electrons that are shaped into a beam by a control grid. The electron beam is then accelerated toward the target but is decelerated by the anode and a wire mesh in front of the target. This arrangement brings the electrons to a near standstill where they are straightened so the beam strikes the target perpendicularly. At the same time the focusing coils bring the electron beam to a point to maintain resolution. Pairs of deflecting coils serve to cause the electron beam to scan the target in a path known as a raster pattern (Figure 38–5). Commercial television uses a 525 horizontal line raster pattern, but high resolution video systems now offer 1,050 line systems. The speed of the electron gun movement is difficult to comprehend. The electron beam scans across the screen nearly 1,000,000 times per minute. However, to avoid flicker each scan is divided into two halves, with the first half scanning even-numbered lines and the second half scanning odd-numbered lines. This permits the 30 scans to be projected as 60 half frames per second and flickering is eliminated. (European systems operate at 25 scans for 50 half frames per second to match the 50 Hz current.) The raster pattern significantly reduces the resolution of the image and is the primary disadvantage of a video viewing system.

Anode

The output phosphor of the image intensification tube is coupled with the face plate of the vidicon tube by fiber optics or optical lenses. This permits the light photons to be transmitted to the signal plate and target. The signal plate consists of a thin film of graphite charged with a positive voltage. It is thin enough to transmit light yet thick enough to conduct the electronic signal out of the tube. The target consists of a thin insulating mica coating in which globules of a light sensitive photoconductive material are suspended in a matrix.

Vidicon tubes use antimony trisulfide (Sb_2S_3) while Plumbicon™ tubes use lead oxide (PbO). The globules are approximately 0.001 inch (0.025 mm) in diameter and their size determines the resolving power of the tube. Each globule is capable of absorbing light photons and then releasing electrons equivalent to the intensity of the absorbed light. The loss of electrons creates a positive charge at the globule, which in turn causes the signal plate to become negatively charged. When the electron gun's beam scans the target, it discharges the globules. This sequential discharging of the globules releases the signal plate's charge as a pulsed signal. This sequential pulsing is

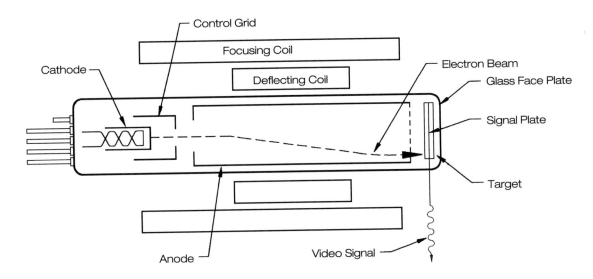

FIGURE 38-4. A video camera tube.

the video signal, which can be translated back into an image via the electron gun of the viewing monitor.

The vidicon tube is connected to the output screen of the image intensification tube by either fiber optics or an optical lens system. Fiber optics are bundles of extremely small, light conducting cable. They are very durable but do not permit the image intensification tube output to be intercepted for spot filming. Spot filming requires an optical lens system similar to the old mirror optical

viewing system. The use of beam splitting mirrors permits the image to be recorded by a spot filming device while being viewed. Other systems use a fully silvered mirror to interrupt viewing while deflecting the image for spot filming. Optical lens systems are considerably larger and are easily distinguished by the large size of the housing on top of the image intensification tube. They must be handled gently to avoid trauma to the lenses and mirrors.

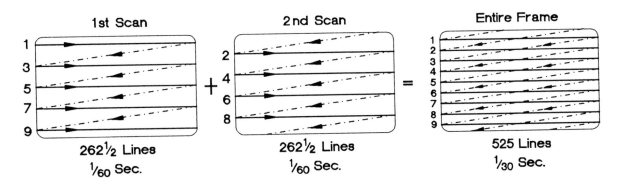

FIGURE 38-5. A video monitor raster scanning pattern. The electron beam scans the diagonal lines as active traces while the horizontal lines are inactive retraces to position for the next active trace. The electron beam scans 262 1/2 alternate lines every 1/60 second and the second set of lines the next 1/60 second. Consequently, the entire 525-line raster pattern is scanned every 1/30 second. This is 30 times per second, which is 15,720 scan lines per second.

Video Camera Charge-Coupled Devices (CCD)

A CCD is a semiconducting device capable of storing a charge from light photons striking a photosensitive surface. When light strikes the photoelectric cathode of the CCD, electrons are released proportionally to the intensity of the incident light. As with all semiconductors, the CCD has the ability to store the freed electrons in a series of P and N holes, thus storing the image in a latent form (see Chapter 4). The video signal is emitted in a raster scanning pattern by moving the stored charges along the P and N holes to the edge of the CCD, where they are discharged as pulses into a conductor. The primary advantage of CCDs is the extremely fast discharge time, which eliminates image lag. This is extremely useful in high speed imaging applications such as cardiac catheterization. Other advantages are that CCDs are more sensitive than video tubes, they operate at much lower voltages, which prolongs their life, they have acceptable resolution and they are not as susceptible to damage from rough handling.

Video Monitor

A video monitor (or television tube) is a cathode ray tube (CRT) that consists of a vacuum tube with a fluorescent phosphor coated on the inside of the front screen and an electron gun with deflecting and focusing electromagnets (Figure 38–6). The electron gun is the cathode while the anode is plated onto the front screen. The monitor creates an image as the gun sprays the pulsed stream of electrons from the camera onto the screen phosphor. The gun follows the same raster pattern used by the camera. The phosphor crystals emit light when struck by electrons and transmit it as a visual image through the glass of the screen to the viewer. The video monitor is the most restrictive element in the fluoro imaging chain resolution. A 525 line monitor is capable of displaying between 1–2 lp/mm. Magnification of this image by the video camera or an optical system can increase resolution significantly. Video monitors often operate in the low kilovoltage range and can emit low energy x-rays.

The video monitor viewing conditions change with viewing distance, raster pattern and screen size. A 525 line pattern on a 9" monitor has a minimum viewing

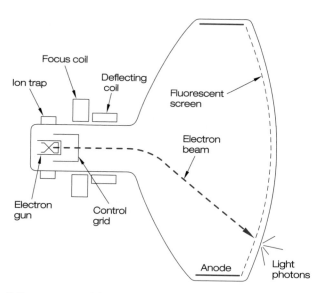

FIGURE 38-6. A video monitor (cathode ray tube [CRT]).

distance of 37" while 70" is suggested for a 17" monitor. High resolution patterns (1,050 lines) may be viewed closer; a 9" monitor has a minimum viewing distance of 17" while 36" is suggested for a 17" monitor. Contrast and brightness can be adjusted with controls on the monitor itself. However, these controls cannot compensate for contrast and brightness problems within the imaging chain. Conversely, the monitor should be checked prior to assuming a problem is in the imaging chain.

Recording The Fluoroscopic Image

Dynamic Systems

Dynamic recording of fluoroscopic images has been limited to cine film and videotape, although laser videodisc would be possible if the recorders were not so expensive.

Cine Film Systems
Cinematic or cine film imaging systems are sometimes referred to as cinefluorography. They consist of a cine (movie) camera positioned to

intercept the image produced by the output screen of the image intensification tube. They require about 90 percent of the image intensity for proper exposure levels. Both 16 mm and 35 mm formats are currently in use. Although they dramatically increase resolution when compared to video systems, they also require significantly greater patient dose.

Cine cameras operate by recording a series of static images at high speed. When the images on processed film are projected at the same high speed, the eye becomes incapable of differentiating the separate images and perceives them as a single image in motion. Cine cameras must be synchronized to ensure that the pulses of radiation from the generator coincide with the opening of the shutter to expose the film. This is usually accomplished by operating the camera at either 30 or 60 frames (images) per second to coordinate with the 60 Hz rectified current operating the x-ray tube. Without synchronization, the output screen intensity would vary during the 1/30 or 1/60 second the shutter was open, resulting in some frames being underexposed. To assist in synchronization, the x-ray tube is grid biased or grid pulsed by placing a negatively charged wire across the cathode focusing cup. When the grid wire is turned off and on in pulses, it permits the cathode to pulse electrons to the x-ray tube anode, thus producing a pulse synchronized x-ray beam.

Cineradiographic film is usually viewed as both movie and stop-action film. It must be shown at 16 frames per second if smooth motion is to be perceived. Because the eye can perceive flicker at up to 50 frames per second, movie projectors operate at 24 frames per second and show each frame twice, thus pulsing the light 48 times per second and eliminating flicker.

The generator and fluoro x-ray tube in a cine system must be able to handle large heat loads. Although individual exposure factors for a single frame are minimal, when multiplied by the 30–60 frames per second required to produce cine, a significant heat load is produced. A 3φ, 12 pulse, 70–80 KW generator and a liquid cooled, 50–60 KW tube with a 0.6 mm focal spot are suggested.

Videotape Recording Both 1/2" VHS and high resolution VHS-S videotape recorders are used to record fluoroscopic images. The VHS-S system requires high resolution cameras, recorders, tape and monitors but

offers a significant increase in resolution that is highly desirable in fluoroscopic systems. All systems utilize tape cassettes and operate the same as home video systems. Magnetic recording and playback heads produce and read a pattern of magnetic particles on the tape, producing a pulsed video signal. In most medical applications only the video track on the tape is used. The audio and synchronization tracks are left empty.

Static Spot Filming Systems

Spot film systems, although part of the fluoroscopic imaging chain, must be considered separately because they are limited to static images. They are necessary when a permanent record of the fluoroscopic examination is desired to document findings. They are therefore used with nearly every fluoro examination.

Spot filming permits a permanent static record to be made when information important to diagnosis (either positive or negative) is observed fluoroscopically. Spot filming remains extremely popular due to the ease with which it can be done, its low cost and the format (transilluminated hard copy films that are easily stored and viewed with other static images).

It is possible to use spot filming equipment to rapidly record a series of static images in a manner that functions as a dynamic record. Angiographic procedures that use serial static exposures can use spot filming when the image resolution is satisfactory.

Spot filming may be accomplished by several methods. Cassettes (radiographic film and intensifying screens in cassettes), 105 mm chip film and 70 mm roll film are the most common formats. Each has its merits.

Cassettes Cassette spot filming uses standard radiographic cassettes equipped with a pair of intensifying screens. Standard sizes are 9" × 9" (24 cm × 24 cm) although some units will accept 8" × 10" (18 cm × 24 cm) cassettes.

The cassette, stored in a lead lined compartment in the fluoroscopic carriage, can be moved into the primary beam field via controls located on the fluoro carriage. The x-ray tube current is simultaneously boosted to radiographic levels (100–1,200 mA). The carriage controls permit selection of the area of the cassette to be exposed, automatically collimate the tube and spot film mask shutters to the appropriate size, and position the cassette properly. Common selections are a full frame exposure, known as 1-on-1, two half frame exposures, 2-on-1 vertical and 2-on-1 horizontal, and four exposures, 4-on-1. The radiographer is usually responsible for replacing exposed cassettes when a radiologist is spot filming with them. In these circumstances the radiographer must observe the exposure selections to anticipate when a new cassette will be required. After the exposure is initiated an AEC terminates it and the cassette is automatically returned to the storage compartment. The process is slow because of the time required to move the cassette into place for exposure.

Cassette spot filming causes the highest dose to the patient. Cassettes may require up to 300 μR per exposure at the entrance to the cassette. This may translate into a 30 mR entrance skin per exposure. It has been estimated that each spot film may be equal to more than a minute of fluoroscopic time. As with any radiographic examination, images should not be produced unless they will contribute significantly to the management of the patient. There is a definite tendency in the United States to overdocument negative findings because of malpractice litigation experiences.

105 mm Chip Film

Chip spot filming uses 105 mm × 105 mm cut film. The process is relatively fast, up to 12 frames per second, as the only movement necessary prior to exposure is the beam splitting of the mirror.

70 mm Roll Film

Roll spot filming uses a roll of film 70 mm wide. As with 105 mm chip film, the process is fast, up to 12 frames per second, as the only movement necessary prior to exposure is the beam splitting of the mirror.

Digital Fluoroscopy

Digital fluoroscopy units process the image coming from the charge coupled device (CCD) by sending an analog signal through an analog-to-digital converter (ADC) microchip. See Chapter 42 (Digital Image Processing) for a complete discussion of this process.

Once the fluoroscopic image has been converted to a digital signal it can be manipulated as desired and transferred repeatedly without loss of quality. Display on a monitor permits changes in density (digital window level), contrast (digital window width), magnification,

filtration enhancements, and other techniques to be applied to the image.

Digitization also permits storage on computer disk, transfer via electronic means such as teleradiology systems or the Internet, and hard copy printing via laser dry image processors.

Mobile Fluoroscopic Equipment

Mobile C-arm fluoroscopic units are extremely popular for surgical procedures (Figure 38–7). When coupled to a videodisc unit, both static and dynamic imaging can be instantly available. The units operate exactly as do stationary fluoroscopic units, although controls may have different labeling. All the cautions and adaptations for mobile radiography are applicable to mobile fluoroscopy.

Radiation Protection During Fluoroscopy

The Patient

Fluoroscopic units operate with the minimum radiation output possible for the efficiency of the imaging system. There is no appreciable difference in the patient dose between an optical mirror viewing system and a video system. The entrance skin exposure for the patient is the surface closest to the source. With an under-table unit the ESE is measured from the surface next to the table top. With an over-table unit it is measured from the surface toward the fluoro carriage. The tabletop exposure rate should not exceed 10 R/min and for most units should range from 1–3 R/min. The minimum source-to-skin distance is 12″ (30 cm) for mobile fluoroscopic equipment and 15″ (38 cm) for stationary equipment.

In the United States, federal law requires an audible five-minute timer. Although it can be reset as many times as necessary to complete a procedure, it is intended to serve as a reminder to the radiologist of how much total exposure time is being used. Fluoroscopy is interrupted when the five minutes have elapsed and the radiographer must reset the timer to continue the procedure.

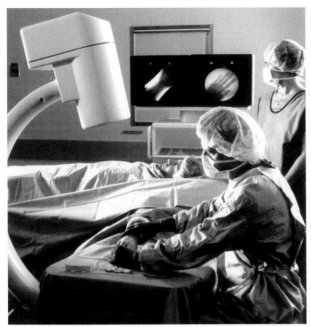

FIGURE 38-7. A mobile C-arm fluoroscopic unit. *(Courtesy of GE Medical Systems)*

Magnification image intensifiers cause increased patient dose because the automatic brightness control (ABC) will increase the tube output to compensate for the loss of electrons within the image intensification tube during magnification. The x-ray tube should have the collimation shutters closed to the viewing image size when in the magnification mode. When magnifying, the output screen of the image intensification tube does not receive the entire image from the input screen so it is possible to irradiate tissue that cannot be viewed. Although these image intensifiers may have interlocks that automatically collimate when magnifying, attention to this detail decreases patient dose.

Patient dose for cinefluorography is significant. The minimum exposure required at the entrance to the image intensification tube is 20 μR per frame. This often translates into an entrance skin exposure of 2,000 μR/frame (2 mR/frame). At 60 frames per second this results in 2 mR/frame × 60 frames/sec = 7,200 mR/min = 7.2 R/min.

Spot film recorders vary in dose to the patient. Cassettes often require 30 mR per exposure while 105 mm or 70 mm film averages about 10 mR per exposure.

Of course, these rates may vary with the sensitivity of the image intensification system and the exact mechanics of and film used in the recording system.

The Radiographer and Radiologist

A lead apron of at least 0.25 mm Pb/eq must be worn by all persons (other than the patient) who are present in the fluoroscopic room during exposure. An apron designed to cover the front and sides of the body is usually sufficient, although a wrap-around apron for both front and back should be considered if the radiographer is required to turn his/her back to the patient and x-ray tube during the procedure. Radiographers assisting during fluoroscopy must develop the ability to back and sidle around the room during exposures, always keeping the front of the body with its lead apron facing the patient and tube. If the hands must be placed within the primary beam, lead gloves of at least 0.25 mm Pb/eq must be worn.

The primary source of exposure to the radiographer and radiologist is the patient. It is worth noting that the highest energy scatter occurs at a 90° angle to the incident beam and that the patient on an x-ray table is usually at the same level (90° from a primary photon angle of incidence) as the gonads of the radiographer. It is also worth remembering that according to the inverse square law, a single step back from the patient will decrease the dose exponentially (Figure 38–8). The slot immediately under the tabletop where the Bucky tray is positioned for diagnostic radiography is also at the gonadal level. Fluoroscopic units must have a lead shield to cover this slot. However, it must be brought into position by moving the Bucky tray to the head or foot of the table prior to beginning fluoro. Strips of lead rubber, forming a drape, are positioned between the fluoroscopist and patient to absorb the majority of the patient scatter. The radiographer has one advantage during fluoroscopy in that he/she may position himself/herself behind the radiologist. This not only adds an additional lead apron, but the entire body of the fluoroscopist is there to protect the radiographer.

Fluoroscopy units with cassette spot filming devices are available in front and rear loading models. The front loading models require the fluoroscopist to eject the cassette and lift the arm to permit the radiographer to remove the exposed cassette and insert an unexposed

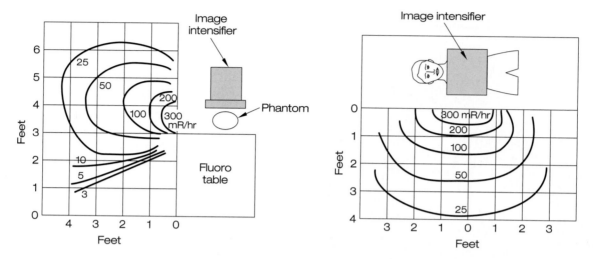

FIGURE 38-8. An isodose curve for a typical fluoroscopic unit. The shape of the curve illustrates areas of lesser dose during fluoroscopic procedures. *(Adapted with permission from Wold, G. J., Scheele, R. V., and Agarwal, S. K. [April 1971] Evaluation of Physician Exposure During Cardiac Catheterization, Radiology, Vol. 99, pp. 188-190)*

replacement. During this procedure it is difficult to operate the fluoroscopic unit, but if it is operated, the radiographer is protected from scatter by a lead drape, the fluoroscopist, and the fluoroscopist's lead apron as well as his/her own lead apron. Rear loading models require the radiographer to lift the exposed cassette from the rear of the carriage. This usually requires stepping onto a platform at the rear of the fluoroscopy table and places the radiographer within inches of the patient (the source of scatter radiation). Fluoroscopy units should not be operated during replacement of spot film cassettes from rear loading units.

Others

The radiographer has a duty to require that anyone present in the fluoroscopy room during an examination wear a lead apron. All persons, regardless of rank or authority, should be informed of this requirement. Fluoroscopy should not be initiated until everyone complies.

Summary

Fluoroscopy (fluoro) is a dynamic radiographic examination that involves active diagnosis during the exami-

nation. For this reason fluoroscopy is primarily the domain of the radiologist. The radiographer's role becomes that of an assistant during an examination. Fluoroscopy is currently used for studies that require observation of dynamic physiological functions, e.g., the flow of barium through the gastrointestinal tract, swallowing, the injection of a contrast medium into the heart, etc.

The fluoroscopic imaging chain consists of a specialized x-ray tube with an image receptor, called the fluoroscopic screen, that can be viewed during an x-ray exposure. The fluoroscopic x-ray tube and image receptor are mounted on a C-arm to maintain their alignment at all times. Fluoroscopic x-ray tubes are very similar to diagnostic tubes except that they are designed to operate for longer periods of time at much lower mA. Where a typical diagnostic tube operates at 50–1,200 mA, the fluoroscopic mA range is 0.5–5.0 mA. An image intensification tube is designed to electronically amplify the brightness of an image. Modern image intensifiers are capable of increasing image brightness 500–8,000 times.

During fluoroscopy, the primary x-ray beam exits the patient and strikes the input screen of the image intensifier tube, which is a vacuum tube with a cathode and an anode. The fluorescent screen is built into the image intensifier as its input screen. The fluorescent screen absorbs the x-ray photons and emits light photons, which immediately encounter the photocathode (the cathode of the tube) that is in contact with the input screen to prevent divergence of the light beam. The photocathode absorbs the light photons and emits electrons. The electrons are then accelerated from the cathode toward the anode and the output screen by the potential difference that exists between the cathode and anode. At the same time, the electron beam is focused onto the output screen, which is much smaller than the input screen. Electrostatic lenses are used to accelerate and focus the electrons. The primary brightness gain occurs from the acceleration and focusing of the electron beam. Brightness gain is a measurement of the increase in image intensity and is determined by minification gain and flux gain. The acceleration of the electron beam increases its energy and its ability to emit light at the output screen. The focusing of the electron beam intensifies the image into a smaller area. The output screen absorbs the electrons and emits light photons, which are then available for viewing or further electronic processing by a video system. The primary factors that affect the quality of the fluoroscopic image include contrast, resolution, distortion, and quantum mottle.

A number of viewing systems have been developed to deliver the image from the output screen to the viewer. These include optical mirror, video, cine and spot film systems. Some of these systems permit dynamic real-time viewing while others are for static images. The viewing time, resolution and processing time vary. During fluoroscopy, it is possible to record either a dynamic or a static image. Dynamic imaging systems include cine film systems and videotape recording. Static spot filming systems include cassettes, 105 mm chip film, 70 mm roll film and videodisc recorders.

Fluoroscopic units operate with the minimum radiation output possible for the efficiency of the imaging system. The entrance skin exposure for the patient is the surface closest to the source. The tabletop dose rate should not exceed 10 R/min and for most units should range from 1–3 R/min.

A lead apron of at least 0.25 mm Pb/eq must be worn by all persons (other than the patient) who are present in the fluoroscopic room during exposure. The primary source of exposure to the radiographer and radiologist is the patient, with the highest energy scatter occurring at a 90° angle to the incident beam. The radiographer has a duty to require that anyone present in the fluoroscopy room during an examination wear a lead apron.

REVIEW QUESTIONS

1. Why is fluoroscopy the domain of the radiologist?

2. What is the typical basic fluoroscopic imaging chain?

3. How does a fluoroscopic x-ray tube differ from a diagnostic x-ray tube?

4. Why is an image intensification system a significant advantage over the conventional screen fluoroscopy?

5. What is the basic function of the fluorescent screen, the photocathode, the electrostatic lenses and the output screen?

6. What is the formula used for determining brightness gain?

7. What is the purpose of the automatic brightness control?

8. What is the primary limitation of resolution of the fluoroscopic image?

9. What are the basic components of the tube used in a video camera?

10. What are the types of dynamic and static filming systems used to record the fluoroscopic image?

11. What radiation protection practices should be adhered to by the radiographer during fluoroscopy?

REFERENCES AND RECOMMENDED READING

Barnes, G. T. & Tishler, J. M. (1981). Fluoroscopic image quality and its implications regarding equipment selection and use. *The Physical Basis of Medical Imaging*. Editors: Coulam, C. M., Erickson, J. J., Rollo, F. D., & James, A. E. New York: Appleton-Century-Crofts.

Beekmans, A. G. (1982). Image quality aspects of x-ray image intensifiers. *Medicamundi. 27*, 25.

Birken, H. & Bejczy, C. I. (1978). A new generation of x-ray image intensifiers. *Medicamundi. 18*(3), 120.

Brink, G. S. (1973). Fundamentals of image intensification: Design and application. *Radiologic Technology. 44*(5), 317.

Bushberg, J. T., Seibert, J. A., Leidholdt, E. M., & Boone, J. M. (1994). *The essential physics of medical imaging*. Baltimore: Williams & Wilkins.

Bushong, S. C. (1997). *Radiologic science for technologists: Physics, biology, and protection* (6th ed.). St. Louis: C. V. Mosby.

Curry, T. S., Dowdey, J. E., & Murry, R. C. (1990). *Christensen's introduction to the physics of diagnostic radiology*. (4th ed.). Philadelphia: Lea and Febiger.

De Voss, D. (1985). *Basic principles of radiographic exposure*. (2nd ed.). Baltimore: Williams & Wilkins.

Fodor, J. & Malott, J. C. (1993). *The art and science of medical radiography*. (7th ed.). St. Louis: C. V. Mosby.

Fuchs, A. W. (1947). Edison and roentgenology. *The American Journal of Roentgenology. 57*(2), 145–156.

Gough, L. (1987). Remote-controlled fluoroscopy in a pediatric hospital. *The Canadian Journal of Medical Radiation Technology. 18*(3), 93.

Gray, J. E., Stears, J. G., Lopez, F., & Wondraw, M. A. (1984). Fluoroscopic imaging: Quantitation of image lag or smearing. *Radiology*. (Feb.), 563.

Gray, J. E., Winkler, N. T., Stears, J. G., & Frank, E. D. (1983). *Quality control in diagnostic imaging: A quality control cookbook*. Baltimore: University Park Press.

Hynes, D. M., Edmonds, E. W., & Baranoski, D. (1981). Reducing fluoroscopic dosage and cause. *Diagnostic Imaging. 3*, 32–37.

Image intensification systems. (1974). *Radiologic Technology. 46*(3), 196.

Morgan, D. (1990). Applying 100 millimetre and digital technology to general radiography. *Radiography Today. 56*(642), 11–13.

Rich, J. E. (1970). *The theory and clinical application of intensified fluoroscopy in the radiology department*. Milwaukee: General Electric Company Medical Systems Division.

Seeram, E. (1985). *X-ray imaging equipment: An introduction*. Springfield: Charles C. Thomas.

Seeram, E. (1978). Some characteristics of the cesium iodide x-ray image intensifier. *The Canadian Journal of Radiography, Radiotherapy, and Nuclear Medicine. 9*(1), 42–43.

Siedband, M. P. (1981). Fluoroscopic imaging. *The Physical Basis of Medical Imaging*. Editors: Coulam, C. M., Erickson, J. J., Rollo, F. D., & James, A. E. New York: Appleton-Century-Crofts.

Skucas, J. & Gorski, J. W. (1976). Comparison of image quality of 105mm film with conventional film. *Radiology. 118*, 433–437.

Stears, J., Gray, J. E., & Frank, E. D. (1989). Radiologic exchange (dose reduction with 105mm spot films). *Radiologic Technology. 60*(6), 515–516.

Thompson, M. A., Hattaway, M. P., Hall, J. D., & Dowd, S. B. (1994). *Principles of imaging science and protection*. Philadelphia: W. B. Saunders.

Tortorici, M. (1992). *Concepts in medical radiographic imaging*. Philadelphia: W. B. Saunders.

Wesenberg, R. L. & Amundson, G. M. (1984). Fluoroscopy in children: Low exposure technology. *Radiology. 153*(1), 243–247.

Wolbarst, A. B. (1993). *Physics of radiology*. Norwalk, CT: Appleton & Lange.

The Case of Do You Know Your Whole Grains?

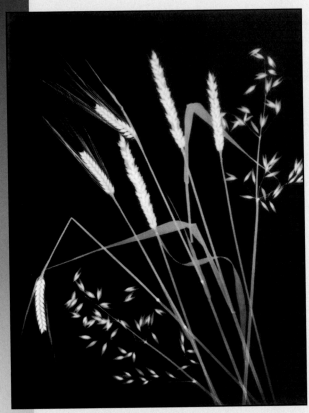

(Reprinted by permission of the International Society of Radiographers and Radiological Technicians from the K. C. Clark Archives, Middlesex Hospital, London, England)

What common grain is this?

Answers to the case studies can be found in Appendix E.

CHAPTER 39

Tomography

> *. . . there exists between (tube and plate), in space, a single fixed plane, in which each point always has a corresponding image point on the plate; hence, only the organs contained in this plane are in focus.*
>
> André-Edmund-Marie-Bocage, from Method of, and apparatus for, radiography on a moving plate.

OBJECTIVES

Upon completion of this chapter, the student should be able to:

▶ Define tomography.

▶ Explain the tomographic principle.

▶ Explain the relationship of tomographic amplitude to exposure amplitude.

▶ Describe the effects of tomographic amplitude, distance from the fulcrum, distance from the image receptor and the orientation of tube motion on image blur.

▶ Explain the causes of tomographic phantom images.

▶ Explain the function of the fulcrum.

▶ Describe the dimensions of the focal plane.

▶ Correlate changes in exposure amplitude with their effect on section thickness.

▶ Describe a section interval.

▶ Evaluate linear tomographic quality parameters.

▶ Compare various types of linear, circular and complex tomographic motions.

▶ Establish a tomographic procedure, including section thickness and interval, for a clinical problem.

▶ Describe the specialized tomographic techniques.

▶ Select appropriate exposure factors for a tomographic examination after a satisfactory preliminary scout radiograph has been produced.

*T*omography is a radiographic technique that employs motion to show anatomical structures lying in a plane of tissue while blurring or eliminating the detail in images of structures above and below the plane of interest. It primarily demonstrates coronal sections, although sagittal sections of most body parts and transverse sections of the head may be accomplished through positioning.

First developed in 1921, and long the premier investigative procedure for removing superimposing structures, tomography is now used in only a few limited areas. Since the advent of modern computerized sectional imaging techniques (i.e., computed tomography and magnetic resonance imaging) its use has declined rapidly, although it is still considered of value for routine examination of the kidneys during intravenous pyelography. Tomography has also been found useful when computerized modalities are too costly or unavailable.

Although many have claimed credit for the development of tomography, only nine investigators actually had a part in its development, beginning with André Edmund Bocage (French dermatologist 1892–1953) and including the American radiographer Jean Kieffer. Tomography has been called planigraphy, stratigraphy and laminography over the years, and it is still sometimes called body section radiography.

The Tomographic Principle

The principle of tomography is based on synchronous movement of two of the three elements in a tomographic system: the x-ray tube, the object and the image receptor. Most tomographic units synchronize the movements of the x-ray tube and the image receptor in opposite directions around a stationary fulcrum (pivot point) during the exposure. Their alignment is maintained by a rigid attachment, such as a metal rod. The object to be examined is placed at the fulcrum (Figure 39–1). The result is a tomographic image in which the area located at the fulcrum is sharp because it has not moved in its relationship to the tube and the image receptor during the exposure (Figure 39–2). However, structures above and below, which would have been superimposed, are now blurred due to the motion. The reduced density

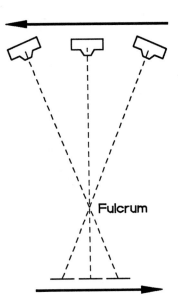

FIGURE 39-1. The tomographic principle—the interrelationships. The x-ray tube and image receptor are attached so they move in opposite directions while maintaining their alignment. The fulcrum, as the point around which the movement occurs, remains the single unmoving point. Objects placed at the fulcrum are imaged sharply, while all other objects are blurred.

permits visualization of the sharp details of the area of interest through their blurred images.

Although tomography is a dynamic process, it can be understood by careful consideration of the tomographic concept. Oblique projections or tube angle projections are used to project objects away from one another. Tomography builds on this geometry in a dynamic manner (Figure 39–3). As the tube proceeds through the tomographic motion, the projected images are first at a severe tube angle, which gradually decreases to a perpendicular beam, which then increases to a severe tube angle in the opposite direction. The resulting projection of superimposed objects first to one side, then to the other, causes their projected image to be streaked, or blurred, across the length of the image receptor. The longer the blurring, the less opportunity to create a sharp image. The shorter the blurring, the sharper the image. Therefore, there is a direct relationship between distance from the fulcrum and blurring. The greater the distance from the fulcrum, the greater the blurring and vice versa.

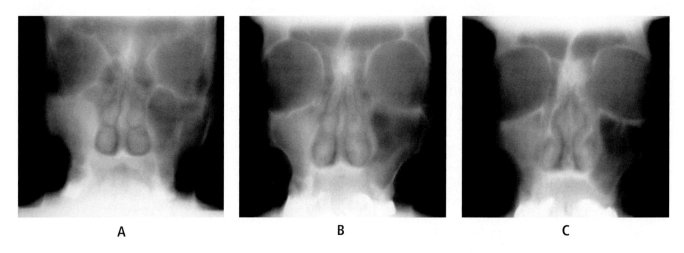

| A | B | C |

FIGURE 39-2. A tomogram of the maxillary sinuses in an AP projection with the fulcrum (A) 19 cm from the table, (B) 20 cm, and (C) 21 cm. The structures that are sharp are located within the fulcrum focal plane. Structures above and below the focal plane are blurred. Note the opacification of the right maxillary sinus and the thickening of the mucosal wall in the inferior left sinus.

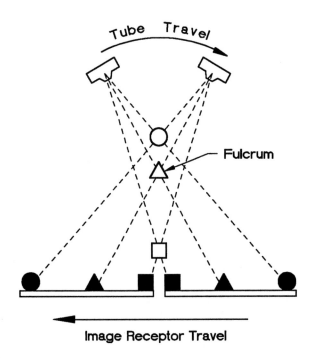

FIGURE 39-3. The tomographic concept. The ball is projected to the right of the triangle as the exposure begins but is blurred completely across the triangle to appear at the left by the end of the exposure. Also note that the box goes through the same blurring, but in the opposite direction.

Those images that lie in the plane of the fulcrum will be projected onto exactly the same location on the image receptor because the image receptor is moving at exactly the proper rate to maintain their location. Objects located above and below the fulcrum will be projected onto varying locations on the image receptor as it moves, thus blurring their images. The further the object is from the fulcrum, the greater the difference between its projected motion and the motion of the image receptor. This causes its image to be projected at various locations. The more its image is blurred, the easier it is to visualize sharp, unblurred structures through the blurring.

Because the creation of a section of sharply defined tissue is similar to cutting slices out of the body for examination, terms such as "cuts" and "slices" have evolved. Because these phrases can easily cause immense distress when overheard by patients, the radiographer should strive to adhere to the term "section," avoiding "cut" and "slice."

Tomographic Quality

Tomographic Amplitude

The tomographic amplitude, arc or angle is the total distance the tube travels (Figure 39–4). The x-ray tube

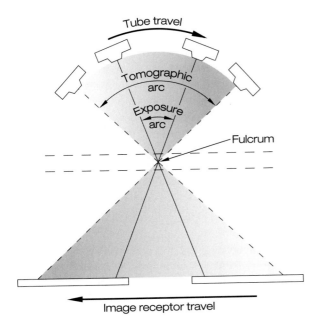

FIGURE 39-4. Tomographic and exposure amplitude, arc or angle.

does not have to be engaged in an exposure for the entire tomographic angle. However, the tomographic amplitude is always greater than or equal to the exposure amplitude. There is an inverse relationship between the tomographic amplitude and the section thickness, as discussed below.

Exposure Amplitude

The exposure amplitude, arc or angle is the total distance the tube travels during the exposure (Figure 39–4). The x-ray tube is engaged in an exposure for the entire exposure angle. The exposure amplitude is always equal to or less than the tomographic amplitude.

Blur

Blur is the streaking or smearing that results in the loss of nearly all recorded detail of objects outside the focal plane. There is an inverse relationship between blurring and the radiographic density of objects. Increased blurring causes decreased density, thus making an object more transparent. This permits objects within the focal plane to be seen through the blurring. Blur is

affected by the tomographic amplitude, distance from the fulcrum, distance from the image receptor and orientation of tube motion.

Tomographic Amplitude The tomographic amplitude has a direct linear relationship to blur width. As the tomographic amplitude increases, blur increases in direct proportion. For example, doubling the tomographic amplitude will double image blur.

Distance from the Fulcrum The distance from the fulcrum has a direct relationship to blur width. As the distance of an object from the fulcrum increases, blur increases.

Distance from the Image Receptor The distance from the image receptor has a direct relationship to blur width. As the distance of an object from the image receptor increases, blur increases. For example, blurring of superimposed structures around a pulmonary lesion is greater when the affected side is positioned down for lateral decubitus tomograms because this positions the unaffected lung farther from the image receptor.

Orientation of Tube Motion The orientation of tube travel has a direct relationship to blur width. As the orientation of tube travel approaches perpendicularity, blur increases. Figure 39–5 shows the difference between an image of a structure that is perpendicular to a linear tomographic motion and one that is parallel.

Phantoms

Phantoms are sometimes called blur edges or blur margins. They are images that do not correspond to existing structures. They are false images and, as such, are dangerous to the diagnostic process. Phantoms are produced during complex tomographic motions, especially circular, when the tube motion is parallel to the long axis of the structure (Figure 39–6). They are also caused by blur overlap (Figure 39–7) and displacement of blur margins due to the tomographic motion. For example, a dense bony structure may have its blur margin projected into a soft tissue area. Especially in cranial and chest tomography, the decreased blur density may simulate a pathological soft tissue condition. Reduced section thickness and increased exposure amplitude decrease phantom images.

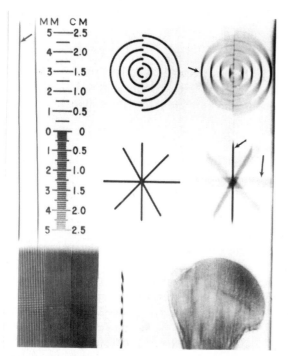

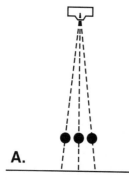

FIGURE 39-5. The effect of the orientation of tube motion on the long axis of the object. The tomographic phantom has a star pattern of wires. When the fulcrum is 1 cm below the wires, blurring occurs. This image was produced with a linear motion from the top to the bottom of the radiograph. Arrows illustrate where the wire perpendicular to the direction of motion is projected wth maximum blurring. The wire parallel to the direction of motion is projected with no lateral blurring. (The linear motion causes blurring only as elongation at the ends of the wire.) The wires at 45° are projected with intermediate amounts of blurring. *(Courtesy of Suellen Chandler, Philips Medical Systems)*

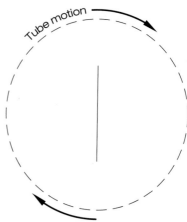

FIGURE 39-6. Phantoms caused by circular tomographic motion. Although the top and bottom of the circle produce motion that is perpendicular to the long axis of the object, the sides produce parallel motion. During the time the parallel motion occurs, the image blurring is decreased, thus producing a sharper and more dense image. This sharper and more dense image is the phantom, blur edge or blur margin.

Fulcrum

The fulcrum is the pivot point around which the motions of the tube and the image receptor are centered. It determines the focal plane and thereby controls the section level. The fulcrum may be fixed so that the patient is moved up and down to change the section level (the Grossman principle). More commonly, the fulcrum is adjustable so that it moves up and down while the patient remains stationary.

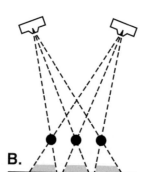
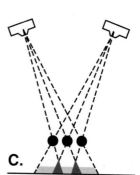

FIGURE 39-7. Tomographic blur overlap phantoms. (A) The sharp image of three wires produced by a static radiograph. (B) The blurred image of three wires produced by a small exposure amplitude. (C) The blur overlap that produces two phantom images from three wires imaged with a large exposure amplitude.

Focal Plane

The focal plane is often referred to as the section, although the terms section level, layer height, object plane and depth of focus have also been used. It is the region within which the image exhibits satisfactory recorded detail and is controlled by the level of the fulcrum. The focal plane is not an exactly defined region. Objects located near the fulcrum are less blurred while objects located further from the fulcrum are more blurred. Consequently, gradually increasing recorded detail eventually reaches a point where it is considered of diagnostic sharpness. This point defines the margins of the focal plane.

Section Thickness

Section thickness is the width of the focal plane and is controlled by the exposure angle (Figure 39–8). Exposure angle is inversely proportional to section thickness. As the exposure angle increases, section thickness decreases. Conversely, as the exposure angle decreases, section thickness increases.

Section thickness occurs in a plane parallel to the image receptor (Figure 39–9). Although there is an increase in magnification due to the increased OID of object C as the x-ray tube moves to the left, there is also a corresponding increase in the SOD and SID. The ratio of SID to SOD, the magnification ratio, remains the same, as do the ratios for objects A and B. Therefore, although magnification has an effect on the detail and sharpness of tomographed objects, tomographic motion does not change the total effect from that seen in a static radiograph of the same area.

Most tomographic images exhibit less contrast than static images of the same regions because of the decreased tissue density that is being imaged with a single section. The decreased difference in subject density also constitutes decreased subject contrast. Additionally, the blurring of structures above and below the fulcrum increases the base density of the image. Increased base

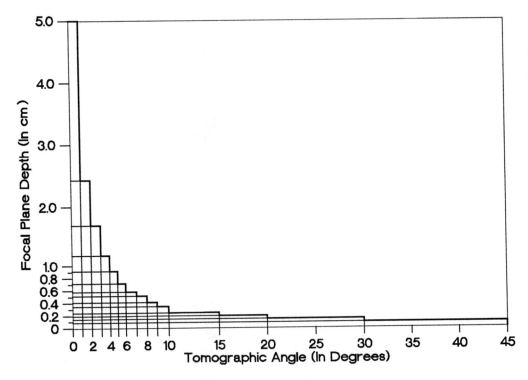

FIGURE 39-8. The effect of exposure angle on section thickness. *(Reprinted with permission from Dowdell, L. C. [1984]. The joy of sectioning, Railfare Enterprises Limited, West Hill, Ontario)*

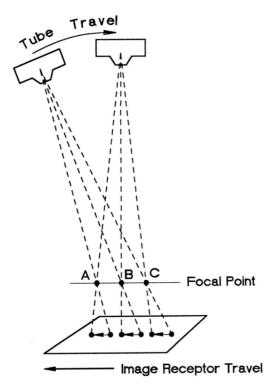

FIGURE 39-9. The effect of tomographic movement on magnification of objects in the focal plane.

density decreases contrast because fewer densities remain within the diagnostically visible range of densities.

Section Interval

The distance between fulcrum levels is the section interval. During tomographic procedures, the section interval should not exceed the section thickness. Tomographing an object with section intervals greater than the section thickness creates gaps of unexamined tissue that may permit misdiagnosis.

A procedure must be planned to establish appropriate section intervals. At least one full section above and below the area of interest is required to prove completion of the sectioning. Careful consideration of section thickness permits the use of section intervals that create a slight overlapping of sections. For example, an exposure amplitude that produces a 0.5 mm section thickness

should be used with fulcrum changes of 0.4 mm to permit a 0.1 mm overlap (0.05 mm at the top and bottom of each section).

Types of Motion

Tomography was first achieved with a linear motion. However, numerous types of complex or pluridirectional tube motions have been developed which provide a total distance of tube travel up to nearly five times that of a linear motion although, to avoid excessive shape distortion, their amplitude does not exceed 48°. In addition, they provide motion significantly different from the shape of the subject, thus increasing perpendicular movement and reducing phantom images. Essentially, these motions add a second dimension to linear tomography (Figure 39–10B–G). Tomographic motion can be visualized by quality assurance pinhole tracings.

Complex motions require equipment that counter-rotates the grid as the tube moves. The image receptor is moved but is not counter-rotated since it must remain aligned to the anatomical structures of the patient. Counter-rotation of the grid eliminates the need for a reciprocating mechanism to blur the grid lines.

Linear

Linear tomography occurs when the movement of the tube and image receptor are along a straight line (Figure 39–10A). Linear motion has a major quality problem because the SID and OID change as the tube moves. Both SID and OID are greater at the extreme left and right positions than at the center position. During the tomographic motion the distances are in constant fluctuation.

Linear tomography also has a significant decrease in image quality because blurring is dependent on the orientation of the structure to the linear motion. Structures that are parallel to the motion are not so much blurred as they are streaked. Figure 39–5 illustrates the blurring of lines perpendicular to linear motion and the streaking (elongating) of parallel lines. Linear streaking causes sharp images from structures as much as several centimeters away from the fulcrum. Elongated linear streaking is not a phantom image; it is the image of structural margins that were not blurred.

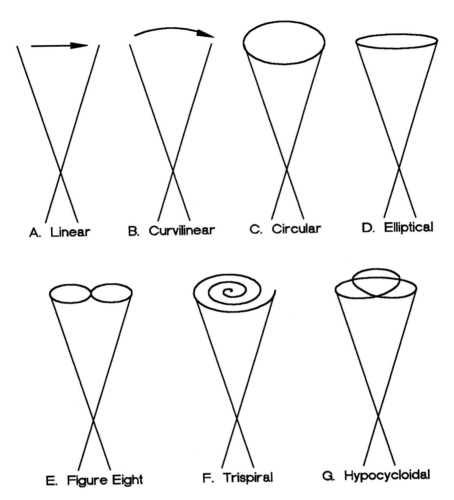

FIGURE 39-10. The tomographic motions.

Linear motion places severe limitations on the total tomographic amplitude. Because the angle of the tube to the object and the image receptor has limits beyond which shape distortion is objectionable, the thinness of the tomographic section is also limited (Figure 39–11). Total tomographic arc is limited to 48°. The only method of decreasing section thickness is to develop complex tomographic motions that permit greater amplitude.

Linear tomography remains popular because it is an inexpensive addition to a diagnostic x-ray unit. It requires a rod to attach the x-ray tube and the Bucky tray, an adjustable fulcrum through which the rod may pivot, and a motor to drive the x-ray tube stand. All other tomographic motions require specialized units designed to provide the desired motion through complicated tracks, gears, pivots, etc.

Because the motion of the tomographic unit creates the tomographic sectional image, it is critical to maximize the motion. This is accomplished by aligning the long axis of the part of interest to the direction of the tube motion. For example, tomograms of the sternum should be done with the long axis of the patient's body perpendicular to the length of the x-ray table. Inability to accomplish this type of positioning for numerous areas of the body is a disadvantage of linear tomography.

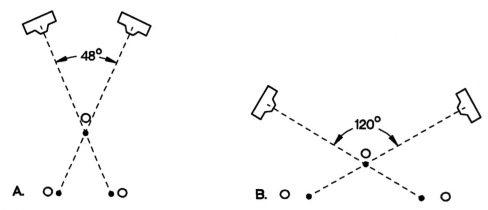

FIGURE 39-11. Limitations to total linear tube amplitude due to excessive distortion produced at the extreme edges of large angles such as 120°.

Curvilinear

Curvilinear tomography improves on the linear motion by maintaining SID and OID and reducing magnification differences (see Figure 39–10B). It is still of limited value due to the single, linear direction of the motion.

Circular

Circular tomographic motions (see Figure 39–10C), although a vast improvement over linear motions, do not eliminate edge phantoms (see Figure 39–6). They require specialized equipment and exposure times of 3–6 seconds. Consequently, they are seldom used because most units capable of circular motions are also capable of more complex motions, as discussed below.

Elliptical

Elliptical tomographic motions (see Figure 39–10D) eliminate some of the edge phantoms of circular motions, especially when the long axis of the ellipse is perpendicular to the long axis of the object of interest. As with circular motions, they are seldom used because most units capable of elliptical motions are also capable of more complex motions.

Figure Eight

Some tomographic units provide a motion that forms a figure eight (see Figure 39–10E) while others are more random in nature. These motions eliminate most phantom images, although their total tomographic amplitude is not as great as that of trispiral or hypocycloidal motions.

Trispiral

The trispiral motion (see Figure 39–10F) provides maximum tomographic amplitude, thus producing the thinnest possible section.

Hypocycloidal

The hypocycloidal motion (see Figure 39–10G) also provides maximum tomographic amplitude, thus producing the thinnest possible section.

Tomographic Procedures

Tomography is most often used to localize objects that are difficult to see due to superimposed structures. Because the section thickness determines how much tissue is visualized for each section, each examination must be evaluated to determine an appropriate series of tomographic sections. Routine procedures often begin with a preliminary scout exposure for diagnostic comparisons. This image is also useful in establishing exact structural locations and verifying exposure factors.

Exposure Factors

Choosing proper technique exposure factors for tomography requires special attention to compensate for the time needed for the tomographic amplitude.

Time It is critical that the time be set first. The exposure time must match the length of time required for the x-ray tube to complete the tomographic amplitude. An exposure time that is less than the amplitude will not permit full blurring and will project erratic phantoms. An exposure time that is greater than the amplitude will increase the density of the image at the final tube position, thus increasing the recorded detail while decreasing the blurring of structures outside the focal plane. Complex tomographic motions often require 3 or 6 second exposures.

Milliamperage Dedicated tomography unit generators provide special stations below 100 mA to permit appropriate mAs to be set with the long times required for complex tomographic motions. Stations of 10, 15, 20, 25, 30, 40 and 50 mA are extremely helpful in these situations. Approximately 30 percent more mAs is required for a wide angle tomogram due to the loss of scatter density caused by the air gap at the extremes of the tomographic motion. Zonographic tomograms usually require the same mAs as static radiographs.

Kilovoltage All fine density adjustments must be accomplished by variations of kVp because of the limitations imposed by the fixed time settings. The 15 percent rule is a critical tool in determining these adjustments. It is also useful to recall that a 5 percent change in kVp is required to produce a visible density difference in most images. Because these adjustments tend to increase kVp to the point where contrast may become a problem, every possible device that will eliminate scatter radiation should be employed. These include maximum collimation (to the exact area of interest), lead masks at the tabletop, high ratio grids and compression bands.

Specialized Techniques

Narrow Angle Tomography or Zonography

Zonography or narrow angle tomography (exposure amplitudes of less than 10°) is used when localization is necessary because the exact location of a structure is unknown or when a survey is being performed, for example, on a lesion of the lung or on the kidneys. A small exposure amplitude is used to produce a thick section (Figure 39–12A). Zonography has reasonable contrast but poor recorded detail because of the thick section.

Wide Angle Tomography

Wide angle tomography is used when a lesion has been localized or a specific structure has been determined to require a more detailed examination. A series of thinner sections may then be used (see Figure 39–12B). Wide angle tomography has inherently low contrast but a reasonable amount of recorded detail because of the thin section. It is useful in the examination of small bone structures, such as the inner ear, although computed tomography now has much to offer in this area of diagnosis.

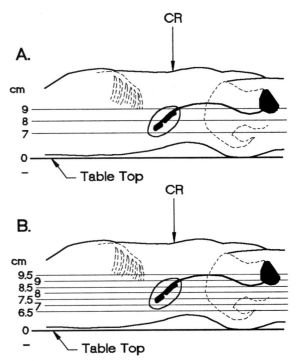

FIGURE 39-12. The effect of exposure amplitude on section thickness. (A) A small exposure amplitude to produce a thick section for localization or as a survey examination. (B) A larger exposure amplitude to produce thin sections for detailed examination. *(Reprinted with permission from Littleton, J. T. [1976]. Tomography: Physical principles and clinical applications, Section 17: Golden's Diagnostic Radiology Series. Baltimore, MD: The Williams & Williams Co.)*

Multifilm Tomography   Multifilm tomography uses a series of films placed at regular intervals by spacers or intensifying screens within a book cassette and uses OID in place of fulcrum changes to achieve the tomographic effect. Although a significantly greater exposure is required to provide sufficient photons for the last film, the single exposure is usually less than the total of the exposures necessary to produce the same information in a series of separate images. Its primary advantage is that the entire series for lung tomography is achieved at the same breathing phase.

Panoramic Tomography   Specialized equipment has been developed to permit slit scan radiography of the curved surfaces of the face and head, especially of the mandible (Figure 39–13). The terms pantomography, orthopantomography and panoramic tomography have been used to describe this type of x-ray unit. Slit scan radiography uses only the perpendicular photons of the primary beam by using a lead mask to collimate the beam to a narrow slit. Both the x-ray tube and the film rotate past the slit during the exposure to lay out the structure of interest, much like rolling paint from a roller onto a wall (Figure 39–14).

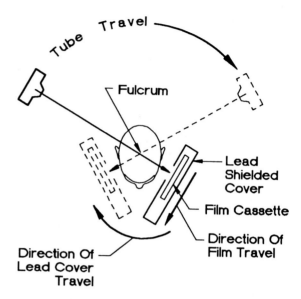

FIGURE 39-14. Panoramic tomographic equipment.

The principle of tomography is based on synchronous movement of two of the three elements in a tomographic system: the x-ray tube, the object and the image receptor. Most tomographic units synchronize the movements of the x-ray tube and the image receptor in opposite directions around a stationary fulcrum during the exposure. Those images that lie in the plane of the fulcrum will be projected onto exactly the same location on the image receptor because the image receptor is moving at exactly the proper rate to maintain their location. Objects located above and below the fulcrum will be projected onto varying locations on the image receptor as it moves, thus blurring their images.

The tomographic amplitude, arc or angle is the total distance the tube travels. The exposure amplitude, arc or angle is the total distance the tube travels during the exposure. The exposure amplitude is always equal to or less than the tomographic amplitude. Blur is the streaking or smearing that results in the loss of nearly all recorded detail of objects outside the focal plane and is affected by the tomographic amplitude, distance from the fulcrum, distance from the image receptor and orientation of tube motion. Blur edges and blur margins are called phantoms.

The focal plane is often referred to as the section, although the terms section level, layer height, object

Summary

Tomography is a radiographic technique employing motion to show structures lying in a plane of tissue while blurring or eliminating the detail in images of structures in other planes. It primarily demonstrates coronal sections, although sagittal sections of most body parts and transverse sections of the head may be accomplished through positioning.

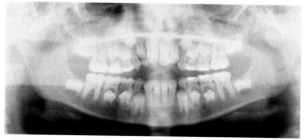

FIGURE 39-13. A panoramic projection of the mandible.

plane and depth of focus have also been used. It is the region within which the image exhibits satisfactory recorded detail and is controlled by the level of the fulcrum. Section thickness is the width of the focal plane and is controlled by the exposure angle. The distance between fulcrum levels is the section interval. During tomographic procedures, the section interval should not exceed the section thickness.

Tomography was first achieved with a linear motion. Complex or pluridirectional tube motions have been developed, which include circular, elliptical, figure eight, trispiral and hypocycloidal.

Choosing proper exposure factors for tomography requires consideration of exposure time, milliamperage and kilovoltage. Specialized tomographic techniques include narrow angle, wide angle, multifilm and panoramic tomography.

REVIEW QUESTIONS

1. Define tomography.
2. How does a basic tomographic system operate?
3. What is the difference between tomographic amplitude and exposure amplitude?
4. What factors affect tomographic blur?
5. What is the function of the fulcrum?
6. How is section thickness controlled?
7. Which of the tomographic motions alters distance during the exposure arc?
8. What are the advantages of complex tomographic motions?
9. Why is it important to establish the exposure time prior to setting the other exposure factors for a tomogram?
10. Differentiate between the uses of narrow-angle and wide-angle tomography.

REFERENCES AND RECOMMENDED READING

Ball, J. & Price, T. (1989). *Chesneys' radiographic imaging.* Oxford: Blackwell Scientific Publishing.

Barnes, G. T. & Moreland, R. F. (1981). A linear tomographic alignment test object. *Radiology.* (Oct), 247.

Bushberg, J. T., Seibert, J. A., Leidholdt, E. M., & Boone, J. M. (1994). *The essential physics of medical imaging.* Baltimore: Williams & Wilkins.

Bushong, S. C. (1997). *Radiologic science for technologists: Physics, biology, and protection.* (6th ed.). St. Louis: C. V. Mosby.

Coulam, C. M., Erickson, J. J., & Gibbs, S. J. (1981). Image and equipment considerations in conventional tomography. *The Physical Basis of Medical Imaging.* Editors: Coulam, C. M., Erickson, J. J., Rollo, F. D., & James, A. E. New York: Appleton-Century-Crofts.

Cullinan, A. & Cullinan, J. (1994). *Producing quality radiographs.* (2nd ed.). Philadelphia: J. B. Lippincott.

Curry, T. S., Dowdey, J. E., & Murry, R. C. (1990). *Christensen's introduction to the physics of diagnostic radiology.* (4th ed.). Philadelphia: Lea and Febiger.

Dowdell, L. C. (1984). *The joy of sectioning.* Toronto: Railfare.

Durzich, M. L. (1978). *Technical aspects of tomography.* Baltimore: Williams & Wilkins.

Forster, E. (1985). *Equipment for diagnostic radiography.* Lancaster: MTP Press.

Littleton, J. T. & Durizch, M. L. (1983). *Sectional imaging methods: A comparison.* Baltimore: University Park Press.

Littleton, J. T. (1976). *Tomography: Physical principles and clinical applications.* Baltimore: Williams & Wilkins.

Lockery, R. M. (1971). Principles of body-section radiography. *Radiologic Technology.* 42(5), 335.

Marlowe, N. A. (1983). The application of blurred undersubtraction in polytomography. *Radiologic Technology.* 54(6), 455.

Milner, S. C. & Case, J. (1984). Tomographic exposure angle: a comparison of two tests. *Radiography.* 50(592), 177.

Moore, C. J., Hopewell, R., Moores, B. M., & Eddleston, B. (1979). Test procedures for conventional tomographic x-ray equipment. *Radiography.* 45(540), 284.

Ramthun, B. (1988). Tomography of the posterior cervical spine fusion: A new concept. *Radiologic Technology. 60*(1), 27–31.

Smith, W. V. J. (1971). A review of tomography and zonography. *Radiography. 37*(433), 5.

Soni, V. P. (1977). A review of tomography. *Canadian Journal of Radiography, Radiotherapy, and Nuclear Medicine. 8*(4), 172–189.

Tomographic exposure angle. (1984). *Radiography. 50*(594), 291.

The Case of the Ghostly plants

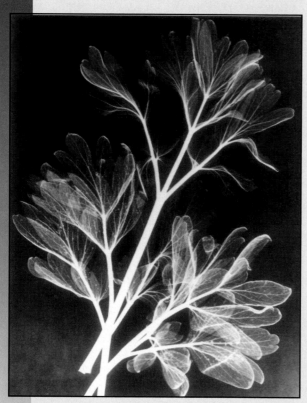

(Reprinted by permission of the International Society of Radiographers and Radiological Technicians from the K. C. Clark Archives, Middlesex Hospital, London, England)

Can you identify this plant?

Answers to the case studies can be found in Appendix E.

CHAPTER 40

Technical Aspects of Mammography

Eugene D. Frank, M.A., R.T.(R), FASRT

Whenever the art of medicine is loved, there is also love for humanity.

Hippocrates

OBJECTIVES

Upon completion of this chapter, the student should be able to:

▶ Explain the development of the regulations and guidelines underlying the performance of mammography.

▶ Describe the unique aspects of the mammography x-ray generator.

▶ Describe the distinctive design and application of the mammography x-ray tube and its associated components.

▶ Specify the accessory components of the mammography machine, detailing their unique design and function in producing quality images.

▶ Assess the critical importance of specialized equipment in producing breast images.

Historical Development

Mammography, in the 1990s, has evolved into one of the most critical and demanding x-ray examinations performed. Every aspect of the examination has to be carried out with the utmost precision. The technical and clinical aspects of the procedure today are guided by strict regulations and specific guidelines. **Mammography is presently the only radiography examination fully regulated by the federal government.** Mammography today requires a team approach. Several professionals, including the radiologist, medical physicist, and most importantly an ARRT registered radiographer, preferably with credentials in mammography.

There is much attention and regulation placed on the technical and clinical aspects of mammography due to the following. The American Cancer Society estimates that 182,000 women will be diagnosed with breast cancer annually and that 46,000 women will die of this disease (about 1,600 men will be diagnosed also). Approximately 1 out of 8 women will develop breast cancer over a lifetime. Until recently, breast cancer was the leading cause of death from cancer among women. Lung cancer has now become the leader. Breast cancer is the leading cause of cancer deaths in females between the ages of 15 and 54. Most notably, the incidence of breast cancer, as a result of participation in screening, has increased 3 to 4 percent, annually, since 1982. The overall age-adjusted incidence rates are higher in white women compared with African-American women. However, for African-American women under age 50, the incidence is nearly three times higher. The size of the population at risk for developing breast cancer is also growing every year.

It is well known that mortality from breast cancer can be reduced significantly through widespread participation in breast screening. As a result, there is great attention placed on breast cancer by the media due to the magnitude of the disease. In addition, the diagnosis of breast cancer is not easily made. **The highest resolution and contrast** attainable has to be brought out in the breast image —more than any other x-ray examination. Remember, from previous chapter readings, that very high resolution and contrast cannot occur in the x-ray image without a corresponding increase in radiation exposure. The risk from ionizing radiation, therefore, is always of concern in mammography.

Although radiation exposures in mammography are relatively safe today as a result of improvements in technology, and certainly due to stringent regulations, one has to recognize that patient exposure is still an important consideration, and the exposure is relatively high in comparison to x-ray examinations of other body parts. In the author's Radiology Department, the entrance skin exposure (ESE) for a 5-cm compressed breast is approximately 1,000 mR, and the ESE for a 21-cm lumbar spine AP projection is 220 mR.

1900s

Mammography has been performed since the early 1900s. In those early years, it was not a technologically well-developed examination. The results were unpredictable, and the technical quality of the images was very poor. Dr. Raul Leborgne of Uruguay was one of the first physicians to perform extended research on mammography, and he published the first textbook on the topic in 1953.

1960

Research into mammography continued at a very low level until about 1960 when Dr. Robert Eagan, then at M. D. Anderson Hospital in Houston, first described the use of a high mA, low kVp exposure technique with direct exposure industrial x-ray film. He introduced the technique of removing the aluminum filter from the port of the x-ray tube so the low-energy x-rays could exit. He also introduced the use of a cylindrical extension cone to reduce scatter radiation. Mammography in the 1960s was performed using a conventional x-ray machine. The x-ray tube at that time had a tungsten anode and a large 2-mm focal spot was common. Typical exposure techniques utilized 28 kVp and 300 mA, with exposure times up to 6 seconds (1,800 mAs). Direct exposure x-ray film was used without a grid. Unfortunately, the exposure to the patient was extremely high. Exposures during this era were between **50 to 100x higher** than exposures applied today. Early mammographers reported exposures greater than **50 R** per projection. If repeat radiographs were performed, erythema of the skin would often occur. Eagan's development of a special technique to optimize the x-ray equipment to image the breast prompted the beginning of widespread research into the use of mammography.

1967

In 1967, CGR (France) introduced the first **dedicated** mammography machine (Figure 40–1). The production model of this machine featured a molybdenum anode, 0.7-mm focal spot, and a beryllium window port. In addition, the unit had a built-in device to compress the breast. As a result of these technical improvements, contrast and resolution in the breast image were greatly enhanced. However, exposure to the patient increased compared to Eagan's technique because of the continued use of direct exposures on industrial x-ray film and a higher mAs was required due to the reduced x-ray output of the molybdenum anode. The radiography community during this time was discovering an uncomfortable tradeoff. High resolution and high contrast breast images could not be produced without introducing high exposure to the patient. It was during this time that the

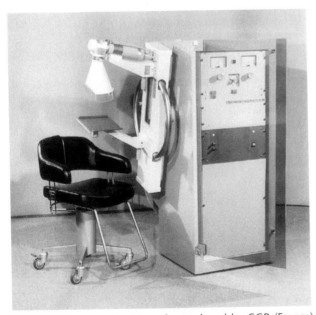

FIGURE 40-1. A 1967 Senograph, produced by CGR (France), became the first commercially available dedicated mammography machine. The unit contained the first molybdenum anode, 0.7-mm focal spot, beryllium window port, and compression device. *(Courtesy of GE Medical Systems)*

benefit-versus-risk debates about mammography practice ensued.

Research continued, and in the early 1970s, Siemens (Germany), Philips (Netherlands), and Picker and General Electric (USA), also introduced dedicated mammography machines. During the early 1970s, nearly every large radiology department in the world was performing mammography.

1971

In 1971, Xerox (USA) introduced a commercially available system of imaging the breast known as xeromammography. The Xerox **dry process** system utilized a conventional overhead x-ray tube with a tungsten anode. However, the filter had to be removed from the port and a low kVp of 40–50, set on the generator. The x-ray exposure was made on an electrically charged imaging plate instead of using screen and film. The imaging plate was then placed in a special development unit and the breast image came out on heavy paper in shades of blue. No film processors or viewboxes were needed. Although a dedicated x-ray machine did not have to be purchased, a special processing machine was needed. Xeromammography was extensively used until the mid-1980s because it produced high contrast images and high resolution (Figure 40–2). Radiation exposures to the patient were lower than Eagan's technique. However, the exposure, which ranged from 2–4 R per projection, was still relatively high. Continued research led to significant improvements in screen/film mammography and lower exposures. Major changes in the design and use of the dedicated mammography machine prompted a major decline in the use of xeromammography for breast imaging by the late 1980s.

1972

In 1972, during the intensive growth and research period in mammography, Du Pont (USA) introduced the first dedicated screen/film system for mammography, **Lo Dose I**. The system utilized a single emulsion film and a single emulsion calcium tungstate screen that was placed in a light-safe polyethylene bag and vacuum sealed. Utilizing a screen for the first time in mammography prompted a major reduction in exposure time and a corresponding reduction in radiation exposure to the

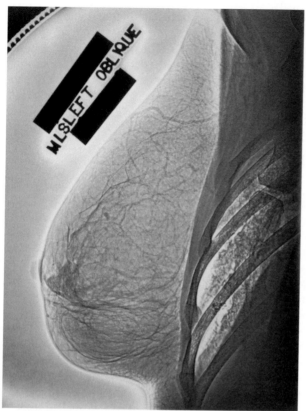

FIGURE 40-2. A 1978 xeroradiographic breast image. Xeromammography produced high contrast and high resolution at doses lower than direct x-ray film exposure. Images were obtained with conventional radiographic equipment, tungsten target, aluminum filter, and 45 kVp.

patient of nearly **20×**. Use of a screen increased the very low inherent subject contrast of the breast in the image. Unfortunately, there was also a corresponding reduction in resolution when compared to direct x-ray exposure and xeromammography. However, the combined effects of a dramatic increase in contrast, reduced motion unsharpness, and corresponding exposure reduction was so significant that screen/film mammography gradually became commonplace. During the 1970s, radiologists debated whether to use the Xerox process or screen/film imaging, and many departments chose to use both.

1975

In 1975, a significant event occurred when Kodak (USA) introduced its specially designed for mammogra-

phy **Min-R** screen, film, and cassette system. The Min-R single emulsion screen, which used the new green emitting rare-earth phosphor, gadolinium oxysulfide, was paired with an orthochromatic (green and blue sensitive) single-emulsion film also called Min-R. The increased screen speed prompted an exposure reduction and there was very negligible loss of resolution. The screen was mounted in a specially designed low-absorption cassette and the screen and film placed so they were as close to the breast as possible (Figure 40–3). Using the cassette saved darkroom time and problems associated with the polyethylene bags. Also during this time, Du Pont introduced an increased speed version of their screen/film — **Lo Dose II**.

1978

The most recent and technologically significant event in mammography occurred in 1978 when Philips (Netherlands) introduced a new generation of dedicated mammography machines (Figure 40–4). This new machine contained the first reciprocating grid. It was also equipped with a foot-pedal; power-driven, breast compression device; aluminum and molybdenum filter selection; automatic exposure control (AEC); a microfocus focal spot; magnification capability; and a high-output generator. Although the introduction of the grid

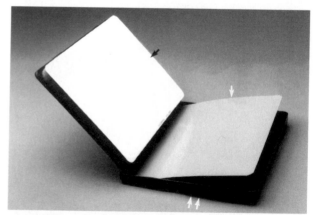

FIGURE 40-3. A 1975 Kodak mammography cassette, the first cassette developed especially for mammography. It contained a Min-R rare-earth phosphor single emulsion screen (black arrow) and green sensitive Min-R single emulsion (white arrow) film. Design of the cassette allowed the screen and film to be placed close to the breast. Top of cassette is indicated by double arrows.

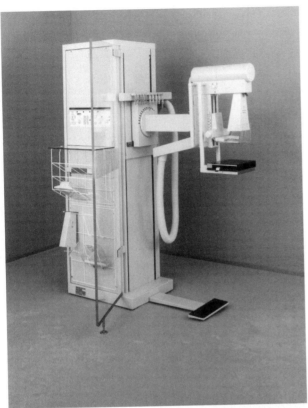

FIGURE 40-4. A 1978 Philips (Netherlands) dedicated mammography machine containing the first reciprocating grid. Introduction of this generation of mammography machines ushered in the modern era of utilizing dedicated machines for mammography. *(Courtesy Philips Medical Systems)*

increased the radiation exposure by a factor of **2 to 3×**, the high contrast image that resulted from the reduction in scattered x-rays, in particular for large and dense breasts, was a dramatic improvement in image quality. Fortunately, at this very same time, Kodak introduced an increased speed version of its Min-R film, Ortho-M, which reduced the radiation exposure by 50 percent, entirely offsetting the increase in exposure from the use of the grid. The modern era of mammography had begun.

1985-1990

In 1985, a nationwide evaluation of x-ray trends (NEXT) study discovered a wide variation in mammographic image quality and in radiation exposures to the patient. Independent studies done later supported the NEXT data and found similar and additional unacceptable variations in image quality. Citations found in the studies included poor processor performance, inexperienced operators of the equipment, improper physician interpretation, poor exposure techniques, and a general inability to perform the examination in a consistent manner.

Concern about the quality of mammography led to the development of the American College of Radiology (ACR) accreditation program in 1987. This voluntary program required mammography sites to meet quality standards to ensure that optimally exposed breast images were being produced at low radiation exposures to the patient. Components of the ACR program included an assessment of both mammographic phantom and actual clinical images for optimal resolution and contrast, measurement of the average glandular dose to the breast, and processor performance. In 1990, additional standards were set forth, which included specific aspects of the equipment and accessory devices, personnel, and the documentation of an effective quality control program. By June 1994, 66 percent of the mammography machines in the United States had passed the ACR voluntary accreditation. Of those that failed, the three most common reasons for failure in descending order were: poor clinical images, failure of the phantom image to demonstrate appropriate contrast and resolution, and poor processor performance.

1991

In 1991, the American Registry of Radiologic Technologists (ARRT) implemented its first **advanced-level** examination specifically for mammography. The examination was designed to ensure that the radiographers who perform mammography have appropriate comprehension of exact positioning techniques, have knowledge of the broad spectrum of mammography projections, understand technical factor selection, and know other specific technical, clinical, and affective aspects related to the performance of the examination. Radiographers who pass the advanced-level mammography examination are formally recognized to perform mammography and use the initial (M) after their radiography credential RT(R).

1992-1994

In 1992, as a result of the American Cancer Society's high visibility public relations campaign that all women over 40 undergo screening mammography, and also because of federal legislation that provided reimbursement for screening mammography in women eligible for medicare, the federal government enacted the Mammography Quality Standards Act (MQSA). The act was written because of lobbying from the ACR due to the great concern about the poor quality mammography being performed. The act went into effect on October 1, 1994, and requires all sites (except VA facilities) that provide mammography service to meet quality standards and become certified for operation by the secretary of the Department of Health and Human Services (DHHS). Enactment of the MQSA marks the first time the use of an x-ray machine and a specific x-ray examination are regulated by the federal government.

1999

On April 28, 1999 the Final Rule of the MQSA went into effect after several years of public comments. MQSA is now officially known as Public Law 105-248. Today, dedicated mammography machines are produced by a variety of manufacturers. These machines are mechanically and electronically designed to meet the stringent radiographic and positioning requirements of breast imaging, and they are used with specially designed screens, film, and cassettes. There are no xeromammography systems in use today. Mammography equipment is presently capable of producing extremely high-contrast images with very high resolution, and the radiation exposures to the patient are reasonably low. However, researchers continue to seek higher contrast and resolution for breast images and methods for lowering the exposure.

This chapter will discuss the current technical aspects of screen/film mammography. The reader should note that every component in the mammography system is modified from conventional radiology. Each component is designed specifically to maximize contrast and resolution while at the same time engineered to keep the radiation exposure to the patient at minimal levels. Table 40–1 illustrates the primary technical differences between mammography and conventional x-ray machines. The

TABLE 40–1. Technical Differences Between Mammography and Conventional Radiography

	Mammography	Conventional
Generator *	1φ high frequency	1φ, 3φ, Capacitor discharge, Falling load
Voltage frequency *	> 10,000 Hz	60 Hz
Voltage ripple	< 4%	4-100%
kVp †	25–28	50–130
mA †	20–160	100–1000
Exposure time (s) †	0.4–4.0	0.01–2.0
Power rating	3–10 kW	50–200 kW
AEC	1 detector	3 detectors
Film density (OD) ††	> 1.30	1.10
Backup timer (mAs)	600 grid, 300 non-grid	600
Focal spot size (mm)	0.1 or 0.3	0.6 or 1.2
SID (cm)	60-65	102–122
X-ray beam utilized	Anode side only	Anode & cathode side equally
Effective target angle ‡	22°–24°	7°–17°
Reference target angle **	7.5°–12°	7°–17°
Anode	Molybdenum or Rhodium	Tungsten
Tube port	Beryllium	Glass
Filter	Molybdenum or Rhodium	Aluminum
HVL (mm AL)	0.3 (30 kVp)	2.3 (80 kVp)
Grid	4:1 or 5:1	6:1–16:1
Screen-film speeds ‡‡	100–320	100–1,200
Resolution (lp/mm)	12–20	5–10

*   Some high frequency generators are being introduced in conventional radiology.

†   Range used in clinical practice.

††   Mammography density measured on the ACR Plexiglas™ phantom.

Conventional density measured on 21-cm Plexiglas™ phantom.

‡   Measured from the vertical central ray.

**   Measured from the reference axis/center of film.

‡‡   Relative speeds of mammography screens are slower than conventional screens with same number.

light-weight (some weigh only 500 lbs.) entirely self-contained mammography unit, which can easily be pushed around a room and simply plugged in, is a relatively sophisticated x-ray machine. Its sole design and purpose is to image the human breast.

Generator Characteristics

Manufacturers of dedicated mammography machines use the new **high-frequency** generators, (Chapter 5) which were introduced by Siemens (Germany) in 1987. There are several reasons for using high-frequency generators in mammography. These generators virtually eliminate voltage regulation problems and allow very precise control of kVp, mA, and exposure time — important considerations in breast imaging. The linearity and reproducibility of the x-ray exposures are excellent. High-frequency x-ray output waveform ripple is much lower than three-phase, 6-pulse ripple at usually less than 4 percent. The high frequency (100 kHz) allows more efficient x-ray production and, therefore, produces a higher effective energy x-ray beam. The result is higher x-ray output for a given kVp and mA setting.

High-frequency generators do not require an auto-transformer, line compensation circuit, or space-charge compensation circuit. This greatly reduces equipment bulk, cost, and space requirements. The high-frequency generator system is uniquely housed within the single-standing mammography unit (Figure 40–5). These new generators operate on single-phase incoming line power, which simplifies installation and greatly reduces cost. High-frequency generators can also be designed to operate from batteries for use in mobile mammography vans. Several manufacturers have designed the high-frequency generator and x-ray tube within the same housing.

kVp

A significant difference between mammography and conventional x-ray machines is the low kVp utilized. The kVp selections on the generator will range from 22 to 40 kVp. The kVp commonly used in clinical practice varies between **25 and 28** kVp. The advantage of using low kVp is its ability to produce a very low-energy (soft) x-ray beam that produces high radiographic contrast. High

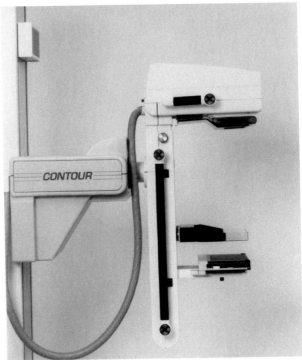

FIGURE 40-5. A 1995 Bennett (USA) current generation mammography machine containing a high-frequency generator, uniquely housed within the standing unit. Operates on single-phase incoming line power. *(Courtesy Bennett Technologies)*

contrast is desirable in breast images because the radiologist must be able to delineate clearly the normal and diseased structures of the breast tissue. Breast tissue is considered **soft tissue** and it is entirely made up of glands, fibers, and fat, which have very low inherent subject contrast (Figure 40–6). The radiologist must have sufficient contrast available in the image to visualize microcalcifications as small as 0.1 to 0.3 mm, and other subtle parenchymal structures. The major disadvantage of using kVp in the twenties range is that there is a high absorption of the low-energy x-rays in the breast, which contributes significantly to patient dose.

Exposure Time, mA, mAs

Mammography generators also utilize low mA settings. Depending on the manufacturer, the mA can vary from about 2 to as high as 180. Generators typically will have a variable mA selection from **20 to 100**, and many

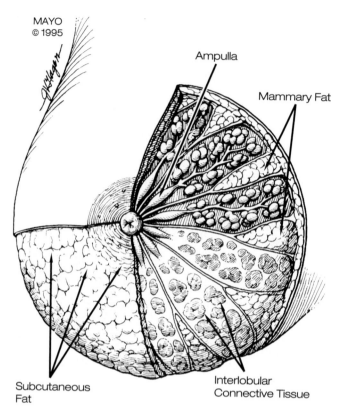

MAYO
© 1995

Ampulla

Mammary Fat

Subcutaneous
Fat

Interlobular
Connective Tissue

FIGURE 40-6. Female breast made up entirely of glands, fibrous tissues, and fat. Creates low inherent subject contrast in the mammographic image. *(Courtesy Mayo Foundation)*

manufacturers design a single mA setting for the small focal spot (e.g., 20 mA) and one for the large focal spot (e.g., 80 mA). Low mA settings are necessary because of the power rating limitations placed on the smaller sized anode and the small focal spot sizes. The power ratings of mammography generators vary between 3 and 10 kilowatts (kW) compared to 50 to 1,200 kW on conventional x-ray generators.

In clinical practice, the specific mA selected is determined based on the principle of keeping exposure times short enough to decrease patient motion. However, the time should not be extremely short, which would cause grid artifacts (textured or structured patterns) to appear in the image. Because the mammography system produces a high-resolution image, grid lines have the potential of being prominently shown and will degrade image quality. Conversely, exposure times that exceed **1 second** will result in **reciprocity law failure**. Typical exposure

times in clinical practice will vary from **0.4 to over 1 second** for standard projections. Exposure times for projections using the magnification technique are much longer, varying from **2 to 4 seconds** due to the low mA used with the 0.l-mm focal spot. When performing magnification studies, mammographers must be very cautious, and explicit instructions must be given to the patient so motion is kept to a minimum during these longer exposures. Unfortunately, the screen response to the long exposure times that occur during magnification studies prompts reciprocity law failure, for which the radiographer must compensate. Additional exposure times from **10 to 30 percent** are required to maintain optimal density at these long exposure times. Fortunately, high-quality mammography machines have sophisticated built-in circuitry that will automatically compensate for reciprocity law failure so that repeat radiographs are kept to a minimum.

Automatic Exposure Control

Automatic Exposure Control (AEC) is an integral component on every dedicated mammography generator. Like the AEC circuitry used on conventional radiography equipment, its design and purpose is to provide consistent film density for the various thickness and density compositions of breast tissues and for the range of kVp used. Because of the high-contrast imaging environment in mammography, there is minimal exposure latitude in terms of film density. Small variations in film density will affect the contrast required to visualize the subtle breast tissue and to diagnose cancer.

Automatic control of exposure techniques is crucial in breast imaging because of the wide range of breast thicknesses and density compositions. A 4-cm compressed breast on a number of similarly aged women can cause a range of x-ray exposure times from **0.05 ms to over 1 second**! It is virtually impossible for the radiographer to determine the exact density composition of breast tissues; therefore, it is difficult to determine the exact exposure time required if AEC were not used. The introduction of AEC on dedicated mammography machines, in particular the current generation machines, prompted a significant reduction in repeat rates for mammography.

The AEC system on most mammography machines utilizes a single radiation-sensitive detector located **behind** the cassette. The detector is capable of moving toward the nipple, from its primary position at the chest wall, to allow for maximum variations in breast size and for critical magnification work (Figure 40–7). Most detectors will have 10 stops between the chest wall and the nipple. The AEC system should be capable of being calibrated for two different screen/film systems and also for non-grid, grid, and magnification options.

The optical density (OD) of the ACR Plexiglas™ mammographic phantom image should not be less than **1.20** and preferably about **1.30 OD**. The film density, as measured using the ACR standardized exposure technique, should be within ±0.15 OD for the range of kVps used and for phantom Plexiglas™ thicknesses from 2 to 6 cm. The generator must contain a **density compensation circuit** that contains at least two + and two − settings. Each setting, or step, should result in a 12% to 15% change in mAs, or approximately a 0.15 change in optical film density to allow maximum flexibility for all

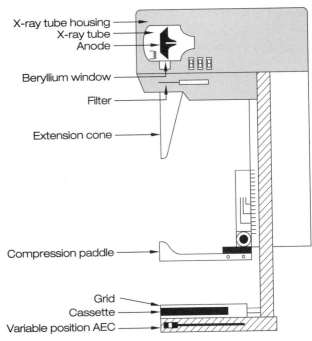

FIGURE 40-7. General design of a mammography machine and its accessory components. Note vertical alignment of the chest wall edge of cassette and compression paddle, straight portion of extension cone, and angle of the anode.

imaging requirements. Mammography generators have a **backup timer** similar to conventional AEC systems. The backup timer for grid techniques must be set at **600 mAs**, and for non-grid and magnification techniques, **300 mAs**. If the backup time is reached during a breast exposure, the radiographer should select a **higher kVp** setting for the repeat radiograph. The density compensation circuit should not be increased as is typically done in conventional AEC imaging. The primary reason backup time is reached in breast imaging is because of the inability of the low-energy photons to penetrate the breast. (This will usually occur on large or dense breasts.) A density compensation circuit increase will only prompt the backup timer to be reached again because the energy of the x-ray beam did not change; therefore, penetration of the breast will not occur. If the AEC system is left on during imaging of a breast with an implant in place, the backup time will also be reached. (Only

manual exposure techniques should be used for implant imaging.)

Quality mammography generators have highly sophisticated microprocessor controlled circuits that provide accurate and reproducible film densities over the entire range of kVp settings required and for the different thicknesses and densities of breast tissue. Well-designed AEC circuitry can automatically compensate for reciprocity law failure during long exposures. Current machines may also contain circuits that can automatically adjust the kVp to a higher level during the actual exposure. This allows the film to be properly exposed and the backup time will not be reached if the breast is large or dense. The circuit adjusts the kVp by sensing the radiation intensity during the first 100 milliseconds of the exposure. If the current is too low, the kVp is automatically increased. When purchasing a new mammography machine, the AEC nomenclature should be carefully checked and tested to ensure that it has accurate density tracking and, therefore, will reproduce film densities for all requirements within ±0.10 OD.

X-Ray Tube

Design

The most distinctive aspect of the mammography machine is the design and application of its x-ray tube and peripheral components. Each component described in this section has a very novel design compared to its counterpart in conventional radiology. The specific design or use of some components will increase contrast, resolution, or radiation exposure. Other components counteract this and cause a decrease in contrast, resolution, or exposure. The production of a high-quality breast image involves many tradeoffs. Taken altogether, however, the x-ray tube design and the components are capable of achieving high resolution and high contrast at moderate radiation exposure levels. First and foremost, the mammography equipment must be engineered to provide the high contrast and resolution required to visualize microcalcifications and the subtle parenchymal structures of the breast. Achieving the right balance of contrast, resolution, and low radiation exposures is a formidable challenge in breast imaging.

Heel Effect

The anode configuration in a mammography x-ray tube produces a prominent heel effect due to the short source-to-image receptor distance (SID) and the use of a narrow target angle. Because the x-ray tube is aligned with the cathode placed directly over the chest wall area and the anode outward toward the nipple end, the heel effect fortunately can be used to maximum advantage (Figure 40–8). Recall that the cathode side of the x-ray beam has a significantly greater intensity of x-rays compared to the anode side. A more uniform-density breast image can be produced because the more intense x-rays are at the chest wall where there is greater tissue thickness (Figure 40–9). The primary reason the cathode end of the x-ray tube is placed directly over the chest wall edge of the image is to take advantage of the prominent heel effect of the anode.

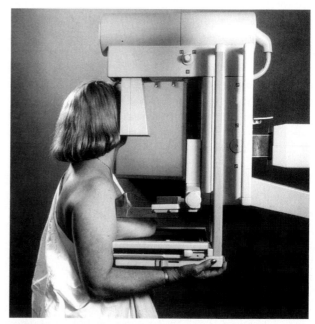

FIGURE 40-8. Patient positioned on a mammography machine. Note short SID of 60 cm, which produces a prominent heel effect. Cathode side of the x-ray tube is placed over patient's head and anode side outward toward nipple. This orientation allows the bulk of the x-ray tube housing to be placed away from the patient's head for ease of positioning.

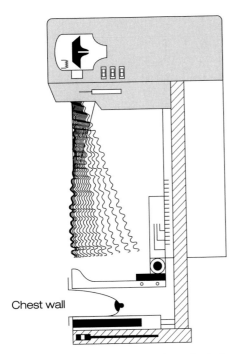

Chest wall

FIGURE 40-9. Mammography x-ray tube oriented with the cathode side placed over the chest wall area and the anode side placed outward toward the nipple end. Heel effect is used to maximum advantage with this orientation. Greater intensity x-rays are placed over the chest wall area where the breast is thicker, producing a more uniform density image.

Cathode

The cathode in a mammography x-ray tube consists of standard helical-shaped tungsten filaments in a focusing cup. Mammography tubes typically utilize a single filament wire for both the large and small focal spots. When the small focal spot is engaged, a negative voltage is applied to the focusing cup, which acts to reduce the size of the electron stream creating the smaller focal spot. This is called **bias focusing** (Chapter 6). Some machines utilize two separate filaments for the small and large focal spots.

The high resolution needed in mammography requires substantially smaller effective focal spot sizes than those used in conventional radiography. In addition, the majority of mammography machines utilize a relatively short SID of only **60 to 76 cm** (24 to 30 inches), which necessitates the use of micro-sized focal spots

to diminish the increased geometric unsharpness. A nominal **0.3-mm large** focal spot is used for the routine contact images and a nominal **0.1-mm small** focal spot is used for magnification images.

In all x-ray tubes, the effective focal spot size varies in length along the cathode-anode axis at the plane of the film due to the line-focus principle. As a result, a larger focal spot size is always projected on the cathode side (Figure 40–10A). Because mammography tubes are oriented with the cathode side placed over the chest wall, the focal spot shape and size phenomenon creates a serious dilemma: resolution is substantially decreased at the chest wall where many lesions are found. The phenomenon is more pronounced for magnification techniques. Another phenomenon that can complicate breast imaging occurs if the actual focal spot and central ray are positioned over the center of the image as in conventional radiology. Due to the short SID, several millimeters of posterosuperior breast tissue will not be imaged (Figure 40–10B). These two negative geometric properties associated with the focal spot in mammography are diminished via the **off-center placement** of the glass x-ray tube unit within the tube housing. The glass tube is moved maximally toward the chest wall so the focal spot on the anode and vertical central ray are positioned **directly over the chest wall** (Figure 40–11A and B). The geometric dilemma is diminished by **eliminating** the entire cathode side of the x-ray beam. Although the effective focal spot size remains larger at the chest wall, utilizing the anode half of the beam provides slightly greater resolution because the projected focal spot sizes at the image plane are smaller on this side. Therefore, a smaller effective focal spot is projected at the important chest wall area (Figure 40–11A). Placing the x-ray tube off center also enables the vertical central ray to enter **straight in** at the chest wall eliminating the possibility of missing the posterosuperior breast tissue in the image (Figure 40–11B). The heel effect continues to be advantageous because there does remain greater intensity at the vertical central ray point than at the anode end. Recall that the x-ray intensity decreases gradually from the cathode toward the anode.

This unique design prompts a change in the orientation of the mammography x-ray beam. Because the vertical central ray is positioned at the chest wall (edge of the film), the x-ray directed to the center of the cassette

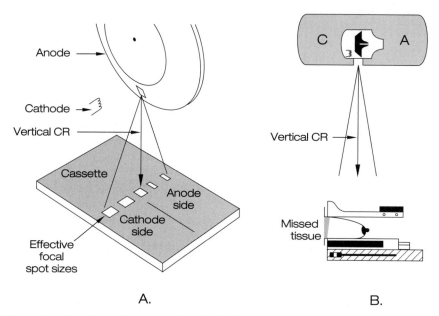

A.   **B.**

FIGURE 40-10. (A) Conventional radiography x-ray tube with focal spot and vertical central ray positioned over center of the cassette. Note focal spot length is projected larger in size toward the cathode end due to the line-focus principle. (B) Conventional focal spot and vertical central ray positioned over center of cassette prompting posterosuperior breast tissue to be missed on the image.

is actually the mid-portion of the anode half of the x-ray beam. This new **angled** central ray is termed the **reference axis** in mammography (Figure 40–11B).

The physical size of the focal spot in mammography is determined and measured by the manufacturers at the **reference axis** point on the film plane, not at the vertical central ray point as in conventional radiography. The target angle will measure smaller from the reference axis perspective, and, therefore, the focal spot will also measure smaller. The nominal 0.30-mm large and nominal 0.10-mm small focal spots measure this size in the center of the film at the reference axis point. Therefore, the projected **length** and overall size of the effective focal spot at the vertical central ray point and chest wall will be at least **2× larger**. This geometric phenomenon results from the line focus principle and cannot be overcome. The high resolution in the image is maintained, in part, via the use of very small focal spot sizes. This may appear to not be an ideal engineering design, however, a tradeoff must be made. Overall, it is more advantageous to have the cathode end over the more dense chest wall structures to take advantage of the **heel effect**. In addi-

tion, this orientation allows the bulk of the x-ray tube housing to be placed away from the patient's head for ease of positioning (see Figure 40–8).

Anode Configuration

Mammography tubes use rotating anodes to take advantage of the increased tube loading. This is particularly important because it enables the use of a higher mA and allows exposure times to be maintained under 1 second.

The **effective target angle** (measured from the vertical central ray point) is **greater** in a mammography tube, varying from **22° to 24°**. The larger effective angle is necessary so the x-ray beam will cover a 24×30-cm cassette at the 60–65 cm SID (Figure 40–12A and B). However, the **reference axis target angle** (measured from the center of the x-ray beam as in conventional radiography) is **smaller** varying from **7.5° to 12°**. The reference axis target angle is specified in mammography tubes because it defines the size of the focal spot as measured in the center of the image.

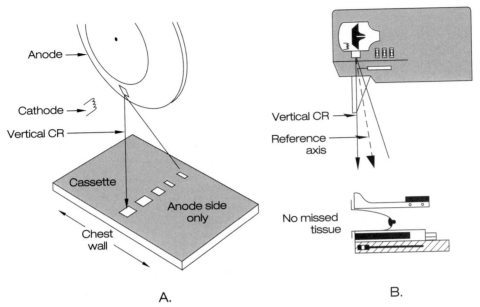

A.

B.

FIGURE 40-11. Off-center placement of the x-ray tube within the tube housing. Cathode side of x-ray beam eliminated. (A) Focal spot and vertical central ray placed directly over the chest wall. (B) Vertical central ray placed directly over chest wall structure allows the posterosuperior breast tissue to be imaged. Note new **central** ray is termed the **reference axis**. Nominal focal spot size is measured at the reference axis point on the film.

Most manufacturers prefer to use a narrow target angle, as measured from the vertical filament, because it allows greater anode heat capacity for a given effective focal spot size. However, to utilize a narrower angle and maintain x-ray coverage on the cassette, the x-ray tube must be **tilted** (Figure 40–12B). One manufacturer utilizes a unique design in which the anode is oriented with the stem placed in a vertical position and the x-ray tube steeply tilted. This allows the **edge** of the anode disk to be used as the actual target rather than the face of the anode (Figure 40–13A and B). The anode edge is designed with two distinct surfaces, one for each focal spot. This design allows radiation coverage of the film with the large focal spot, achievement of maximum anode heat capacity, capability of producing a small effective focal spot, and placement of the effective small focal spot closer to the chest wall allowing greater resolution. Designing the anode configuration to achieve a small effective focal spot size, allowing maximum x-ray coverage of the cassette, and producing optimal resolution at a short SID are engineering challenges.

Anode Material

The anode in mammography x-ray tubes is made of **molybdenum**. Some manufacturers use a solid molybdenum disk and others design the molybdenum anode with graphite backing similar to conventional radiography. In order to prevent anode surface roughness and pitting, which could ultimately decrease x-ray output, the molybdenum may be doped with about 3 percent vanadium. Like tungsten, molybdenum has a high melting point, and conducts heat well.

Molybdenum is used as the anode material of choice over tungsten for several reasons. Studies indicate that x-ray energies ranging between 17–25 keV are required to differentiate the inherent low contrast structures of all types of breasts. Specifically, x-ray energies between the narrow range of **17–20** are preferred. These specific x-ray energies must be present in the mammography x-ray beam to maximize subject contrast and visualize microcalcifications. If the x-ray beam contains energies higher than this narrow range, the x-rays will over-penetrate,

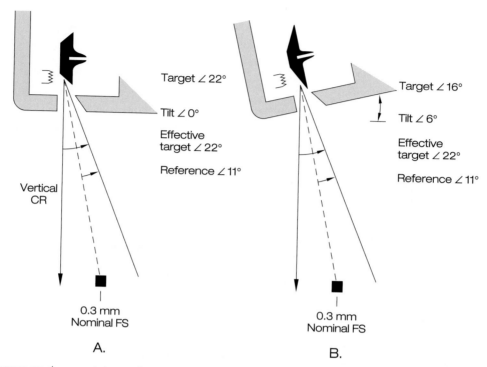

FIGURE 40-12. Mammography x-ray tube configurations. (A) Horizontal tube placement and 22° target angle. Large **effective** target angle of 22° allows x-ray coverage of cassette at a short SID. **Reference axis** target angle of 11° creates a 0.3-mm focal spot size in the center of the image. (B) Tilting the tube 6° allows use of a smaller target angle of 16° and prompts the same **effective** angle of 22° and **reference axis** angle of 11° as horizontal tube. Tilting allows greater anode heat capacity due to the smaller target angle.

scatter, and decrease radiographic contrast. A relatively large number of **photoelectric absorption** interactions is needed to produce the high radiographic contrast that will improve the visibility of detail in the image. Low kVp is necessary to produce the 17–20 keV range of x-ray photons that will create the photoelectric interactions. Unfortunately, this will introduce a higher radiation exposure to the patient. As in all areas of mammography, a tradeoff must be made. Without low kVp x-rays and high photoelectric absorption, radiographic detail of the breast structures cannot occur.

The three primary breast tissues — adipose, fibrous, and glandular — have very low atomic numbers ranging from 6 to 8. Approximately 40 percent of cancers in the breast contain microcalcifications that have an atomic number of 20. Therefore, kVp settings around 25 are necessary. One must set the generator kVp slightly higher than the atomic number of the tissues being imaged so there is adequate penetration. Figures 40–14A and 40

–14B illustrate an x-ray emission spectrum for a conventional tungsten anode x-ray tube and a molybdenum anode mammography tube operating at 26 kVp. Note that the tungsten anode will produce x-ray photons with energies in the preferred 17–20 keV range. It also produces a high volume of photons above this range and a relatively large number below the range. The x-ray photons above the preferred mammography range will produce Compton interactions that decrease contrast, and the x-ray photons below this range will be virtually all absorbed via the photoelectric process and only contribute to patient dose. The entire tungsten produced x-ray beam consists of bremsstrahlung x-rays.

The x-ray emission spectrum produced from the molybdenum anode has a drastically different shape. Note that the most prominent x-ray photons are **characteristic**. The characteristic x-rays are created from displacement of the K-shell binding electrons in the molybdenum atom (Table 40–2). Characteristic x-rays will

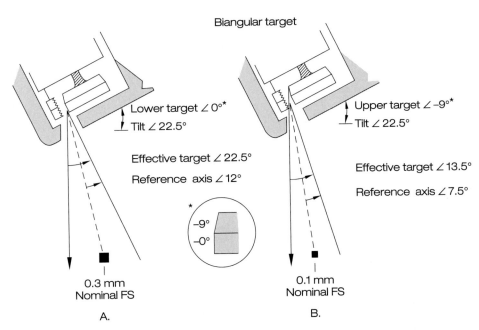

FIGURE 40-13. Anode oriented with stem placed in a vertical position, a biangular anode disk **end** used as the target, and the tube steeply tilted. Circled inset shows anode end in true vertical position with 0° lower edge and -9° upper edge. (A) Lower edge of anode disk used for large focal spot. Steep 22.5° tube tilt produces a 22.5° **effective** target angle to allow x-ray coverage of the cassette and a 12° **reference axis** angle creates a 0.30 nominal focal spot. (B) Upper edge of anode disk used for small focal spot and magnification studies. The 22.5° tilt produces a 13.5° **effective** target angle, which allows adequate coverage for magnification images. The 7.5° **reference axis** angle creates a 0.10 nominal small focal spot. The small focal spot is projected closer to the chest wall structure, allowing greater resolution.

account for approximately 30 percent of the total x-rays in the molybdenum beam at 30 kVp. Most importantly, there is an increased volume of characteristic x-ray photons produced at exactly 17 and 20 keV in the preferred range, which creates a nearly perfect x-ray beam for breast imaging. When properly filtered, the molybdenum anode produces very few x-ray photons above the preferred mammographic energy range. The x-ray photons below this range are photoelectrically absorbed and aid in producing high subject contrast. Unfortunately, they also contribute to dose. Many textbooks refer to the molybdenum x-ray emission spectrum as being essentially homogeneous due to the high concentration of x-rays in a very narrow range.

The advantages of using molybdenum for the anode material in mammography tubes are:

- **Increased number of low-energy photons** are produced.

- **High radiographic contrast** is achieved in the image.
- **Production of specific x-ray energies** required for breast imaging.

The disadvantages of molybdenum are:

- **Less x-ray photon output** due a to lower atomic number—42.
- **Increased mAs required** to maintain film density.
- **Increased dose** to the patient.

The higher contrast image produced by the molybdenum target is illustrated in Figure 40–15.

Recently, a new anode material, **rhodium**, was introduced for use in mammography. The slightly higher atomic number of rhodium, 45, creates higher energy x-ray photons (Table 40–2). The primary advantage of

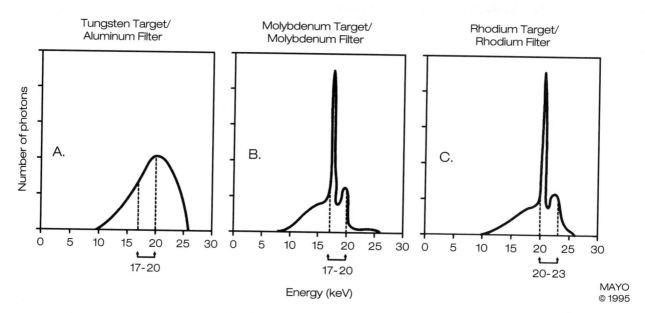

FIGURE 40-14. X-ray emission spectrums produced at 26 kVp. (A) Conventional tungsten target with aluminum filter. High volume of photons produced above the preferred mammography range of 17 to 20 keV and high volume below this range. Note entire x-ray beam is bremsstrahlung photons. (B) Mammography molybdenum target and molybdenum filter producing prominent characteristic photons at 17 and 20 keV in the preferred energy range. Very few photons produced above this range. (C) Mammography rhodium target and rhodium filter. Spectrum shape is identical to B but produces a **higher** average energy x-ray beam than molybdenum. Note prominent characteristic photons at 20 and 23 keV, which provide better penetration for larger or more dense breasts at a lower dose to the patient.

TABLE 40–2. Characteristic X-Rays From Mammography X-Ray Targets

Electron Shells	Molybdenum (Z-42)	Rhodium (Z-45)
	keV*	
L to K	17	20
M to K	20	23

using rhodium is that the characteristic x-rays it produces have energies that are **2–3 keV higher** than molybdenum. In the rhodium x-ray emission spectrum, the x-ray photon energies shift slightly to the right and the characteristic x-rays are prominent at **20 and 23 keV** (Figure 40–14C). This provides better penetration of large breasts or those breasts that are very dense. Of significance, also, is that rhodium's higher average energy x-

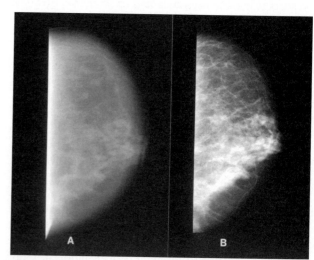

FIGURE 40-15. Craniocaudal projection of the same patient's breast produced at 30 kVp showing effect of molybdenum anode on radiographic contrast. (A) Tungsten anode produces suboptimal radiographic contrast. (B) Molybdenum anode produces significantly higher contrast and greater visibility of detail. *(Images courtesy of C. Vyborny, M.D., Ph.D.)*

ray beam prompts a reduction in exposure time of approximately 25 percent. When used with the appropriate filter, use of a rhodium anode can decrease x-ray exposure by 50 percent or more. The primary disadvantage of rhodium as an anode material is that its higher energy beam is not appropriate for use on small to regular sized breasts, or those breasts that are not dense. Therefore, it cannot be the sole anode material. To take advantage of the inherent properties of rhodium, one manufacturer has designed a **biangular** anode, similar to Figure 40–13, in which the same disk contains a track for molybdenum and a separate track for rhodium, selectable by the operator. The x-ray tube can be moved in one of two positions, one for each of the two focal spots. This allows both focal spot sizes to be available for each track. Interestingly, another manufacturer has recently introduced a dual-track anode that contains molybdenum and **tungsten,** selectable by the operator also. The tungsten anode is used with a rhodium filter and, like the rhodium anode, is designed to be used on the larger or more dense breasts at a significantly reduced exposure. While molybdenum is the primary anode material used, all machines will have either rhodium or tungsten as an alternate choice.

Filtration

The port of the x-ray tube in mammography is specially designed. **Beryllium**, with an atomic number of 4, is used in the port of all mammography x-ray tubes to allow the low-energy x-rays to exit. Glass cannot be used because it would attenuate most of the low-energy x-rays needed to produce the breast image.

Filtration must be used at the tube port on all mammography machines. As in conventional radiography, the primarily purpose of filtration is to attenuate the very low energy x-rays that are not needed to produce the breast image. Without filtration, a relatively large number of 5–10 keV x-rays would exit the tube. In addition, a larger number of 20–30 keV x-rays at the higher energy end of the spectrum would also exit. The 5–10 keV x-rays would all be absorbed in the breast and drastically increase the dose. The 20–30 keV x-rays would degrade image quality by decreasing radiographic contrast. A specific function of the filter in mammography, therefore, is to decrease most of the low and some high-energy bremsstrahlung x-rays to maximize subject contrast. To accom-

plish this, mammography filters are made of the **same element** as the anode material. For a molybdenum anode the filter is **0.03-mm molybdenum** and for the rhodium target, **0.025-mm rhodium**. The x-ray emission spectrums for molybdenum and rhodium in Figure 40–14 show the effect of this filtration. Eliminating much of the high 20–30 keV photons provides a nearly perfect x-ray beam for breast imaging.

Many mammography machines provide a selectable molybdenum or rhodium filter that can be used with the molybdenum anode. Selection of the rhodium filter with the molybdenum anode will produce an emission spectrum that lies half-way between the molybdenum and the rhodium configurations. The rhodium filter used with the molybdenum anode will produce a higher energy x-ray beam that is more desirable for larger or dense breasts. Use of the rhodium filter will also reduce radiation exposure by about 38 percent. Caution must be exercised to ensure that the rhodium filter is not used with small and regular sized breasts or non-dense breasts, because it will produce a lower contrast image that would not provide the appropriate visibility of detail.

The half-value-layer (HVL) is an indirect measurement of the total filtration in the path of the x-ray beam. It is expressed in millimeters of aluminum (mm-Al). In a mammography machine, the HVL will include the attenuation properties of the beryllium window, molybdenum filter, mirror, and the plastic compression paddle. The minimum HVL is specified by government regulations and should not measure less than **0.30-mm Al** at 30 kVp or **0.25-mm Al** at 25 kVp. This will ensure that adequate filtration is present in the x-ray beam, and the patient will not receive excessive radiation exposure. If the HVL is too high, image quality can be degraded. Excessive filtration, although it would reduce exposure, will decrease overall radiographic image contrast. Therefore, the HVL should not exceed **0.40-mm Al** at 30 kVp. It is recommended that the HVL be maintained as close as possible to the minimal level to ensure that image contrast is maintained at a high level.

Magnification

Magnified projections of the breast are additionally requested when the visibility of detail in very small breast structures and when microcalcifications need to be enhanced. They are also requested when breast structures that lie close together and overlap have to be separated. As many as 10 percent of patients require additional projections using the magnification technique.

The magnification factor on the mammography machine varies slightly among manufacturers and is standardized between 1.5× and 1.8×. Some manufacturers design their equipment with two magnification selections — the second may be as high as 2.0×. To magnify the breast, a raised platform is placed on the cassette holder unit and the breast is placed on top of the platform for the exposure (Figure 40–16).

Magnified projections of the breast provide the following enhancements:

- **Increased resolution** due to the small focal spot and reduced quantum mottle.

- **Reduction in scatter radiation** reaching the film due to the air gap.

- **Improved visibility of detail** due to the larger field of view.

Magnifying the breast will technically reduce resolution in the image due to an increase in geometric unsharpness. A magnification of 1.5× will reduce resolution by at least 50 percent from about 20 lp/mm to 10 lp/mm. To regain the lost resolution, a very small 0.10-mm focal spot is utilized, which returns the resolution to the 20 lp/mm level. This is the smallest focal spot size employed anywhere in radiology. Effective resolution may even be improved in magnified images due to a **reduction in noise**. Recall that noise is primarily a product of the screen/film combination (quantum mottle). The screen/film combination typically is not changed for magnification techniques. Noise is, therefore, reduced by about 30 percent for 1.5× magnification because significantly more x-ray photons are used per unit volume of tissue to produce the image. This is due to the breast being placed closer to the x-ray tube where there is a higher volume of x-rays available to form the image. For 1.5× magnification, a given square of tissue covers approximately 2.25× more area on the film compared to the contact image, and many more screen phosphors are utilized to form the image.

Scattered radiation is reduced somewhat as a result of the air-gap between the cassette and breast. The reduced scatter increases radiographic contrast and, fortunately, a grid does not have to be used. The breast structures are seen much better when the magnification technique is used due to a combination of the micro-sized focal spot, the reduction in noise, and the reduction in scatter radiation. When the breast structures are magnified, they are spread apart and the anatomical field of view is enhanced (Figure 40–17A and B).

Radiation exposure to the patient is a major concern in magnification radiography of the breast. Radiation to the breast can increase **2–3X** during a single exposure, even without the use of a grid. This results from the breast being placed much closer to the x-ray source where the radiation intensity is greater. The exact exposure increase will vary among different manufacturers' units depending upon their specific design and magnification factor. The increase in radiation is due also to the additional exposure required because of reciprocity law failure. Use of the 0.10 focal spot requires that the mA

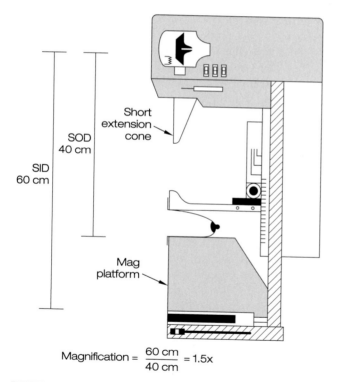

Magnification = $\dfrac{60\ cm}{40\ cm}$ = 1.5x

FIGURE 40-16. Breast in position on a raised platform to produce a 1.5x magnification image. There is greater intensity of radiation at the breast when placed closer to the x-ray tube. Magnification technique requires the use of a 0.10 focal spot to maintain resolution.

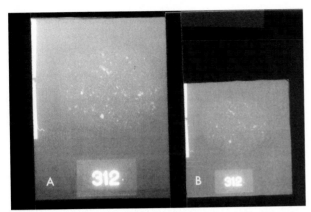

FIGURE 40-17. (A) Magnification image of calcifications in a Plexiglas™ breasts phantom at 1.5x and 26 kVp. (B) Non-magnified image of same phantom as A.

be reduced considerably (e.g., 100 mA to 25 mA) due to tube loading. The reduction in mA will prompt exposure times to be increased to **2–4 seconds**. The long exposure time will require the mammographer to explain the procedure carefully and to watch the patient during the exposure so motion does not degrade image quality.

Accessories

Grids

Scatter control plays an important role in the production of a high-quality mammographic image. Scatter radiation is produced from the breast during the exposure which contributes to the overall film density, and the effect is a reduction in radiographic contrast. Scatter increases significantly for larger and more dense breasts and with higher kVp settings. With the introduction of the grid on dedicated mammography machines in 1978, scatter and secondary radiation reaching the film has been reduced and high contrast maintained in the image. Use of a grid in mammography greatly improves radiographic quality and today grids are used for all mammographic images. The use of a grid will, however, increase radiation exposure to the patient by a factor of **2–3x**.

Mammography grids are the linear type with a very low ratio of 4:1 or 5:1. The grid frequency will range from 30–50 lines/cm. The grid strips are made of lead as in conventional radiography. However, wood or carbon-fiber are used as the inner space material instead of aluminum in order to keep the bucky factor as low as possible. All mammography grids in use today are a moving type —moving in one direction only. They do not reciprocate. A separate grid device is used for each of the two film sizes used.

Grids are capable of producing artifacts in the image. Typically this occurs with the use of ultra-short exposure times which can be controlled by using an appropriate mA setting that will prevent short exposure times. Grids can also contain inherent artifacts. Upon purchase, mammography grids should be carefully checked before use to ensure they are free of artifacts. A basic quality control check can be performed by making a lighter density film exposure with the grid stationary and another lighter density exposure with the grid moving. If artifacts appear on the image made with the moving grid, the grid should probably be replaced.

Compression Device

All mammography machines contain a compression device that is used to compress the breast (Figures 40–7 and 40–8). Improvements in breast compression technology in recent years has greatly improved the visibility of detail in breast images. Appropriately applied compression is one of the critical components in the production of a high quality mammogram. The overall function of compression is to decrease the thickness of the breast, bring the breast structures as close to the film as possible, and increase radiographic contrast (Figure 40–18). The specific advantages of this technique are:

- **Reduced magnification** lessens geometric unsharpness and increases resolution.
- **Reduced tissue thickness** requires less kVp prompting a reduction in scattered radiation and an increase in radiographic contrast.
- **Reduced radiation exposure** because less exposure time is required due to the decreased tissue thickness.
- **Reduced motion unsharpness** occurs because the breast is completely immobilized.

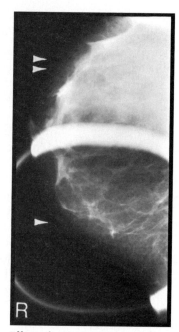

FIGURE 40-18. Effect of compression on the breast image. Spot compression on half of the breast (arrow) shows excellent contrast and resolution. Noncompressed side (double arrows) shows decreased density due to a thicker breast when no compression is applied. Significantly increased technical factors would be required to penetrate and achieve appropriate film density if compression were not applied and dose would be considerably higher.

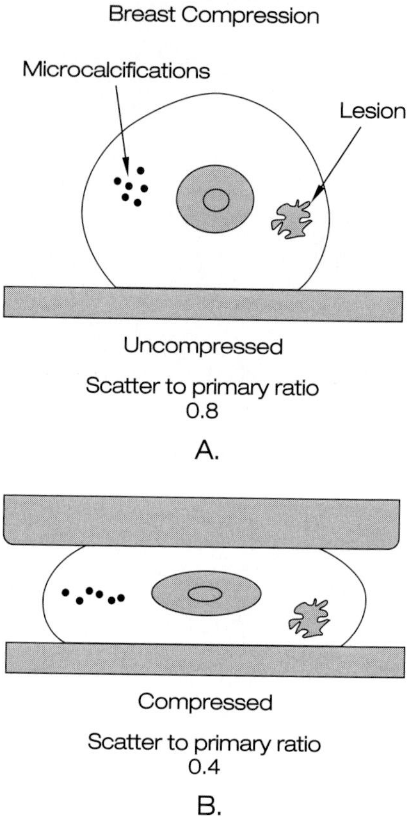

- **Improved visualization** of breast structures because the structures are spread out over a larger area. There is also less superimposition of overlying structures.

- **More uniform film density** occurs due to the flattening effect of compression permitting optimal exposure of the entire breast.

The effect of scatter and contrast is dramatic. A 6-cm thick breast measuring 9 cm in diameter will have a scatter-to-primary ratio of about 0.8, or 80 percent of the film density results from scatter. If the breast thickness is reduced to 3 cm with the breast area increased to 12 cm due to vigorous compression, the scatter-to-primary ratio is reduced to 0.4, or only 40 percent of the film density results from scatter. Radiographic contrast would increase two-fold (Figures 40–19A and B).

Breast Compression

Microcalcifications

Lesion

Uncompressed

Scatter to primary ratio
0.8

A.

Compressed

Scatter to primary ratio
0.4

B.

FIGURE 40-19. Breast compression. (A) No compression and scatter to primary ratio of 0.8. Note location of microcalcifications and lesion. (B) Compression decreases scatter to primary ratio to 0.4, breast structures are brought closer to the film and spread out. Decreased tissue thickness and reduction in scatter radiation prompts greater radiographic contrast. Decreased magnification of structures creates greater resolution.

The compression device is made of a plastic that allows transmission of the low energy x-rays. The device should have a straight chest wall edge to allow the compression to grasp the breast tissues close to the chest wall edge. Compression is controlled by the radiographer and must be capable of being applied at 25–45 lbs. of force. In addition to the standard compression devise, a smaller "spot" device is used to compress localized areas. The device should be checked regularly to ensure that it is working properly and applying the correct amount of pressure.

Cassettes

Like many of the previously described components of the mammography unit, the cassettes and screen/film combination used are also designed specifically to image the breast. The use of direct exposure x-ray film for mammography ended in the early 1970s because of the high exposure involved, and intensifying screens have been used ever since. Today, specially designed cassettes containing a single emulsion screen and used with a single emulsion film are the standard.

Mammography cassettes are manufactured of plastic or low attenuation carbon-fiber. Carbon-fiber enables the maximum number of x-rays to reach the intensifying screen, thereby keeping exposures at minimum levels. The screen is mounted on a foam pressure pad, and when closed, is placed at the extreme top of the cassette as close to the breast as possible (Figure 40–3). The single screen is placed **behind** the film so there is high x-ray absorption of the screen phosphors closest to the film emulsion, thereby reducing the diffusion of light emitted from the screen (line-spread function). This arrangement prompts less image noise and greater resolution (Figure 40–20). The x-ray photons that exit the breast enter the top of the cassette and go through the film before reaching the screen phosphor.

Screens

Mammography screens are manufactured by a variety of companies and they are all very similar in design. Each company offers at least two different screen speeds— typically one screen will be twice as fast as the other. The majority of manufacturers use green emitting **gadolinium oxysulfide** as the screen phosphor material. Mammography screens are much slower than those used in conventional radiography. A slow screen offers reduced noise and increased resolution. Using a screen in mammography instead of direct x-ray exposure offers two distinct advantages — a major reduction in radiation exposure to the patient and a dramatic increase in radiographic contrast. The disadvantage of using a screen is the decrease in resolution and increased image noise. However, a tradeoff must once again be made due to the unacceptably high radiation exposure from the direct exposure technique. Recall that direct exposure required from 50 to 100 times more radiation than screen technique. Fortunately, the overall design of the dedicated mammography machine and its specially engineered components allows high resolution to be maintained despite the use of a screen.

Uniformity of the speed of all the screens used is important. The difference between the minimum and maximum optical densities in all the screens shall not exceed 0.30 OD.

Film

Mammography film is designed to be very high in contrast and resolution. When used with a mammography screen, it is the highest contrast and highest resolution imaging system used in diagnostic radiology. Because the breast structures contain very low inherent subject contrast, a high contrast film is needed to enhance the anatomical structures. Mammography film, like the screen, is single emulsion and designed to be slow in speed. The slow speed prompts low image noise and high resolution. Mammography film is green sensitive to match the spectral characteristics of the green emitting screen. Manufacturers offer at least two different film speeds and two films with different contrast levels. An

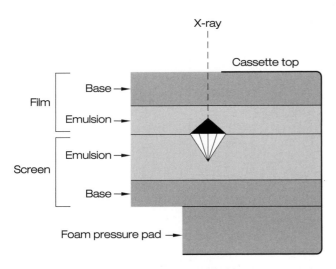

FIGURE 40-20. Cross-section of mammography screen and film in cassette. Single screen is placed behind film as a back screen. Single-emulsion film is placed in contact with single-emulsion screen. Design allows high absorption of x-rays in the screen phosphors closest to the film emulsion, which reduces diffusion of light emitted from the screen.

antihalation coating is placed on the non-emulsion side of the film. The coating prevents screen light from going through the film and scattering back to the film, which would decrease resolution. Caution must be exercised so the non-emulsion side of the film (shiny side) is not placed in contact with the screen. The screen and film emulsions must always be in direct contact with each other.

Most manufacturers also offer a special film, referred to as "extended film," which is designed to provide the same results as using standard mammography film and **extended cycle** processing. Extended cycle processing is a technique whereby the speed of a standard film can be increased up to 35 percent and radiographic contrast increased measurably, by **doubling the time the film is in the developer solution** (Figure 40–21). With some extended cycle techniques, the developer temperature is increased along with the immersion time. The intent of extending the development portion of the processing cycle is to allow the developer solution more time to fully process the silver halide crystals. Single emulsion film

contains a thicker emulsion layer and can benefit from increased development. The advantages of extended film processing are increased radiographic contrast and reduced radiation exposure to the patient. The disadvantage of extended processing is that the increased speed of the film increases radiographic noise and resolution is decreased. In addition, the longer development time also decreases film throughput in high volume mammography departments. The special "extended look" film described earlier was designed specifically to provide the faster speed and higher contrast without increasing the developer time and without reducing film throughput. Mammographers should exercise caution and use the correct film with the appropriate processor set-up.

Screen/Film Combination

The relative speed of a mammography screen/film combination should not be associated directly with a conventional screen/film system. A **100-speed** mam-

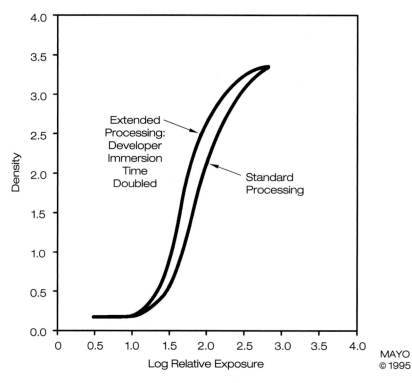

FIGURE 40-21. H and D curve showing effect of extended processing with standard mammography films. Speed and contrast of mammography film is increased when developer immersion time is doubled.

mography system will typically be **50 to 75 percent slower** than a 100-speed conventional system. The stated speed will depend primarily upon the specific speed of the screen, the type and specific speed of film, and whether extended or regular 90-second processing is used. The mammography speed of 100 was arbitrarily assigned to the original Kodak Min-R screen and film developed in 1975. Today mammography screen/film systems range in relative speed from 100 to as high as 320 (Table 40–3).

Researchers continue to work on improving screen/film systems in an effort to keep radiation exposures low and resolution high. Recently, a dual screen and dual emulsion film was introduced by Kodak. The back screen is standard thickness and the front screen is one-half the thickness of the back screen. The quantity of light reaching the film emulsion is equal from both screens. The film has anti-crossover light properties, which helps to maintain resolution. The primary advantage of this dual emulsion system is that the effective speed is doubled compared to using a single screen and film. The disadvantage is that the increased speed produces an increase in image noise thereby decreasing resolution which may be unacceptable for routine mammography images. In addition, it may be difficult to pass the ACR accreditation phantom test with reduced resolution. The shorter exposure time and reduced radiation exposure achieved from this system may, however, be an advantage for magnification techniques.

Resolution

Dedicated mammography systems are capable of producing very high-image resolution compared to conventional radiography. In conventional radiography, limit-

TABLE 40–3. Screen/Film Characteristics*

Screen	Film (Min-R)	Process	Relative Speed	Mean Glandular Dose (mrad)	Contrast††	Resolution‡ lp/mm	Noise
Min-R	M	Standard	100	250†	2.95	21	Low
Min-R	E	Extended	140	175	3.25	21	
Min-R Medium	M	Standard	170	150	2.95	19	
Min-R	H	Standard	180	150	3.20	21	
Min-R Medium	E	Extended	240	100	3.25	19	
Min-R Fast	T	Standard	280	125	2.90	18	
Min-R Medium	H	Standard	320	75	3.20	19	High

* Screens and Film are Eastman Kodak. From Haus, A.G., *Screen-Film Processing Characteristics and Quality Control in Mammography* (KODAK Publication #N-314)

† Average two-view dose from ACR accreditation program data. Measured on RMI 156 phantom.

†† Contrast — measured as the average gradient between densities 0.25 and 2.00 above base + fog.

‡ Limiting resolution — based on 5 percent value of modular transfer function.

ing resolution will range from a low of about 2 lp/mm in fluoroscopy, to 5 lp/mm for a 300 speed screen/film system, and as high as 10 lp/mm for a 100-speed extremity system. Current mammography systems are capable of producing limiting resolutions as high as 22 lp/mm. Few mammography systems are set up to produce the maximum resolution that is capable in the system in order to keep radiation exposures at minimal levels. The mammography system must provide a minimum of **11 to 13 lp/mm.** Many components, used altogether, play a role in achieving this high resolution. Most notably, the micro-sized focal spots, compression, low kVp, and the slow speed screen/film system. Radiologists are relatively comfortable with the current levels of resolution. Cancer and other pathology can be identified although a magnifying glass is often required to view the small structures in the images and to actually see the high resolution.

Mammography images today are the best ever produced (Figure 40–22). Federal government regulation has mandated that consistent high quality images be pro-

duced wherever mammography machines have met the MQSA standards. Mean glandular dose (MGD) provides the best indicator of risk to the patient instead of ESE. According to the federal government's MQSA program, in 1997 the average MGD for a single screen/film/grid study was 160 mrads (1.6 mGy). The risk from mammography at these levels is low when compared to the decreased deaths that result through screening. The lifetime risk of death from mammography is 5 in 1 million. With doses at their current levels, image noise and resolution are greater considerations than dose.

Quality Control

The production of an optimal quality breast image may be the most technically challenging of all radiographic examinations. Quality control tests are required under the rules of the MQSA to ensure that high standards of image quality are achieved daily. Some states may require additional tests. The ACR provides a quality control manual for medical physicists that contains a section for radiographers. The manual describes the quality control tests that should be carried out along with their frequency (Table 40–4). The tests must be carried out accurately and at the **minimum** frequency stated. If problems occur in the production of images, the tests may need to be done more frequently. Regular quality control testing is the only means of assuring that high image quality is always maintained. Slight changes in equipment performance, in particular the film processor and the accessory devices, can affect the contrast, resolution, or radiation exposure.

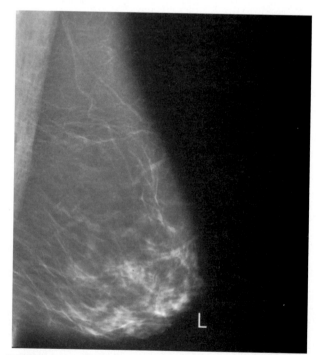

FIGURE 40-22. Mediolateral oblique projection of the breast produced on a current generation mammography machine. High quality image demonstrates optimal resolution and contrast. Radiation dose is low.

Summary

Early detection of breast cancer depends on consistently reliable high-quality images. Image quality standards have been set forth by the American College of Radiology and the federal government's Mammography Quality Standards Act. The imaging requirements needed for mammography are more demanding than for other x-ray examinations. Mammography requires very

TABLE 40–4. Mammography Quality Control Minimum Test Frequencies*

Test	Minimum Frequency
Darkroom cleanliness	Daily
Processor quality control	Daily
Screen cleanliness	Weekly
Viewboxes and viewing conditions	Weekly
Phantom images	Weekly
Visual check list	Monthly
Repeat analysis	Quarterly
Analysis of fixer retention in film	Quarterly
Darkroom fog	Semiannually
Screen/film contact	Semiannually
Compression	Semiannually

* *From* Mammography Quality Control for Medical Physicists. ACR, Reston, VA

high radiographic contrast and resolution so microcalcifications as small as 0.1 mm or less can be visualized along with the inherently low-contrast breast tissues. It is essential to use an imaging system that produces low noise. The radiation exposures associated with the examination must be sufficiently low to ensure that there is minimal risk to the patient.

The high subject contrast needed for effective mammography requires the use of low kVp techniques along with a molybdenum anode and a molybdenum filter. The low x-ray energy range will enhance the breast structures and improve the visibility of detail. Two new options for imaging large and dense breasts have recently been introduced. These include the use of rhodium anodes with rhodium filtration and tungsten anodes with rhodium filtration.

Geometric unsharpness is minimized and resolution increased during mammography by using micro-focus focal spots, uniquely designed x-ray tube configurations, the heel effect to advantage, low magnification, and firm breast compression. Although the breast structure is

small and low energy is utilized, there is still a significant component of scatter radiation that can obscure contrast. Therefore, low ratio grids are required, along with breast compression, to reduce scattered radiation.

Slow speed single emulsion screens and film, along with special cassettes, are required in mammography. Resolution in a mammography system is typically 11 to 13 lp/mm.

REVIEW QUESTIONS

1. What advantage did xeromammography have over direct exposure mammography?

2. List three advantages screen/film mammography has over direct exposure mammography?

3. List at least two reasons why high-frequency generators are used in mammography.

4. What is the kVp range for mammography?

5. What is the AEC backup time for a grid technique?

6. Which end of the mammography tube is placed over the chest wall area?

7. What are two focal spot sizes used in mammography tubes?

8. Which side of the x-ray beam, anode or cathode, is eliminated in mammography?

9. What is the most common anode material used in mammography?

10. List two reasons why x-ray tubes are tilted.

11. Of what material is the port of the x-ray tube in mammography made?

12. List two advantages of producing magnified images of the breast.

13. State the two common grid ratios used in mammography.

14. List three advantages of using breast compression in mammography.

15. Why is the single-emulsion film placed behind the single-emulsion screen in a mammography cassette?

16. Describe extended processing.

REFERENCES AND RECOMMENDED READING

American Cancer Society. (1994). *Cancer facts and figures—1994.* Atlanta: American Cancer Society.

American College of Radiology. (1999). *Mammography quality control for medical physicists.* Reston, VA: American College of Radiology.

American College of Radiology. (1999). *Mammography quality control for technologists.* Reston, VA: American College of Radiology.

Barnes, G. T. & Brezovich, I. A. (1978). The intensity of scattered radiation in mammography. *Radiology. 126,* 243–247.

Barnes, G. T., Wu, X., Wagner, A. J., & Rubin, E. (1989). Scatter control in mammography: Past, present and future (abstr). *Radiology. 173,* 472.

Bassett, L. W. & Gold, R. H. (1988). Evolution of mammography. *American Journal of Roentgenology. 150,* 493.

Buchanan, R. A., Finkelstein, S. I., & Wickersheim, K. A. (1976). X-ray exposure reduction using rare earth oxysulfide intensifying screens. *Radiology. 118,* 183–188.

Bushberg, J. T., Seibert, J. A., Leidholdt, E. M., & Boone, J. M. (1994). *The essential physics of medical imaging.* Baltimore: Williams & Wilkins.

Conway, B. J., McCrohan, J. L., Reuter, F. G., & Suleiman, O. H. (1990). Mammography in the eighties. *Radiology. 177,* 335–339.

Egan, R. L. (1964). *Mammography.* Springfield, IL: Thomas, 3–16.

Egan, R. L. McSweeney, M. B., & Sprawls, P. (1983). Grids in mammography. *Radiology. 146,* 359–362.

Feig, S. D. & Ehrlich, S. M. (1990). Estimation of radiation risk from screening mammography: Recent trends and comparison with expected benefits. *Radiology. 174,* 638–647.

Gray, J. E. (1991). Acceptance testing of diagnostic x-ray imaging equipment: Considerations and rationale. In: Siebert, J. A., Barnes, G. T., & Gould, R. G., eds. *Specification, acceptance testing and quality control of diagnostic x-ray imaging equipment.* New York: American Association of Physicists in Medicine, 1–9.

Gray, J. E., Winkler, N. T., Stears, J. G., & Frank, E. D. (1983). *Quality control in diagnostic imaging: a quality control cookbook.* Baltimore: University Park Press.

Haus, A. G. (1990). Technologic improvements in screen-film mammography. *Radiology. 174,* 628–637.

Haus, A. G., Cullinan, J. E. (1989). Screen film processing systems for medical radiography: a historical review. *Radiographics. 9,* 1203–1224

Haus, A. G., Metz, C. E., Chiles, J. T., & Rossmann, K. (1976). The effect of x-ray spectra from molybdenum and tungsten target tubes on image quality in mammography. *Radiology. 118,* 705–709.

Haus, A. G., Paulus, D. D., Dodd, G. D., Cowart, R. W., & Bencomo, J. (1979). Magnification mammography: Evaluation of screen film and xeroradiographic techniques. *Radiology. 133,* 223–226.

Haus, A. G., Rossmann, K., Vyborny, C., Hoffer, P. B., & Doi, K. (1977). Sensitometry in diagnostic radiology, radiation therapy and nuclear medicine. *Journal of Applied Photographic Engineering. 3,* 114–124.

Hendrick, R. E. (1990). Standardization of image quality and radiation dose in mammography. *Radiology. 174,* 648–656.

Hendrick, R. E. (1992). Quality assurance in mammography: Accreditation, legislation, and compliance with quality assurance standards. *Radiological Clinics of North America. 3,* 243–255.

Kimme-Smith, C., Bassett, L. W., Gold, R. H., Roe, D., & Orr, J. (1987). Mammographic dual screen, dual emulsion film combination: Visibility of simulated microcalcifications and effect on image contrast. *Radiology. 165,* 313–318.

Kimme-Smith, C., Rothchild, P. A., Bassett, L. W., Gold, R. H., & Moler, C. (1989). Mammographic film processor temperature, development time, and chemistry: Effect on dose, contrast and noise. *American Journal of Roentgenology. 173,* 65–69.

Kimme-Smith, C., Wang, J., Debruhl, N., Basic, M., & Bassett, L. W. (1994). Mammograms obtained with rhodium vs molybdenum anodes: Contrast and dose differences. *American Journal of Roentology. 162.* 1313–1317.

Logan, W. W. & Norlund, A. W. (1979). Screen-film mammography technique: Compression and other factors. In: Logan, W. W., Muntz, E. P., eds. *Reduced dose mammography*. New York: Masson, 415–431.

National Council of Radiation Protection and Measurements. (1988). *Quality assurance for diagnostic imaging. NCRP Report No. 99*. Bethesda, MD: NCRP.

Ostrum, B. J., Becker, W., & Isard, H. J. (1973). Low-dose mammography. *Radiology. 109*, 323–326.

Sickles, E. A., & Feig, S. A. (1993). American College of Radiology statement on screening mammography for women 40–49. *ACR Bulletin. 49*, 5.

Tabar, L. & Haus, A. G. (1989). Processing mammographic films: Technical and clinical considerations. *Radiology. 173*, 65–69.

Vyborny, C. J. & Schmidt, R. A. (1989). Mammography as a radiographic examination: An overview. *RadioGraphics. 9*, 723–764.

Vyborny, C. J. & Schmidt, R. A. (1992). Technical image quality and the visibility of mammographic detail. In: Haus, A. G., Yagge, M. J., eds. *Syllabus: A categorical course in physics: technical aspects of breast imaging*. Oak Brook, IL: Radiological Society of North America, 85–93.

Weiss, J. P., & Wayrynen, R. E. (1976). Imaging system for low-dose mammography. *Journal of Applied Photographic Engineering. 2*, 7–10.

Wolfe, J. N. (1987). History and recent developments in xeroradiography of the breast. *Radiologic Clinics of North America. 25*, 929–937.

Yaffe, M. J. (1990). Physics of mammography: Image recording process. *RadioGraphics. 10*, 341–363.

CHAPTER **41**

Vascular Imaging Equipment

Joseph R. Bittengle M.Ed., R.T.(R) and Donna C. Davis M.Ed., R.T.(R)(CV)

During World War I the demand for x-ray technicians in military hospitals was so great that a shortage of technical workers became acute at home. The value of the well-trained technician was emphasized, and the radiologist was no longer satisfied with someone who knew only how to throw the switch and develop films.

Margaret Hoing (The First Lady of Radiologic Technology)
from A History of the American Society of X-Ray Technicians, 1952.

OBJECTIVES

Upon completion of this chapter, the student should be able to:

▶ Explain the various operational parameters of x-ray generating systems utilized for vascular imaging.

▶ Discuss the construction and operational parameters of x-ray tubes utilized for vascular imaging.

▶ Describe the structure and function of the C-arm assembly.

▶ Describe the essential operational characteristics of the angiographic table.

▶ Describe the operation and use of roll film and cut film changers.

▶ Explain the biplane imaging technique.

▶ Identify the advantages of biplane imaging technique.

▶ Describe the use of programmers during a vascular imaging procedure.

▶ Discuss the structure and operation of cineangiographic cameras as used during vascular imaging procedures.

▶ Describe the structure and operation of contrast medium injection devices.

▶ Identify quality control procedures specific to vascular imaging equipment.

The equipment in the vascular imaging suite is different from the imaging equipment found in the radiographic or fluoroscopic room. Vascular imaging requires rapid film changers and sequential filming. To accommodate rapid sequence filming, however, specialized generators and x-ray tubes must be available. The equipment found in a vascular imaging suite includes specialized programmers, which control the filming sequence with the flow of contrast medium through the anatomical part. Biplane imaging is used in some institutions to achieve two right angle projections with one contrast medium injection. Cineangiographic equipment is also available and most commonly utilized for cardiac catheterization procedures. A contrast medium injection device for the delivery of the contrast medium during the imaging procedure is also necessary.

No matter how specialized or sophisticated the imaging equipment may be, without a dedicated quality control program to ensure high-quality images and optimum on-demand operation, the execution of the imaging procedure could be ruined if proper preventative maintenance is ignored and a piece of equipment becomes inoperative. This chapter will discuss these issues as they pertain to vascular imaging equipment and vascular imaging procedures.

Generators

High-frequency generators offering high-performance capabilities are typically chosen for use during cardiovascular and interventional angiographic procedures. These generators should have a capacity of delivering 800 to 1,500 milliamperes (mA). These high mA stations permit the use of lower kilovoltage settings, which in turn improve the visibility of the contrast medium against the surrounding soft tissue structures. A generator that is capable of delivering a kilovoltage range of 50 to 100 peak kilovolts is desirable. Most angiographic studies are produced at kilovoltage peaks (kVp) in the range of 70 to 80 kVp to produce images exhibiting high radiographic contrast. Some special applications may require kVp values outside this range. Vascular procedures of the extremities may require lower kVp values, while magnification studies of the cerebral vessels may require higher kVp values.

The generator, in multiphasic or three phase format, offering the constant potential of 12 pulses per second provides the very short exposure times of at least one millisecond (0.001 second) as required during many cardiovascular and cineangiographic exposures.

Other advantages of this constant potential generator include the production of a nearly homogeneous radiation output and the resultant reduction in patient absorbed dose. (See Chapter 5 for additional discussion of these advantages.)

X-Ray Tubes

General Vascular

Angiographic x-ray tubes are different from general diagnostic imaging x-ray tubes in that the angiographic x-ray tubes must be able to withstand increased heat units while providing excellent detail. During angiography, fluoroscopy may be used for extended periods and many exposures may be made in rapid sequence in a short period of time, thus increasing the amount of heat generated at the anode. The amount of heat an anode can tolerate for a sequence of exposures is known as its **short-term loading ability**. The amount of heat the anode can tolerate during a fluoroscopic exposure is termed its **continuous heat loading ability**.

Short-term heat loading in the range of 15 to 50 kilowatts and a continuous heat loading of approximately 300 kilowatts are typical for a conventional angiographic x-ray tube constructed with a glass envelope and an 11° tungsten-rhenium-molybdenum alloy anode. Some angiographic x-ray tubes with an 11° tungsten-rhenium-molybdenum alloy anode and incorporating ceramic insulation technology with a metal tube envelope can withstand short-term heat loading in the range of 40 to 85 kilowatts and a continuous heat loading of approximately 750 kilowatts.

The maximum heat loading characteristics of an x-ray anode are measured by a calculation of the **heat units** generated at the anode. The equation to calculate heat units is:

$$H.U. = kVp \times mA \times s \times c \times exposures$$

where: H.U. = heat units
         kVp = peak kilovoltage
          mA = milliamperage
           s = time in seconds
           c = rectification constant
                single phase = 1
                three phase, six pulse = 1.35
                three phase, twelve pulse = 1.41
   exposures = number of consecutive exposures

Example: How many heat units are generated by a series of twelve exposures using 70 kVp, 300 mA, 0.1 second on a three phase, 6 pulse unit?

Answer: H.U. = 70 × 300 × 0.1 × 1.35 × 12
             H.U. = 34,020

34,020 heat units represent the total amount of heat generated at the anode for these twelve exposures.

Each angiographic x-ray tube is accompanied by a **tube rating chart** that indicates the safe maximum combination of kVp, mA, and time for a given exposure (Figure 41–1). The cardiovascular interventional technologist should consult the tube rating chart when there is a suspicion of exceeding the safe operating parameters of the x-ray tube for any given sequence of exposures.

The cardiovascular interventional technologist must consult the anode cooling and tube housing cooling charts, which indicate the amount of time one must wait between exposures, for cooling purposes, to be sure the maximum heat generated in the tube at the anode, or in the tube housing, does not exceed safe parameters

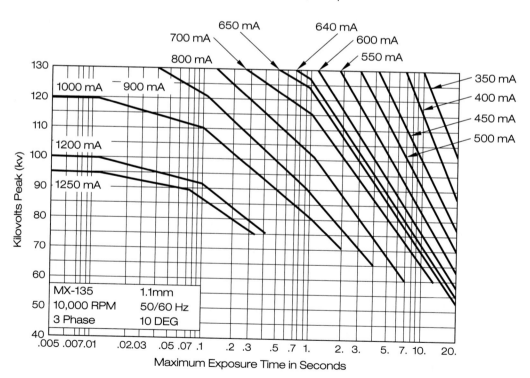

FIGURE 41-1. Single load tube rating chart for the Maxiray 135 Hexagraph x-ray tube. *(Courtesy of GE Medical Systems)*

(Figures 41–2 and 41–3). A detailed discussion of these charts may be found in Chapter 6.

The anode heating chart, also known as an input chart, combines the familiar cooling curve with curves indicating the rate of heat generated at the anode for a set of technical factors. One of the distinguishing characteristics of an input chart is the additional designation of joules along side heat units on the vertical axis. Another distinguishing characteristic is the numerous heat input curves with designated values in units of watts. For a known set of technical factors, the cardiovascular interventional technologist can determine the quantity of heat generated at the anode over a given time period (Figure 41–4).

The following equation may be used to determine the number of watts/second (heat units/second) that will be generated at the anode given these tehcnical factors:

400 mA   .10 second   75 kVp

$$400 \times 75 \times .1 = 3,000 \text{ W/sec}$$

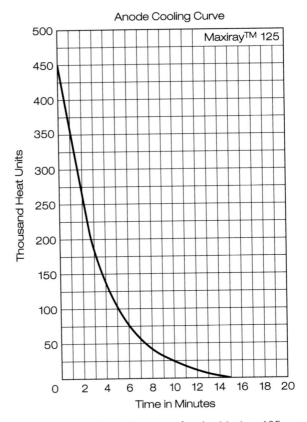

FIGURE 41-3. Anode cooling curve for the Maxiray 125 x-ray tube. *(Courtesy of GE Medical Systems)*

For example, the anode heating chart (Figure 41–4) indicates that at an input rate of 3,000 W/sec, after one minute of heating, 200,000 joules of energy will be delivered to the anode.

The heat loading capacity of an x-ray tube is dependent upon many factors, such as the focal spot size, the anode angle, the anode rotational speed, and the configuration of the generator. For example, larger focal spot sizes, larger target angles, higher anode rotational speeds, and the use of three phase, twelve pulse, or high-frequency generators would permit a greater heat loading capacity at the anode. It must be mentioned here that the use of a large focal spot during angiographic procedures is not always advisable. Large focal spot sizes render less recorded detail in the angiographic image. While using a small focal spot or small target angle does provide

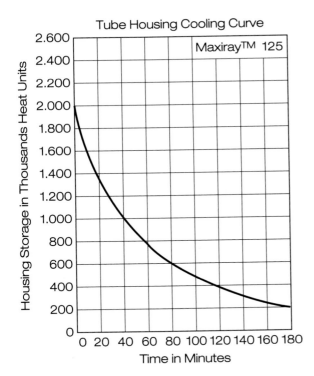

FIGURE 41-2. Tube housing cooling curve for the Maxiray 125 x-ray tube. *(Courtesy of GE Medical Systems)*

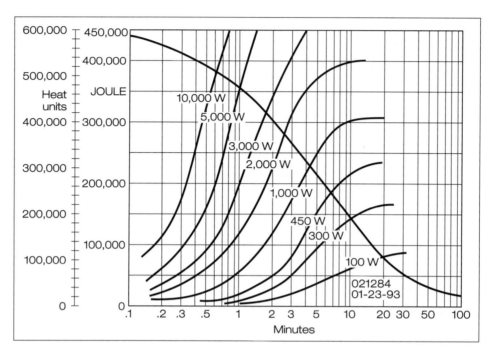

FIGURE 41-4. Anode heating and cooling chart. *(Courtesy of Eureka X-Ray Tube Corp.)*

greater detail in the image, there are some drawbacks to the use of a small target angle that the technologist must be aware of during imaging. These disadvantages include greater heat generated at the anode as previously mentioned, but additionally the small target angle provides a smaller field of coverage, also known as field of view (FOV) (Figure 41–5). In addition, the anode heel effect becomes more noticeable. There are situations when a small focal spot is advisable, such as magnification angiography of the cerebral vessels, during which a 0.3 mm focal spot or smaller is suggested. For other routine angiographic studies, radiographic tubes with focal spot sizes of 0.6 mm to 1.2 mm are generally satisfactory.

Another characteristic of the general vascular x-ray tube is found in the construction of the anode. Anodes, which must withstand greater heat loads, are constructed with a thicker molybdenum disk and a graphite backing. The thicker molybdenum disk allows the anode to withstand greater heat loading. The graphite backing helps to dissipate this heat more efficiently.

Cineangiographic Tubes

X-ray tubes used for cineangiography have many of the same characteristics as the general vascular x-ray tube. A notable difference is the introduction of a third electrode in the x-ray tube giving the cineangiographic x-ray tube its common names of either a **biased x-ray tube** or a **grid-controlled x-ray tube**. In a grid-controlled x-ray tube, the third electrode, or grid, is energized in an alternating sequence during the exposure, which results in a pulsing of the x-ray beam. The pulsation rate of the x-ray beam corresponds to the shutter speed of the cineangiographic film camera. The pulsing of the beam during a cineangiographic procedure, such as a left coronary arteriogram, has several advantages including a reduction in the exposure to the patient, a reduction in the amount of heat that is generated at the anode, and the delivery of extremely short exposure times.

Some cineangiographic x-ray tubes incorporate ceramic insulation technology and liquid metal lubricat-

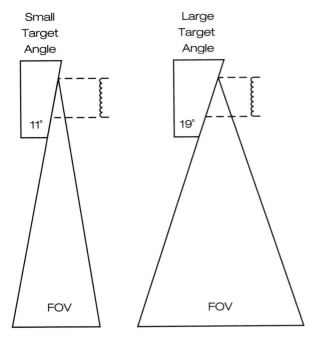

FIGURE 41-5. Comparison of field coverages at the same source-image distance for an 11° and a 19° target angle.

ed spiral groove bearings with a 9° tungsten-rhenium-molybdenum anode. This technology permits the cineangiographic x-ray tube to accommodate short-term loading in the range of 40 to 85 kilowatts and continuous loading of approximately 3,200 kilowatts (Figure 41–6). These loading characteristics permit the use of high mA techniques with extremely short exposure times for extended cineangiographic procedures. Additionally, delays in the cineangiographic procedure due to tube cooling purposes are reduced.

Special tube rating and anode cooling charts are also available for cineangiographic x-ray tubes. These charts are typically known as a **percent duty factor** or **percent duty cycle charts** and generally indicate the maximum amount of time the x-ray tube may be energized for any given sequence of exposures (Figure 41–7).

Because cooling does not occur between exposures during rapid serial imaging, a special rating chart is required for vascular and cineangiographic x-ray tubes. Since severe demands are placed on the x-ray tube, three factors are considered in the use of this chart: **percent duty cycle, series duration, and the product of kilovoltage times milliamperage.**

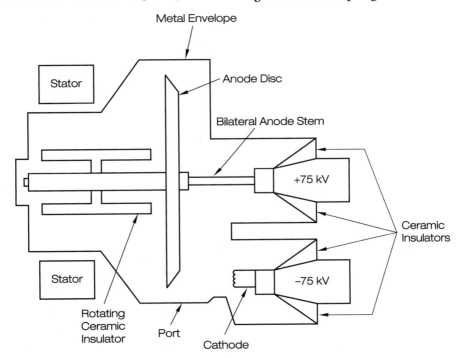

FIGURE 41-6. A bilateral-bearing, ceramic-insulated, high load x-ray tube with metal envelope

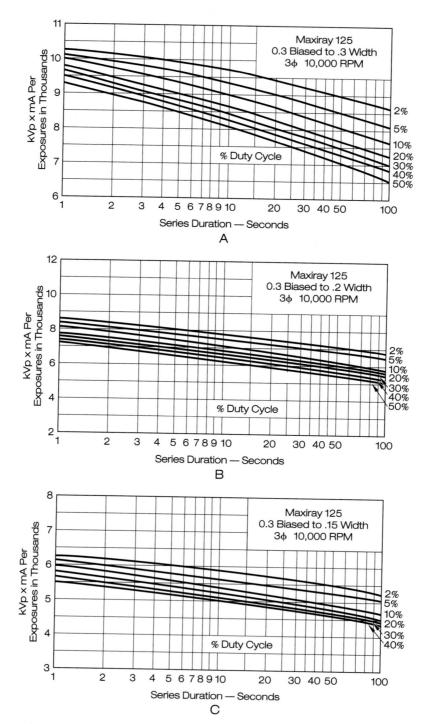

FIGURE 41-7. These percent duty cycle charts are used for three different focal spots available with the Maxiray 125 x-ray tube: (A) 0.3 mm focal spot, (B) 0.2 mm focal spot, and (C) 0.15 mm focal spot. *(Courtesy of GE Medical Systems)*

The following equations may be used to determine if an exposure series can be safely made within the rating of the particular focal spot:

$$\text{percent duty cycle} = t \times f \times 100$$

where: t = exposure time
f = maximum frame rate in the series

Example: What is the percent duty cycle if the desired imaging series is 2 films/second for 3 seconds and 4 films/second for 2 seconds (a total of 14 exposures) with a technique of 100 mA, 95 kVp, and 0.04 second?

Answer: Percent duty cycle = 0.04 × 4/second × 100 = 16 percent.

The percent duty cycle is 16 percent.

Most manufacturers provide a duty cycle chart that provides the percent duty cycle at a given exposure time and film frame rate (Figure 41–8).

The series duration can be calculated by the following equation:

$$\text{series duration} = \frac{E}{F}$$

where: E = total number of exposures in series
f = maximum frame rate in the series

Example: What is the series duration for the imaging parameters given in the previous example?

Answer:

$$\text{series duration} = \frac{16 \text{ exposures total}}{4 \text{ films/second}} = 4 \text{ seconds}$$

The series duration is 4 seconds.

In this same example of 100 mA, 95 kVp, and 0.04 second the product of kilovoltage and milliamperage equals 9,500.

$$kVp \times mA$$
$$95 \times 100 = 9,500$$

Using the 0.3 mm, 10° (175 mRad) percent duty cycle chart (Figure 41–9), enter the chart at 9,500 on the vertical axis for 4 seconds on the horizontal axis. The intersection of these factors is greater than the 50 percent duty cycle curve. Therefore, this exposure series is within the safe ratio of the focal spot. If the percent duty

Exposure Time	Film Frame Rate			
Seconds	2/sec.	4/sec.	6/sec.	8/sec.
.005	1.0%	2.0%	3.0%	4.0%
.0063	1.26%	2.52%	3.78%	5.04%
.008	1.6%	3.2%	4.8%	6.4%
.010	2.0%	4.0%	6.0%	8.0%
.013	2.6%	5.2%	7.8%	10.4%
.016	3.2%	6.4%	9.6%	12.8%
.020	4.0%	8.0%	12.0%	16.0%
.025	5.0%	10.0%	15.0%	20.0%
.032	6.4%	12.8%	19.2%	25.6%
.040	8.0%	16.0%	24.0%	32.0%
.050	10.0%	20.0%	30.0%	40.0%
.063	12.6%	25.2%	37.8%	50.4%
.080	16.0%	32.0%	48.0%	
.10	20.0%	40.0%	60.0%	
.13	26.0%	52.0%		
.16	32.0%	64.0%		

FIGURE 41-8. A duty cycle chart. (Courtesy of GE Medical Systems)

cycle interpolated from the chart is less than the calculated percent duty cycle (for example, 16 percent on the chart: 16 percent calculated) the exposure series is not within the safe ratio of the focal spot.

One of the following factors must be reduced to permit a safe series of exposures: mA, kVp, total number of exposures, or maximum frame rate.

C-Arm Assembly

The typical design of the dedicated angiographic imaging system uses either a C-arm or U-arm configuration (Figure 41–10).

The image intensifier, TV camera, and rapid film changer are mounted on one end of the C-arm. The angiographic x-ray tube is mounted on the opposite end.

The imaging assembly is capable of rotating at the point of attachment to the gantry. This allows the use of angled projections, such as the craniocaudal projection utilized for imaging the coronary arteries, and oblique projections, such as the left anterior oblique projection utilized for imaging the aortic arch, without needing to move the patient.

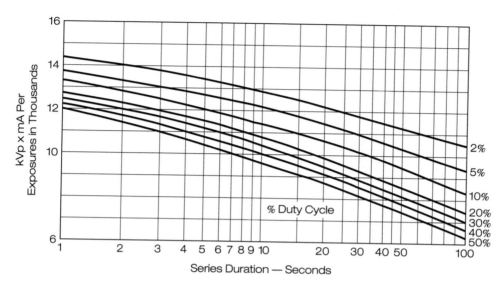

FIGURE 41-9. A percent duty cycle chart for a 0.3 mm, 10° (175 mRad), 3 phase, 10,000 rpm, 50/60 Hz Maxiray 125 x-ray tube. *(Courtesy of GE Medical Systems)*

An important design consideration of the C-arm is that the alignment of the angiographic x-ray tube to the image intensifier is such that the central ray of the x-ray beam is always perpendicular to the input phosphor of the image intensifier (Figure 41–11).

Angiographic Tables

The table used for angiographic procedures must contribute ease and convenience for the angiographer performing the procedure, must provide support and comfort to the patient, and must not degrade the diagnostic quality of the image.

The angiographic table must be capable of freely floating in all directions and should be capable of being raised and lowered. The table must be able to accommodate the attachment of manual controls, IV poles, restraining devices, contrast medium injection devices, and hemodynamic monitoring transducers.

The angiographic table may be floor mounted or suspended from the ceiling and is typically cantilevered to permit flexibility in positioning the patient in reference to the x-ray beam. Additionally, the angiographic table may be shaped to accommodate special procedural

needs. For example, the table used for cerebral angiography is narrower at the head end.

For ease and comfort of the patient, most angiographic tables are equipped with a foam pad. Arm boards

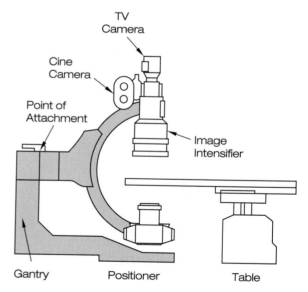

FIGURE 41-10. A typical C-arm configuration demonstrating the relationship of the cantilevered angiographic table to the tube-image intensifier axis. *(Courtesy of GE Medical Systems)*

can also be attached to the angiographic table to support the patient's extremity during the angiographic procedure (Figure 41–11).

Finally, the angiographic table should be composed of a low x-ray attenuation material. A composite of low radiation-absorbing plastic and carbon fiber is ideal. The quality of the diagnostic image is not compromised, and the exposure to the patient and the angiographic team is kept to a minimum when low attenuation tables are utilized.

A programmable **stepping device** may be attached to the angiographic table. This device is primarily used for angiography of the arterial structures of the lower extremities. This stepping device will permit movement of the angiographic table during contrast medium injection resulting in a sequential series of images from the pelvis to the feet. The technologist must be aware that the technical factors (mAs or kVp) should be appropriately adjusted for each anatomical segment of the lower extremity. For example, the technique required for the pelvis will be greater than that required for the feet.

Some institutions still use angiographic tables that permit full-length angiography of the lower extremity. This technique is performed using cassette changers or by using a single long-field cassette. This cassette changer utilizes three or four 14" × 51" cassettes with varying intensifying screen speeds. Images of the abdomen and pelvis require a higher speed screen than images of the legs and feet. A disadvantage to this graduated screen technique is the high radiation exposure received by the patient. An alternative method used with the cassette changer incorporates the use of a wedge-shaped compensatory filter attached to the tube collimator and rare-earth intensifying screens in the cassette. This combination effectively reduced patient exposure.

The use of the wedge filter coupled with the use of a long source-image distance (usually in excess of 72") and a single long-field cassette can also be used to produce an image of the lower extremity with a single exposure. The wedge filter compensates for various anatomic thicknesses and must be correctly placed on the x-ray tube such that the thinner section of the filter is positioned over the thicker portion of the anatomy.

Image Recording Devices

Since angiographic procedures typically evaluate the anatomy and physiology of the vascular structures under investigation, a method of recording dynamic events is required. The rapid film changer is a device that is able to record many images of the contrast medium flowing through the anatomy in a rapid sequence during angiography. There are generally two configurations for rapid film changers. They include roll film and cut film rapid changers.

Rapid Film Changers

Types **Roll film changers** were developed as early as 1925. Since 1925, there have been many improvements made to the roll film changer. The roll film changer operates on the same basic principle as that of the cine camera.

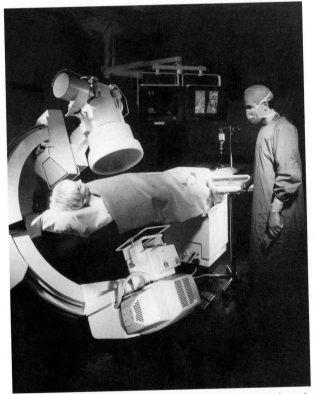

FIGURE 41-11. Advantx AFM C-arm assembly. Note that the central ray of the x-ray beam remains perpendicular to the image intensifier regardless of the C-arm angle. *(Courtesy of GE Medical Systems)*

Although roll film changers are no longer manufactured, it is still important to understand their basic operational parameters because they may still be used in some medical facilities.

The important components of the roll film changer are the **grid**, incorporated in the changer; the **upper and lower intensifying screens**; the **pressure plate**; the **film cutter**; and the **supply** and **receiving magazines** (Figure 41–12).

A linear, focused grid is located between the patient and the upper intensifying screen and is usually incorporated into the surface structure of the changer. The grid ratio and the grid frequency are dependent on the manufacturer's specifications and the angiographer's needs. The function of the grid is to absorb scattered radiation generated in the patient before it reaches the film thus reducing the amount of scatter on the angiogram.

The upper and lower intensifying screens function to enhance the ability of the x-ray beam to produce a diagnostic image on the film. During operation, the pressure of the screen against the film is relaxed as the film is moved into exposure position. Once the film is in the exposure position, the pressure plate is activated and compresses the upper and lower intensifying screens against the film ensuring uniform film/screen contact.

The film cutter is located near the receiving magazine. It permits the cardiovascular interventional technologist

to manually cut the roll film after the desired images have been obtained.

The supply magazine houses the unexposed roll film in a light-tight, lead-lined container. The roll film system is said to be in the ready position when the unexposed film is contained within the supply magazine prior to being moved into the exposure position. The supply magazine is capable of accommodating approximately 60 feet of unexposed roll film, which will permit approximately 60 exposures.

The receiving magazine is also a light-tight, lead-lined container. It receives the exposed roll film and permits the cardiovascular interventional technologist to remove the receiving magazine assembly for processing of the exposed roll film. The roll film system is said to be in the park position when exposed roll film is contained within the receiving magazine after exposure by radiation.

Cut film changers allow real-time monitoring of angiographic exposures. These see-through cut film changers permit the angiographic team to view the vascular anatomy during both the fluoroscopic and angiographic phases of the procedure. They consist of **a grid, two intensifying screens, compression plate, compression table, supply magazine, and a receiving cassette** (Figure 41–13).

The grid is situated between the patient and the compression plate and again functions to absorb scattered

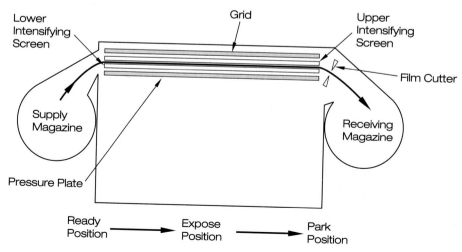

FIGURE 41-12. The roll film changer. Note film travels from the supply magazine (ready position) between the intensifying screens (expose position) into the receiving magazine (park position).

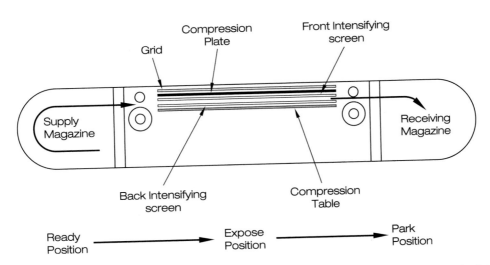

FIGURE 41-13. The cut film changer. Note film travels from the supply magazine (ready position) between the intensifying screens (expose position) into the receiving magazine (park position).

radiation before it strikes the film. The compression plate is composed of reinforced plastic and carbon fiber. It is located above the upper intensifying screen. The upper and lower intensifying screens again function to enhance the effects of the x-radiation in producing the diagnostic image. The compression table is situated below the lower intensifying screen.

The supply magazine is capable of holding 20 to 30 cut sheets of unexposed film depending on the manufacturer. The receiving cassette accepts the exposed cut film and permits the cardiovascular interventional technologist to easily transport the exposed cut film to the darkroom for processing.

Some cut film systems, when in the ready position, usually have 30 sheets of film in a curved pattern (film stack) within the supply magazine. The leading edge of the inside film is pulled between the intensifying screens and is in the exposure position. The compression table raises to ensure uniform film/screen contact. Following exposure, the compression plate relaxes and the exposed cut film is pulled into the receiving cassette and the system is now in the park position.

Table 41–1 discusses the differences between roll film and cut film changers.

Rapid film changers can be used in either the monoplane or biplane modes. The term **biplane** refers to the simultaneous production of angiographic images in two

planes. Ordinarily, the posteroanterior or anteroposterior and lateral projections are utilized (Figure 41–14).

Biplane imaging techniques during angiographic procedures have several advantages over monoplane imaging techniques. These advantages include the following: simultaneous imaging of vascular structures in two different planes; two projections of the anatomy can be obtained with a single injection of a contrast medium thus increasing the safety of the procedure for the patient; and the overall duration of the procedure can be shortened also making the procedure safer for the patient.

There are several technical considerations the cardiovascular interventional technologist must anticipate when using biplane imaging techniques. These considerations include: control of scattered radiation, limited filming rate, and appropriate selection of technical exposure factors.

TABLE 41–1. Comparison Of Roll And Cut Film Changers

Changer Type	Minimum Exposures/ Second	Maximum Exposures/ Second	Usual Filming Rate	Film Size
Roll	1 film/sec.	12 films/sec.	6 films/sec.	11" × 14"
Cut	1 film/sec.	6 films/sec.	3 films/sec.	14" × 14"

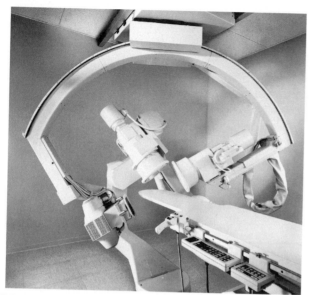

FIGURE 41-14. Advantx L/C-LP biplane C-arm assembly. (Courtesy of GE Medical Systems)

With simultaneous biplane imaging, scattered radiation is generated in two planes. With the additional scatter thus generated, the fogging effect on the angiographic image can be detrimental to the overall diagnostic quality of the image. There are several options for controlling this excess scattered radiation.

The use of a cross hatch (criss-cross) grid in the vertical changer will reduce the amount of scattered radiation reaching the vertical changer for the lateral projection. The technologist is reminded, though, the tube must remain perpendicular to the center of the vertical criss-cross grid thus allowing no tube angulation to the vertical film changer. A linear grid in the horizontal changer will reduce the amount of scattered radiation reaching the horizontal changer during the posteroanterior projection. The lead strips in the linear grid must be oriented parallel to the long axis of the angiographic table so angled tube techniques can be employed during selected angiographic procedures, such as cerebral arteriography.

An option for limiting the production of scattered radiation is the alternating of exposures between the horizontal and vertical planes. For example, the first film is exposed with a posteroanterior projection and the second film is exposed with a lateral projection. This pulsing of the x-ray beam effectively reduces the amount of scattered radiation produced.

Another option available for reducing the effects of scattered radiation is the use of ancillary devices such as the collimator keyhole aperture and scatter absorbing masks. A discussion of these optional devices can be found in Chapter 15.

An additional consideration the cardiovascular interventional technologist must anticipate is a limited filming rate in the biplane imaging mode. Typically, the maximum filming rate utilized for biplane angiography is 1.5 films/second. This limited filming rate results in the recording of less physiologic information.

The final consideration involves the manipulation of the technical exposure factors for the simultaneous biplane projections. A separate set of technical factors must be selected for the posteroanterior and lateral projections. When selecting technical factors, the cardiovascular interventional technologist must account for the difference in grid configuration and patient thickness in each plane.

Programmers
The programmer controls the duration of the exposure and the pulsing of the beam in synchronization with the transportation of the angiographic film through the rapid film changer.

Operational parameters manipulated by the programmer include: **maximum exposure time, total films exposed, filming rate, monoplane or biplane modes, stepping motion, filming pauses,** and **injector start.**

The operation of programmers that control the generator and the filming device are characterized by the concepts of **cycle time, time-in-motion (TIM), stationary time, zero time,** and **phase-in-time (PIT)** (Figure 41–15).

The cycle time is the total amount of time a particular rapid film changer requires for a film to leave the supply magazine, be transported into the exposure position, and be pulled into the receiving cassette.

The time-in-motion (TIM) is the total amount of transport time as stated as a percentage of the cycle time. A time-in-motion value of 60 percent is common.

Stationary time is the total amount of time the film is not moving and is also stated as a percentage of the cycle time. A stationary time of 40 percent is common. During a portion of the stationary time, the film is actually being exposed.

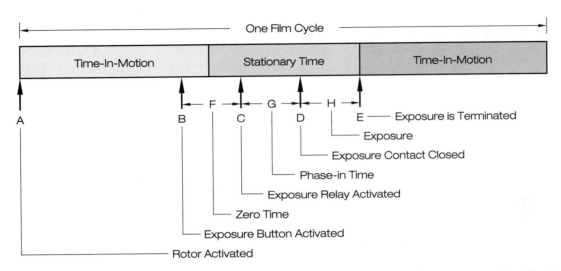

FIGURE 41-15. The relationship between the activation of the exposure by the generator to the movement of the film through the film changer: (A) rotor activated; (B) exposure button activated; (C) exposure relay activated; (D) exposure contact closed; (E) exposure terminated; (F) zero time; (G) phase-in time; (H) exposure.

Zero time is the time between the activation of the exposure button and the activation of the exposure relay in the exposure switch circuit. The zero time does not vary as it is constant for a particular imaging system. The zero time represents the time required for the circuitry to respond to the depression of the exposure switch.

The phase-in-time (PIT) is the time between the activation of the exposure relay and the actual closure of the exposure contact and initiation of the exposure. The phase-in-time can vary from 0 to 16 milliseconds since the exposure can only be initiated when the line voltage is zero.

The maximum exposure time is generally dependent upon the x-ray generator specifications, and most manufacturers provide maximum exposure time values in their operating instruction manuals. If such values are not given, the following equation may be used to calculate the maximum exposure time per film in the monoplane mode:

$$\text{max. exposure time/film} = \\ [\text{msec/film} \times (1 - \text{TIM})] - \text{max. PIT}^*$$

where: TIM = time in motion
          PIT = phase in time

Example: With a given time-in-motion value of 60 percent for a rapid film changer, what is the maximum

exposure time for each film with a filming rate of 3 films/second?

where: TIM = 60 percent
          max. PIT = 16 msec (constant)

1,000 msec/3 films = 333 msec/film

Answer: [(333)(1-60%)] − 16
          [(333)(40%)] − 16
          133.2 − 16 = 117.2 msec

The maximum exposure time for each film is 117 milliseconds.

The total number of images obtainable in a given filming run is calculated with the following equation:

$$\text{max. number of images} = \frac{d^*}{t + [t(\text{PIT})]}$$

where: d = duration of filming in
               milliseconds
          t = exposure time in milliseconds
               for each film
          PIT = phase-in time

Example: With a given phase-in time value of 40 percent for a rapid film changer, what is the maximum

*© 1994, J. Bittengle and D. Davis

number of images that can be obtained with a 200 millisecond exposure time with a 6 second filming run?

where: d = 6,000 msec
               t = 200 msec
         PIT = 40 percent

Answer:

$$\frac{6,000}{200 + [200(40\%)]} = \frac{6,000}{200 + 80} = \frac{6,000}{280} = 21.4$$

The maximum number of images that can be obtained is 21.

The filming rate is the number of images produced each second. Typical filming rates include: 1 film/sec., 1.5 films/sec., 2 films/sec., 3 films/sec., and 4 films/sec. The higher filming rates are capable of imaging more dynamic physiologic information. The total number of images produced in a given angiographic run can be calculated with the following equation:

$$\text{Total films} = [(\text{films/sec}) \times r]$$

where: films/sec. = the filming rate
                      r = duration of the filming run
                             in seconds

Example: If the filming rate is 2 films/sec. and the duration of the filming run is 5 seconds, how many total images will be produced?

where: films/sec. = 2
                      r = 5

Answer: (2)(5) = 10 films

The total number of images produced is 10.

The programmer also permits the cardiovascular interventional technologist to choose between monoplane imaging (as may be used for an aortofemoral runoff [AFRO]) or biplane imaging (as may be used for cerebral angiography). If the imaging table is equipped with a stepping device, the motion of the stepping device during the exposure can also be controlled by the programmer. Additionally, the initiation of the injection of the contrast medium by the automatic injection device can be controlled by the programmer.

Cineangiographic Cameras

Cineangiographic imaging systems are typically used for cardiac catheterization procedures to provide detailed images of fast moving anatomic structures, such as the beating, contrast medium-filled heart. Cine film systems generally provide better spatial image detail than electronic or magnetic recording devices but at a higher radiation dose to the patient. Digital imaging systems, however, generally provide better contrast resolution due to post-procedural computer enhancement.

In the United States, cine images are usually recorded on 35 mm roll film. The 16 mm roll film is seldom used today in this country (Table 41–2).

To properly expose cine film, a pulsed x-ray beam and special camera are required. The x-ray beam is pulsed and synchronized with the movement of the shutter and the transportation of the film in the cine camera.

The x-ray beam is pulsed or synchronized by using a grid-controlled x-ray tube and a constant potential generator. The x-ray beam is activated when the shutter is open and the film has been transported to proper position. At the termination of the exposure, the shutter is closed and the film is transported so the next frame is in position for exposure. Because the x-ray tube is not energized when the film is being advanced into the exposure position, this pulsed, intermittent beam delivers a lower dose to the patient than the older continuous beam models.

With a single phase generator, filming rates of 7.5 frames/second, 15 frames/second, 30 frames/second, and 60 frames/second, are common. The technologist must be aware that the patient exposure is higher with increased filming rates. These filming rates are dependent upon the 60 Hz voltage frequency available with single-phase generators.

TABLE 41–2. Comparison Of Cine Films

	35 mm	**16 mm**
Frames/foot	16	40
Radiation dose	higher	lower
Image quality	higher	lower
Frame size	22 mm × 18 mm	10.5 mm × 7.5 mm

The filming rate with three phase, twelve pulse generators is not dependent on the voltage frequency. Therefore, other filming rates, such as 12 frames/second, 24 frames/second, 48 frames/second, and faster, are possible.

When viewing cineangiographic images, slow motion can be achieved by using a higher filming rate (60 frames/second) and projecting the images at a slower viewing rate (30 frames/second). Normal motion is achieved by viewing the images at the same rate as the filming rate. Filming rates less than 30 frames/second generally produce a noticeable "flicker" during the angiographic procedure.

Three important subsections of the cineangiographic imaging system are the **automatic brightness control**, the **beam-splitting mirror**, and the **cine camera**. The automatic brightness control (ABC) device adjusts the kVp, mA, or both to compensate the beam quality and/or quantity for differences in anatomic thickness or density. The beam-splitting mirror converts approximately 10 percent of the image to the television viewing system and directs approximately 90 percent of the image to the cine camera. The beam-splitting mirror permits simultaneous cine recording and television viewing during the procedure. This simultaneous cine and television viewing increases patient exposure compared to cine recording without simultaneous television viewing.

The cine camera is similar to a motion picture camera. The major components of the cine camera include: **lens, iris diaphragm, shutter, aperture, pressure plate, transport mechanism**, and **film supply** and **take-up reels** (Figure 41–16).

The optical lens focuses the light from the output phosphor of the image intensifier tube onto the cine film.

The iris diaphragm is located between the lens and the shutter and restricts the divergence of the light from the lens. The shutter is a rotating half-disc situated in front of the aperture (Figure 41–17). As the shutter rotates, it interrupts the flow of light to the film. The shutter opening is approximately 160° to 180°. The aperture is a rectangular opening in the front of the camera that further restricts the amount of light entering the camera.

The pressure plate is behind the aperture, in the cine camera, and assures the film is in firm contact with the aperture.

A synchronous motor transports the cine roll film from the supply reel, past the aperture, and to the take-up reel. As the shutter closes, a pulldown arm advances the next frame of the cine roll film into position for exposure. When the shutter opens, the cine film is stationary and the frame is exposed (Figure 41–18).

Some newer synchronized cineangiographic systems using a pulsed beam and constant potential generators have eliminated the need for a shutter.

The required minimum exposure time and film frame advance-time are dependent upon the size of the shutter opening and the filming rate. The following equation can be used to calculate the amount of time required for the exposure to occur and the transportation of one frame by the pulldown arm:

$$\text{total exposure plus transport time} = \frac{(s/360°)^*}{f}$$

where: s = shutter opening in degrees
f = filming rate in frames/second

Example: What is the total exposure and pulldown time for a 180° shutter opening with a filming rate of 30 frames/second?

Answer: $s = 180°$
$f = 30$ frames/second

$$\frac{(180/360)}{30} = \frac{0.5}{30} = 0.0166 \text{ or } 1/60 \text{ second}$$

The total exposure and pulldown time is 1/60 second.

Cine framing is defined as the amount of film surface used to generate the image. The framing is controlled by the optic lens and is usually set to manufacturer specifications. Two types of framing are exact framing and over-framing. A comparison of exact framing and over-framing is discussed in Table 41–3.

Cineangiographic film should have a relatively high speed, have a high inherent contrast level, and be capable of recording fine detail. The resolving power of a cine system is primarily dependent on the size of the image intensifier input phosphor, the resolving power of the input phosphor, and the film dimension utilized. The following equation may be used to calculate the resolution of a given cine imaging system:

*© 1994, J. Bittengle and D. Davis

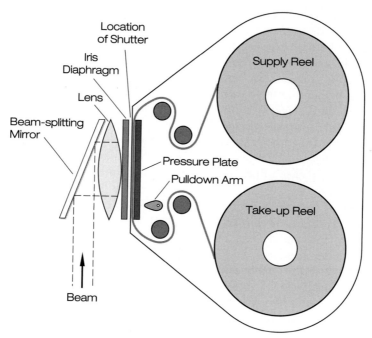

FIGURE 41-16. A typical cine camera

$$\text{cine resolution} = (a) \ \frac{(b)(2.54)^*}{f}$$

where: a = input phosphor resolving power in lines/mm

b = input phosphor diameter in inches

f = frame dimension utilized in centimeters

Example: What is the resolution of the cine imaging system when exact framing is used with a 35 mm cine film and a 9 inch input phosphor with a resolving power of 3 lines/mm?

Answer:

a = 3

b = 9

f = 1.8

$$\frac{(9)(2.54)}{1.8} = 38 \text{ lines/mm}$$

The resolving power of this cine system is 38 lines/mm.

*© 1994, J. Bittengle and D. Davis

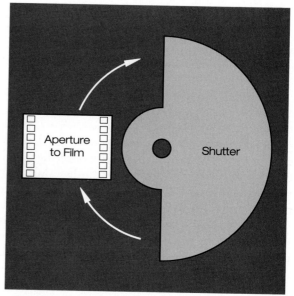

FIGURE 41-17. The relationship of the shutter to the aperture in a cine camera with the shutter open.

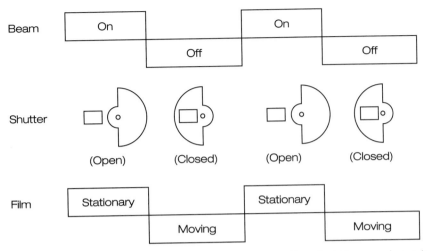

FIGURE 41-18. Synchronization of the x-ray beam, shutter, and film transport. Note that the x-ray beam is off and the shutter is closed during transportation of the film.

Contrast Medium Injection Devices

Pressure injector devices are used to deliver a safe, uniform quantity of contrast medium under controlled conditions into a vascular structure during some angiographic procedures (Figure 41–19). Other angiographic procedures, such as coronary arteriography, generally require a hand injection by the physician.

The major components of the contrast medium injection device include the **control panel, syringe, warming device** and **pressure mechanism** (Figure 41–20).

The control panel permits the cardiovascular interventional technologist to manipulate the injection

parameters. New computerized control panels can store injection parameter protocols in their memory and also can provide an injection history of the patient.

The syringe is most commonly a disposable type that is removable from the injection device. Depending on the manufacturer, the capacity of the syringe may vary from 40 to 260 cc. The contrast medium filled syringe is placed inside the syringe-loading assembly for procedural use.

The warming device is a thermal sleeve located near the syringe loading assembly. The function of the warming device is to maintain the temperature of the contrast medium at or near body temperature (37°C, 98.6°F). The warming device should not be used to bring the contrast medium from room temperature up to 37°C. The contrast medium, therefore, must be warmed prior to being drawn into the syringe.

The pressure mechanism consists of an electro-mechanical motor attached to a jackscrew. The pressure mechanism is capable of moving the injector piston, which in turn moves the syringe plunger forward or backward as desired.

Injection parameters which are controlled by the contrast medium injection device include **flow rate, total volume, pressure (psi), rate rise**, and **delay**.

Flow rate is the number of cubic centimeters of contrast medium delivered every second (cc/sec.). Five fac-

TABLE 41–3. Comparison Of Exact Framing And Overframing

	Exact Framing	Over-Framing
Film area covered	~79%	100%
Film dimension utilized	18 mm	22 mm
Image size	smaller	larger
Patient exposure	lower	higher

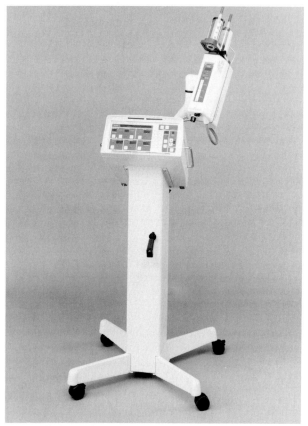

FIGURE 41-19. MedRad Mark V Plus Pedestal Injector. *(Courtesy of MedRad)*

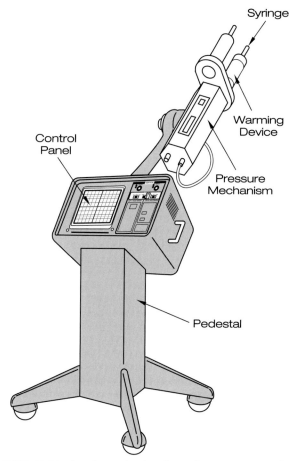

FIGURE 41-20. A schematic drawing of a contrast-medium injection device demonstrating its major components.

tors affect the flow rate: viscosity of the contrast medium, length of the angiographic catheter, internal diameter of the angiographic catheter, injection pressure, and number of side holes in the angiographic catheter.

The viscosity of the contrast medium can be altered by either warming the contrast medium to body temperature or by choosing a contrast medium with reduced iodine content. The effects of viscosity and the other four factors are discussed in Table 41–4.

The total volume of contrast medium injected is calculated by the following equation:

$$V = (cc/sec.)s$$

where:
V = total volume
cc/sec. = flow rate
s = injection time in seconds

Example: What is the total volume if a 2 cc/sec. flow rate is used during a 5 second injection?

Answer: cc/sec. = 2
$$s = 5$$
$$(2)(5) = 10$$

The total volume of contrast medium injected is 10 cc.

The pressure of the injection is measured in pounds per square inch (psi). The common range of pressure values is 100 to 1,000 psi. For example, a typical psi setting for cerebral angiography may be 600 psi. The cardiovas-

TABLE 41–4. Factors Affecting Flow Rate

Viscosity	Lower viscosity permits higher flow rates
Catheter Length	Shorter catheters permit higher flow rates
Catheter Internal Diameter	Larger internal diameters permit higher flow rates
Injection Pressure	Higher PSIs permit higher flow rates
Catheter Sideholes	The presence of sideholes in the catheter permits higher flow rates

cular interventional technologist should consult the manufacturer insert information in determining the safe pressure limits of the particular catheter in use.

Rate rise or acceleration regulation permits the injection pressure or flow rate to slowly rise to the desired level over 0.2 to 2.0 seconds. For example, if 200 psi is selected at a rate rise of 0.4 seconds, the psi will slowly rise to the desired level of 200 psi exactly 0.4 second after the initiation of the injection. The rate rise feature permits biphasic and multiphasic injections.

The delay control permits a pause in the initiation of the injection and/or the exposure. For example, when performing a lower extremity arteriogram via a femoral puncture, a delay in exposure may be necessary to image only the vessels distal to the knee.

Safety features of the contrast medium injection device include a mechanical volume limit and a pressure limit. The mechanical volume limit prevents the delivery of more contrast medium than selected for the procedure. The pressure limit allows the selection of the maximum pressure that can be developed during the procedure.

An optional feature of the contrast medium injection device is the incorporation of cardiac gating (ECG triggering). Cardiac gating may be utilized during a cardiac catheterization procedure while performing a left ventriculogram. The cardiac gating device synchronizes the injection of contrast medium with the r wave impulse of the patient's cardiac cycle. This gating technique results in lower incidence of cardiac arrhythmias and tends to reduce the volume of contrast medium required.

Other contrast medium injection devices have been specially designed for computed tomography and lymphography which incorporate features specific to these imaging procedures.

Quality Control

Quality control procedures in a cardioangiographic suite are important components of an institution's ongoing commitment to ensure the safe utilization of imaging equipment and to produce the highest quality image with the least amount of radiation exposure and at the lowest cost.

The various types of imaging equipment in the angiographic suite and the cardiac catheterization laboratory are typically some of the more expensive pieces of equipment in the medical facility. The condition of patients examined with this equipment tends to be more critical. The radiation dose received by the patient and the members of the angiographic team tends to be higher than for other imaging modalities. For these three reasons, a dedicated quality control program is essential to the continual operation of the vascular imaging department.

Components of the vascular quality control program should include periodic monitoring of the film processing and viewing systems, evaluation of the external beam, and assessment of ancillary equipment. (A discussion of processor monitoring and external beam evaluation can be found in Chapter 30 of this text.) Evaluative techniques used to monitor angiographic and cineangiographic equipment are similar to the monitoring techniques used for general radiographic, fluoroscopic, and film processing equipment. An additional schedule for monitoring the operation of the cine camera, film changer, cine projector, contrast medium injection device and cardiac monitoring device must be incorporated into the cineangiographic quality control program.

Specifically, the lenses of the cine camera should be inspected and cleaned with a fine hair brush every month. The cine camera magazine should be inspected for emulsion build-up, smooth operation of the take-up arm, and the accumulation of flecks of broken film every day. The intensifier screens of the film changer should be inspected and cleaned with a fine hair brush every month. The lenses of the cine projector should be inspected and cleaned with a fine hair brush every month. The uniformity of the intensity of light output of the cine projector viewing screen should be evaluated monthly. The safety devices of the contrast medium injection device (volume limiter and pressure limiter) should be tested monthly. The cardiac monitoring device should be inspected prior to each use.

In all cases, the cardiovascular interventional technologist should consult the manufacturer's recommended schedule for preventative maintenance and service for each piece of equipment used in the angiographic and cardiac catheterization suites. Contracts with service personnel specifically trained to monitor and correct faulty imaging equipment or the establishment of an in-house biomedical instrumentation department are of utmost importance in ensuring an imaging department, which consistently produces the highest quality images at the lowest radiation dose and at the lowest cost.

Summary

The angiographic and cineangiographic imaging suites contain specialized equipment for producing high quality images of contrast-filled vascular structures in the body.

A three-phase or high-frequency, constant potential generator capable of delivering 800 to 1,500 milliamperes and 50 to 100 peak kilovolts is advisable. The conventional general vascular x-ray tube should have a short-term heat loading rating of 15 to 50 kilowatts and a continuous heat loading rating of 300 kilowatts. A grid controlled x-ray tube is used for cineangiographic procedures. Tube rating, anode cooling, tube housing cooling, and percent duty cycle charts should be consulted prior to the formulation of exposure techniques during a vascular procedure. A C-arm assembly with a cantilevered table and biplane film changers are often available.

Programmers that coordinate the synchronization of the x-ray beam with the transportation of the film through the rapid film changer are also utilized for vascular procedures. Specialized cineangiographic cameras are used for cardiac catheterization procedures to produce a motion picture image of the flow of contrast medium through a vessel.

The contrast medium may be injected by hand or by the use of a contrast medium injection device. This device is capable of delivering a uniform injection at a constant flow rate and pressure.

A quality control program for a vascular or cineangiographic suite should incorporate an evaluation schedule of the film processing and viewing systems, the external x-ray beam and ancillary equipment used during the procedure. The goals of the quality control program should be to ensure the safe operation of the imaging equipment, to produce the highest quality image, to reduce radiation exposure to the patient and staff, and to maintain costs as low as achievable.

REVIEW QUESTIONS

1. What are two important characteristics of the x-ray generator used for vascular procedures?

2. What is the total heat units generated by a vascular x-ray tube for a series of ten exposures using 400 mA, 0.1 second, 74 kVp, on a three phase, twelve pulse unit?

3. What is the percent duty cycle for a cineangiographic tube operated at 100 mA, 90 kVp, 0.03 second for a series of 2 films/second for 2 seconds and 3 films/second for 3 seconds?

4. What is the most important design consideration of the C-arm assembly?

5. What materials should be used in the construction of the angiographic table?

6. What is the function of the compression table in a cut film changer?

7. What is the maximum exposure time for each film if the time-in-motion of the film changer is 60 percent and the filming rate is 4 films/second?

8. What is the total number of angiographic images exposed if the duration of the filming run is 6 seconds with a 3 film/second filming rate?

9. Define biplane imaging.

10. What are the advantages of biplane imaging techniques over monoplane imaging techniques?

11. How is the x-ray beam pulsed during a cineangiographic exposure?

12. What device in the cineangiographic imaging system adjusts the brightness of the image?

13. List the operational parameters of a contrast medium injection device.

14. List the major components of a quality control program for vascular imaging equipment.

REFERENCES AND RECOMMENDED READING

Behling, R. (1990). The MRC 200: A new high-output x-ray tube. *Medica Mundi. 35*, 49–56.

Bushong, S. C. (1997). *Radiologic science for technologists: Physics, biology, and protection.* (6th ed.). St. Louis: C. V. Mosby.

Cullinan, A. & Cullinan, J. (1994). *Producing quality radiographs.* (2nd ed.) Philadelphia: J.B. Lippincott.

Curry, T. S., Dowdey, J. E., & Murry, R. C. (1990). *Christensen's introduction to the physics of diagnostic radiology.* (4th ed.). Philadelphia, PA: Lea & Febiger.

Grossman, W. & Baim, D. S. (1991). *Cardiac catheterization, angiography, and intervention.* (4th ed.). Philadelphia, PA: Lea & Febiger.

Kandarpa, K. (1989). *Handbook of cardiovascular and interventional radiologic procedures.* Boston, MA: Little, Brown & Co.

Laudicina, P. & Wean, D. (1994). *Applied angiography for radiographers.* Philadelphia, PA: W. B. Saunders Co.

Schreiber, P. (1990). Heat management in x-ray tubes. *Medica Mundi. 35*, 57–64.

Snopek, A. M. (1999). *Fundamentals of special radiographic procedures.* (4th ed.). Philadelphia: W. B. Saunders.

Tortorici, M. (1992). *Concepts in medical radiographic imaging.* Philadelphia: W. B. Saunders.

CHAPTER **42**

Digital Image Processing

. . . the digital computer has revolutionized virtually every element of diagnostic imaging . . . diagnostic imaging is one of the most exciting and rapidly evolving fields of medicine, and without question is leading all of medicine into the computer-electronic era.

William R. Hendee, Preface to Christopher C. Kuni's
Introduction to Computers and Digital Processing in Medical Imaging.

OBJECTIVES

Upon completion of this chapter, the student should be able to:

▶ Describe the differences between analog and digital computers.

▶ Describe the differences between programs and data.

▶ State reasons why binary machine code is used in place of other languages.

▶ Describe the basic function of a central processing unit, read only memory and random access memory.

▶ Describe the basic function of various memory storage, input and output devices.

▶ Explain the basic function of an array processor.

▶ Describe the process of digital image data acquisition.

▶ State reasons why Fourier transformation and inverse Fourier transformation are used in digitization of imaging data.

▶ State the function of convolution and deconvolution.

▶ Describe the effects of frequency, contrast and noise on digital image quality.

▶ Explain the function of digital image window level and width controls.

▶ Describe various factors that directly affect digital image resolution.

▶ Explain the digital subtraction process and various filtering techniques.

▶ Describe a digital picture archiving and communication system (PACS).

*T*he future of medical imaging lies unquestionably in computerized applications of the numerous modalities that currently exist, as well as in the integration of those now on the horizon. The explosion of the imaging sciences that took place between the early 1970s and the 1990s was caused by the first wave of digital computerization in computed tomography (CT) and ultrasound. Computed tomography has captured the imagination of the public; digital processing has now been successfully applied to nuclear medicine, cardiovascular imaging and magnetic resonance imaging (MRI), and is now beginning to predominate in diagnostic imaging as well.

The method by which these imaging modalities have been computerized is digital processing of imaging information. The resulting images have enabled radiographers to understand anatomy from transverse, sagittal and coronal perspectives. Those who work in the digital computerized modalities must often visualize anatomy as a dynamic three-dimensional tilting, rotating and tumbling process due to computer manipulation of imaging data.

The Computer

Computers are devices that process information. The earliest computer device, the abacus, dates to around 3,000 B.C., and calculating machines were developed in the 1600s. The modern electronic computer, ENIAC, was developed in 1945 at the University of Pennsylvania. The addition of the mathematical theories of Baron Jean Fourier (1768–1830) and George Boole (1815–1864), solid state electronics in the 1940s, and microchip technology in the 1960s were all required prior to the first digital computer applications in medical imaging.

Analog and Digital Computers

Analog computers handle data composed of continuously varying electrical currents. Digital computers handle data composed of definite quantities of current (i.e., current on versus current off). For example, an analog watch displays time with hands while a digital watch uses a numerical readout. All medical imaging is achieved with digital computers, often from information that has been processed by an analog-to-digital converter (ADC). Digitization of analog information, such as the vast number of incident photons that comprise a radiographic image, always reduces the quantity and quality of the remaining information. Figure 42–1 illustrates the digitization process. Digital-to-analog converters (DAC) are sometimes used to permit faster transmission of data. After transmission, an ADC is used to convert the data for digital display or processing.

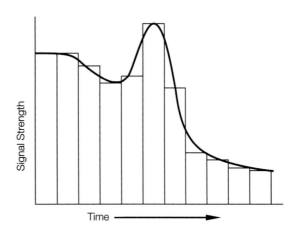

FIGURE 42-1. Analog-to-digital conversion of imaging information. The line represents the input data; the blocks represent the digitization of the data.

Programs and Data

Computers use two types of information: operating instructions, called the **program** and collected facts, called **data**. Programs provide specific instructions for calculations and sequential steps to be followed. Special computer languages are used for programming. Programs are called **software** while computer equipment is called **hardware**. One of the most useful programming techniques is the ability to program a computer to do problem solving, such as an if-then statement in which a computer can determine if a condition has been met, and then perform various operations depending on the exact conditions.

1	read memory 1
2	if memory 1 is less than 5 then go to line 5
3	if memory 1 equals 5 then go to line 6
4	if memory 1 is greater than 5 then go to line 7

For example, this program provides three alternative actions depending on the value of the information stored in memory 1. Complex programs have many alternative functions that can be performed as variables are processed by the computer.

Binary Machine Language

Computers operate from a **binary machine language**. Just as English has a 26 letter symbol alphabet, the binary system operates with a two symbol alphabet. Because electrical currents are most easily understood as being either on or off, the binary system consists of information recorded as either a zero for off or a one for on. Each binary number is called a **bit**, for **b**inary dig**it**s. Nominal numbers function on a base 10 system instead of base 2. Table 42–1 illustrates how the numbers 1 through 10 are written in binary code. An eight bit word is required to form the 26 letters of the English alphabet. As a convenience, an eight bit word is called a **byte**. Computer mem-

TABLE 42–1. Binary Code Numbers

Arabic	Binary
1	1
2	10
3	11
4	100
5	101
6	110
7	111
8	1000
9	1001
10	1010
.	.
.	.
.	.
16	10000
.	.
.	.
32	100000
.	.
.	.
.	.
etc.	

ory is often rated in terms of the total byte memory (rounded off). For example, a 10 megabyte magnetic hard disk will store over 10,000,000 bytes (80,000,000 bits) of information.

Central Processing Unit (CPU)

The CPU is the heart of every computer. It directs information to and from the various components that make up the computer system. For example, when a computer is turned on, the CPU may extract information from a permanent memory that loads an operating system program into the working memory. This operating system may then display instructions on a cathode ray tube (CRT) monitor. When a keyboard is used to input information, the CPU may then extract a program from memory and begin to carry out its instructions to operate imaging equipment.

The electrical connections between the CPU and the components run along a system of parallel or series conductors called a **bus**. Parallel connections permit simultaneous transmission of information but they are expensive because a separate conductor must exist for each channel of information. Serial connectors are less expensive but require significantly more transmission time because information must be transmitted sequentially instead of simultaneously. Peripheral devices, such as memory storage units, printers, modems and imaging systems, also use parallel and serial connectors.

Memory

Information can be stored in a computer's memory as magnetic variations and can be transferred as voltage. Magnetic field direction or greater and lesser voltage represent "on," or 1, and "off," or 0 indications. Memory is also classified as **read** memory or **write** memory. Read memory simply extracts information without alteration. Write memory replaces (deletes) old memory with new information.

ROM AND RAM Memory is classified as read only memory (ROM) or random access memory (RAM). Both standard ROM and programmable ROM (PROM) usually contain basic operating instructions that are rarely, if ever, changed. The RAM usually functions as temporary storage for programming and operating instructions during their use and is constantly changed. When the main power to the computer is turned off, RAM is erased while ROM is maintained.

Bus

A bus is the system of conductors that connects the various components of a computer system. It functions in a manner similar to a city bus route in that it permits the computer processing system to accept inputs from any point along the conductor, as if it were a bus picking up jobs to do instead of people to carry. The bus speed is critical to how fast the computer system can function. For example, a 120 MHz system is significantly more efficient than an old 12 MHz system.

Peripherals

Peripheral devices permit input and/or output of information to and/or from the CPU. Some peripherals may appear to be a physical part of the computer, such as an input memory disk drive, while others may appear to be separate devices, such as a paper printer.

Memory Storage Devices   A number of memory storage devices for data have become popular. These include **magnetic** and **optical** recording on both **tape** and **disk**. Information can be stored by optical (laser) recording and reading as well as by electronic and magnetic fields. Magnetic tape is often called mag tape and, although inexpensive, is difficult to access because data is stored serially. Consequently it is seldom used today. Magnetic disks have evolved from large (8") to small (5¼") **floppy disks** and finally to even smaller (3½") **diskettes**. For large amounts of data a **hard disk** is required. Optical tape and disks permit the storage of significantly more data. Medical imaging modalities have used all of these devices for storing images and their associated data. Table 42–2 illustrates typical memory requirements for various imaging modalities.

Input Devices   The most familiar computer input device is a keyboard with a CRT for visualization of information before it is sent into the CPU. For example, a CT unit may wait for an entire examination protocol to be entered before it is sent to the CPU. In addition to keyboards, some units provide a visual marker known as a **cursor** on the CRT screen. The cursor can be moved by keyboard arrows, a joystick, track ball, pad and pen, light or ultrasonic pen or a specialized sliding control unit called a **mouse**. Some radiographic equipment uses a CRT touch screen for input, and voice-activated units will be feasible eventually. Input via these devices can be remarkably simple. For example, ultrasound units will place a centimeter ruler through the anatomical image from a cursor location and CT units will provide radiation attenuation coefficient numbers (CT numbers) for the tissue at the cursor location. Image receptors, such as television cameras, ultrasonic transducers, CT ion detectors and MRI radiofrequency detectors also input information signals to CPUs for processing into visual images.

Output Devices   The most familiar output devices are CRT screens and paper printers. Computerized

TABLE 42–2. Typical Memory Requirements for Various Imaging Modalities

Imaging Modality	Typical Image Memory Size	Images Per Typical Exam	Total Memory Requirements
Mammography	50 Mb	7	350 Mb
Digital Radiography	10 Mb	4	40 Mb
Digital Fluoroscopy	2 Mb	15	30 Mb
Computed Tomography	500 Kb	120	60,000 Mb (60 Gb)
Computed Tomography Spiral	500 Kb	200	100,000 Mb (100 Gb)
Ultrasound	250 Kb	24	6,000 Mb (6 Gb)
Magnetic Resonance Imaging	125 Kb	70	1,050 Mb (1 Gb)
Nuclear Medicine	10 Kb	20	200 Mb

imaging systems often send output information directly to CRT or laser film recording systems for the production of visual images. Most computerized imaging systems incorporate both input and output CRTs into their control consoles. Some computers use a single CRT for both input and output information.

Array Processors　　An array processor is a specialized computer that functions as a peripheral. It uses its CPU memory to perform simultaneous mathematical operations in a parallel fashion at extremely high speed instead of performing them sequentially. Array processors are useful when vast numbers of repetitive calculations are required, as in the processing of image detector data from CT or MRI equipment.

Image Processing

Digital Image Acquisition

A digital image is one that has been converted into numerical values for transmission or processing. A detector of some type must be used to acquire the image information. There are many types of detectors for various types of input information — ionizing radiation,

ultrasonic waves, radiofrequencies, etc. Detectors acquire information either by **scanning** an area for information or by area or **array** detection, in which information is received from an entire area at once. For example, a fluoroscopic image is digitized by the plumbicon™ camera for transmission to the display monitor CRT. Although the CRT image is of significantly less resolution than the original image, it is simply a matter of numbers. The CRT is limited to 525 or 1,050 lines of resolution while the primary photon beam has millions of incident photons. If the CRT could display millions of lines of data, the image would exhibit comparable resolution. Most CRTs are capable of only 1–2 lp/mm.

Although digital images currently have diagnostic limits due to resolution, as display capabilities increase diagnostic confidence will also increase. Computerized digital images are described in terms of the number of values displayed per image side. A **matrix** is a square series of boxes that gives form to the image (Figure 42–2A). Each box of an image matrix will display a numerical value which can be transformed into a visual brightness or density level (Figure 42–2B & C). The individual matrix boxes are known as picture elements or pixels. The greater the matrix size the better the resolution because a larger matrix provides smaller **pixels**. Pixel size determines resolution (Figure 42–3). Each pixel

A.

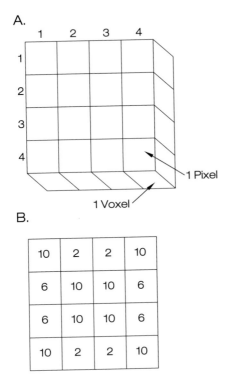

B.

10	2	2	10
6	10	10	6
6	10	10	6
10	2	2	10

C.

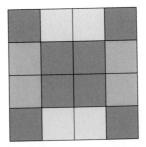

FIGURE 42-2. Digital image matrix expressions: (A) a matrix, (B) a matrix with numerical values, and (C) a matrix with visual density values corresponding to the numerical values in B.

TABLE 42–3. Typical Matrix Sizes for Various Imaging Modalities

Imaging Modality	Typical Image Matrix Size
Mammography	$4,000 \times 4,000$
Digital Radiography	$2,000 \times 2,000$
Digital Fluoroscopy	$1,000 \times 1,000$
Computed Tomography	512×512
Computed Tomography Spiral	512×512
Ultrasound	512×512
Magnetic Resonance Imaging	256×256
Nuclear Medicine	64×64

location is determined by its address. (For example, in Figure 42–2A the address of the labeled pixel is 4-4.) In medical imaging each pixel value corresponds to a three-dimensional volume of tissue known as a voxel (Figure 42–2A). Typical matrix sizes are shown in Table 42–3.

The radiologic community has promulgated a digital standard for imaging known as the Digital Imaging and Communication in Medicine (DICOM) standard. It is designed to ensure that all equipment from all manufacturers who choose to adhere to the standard are speaking the same computer language that can be understood across manufacturer and device lines. For example, a central display or printing unit needs to be able to understand how to handle a CT image from one manufacturer's scanner as well as a digital fluoroscopy image from a different manufacturer and be able to send both to a teleradiology system if necessary. The original DICOM standard was for output devices while the more recent DICOM2 standard requires both input and output data meet the same compatibility standards.

Fourier Transformation

The primary mathematical method used in the creation of computerized medical images is the Fourier transformation. Transformations are simply conversions of data to more useful forms, as when radiation doses are changed from rems to mSv. Visual transformations can also be useful, as when a decubitus abdomen radiograph is viewed horizontally to facilitate detection of air-fluid levels.

Fourier's mathematics accomplishes transformations of extremely complex functions into separate but simpler functions. For example, a Fourier transform can be

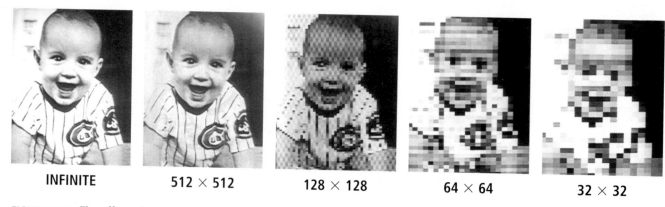

| INFINITE | 512 × 512 | 128 × 128 | 64 × 64 | 32 × 32 |

FIGURE 42-3. The effect of matrix size on resolution. *(Photographs courtesy of Doug Raver, Lima Technical College)*

applied to separate music into functions of varying amplitudes, frequencies and timing phases. This data can then be recorded for use in a magnetic tape player or CD-Rom. The Fourier transform permits the reconstruction of portions of the data when the other portions and their relationships are known. It is also possible to use the inverse Fourier transform to change back to the original data.

In digital imaging, the Fourier transform is used on data representing image intensities at specific locations. For example, Figure 42–4 demonstrates different attenuation coefficients at specific image receptor locations.

The information received by the image receptors can be processed through a variety of mathematical formulas (often referred to as algorithms or kernels). The Fourier algorithm is a fundamental formula used in image reconstruction.

It is based on algebraically adding several sets of incoming data from the image receptor. For example, in Figure 42–5, the top two waveforms have been combined to produce the bottom wave. Figure 42–6 illustrates how several different additions would change to combined waveform. Finally, Figure 42–7 shows how numerous additions would produce a square waveform. Various mathematical algorithms can change or transform the amplitude and time domain to the frequency domain and vice versa. This transformation process is called a Fourier transform or fast Fourier transform (FFT).

The inverse Fourier transformation can be used to mathematically back-project an image of the structures

that produced the attenuation coefficients as demonstrated in Figure 42–8.

Convolution and Deconvolution

It is sometimes useful to modify the value of each pixel to enhance or suppress a visual characteristic of the image. This process is actually mathematical filtering.

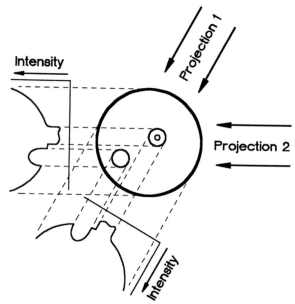

FIGURE 42-4. Image receptor data correlated to specific spatial locations. *(Reprinted with permission from Greenfield, G. B. & Hubbard, L. [1984]. Computers in radiology, New York: Churchill Livingstone)*

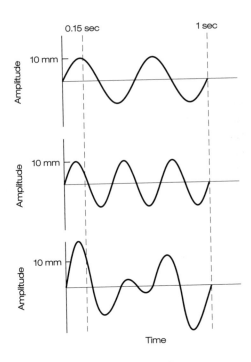

FIGURE 42-5. Basic Fourier algorithm. The top two waveforms have been combined to produce the bottom wave. *(Used by permission from Hedrick, W. R. & Hykes, D. L. [1992]. A simplified explanation of Fourier analysis, Journal of Diagnostic Medical Sonography. J. B. Lippincott, Philadelphia, PA, 8[6], 302-303.)*

Convolution is the process of modifying pixel values by a mathematical formula. It is sometimes called a **mask** because a set of mathematical operations is placed over each pixel, the pixel value is changed, the mask is then applied to the next pixel and so on. The total process is one of sliding the mask over all the pixel data and then displaying the modified image. **Deconvolution is the process of returning the pixel values to their original level by a reverse process.**

Digital Image Quality

Data Characteristics

The quality of the data acquired from the image receptor is measured by its frequency, contrast and noise.

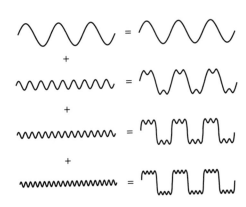

FIGURE 42-6. Basic Fourier algorithm. Several different additions changed to a combined waveform. *(Used by permission from Hedrick, W. R. & Hykes, D. L. [1992]. A simplified explanation of Fourier analysis, Journal of Diagnostic Medical Sonography. J. B. Lippincott, Philadelphia, PA 8[6], 302-303.)*

Frequency The frequency data is the raw data to which a Fourier transformation is applied to create the digital image. The acquired frequency is a measure of the

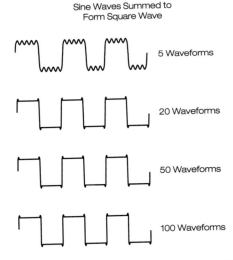

FIGURE 42-7. Basic Fourier algorithm. Numerous additions producing a square waveform. *(Used by permission from Hedrick, W. R. & Hykes, D. L. [1992]. A simplified explanation of Fourier analysis, Journal of Diagnostic Medical Sonography. J. B. Lippincott, Philadelphia, PA, 8[6], 302-303.)*

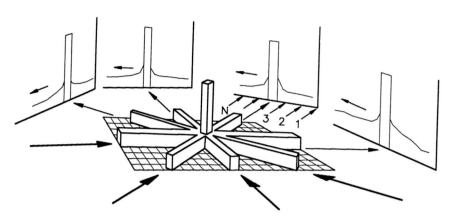

FIGURE 42-8. The concept of back-projection. *(Reprinted with permission from Coulam, C. M. & Erickson, J. J. [1981]. Equipment consideration in computed tomography,* The Physical Basis of Medical Imaging. *New York: Appleton-Century-Crofts, 213-229)*

total amount of contrast within the image. A high contrast image has high frequency, while a low contrast image has low frequency.

Contrast

As with any image contrast, the acquired contrast is a measure of the differences between the data values. A **direct** relationship exists between subject contrast and acquired data contrast. When the subject contrast is high, the acquired data contrast will be high.

Noise

Image noise is random background information that is detected but does not contribute to image quality. It is congruent with audio noise, such as the static "white noise" heard on frequencies between radio stations. White noise is visualized as "snow" on frequencies between television stations. It is measured as the **signal-to-noise ratio** (S/N). A high S/N indicates little noise in the image. Most fluoroscopic image noise is from electronic sources (i.e., the television chain). Background noise can be seen when the unit is used without a subject, although static digital images also contain visual noise. The noisiest component of most digital systems is the television camera. Commercial systems often have an S/N of 200 but the high resolution systems used in digital fluoroscopy have an S/N between 500 and 1,000.

Although noise looks like quantum mottle, the effect of the noise level on the digital image is more like the effect of base plus fog on radiographic film. Image noise has an **inverse** relationship to contrast. Increased noise decreases image contrast. Conversely, increased image contrast tends to obscure or decrease noise. The effect of

image noise on density is irrelevant in digital imaging because the computer can easily compensate for lack of density as long as sufficient contrast exists to differentiate diagnostic data from noise.

Display Qualities

The density and contrast of the digital image are controlled by varying the numerical values of each pixel. The human visual range encompasses 32 or fewer shades of gray, while the photon beam that exits the patient encompasses over 1,000 shades. Most digital image detectors are sensitive to the majority of these 1,000 differences. Because the range of stored densities is so much wider than the visual range, any digital image is only a small part of the total data obtained by the computer. Each image is only a "window" on the total range of data (Figure 42–9). The computer can easily change the level and width of the display window by mathematical recalculations.

The quantity of information stored for each pixel varies depending on the gray scale imaging abilities of the system. For example, if a black and white image is desired with no intermediate shades of gray, each pixel will require a single bit. Each pixel will either be turned on for white or off for black. When shades of gray are required, as for all diagnostic images, as many as 12 bits may be required per pixel. A 512 × 512 CT image could require 3,145,728 bits (393,216 bytes or 394 Kb).

The radiographer usually controls which portion of this vast amount of information will be seen by control-

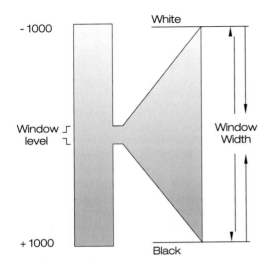

FIGURE 42-9. Digital image windows. The window level can be moved up and down the density scale. The window width can be expanded and contracted.

ling the display image density and contrast recorded on the hard copy from which many radiologists diagnose. Although argument has been made for encouraging diagnosis from CRT displays, the majority of radiologists continue to read transilluminated film hard copy images for most examinations. This practice makes the radiographer responsible for choosing the appropriate density and contrast ranges to be displayed. It is critical that radiographers who are required to produce digital images be familiar with the manner in which the computer determines what portion of the image information will be displayed. Careful image processing is critical to avoid obscuring diagnostically critical information from the radiologist.

Window Level

When the values of each pixel are changed by addition or subtraction, the total value of the entire image changes. Because a computer can express a vast range of values, it can "see" image densities far below and beyond the range of human vision. One of the most important values of digital imaging is the ability of the computer to mathematically bring density differences into the visual range from extremely low input doses that would produce densities far below the normal range of vision.

The window level controls image density. There is a **direct** relationship between window level and image density (see Figure 42–9). When the window level is increased, image density increases. The window level must be adjusted to the proper level to display diagnostically relevant information. Information outside the chosen window level is lost from diagnosis. In some instances two images may have to be produced to visualize an appropriate range of densities. For example, in routine chest CT an image with appropriate densities for the mediastinum and chest wall must be recorded in addition to a second image with appropriate densities for the lung fields (Figure 42–10).

Window Width

When the values of each pixel are changed by multiplication or division, the value range of the entire image changes. A computer can expand or compress image densities to fill the range of human vision. Window width changes are sometimes called gray scale expansion or compression. Another important value of digital imaging is the ability of the computer to mathematically expand the visual density differences from similar input doses that would produce contrast far below the normal range of vision.

The window width controls image contrast. There is an **inverse** relationship between window width and image contrast (see Figure 42–9). When the window width is increased, image contrast decreases. Figure 42–11 illustrates different window levels and widths. An extremely wide window width requires the computer to ignore fine contrast differences in order to display the entire range of data. An extremely narrow window width requires the computer to ignore a large amount of data outside the chosen range. For this reason, **window width can be said to control visibility of detail.** Extremely narrow window widths may cause an objectionable increase in the image noise level. Information outside the chosen window width is lost from diagnosis. The window width must be adjusted to display a maximum amount of diagnostically relevant contrast.

Resolution

Resolution is controlled by the matrix size, as discussed above. There is a direct relationship between matrix size and image resolution (see Figure 42–2). When matrix size is increased, image resolution increases. Matrix size is not variable within a system. It is

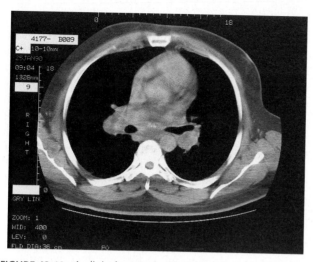 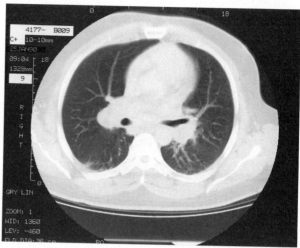

FIGURE 42-10. A clinical example of window level and width changes. Computed tomography of the chest requires two images to demonstrate the entire range of diagnostic densities. (A) High window level and narrow window width demonstrate the mediastinum and chest wall. (B) Low window level and wide window width demonstrate the lung fields. *(Courtesy of Van Wert County Hospital, Van Wert, OH)*

controlled by the quantity of image detectors and the accompanying electronics built into the system.

As discussed previously, the primary limitation on digital images is the raster scan pattern of the display CRT. Commercial units achieve only 525 lines of interlaced scanning in which only 262.5 lines are scanned in one pass. This produces only 1–2 lp/mm for diagnostic imaging. The frequency response of the incoming signal is termed the **bandwidth**. The bandwidth also affects the resolution. In the United States, commercial television is broadcast at 4 MHz, which produces about 320 lines of resolution.

Progressive scanning increases resolution slightly by scanning all 525 lines in order. **Slow scanning** also increases resolution but cannot be used in real-time dynamic studies with digital fluoroscopy. High resolution video is now available commercially and has been used in radiological applications for some time. The raster pattern is increased to 1,050 lines (often called a 1,000-line system) and the bandwidth is increased to 20 MHz, which produces about 800 lines of resolution. The result is a resolving ability of about 5–7 lp/mm.

Filtering

Digital filtering of images utilizes the computer to extract more diagnostic information. It is usually accomplished by transforming the image into frequencies, mathematically altering the frequency by convolution and then using deconvolution and an inverse Fourier transformation to reproduce the image. The computer either accentuates or suppresses selected frequencies during the filtering process. Digitized image filters are classified as low-pass, band-pass or high-pass although various equipment manufacturers have developed trade names and added unique modifications to many of them. The term **masking** is sometimes applied to the filtering process to indicate which frequencies have been suppressed. Masking of high frequencies produces low-pass filtering and vice versa.

Low-pass filtering either amplifies or deletes all but the low frequencies. It frequently appears to reduce image contrast and is often used to remove high frequency noise, especially when very little data is available (Figure 42–12). Low-pass filtering can also be accomplished by averaging each pixel's value with that of adjacent pixels. This type of low-pass filtering is sometimes called **smoothing**. Nine point smoothing averages each pixel with the eight adjacent pixels to accomplish a nine pixel average. Low radiation count nuclear medicine studies often use smoothing techniques.

Band-pass filtering either amplifies or deletes all but a selected range or band of frequencies. It is useful in the elimination of characteristic emission peaks, or in

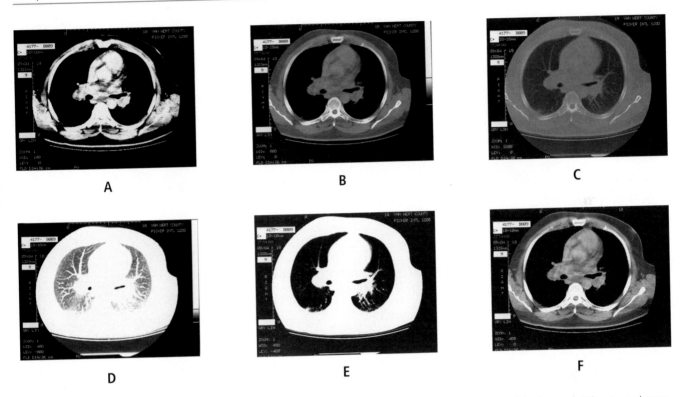

FIGURE 42-11. Window levels and widths. The same chest CT as in Figure 42-10 with window width changes: (A) extremely narrow, (B) moderate, and (D) extremely wide. The same chest with window level changes: (D) extremely low, (E) low, and (F) normal. The gray scale at the right of each image has a line to demonstrate where the high and low densities are extracted from the available data, illustrating both the window width and level. It is advisable to set the window level (density) first and then determine an appropriate window width (contrast). *(Courtesy of Van Wert County Hospital, Van Wert, OH)*

nuclear medicine, when a particular characteristic emission permits the localization of an injected radioisotope.

High-pass filtering either amplifies or deletes all **but** the high frequencies. It often appears to increase image contrast and is sometimes called **edge enhancement** filtering or **sharpening** (Figure 42–13). When the frequencies that represent structures of interest can be identified, as in contrast medium filled vessels, amplification of their frequencies can produce an edge enhancement effect while other frequencies are actually suppressed. The result is an image with edge enhancement and greatly increased contrast. This type of high-pass filtering is useful in digital vascular imaging and in digital mammography. However, extremely small structures can

sometimes be buried in an edge, and undesirable edges are usually enhanced as well as those that are of diagnostic value.

Digital Subtraction Radiography

Digital subtraction radiography (DSR) combines the digitization of an image with subtraction techniques. The most common use of DSR is with fluoroscopic angiography as a substitute for static serial angiographic films produced by a rapid film changer. As a result of this primary use, DSR is also known as digital subtraction angiography (DSA), digital subtraction imaging (DSI), digital vascular imaging (DVI) and digital fluoroscopy

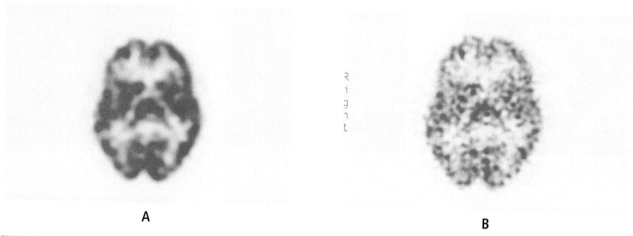

FIGURE 42-12. Low-pass filtering or smoothing. Transverse brain sections from a nuclear medicine study: (A) smoothed, and (B) noisier filter. *(Courtesy of Mike Ballistrea, Department of Nuclear Medicine, Meridia Hillcrest Hospital, Mayfield Heights, OH)*

(DF), although the last two do not necessarily use subtraction.

Imaging Procedure

The x-ray tube used for digital fluoroscopy operates in pulses at diagnostic range mA (100–300 mA) to avoid quantum mottle. A high-resolution image intensifier with a low lag plumbicon™ tube or CCD camera is used as the image receptor in a DSR system. Its function is to digitize the incoming photon beam. Formation of the DSR image requires that a scout image be obtained. The scout image is then reversed to form a **mask**. The mask is then superimposed on subsequent images containing an injected contrast medium. The result is subtraction of all the densities that were present in the scout image, leaving only the densities that were added by the injected contrast medium. For example, a cerebral angiogram can be modified by DSR to produce dynamic images of the cerebral vasculature with

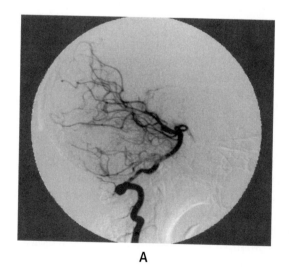
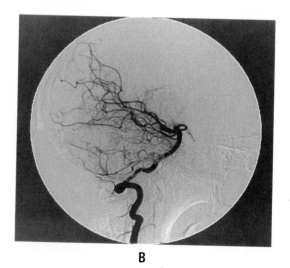

FIGURE 42-13. High-pass filtering or sharpening. Edge enhancement is demonstrated on these digital subtraction angiograms: (A) normal image, and (B) with high-pass filtering. *(Courtesy of Rick Halker, Lima Memorial Hospital, Lima, OH)*

the cranial structures removed. The technique is particularly useful in demonstrating small vessels that would otherwise be obscured by superimposed bony structures.

A DSR system does not use mathematical reconstruction such as the Fourier transformation. Instead it simply manipulates the digitized information mathematically. Because manipulation must be accomplished very quickly (about 30 images per second), an array processor is required.

Temporal subtraction is the basic subtraction procedure discussed above but within a limited time. It is used to reduce subject noise, thus increasing contrast between opacified vessels and other structures. The term **mask subtraction** is applied to the simplest form of temporal subtraction, which consists of real-time display and storage of subtracted images.

Time interval difference (TID) subtraction is designed to permit visualization of the difference between two different phases of vascular injection. It is accomplished by setting a time interval that is maintained between the mask and the injection image. Consequently, the mask continues to change. For example, if the time interval corresponds to the difference between 5 images, exposure 1 would become the mask for exposure 6, exposure 2 would mask exposure 7, etc. The resulting image can demonstrate early vascular filling in one color (usually black) and late filling in another color (usually white). TID subtraction presents an abbreviated dynamic study. The primary advantage of the technique is that motion is often eliminated because the time interval between the mask and the injection image is very short.

Matched filtering uses the sum of several images obtained when the contrast medium is at its maximum (during the arterial phase of an injection). The mask is then subtracted from the combined image of maximum contrast material.

Recursive filtering combines several injected images to form a subtraction, as with matched filtering. Recursive filtering is much more sophisticated in that the images are density weighted, or given greater emphasis according to a time scheme. The time scheme or **time filter** can be set by the operator to enhance structures of interest.

Dual energy subtraction techniques can be used to separate the K-shell characteristic edge of iodine (at 33 keV) from surrounding bone and soft tissue. Essentially the technique subtracts a high kVp image and a low kVp image. Dual energy subtraction is useful because all images can be acquired during the injection phase, thus sufficiently reducing the time between exposures to eliminate most motion. It is of little value by itself, but it is useful in hybrid subtraction.

Hybrid subtraction is a combination of energy subtraction with one of the temporal subtraction techniques. It has the advantage of reducing patient motion while providing a more normal image than with time interval difference subtraction.

Pixel shifting or linear translation, is a computer shifting of pixel values. It is used to help overcome patient motion, which is especially a problem with temporal subtraction. Motion disrupts the alignment, or registration, of the mask and renders the image useless.

When high pressure injection techniques are used, as in most angiographic studies, it is extremely difficult for patients to avoid movement. Pixel shifting is possible when attempting to resolve motion problems. The computer can compare pixel values while shifting either the mask or the injected image until overall pixel values are as close to one another as possible to create the closest possible visual alignment. Pixel shifting is effective only for linear motion; it is not effective with rotary motion, such as swallowing.

Picture Archiving and Communication Systems (PACS)

Picture archiving and communication systems (PACS) are computerized storage and transmission systems for digitized images of all types, including computed and digital radiography, mammography, ultrasound, CT, MRI, DSR, etc. The first advances in PACS technology were made with long distance transmission systems for clinics in remote areas (such as northern Canada) and for specialist consultations in rural areas. Most hospitals use PACS-style teleradiology image transmission systems via telephone lines so radiologists can receive images and provide immediate consultation at satellite centers and when on call at home.

In addition, PACS images can be manipulated by window level and width adjustments, enlargements, tissue density readings and subtractions, permitting the radiologist to obtain more information than any film image can provide and without additional exposure to the patient.

Archiving

A major problem for all radiology departments is the storage of film as required by local legal precedents. Many institutions store all films for five to seven years, with pediatric and litigation films retained indefinitely. Many hours of staff time and immense amounts of space are required to maintain these files. A PACS system eliminates the need for most of the space for storage and reduces the time requirements. Misfiling becomes much less likely and acquisition time can be reduced tremendously. In addition, PACS terminals permit access to images from remote locations (for example, surgery, emergency units, etc.).

Image storage requires immense amounts of memory. Digital storage of images for a typical large radiology department that does 150,000 examinations per year (with about 100,000 of these diagnostic radiography and the other 50,000 divided among CT, ultrasound, MRI, nuclear medicine, mammography, and vascular procedures) has been estimated at about 3.2 terabytes of computer memory per year. Considering a normal 3–5 year image storage requirement, a total memory of 10–16 terabytes (10,000–16,000 Gb or 10,000,000–16,000,000 Mb) would be required for a complete digital PACS system. With gigabytes and terabytes of memory now readily available, many radiology departments are beginning digital storage of many procedures.

Communication

Communication of PACS images involves transmitting images with voice and/or word processing to distant locations. Whether the location is removed from the radiology department by a floor, a building, a block or hundreds of miles, radiologist consultation becomes available more efficiently than before.

Thinking has also begun on linking PACS images to programming that would permit radiological diagnosis. In the early 1960s a radiological diagnostic program was proven to be accurate, but no method has yet been accomplished to acquire the complex pattern recogni-

tion that is necessary. This development is in the distant future, after artificial intelligence programming has been developed.

Laser Film Printers

Laser film printers use either an **infrared laser diode** or a **helium neon laser** to produce transilluminated hard copy film images from computerized digital information. Images are created by the laser beam exposing the film emulsion according to the digital information arriving from the computer. The laser beam does not burn the emulsion. It simply exposes the silver halides in the film to the light photons of the laser beam.

Transferring the digital image to film permits it to be viewed on a radiographic illuminator (viewbox) instead of from a cathode ray tube (CRT) screen. Laser film printers are popular because they provide excellent resolution, good text reproduction, and have high productivity with low maintenance. Laser printers can produce up to 180 films per hour (2 per minute) and can be connected to multiple imaging units. (For example, one printer can simultaneously serve a digital fluoroscopy unit as well as a CT and MRI scanner.)

Summary

The future of medical imaging lies in computerized applications of the numerous modalities. The method by which these imaging modalities have been computerized is digital processing of imaging information.

Computers are devices that process information. Analog computers handle data composed of continuously varying electrical currents. Digital computers handle data composed of definite quantities of current (for example, current on versus current off). All medical imaging is achieved with digital computers, often from information that has been processed by an analog-to-digital converter (ADC). Computers use two types of information: operating instructions, called the program and collected facts, called data. Programs are called software while computer equipment is called hardware.

Computers operate from a binary machine language with a two symbol alphabet. Because electrical currents are most easily understood as being either on or off, the binary system consists of information recorded as either a 0 for off or a 1 for on. Each binary number is called a bit, for **b**inary dig**its**. An eight-bit word is called a byte. Computer memory is often rated in terms of the total byte memory.

The CPU directs information to and from the various components that make up the computer system. Information is stored in a computer's memory and is classified as read only memory (ROM) or random access memory (RAM). Peripheral devices permit input and/or output of information to and/or from the CPU and include memory storage devices, along with a variety of input and output devices.

A digital image is one that has been converted into numerical values for transmission or processing. A detector of some type must be used to acquire the image information. A matrix is a square series of boxes that gives form to the image. The individual matrix boxes are known as picture elements or pixels. Pixel size determines resolution. In medical imaging each pixel value corresponds to a three-dimensional volume of tissue, known as a voxel.

The primary mathematical method used in the creation of computerized medical images is the Fourier transformation. Convolution is the process of modifying pixel values by a mathematical formula. Deconvolution is the process of returning the pixel values to their original level by a reverse process.

The quality of the data acquired from the image receptor is measured by its frequency, contrast and noise. The density and contrast of the digital image are controlled by varying the numerical values of each pixel. The window level controls image density. Window width changes the gray scale expansion or compression and therefore controls contrast. Resolution is controlled by the matrix size.

Digital filtering of images is usually accomplished by transforming the image into frequencies, mathematically altering the frequency by convolution and then using deconvolution and an inverse Fourier transformation to reproduce the image. The computer either accentuates or suppresses selected frequencies during the filtering process. Digitized image filters are classified as low-pass, band-pass or high-pass.

Digital subtraction radiography (DSR) combines the digitization of an image with subtraction techniques. The most common use of DSR is with fluoroscopic angiography as a substitute for static serial angiographic films produced by a rapid film changer.

Picture archiving and communication systems (PACS) are computerized storage and transmission systems for digitized images of all types.

Laser film printers use either an infrared laser diode or a helium neon laser to produce transilluminated hard copy film images from computerized digital information. The laser beam exposes the silver halides in the film to the light photons of the laser beam. Laser film printers provide excellent resolution, good text reproduction, have high productivity with low maintenance, and can be connected to multiple imaging units.

REVIEW QUESTIONS

1. What is the difference between analog and digital computers?

2. Why do computers operate from a binary machine language?

3. What is the function of the central processing unit?

4. What is the most common input device?

5. How is a digital image acquired?

6. What is image noise?

7. How do the window level and the window width affect the digital image display?

8. What are the three types of digital image filtering methods?

9. What is the principle application of digital subtraction radiography?

10. What is the purpose of pixel shifting during digital subtraction?

11. What are the advantages of PACS?

12. How does a laser film printer create an image?

REFERENCES AND RECOMMENDED READING

Bedard, L. & Delisle, C. (1992). Image digitizing in conventional radiology. *Canadian Journal of Medical Radiation Technology.* 23(2), 67–70.

Berland, L. L. (1987). *Practical CT technology and techniques.* New York: Raven Press.

Brody, W. R. (1984). *Digital radiography.* New York: Raven Press.

Brody, W. R. & Macovski, A. (1981). Dual-energy digital radiography. *Diagnostic Imaging. 3,* 18–25.

Burns, C. (1993). Using computed digital radiography effectively. *Seminars in Radiologic Technology. 1*(1), 24–35.

Bushberg, J. T., Seibert, J. A., Leidholdt, E. M., & Boone, J. M. (1994). *The essential physics of medical imaging.* Baltimore: Williams & Wilkins.

Bushong, S. C. (1997). *Radiologic science for technologists: Physics, biology, and protection.* (6th ed.). St. Louis: C. V. Mosby.

Coulam, C. M. & Erickson, J. J. (1981). Equipment considerations in computed tomography. *The Physical Basis of Medical Imaging.* Editors: Coulam, C. M., Erickson, J. J., Rollo, F. D., & James, A. E. New York: Appleton-Century-Crofts.

Curry, T. S., Dowdey, J. E., & Murry, R. C. (1990). *Christensen's introduction to the physics of diagnostic radiology.* (4th ed.). Philadelphia: Lea and Febiger.

De Brusk, P. D. (1983). Digital x-ray imaging: The basics. *Radiologic Technology. 54*(4), 280.

Dobbins, J. T. & Powell, A. O. (1989). Variable compensation technique for digital radiography of the chest. *Radiology. 157,* 451.

Forster, E. (1985). *Equipment for diagnostic radiography.* Lancaster: MTP Press.

Glazer, H. S., Muka, E., Sagel, S. S., & Jost, R. G. (1994). New techniques in chest radiography. *Radiologic Clinics of North America. 32*(4), 711–729.

Gould, R. G. (1984). Digital hardware in radiography and fluoroscopy. *Applied Radiology. 13,* 137–140.

Hindel, R. (1983). Digital imaging: The technology of the future. *The Canadian Journal of Medical Radiation Technology. 14*(4), 128.

Hedrick, W. R. (1993). Digital image acquisition and processing in computed radiography. *Seminars in Radiologic Technology. 1*(1), 6–15.

Huda, W. & Szeverenyi, N. M. (1999). The filmless radiology department: A primer. *Applied radiology.* (February). 30–34.

Kuni, C. C. (1988). *Introduction to computers and digital processing in medical imaging.* Chicago: Year Book Medical Publishers.

Kushner, D. C. (1986). Radiation dose reduction in the evaluation of scoliosis: An application of digital radiography. *Radiology. 154,* 175.

Long, B. W. (1989). Computed radiography: Photostimulable phosphor image plate technology. *Radiologic Technology. 61*(2), 107–112.

Malott, J. C. & Fodor, J. (1982). Digital video angiography. *Radiologic Technology. 54*(2), 83–89.

Marjois, J. D. (1985). Minimizing dose associated with digital subtraction angiography. *The Canadian Journal of Medical Radiation Technology. 16*(4), 141.

Mistretta, C. A. & Crummy, A. B. (1981). Digital fluoroscopy. *The Physical Basis of Medical Imaging.* Editors: Coulam, C. M., Erickson, J. J., Rollo, F. D., & James, A. E. New York: Appleton-Century-Crofts.

Mistretta, C. A., Crummy, A. B., Strother, C. M., & Sackett, J. F. (1982). *Digital subtraction arteriography: An application of computerized fluoroscopy.* Chicago: Year Book.

Nishitami, H. (1986). Dual energy projection radiography using a condenser x-ray generator and digital radiography apparatus. *Radiology. 154,* 533.

Schaefer, C. (1989). Improved control of image optical density with low-dose digital and conventional radiography in bedside imaging. *Radiology. 153,* 713.

Sherrier, R. & McAdams, H. P. (1986). Digital processing of portable films can reduce need for repeat studies. *Diagnostic Imaging.* (July), 117.

Smith, C. B. (1984). Physical principles of digital radiography. *Radiography. 50*(590), 41–44.

Toth, B., Edmonds, E.W., Rowlands, J. A., Porter, A. J., & Hynes, D. M. (1985). The 'digital' compromise. *The Canadian Journal of Medical Radiation Technology. 16*(2), 28.

Wilson, P. (1984). Digital imaging: An introduction. *Radiography. 50*(590), 449.

The Case of the Deep Sea Rodeo

This creature was radiographed after a sojourn in the deep. What is it?

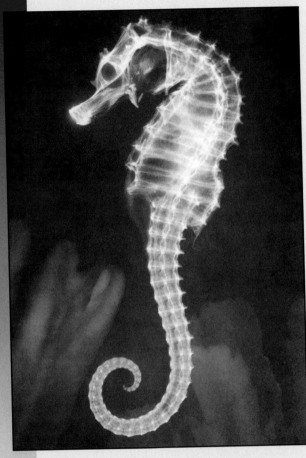

(Reprinted by permission of the International Society of Radiographers and Radiological Technicians from K. C. Clark Archives, Middlesex Hospital, London, England)

Answers to the case studies can be found in Appendix E.

CHAPTER 43

Digital Radiography

Barbara Smith, Barry Burns, Richard R. Carlton

My body is the frame wherein 'tis held,
And perspective it is the painter's art.
For through the painter must you see his skill,
To find where your true image pictured lies;

Shakespeare, Sonnet 24, XXIV

Objectives

Upon completion of this chapter, the student should be able to:

▶ Describe various digital radiography image receptor and detector systems.

▶ Explain critical elements used in the different digital radiography systems.

▶ Discuss limitations inherent in each of the currently available digital radiography systems.

▶ Describe the process by which the digital radiography histogram is acquired and the display algorithm is applied to the collected data.

▶ Explain why digital radiography systems have significantly greater latitude than conventional film-screen radiography systems.

▶ Analyze elements of digital radiography systems that make them prone to violation of ALARA radiation protection concepts.

▶ Explain the causes of several digital radiography artifact problems.

Introduction

Digital radiography systems replace traditional film with a reusable detector. The more recent DICOM2 standard requires that both input and output data meet the same compatibility standards. Detectors currently used to acquire radiographic images include photostimulable storage phosphor imaging plates (IP), charged coupled devices (CCD), and silicon and selenium receptors. These detectors are commonly divided into two types, indirect conversion and direct conversion. However, the silicon and selenium receptors are also known as flat panel detectors. Table 43–1 provides an outline of currently available CR systems.

Indirect conversion systems use a two-part process involving a scintillator (which converts incoming x-ray photons to light) and a photodetector (which converts light into an electronic signal). Indirect systems include those that use photostimulable storage phosphor imaging plates (IP), charged coupled devices (CCD), and silicon.

Direct conversion systems directly convert incoming x-ray photons to an electronic signal. These systems use selenium and are sometimes referred to as **direct radiography (DR) systems.**

The term **flat panel** (or **flat field**) **detectors** is also being used to describe both the indirect amorphous silicon and the direct amorphous selenium plates that are being used in some digital systems.

Historical Development

Computed radiography first became available in the early 1980s when it was introduced by Fuji but, as happens with many new technologies, there were problems with high cost and poor image quality. As computer technology has advanced, so too has the ability of CR to produce images comparable to, and in many instances better than, film. Currently, a number of manufacturers produce CR plates and processor systems. Many of them have Internet web sites with a considerable amount of information on the advantages of their particular systems. (Commercial web sites with information on computed radiography include www.fujimed.com, www.kodak.com, www.agfaus.com, www.ge.com, www.lumisys.com).

Indirect Photostimulable Phosphor Imaging Plate Systems

Photostimulable Imaging Plates

A photostimulable phosphor imaging plate is a rigid sheet with several layers that are designed to record and enhance transmission of the image from a beam of ionizing radiation. The layers include a protective layer, a phosphor layer, a support layer made of polyester, a conductor layer, and a light shield layer (Figure 43–1). The protective layer simply insulates the imaging plate from handling trauma. The phosphor layer holds the photostimulable phosphor, which is the active component in the plate. The support layer is simply a base on which to coat the other layers. The conductor layer grounds the plate to eliminate electrostatic problems and absorb light to increase sharpness. Finally, the light shielding layer prevents light from erasing data on the imaging plate or leaking through the backing, decreasing the spatial resolution. The imaging plate is loaded into a cassette that

TABLE 43–1. Most Common CR Systems

Type		Detector	Scintillator	Charge Reader	Company
Indirect		Photostimulable phosphor		Laser	Fuji
Indirect	Flat panel	Amorphous silicon	CsI	TFT	Philips, Siemens, GE
Direct	Flat panel	Amorphous selenium		TFT	Canon
Indirect		Rare earth intensifying screen		CCD	Swiss ray

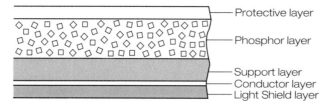

FIGURE 43–1. Photostimulable phosphor imaging plate showing layers.

looks much like a radiographic film and intensifying screen cassette. Consequently, computed radiography cassettes are sometimes referred to as "filmless cassettes."

In order for CR to function, the imaging plate material must have the ability to store and release the image information in a usable form. The most common phosphor with characteristics favorable for CR is barium fluorohalide bromides and iodides with europium activators (BaFBr:Eu and BaFI:Eu). The halides are approximately 85 percent bromide and 15 percent iodine. Due to the lower atomic number of barium, the K-edge attenuates best between 35 to 50 keV, somewhat lower than the typical K-edge for rare earth intensifying screens, but well within the diagnostic range (35 keV is a typical average energy production from an exposure of 80 kVp). However, **the absorption efficiency above and below 35 to 50 keV is below that of rare earth intensifying screens.** This means that more exposure may be needed in order to have similar quantum noise outside the optimal energy range. Also, the imaging plate phosphor will absorb more low energy scatter than the rare earth phosphor and film, which means appropriate kVp and masking must be used to achieve optimal images. **This also makes the imaging plate more sensitive to scatter both before and after it is sensitized through exposure to the x-ray beam.**

Latent Image Production

The incident x-ray beam produces a latent image within the photostimulable fluorohalides that comprise the active layer of the imaging plate (IP) in the cassette. When the fluorohalides luminesce, they do not release all the energy absorbed from the incident x-ray beam. Although some light is emitted, the phosphors retain sufficient energy in the form of a latent image. It is this latent image that will be used to create a digital image for the computer to record and display.

This latent image is actually created by energy transfer during photoelectric interactions. The photoelectrons that are produced then excite a number of low energy electrons to create "holes" in the crystal phosphor. Although about half of the electron holes will recompose and emit light photons, the fluorohalides will hold the other half of the electrons, thus creating the "holes" at the Europium sites. These Europium electron holes are the actual latent image. **The latent image will lose about 25 percent of its energy in 8 hours, so it is important to process the cassette shortly after exposure.** Cassettes stored for several days after exposure and before processing lose most of their latent image.

The latent image is processed by loading the cassette into an image reader device (IRD) where the imaging plate is scanned by a helium-neon laser beam. These laser beam scans cause the phosphors to emit the stored latent image in the form of light photons, which are detected by photosensitive receptors converted to an electrical signal, which is in turn converted to a unique digital value for that level of luminescence. Once the plate is read, it is erased to remove all vestiges of the latent image.

Image Acquisition

Image acquisition begins with x-ray exposure to the imaging plate. Since the imaging plate is placed in a cassette it can be used tabletop or with a grid, similar to the use of film screen. The rules of positioning hold true for CR, areas that are clipped or poorly positioned cannot be corrected with this or any other system. It is the responsibility of the radiographer to select proper technique; chronic overexposure should be avoided. Radiation exposure causes fluorescence of the imaging plate but some of the energy of the beam is also stored in the plate. It is this stored energy that is used to create an image during reading and processing. Some of the electrons, which are excited by the absorbed energy, are trapped in the crystal structure of the phosphor at higher energy levels. Thus a latent image is stored in the imaging plate, similar to a latent image on film, but with wider latitude. The imaging plate then needs to be read to release the stored information, which can be manipulated by the computer and used in either soft or hard copy form.

Reading Digital Radiography Data

Reading the imaging plate involves a finely focused laser beam that frees the trapped electrons, allowing them to return to a lower energy state, referred to as photostimulated luminescence (PSL). Electrons moving to a lower energy state release blue-purple light photons in proportion to the absorbed radiation. The laser light beam is directed to the imaging plate through a series of components; this beam must be monitored since the intensity of the blue light from the imaging plate is dependent on the power of the laser beam. Scanning of the imaging plate by the laser occurs in a raster pattern as the plate is fed through the processor. The light liberated from the imaging plate is emitted in all directions and is collected by an optical system that directs it to one or more photomultiplier (PM) tubes, which are sensitive only to the blue light. The PM tube converts the visible light into an electronic signal whose output is in analog form. This analog signal must be converted into a digital signal before the computer can work with the image information. This is accomplished with an analog to digital converter (ADC). The entire reading process is illustrated in Figure 43–2. The PM tubes adjust the output signal range so it can be optimally handled during the digitization process. Any residual image left on the imaging plate is erased by exposure to an intense light to release any remaining trapped electrons. The reading and erasing of an imaging plate can occur in a single processor unit as seen in Figure 43–3 or can be accomplished with separate desktop processor and erasure units. The larger units typically allow stacking and loading of multiple cassettes, whereas a desktop processor requires the imaging plate to be removed from the cassette and fed into the processor. Plate throughput can average anywhere from 30 plates/hour up to 110 plates/hour depending on the type of processor used. Workload and cost will determine which unit will best serve department requirements.

The finely focused laser beam that scans each line of the imaging plate correlates to one line spacing or pixel dimension. The analog signal emitted by the PM tube has an infinite range of values that the ADC must con-

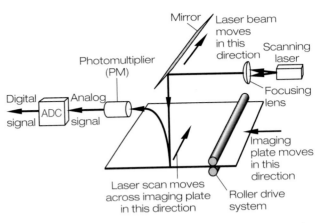

FIGURE 43–2. Photostimulable phosphor imaging plate reader. The plate is moved through the system while a focused laser scans the surface in a raster pattern. When the laser strikes the surface of the imaging plate, the emitted light is detected by the PM tube, which sends an analog signal to the ADC for conversion into a digital signal, which is then sent to the computer for processing and display.

vert into limited discrete values that can be stored as digital code. Pixel depth or the number of bits that represent an analog signal will determine the number of density values. Typically there are 10 (2^{10} = 1,024), 12 (2^{12} = 4,096), and 16 (2^{16} = 65,536) bit ADCs, which will determine the density values for the analog signal and so the gray scale of the system. Therefore, the number of bits/pixels will determine how many density values can be present and so affect the density and contrast of an imaging system. Another important variable related to pixels is spatial resolution. **The smaller the pixel the higher the spatial resolution.** Pixel size is dependent on the sampling frequency, which is expressed in pixels/mm.

The matrix size is dependent on the sampling frequency and the image receptor size. At 10 pixels/mm a 14 x 17" plate would have a matrix of ~3,500 x 4,200, while at 5 pixels/mm the 14 x 17 would have a matrix of ~1,750 x 2,100. Pixel size, matrix, and bit depth determine the size of the computer file for a given image.

To accomplish the task of changing the analog signal into the correct components for digital manipulation, the analog signal must be sampled in order to find the location and size of the signal. It must then be quantitized to

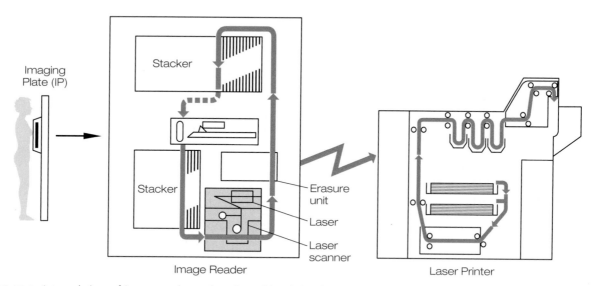

FIGURE 43–3. Internal view of image reader and stacker with relationship to a chest unit and laser printer. *(Courtesy of Fuji Photo Film Co., Ltd.)*

determine the average value of the signal in the sample. During preprocessing, the CR system must also determine the orientation of the part on the plate as well as the number of projections present per plate. Locating the image data on the plate allows the system to sample and manipulate only the clinically useful information. The method used by Fuji to recognize the clinically useful area on the imaging plate is known as exposure data recognition (EDR), which has three modes: automatic (auto), semiautomatic (semi), and fixed. Automatic mode adjusts latitude and sensitivity for the image. It is also used when placing more than one image on a cassette.

There are certain expectations that need to be met when placing more than one image per plate. The plate can be programmed and then used for a number of different scanning detection patterns (Figure 43–4). **The beam and part need to be centered within each pattern and collimation must be parallel and equidistant from the edges of the imaging plate** (Figure 43–5). The semiautomatic mode automatically adjusts only sensitivity while the reading latitude is fixed. It is used when the image is centered, but the collimation borders are not parallel or equidistant from the plate edges. **Fixed mode is similar to film screen processing in that latitude and sensitivity are fixed, requiring correct technique factors**

to be used to obtain a diagnostic image since this mode will not correct density problems.

During initial processing a histogram is generated from the image data that allows the CR system to find the useful signal by locating the minimum and maximum signal within the anatomical regions of interest in the image. To generate a histogram the scanned area is divided into pixels and the signal intensity for each pixel is determined. An example of a histogram is shown in Figure 43–6.

The histogram is associated with specific examinations that will produce digital images that are consistent, regardless of variations in kVp and mAs. This helps determine the shades of gray. The appropriate histogram is selected by body part by the radiographer when the imaging plate is loaded into the reading unit. Histograms are also used to eliminate unnecessary information outside the collimated field, like scatter radiation, which degrades the final image. The computer compares the histogram from the imaging plate to an existing histogram for the programmed body part. This is when exposure errors are corrected. Algorithms, which are unique for each manufacturer, process the data once the exposure area is determined and the signal histogram is established. Fuji uses gradation processing, tonescaling

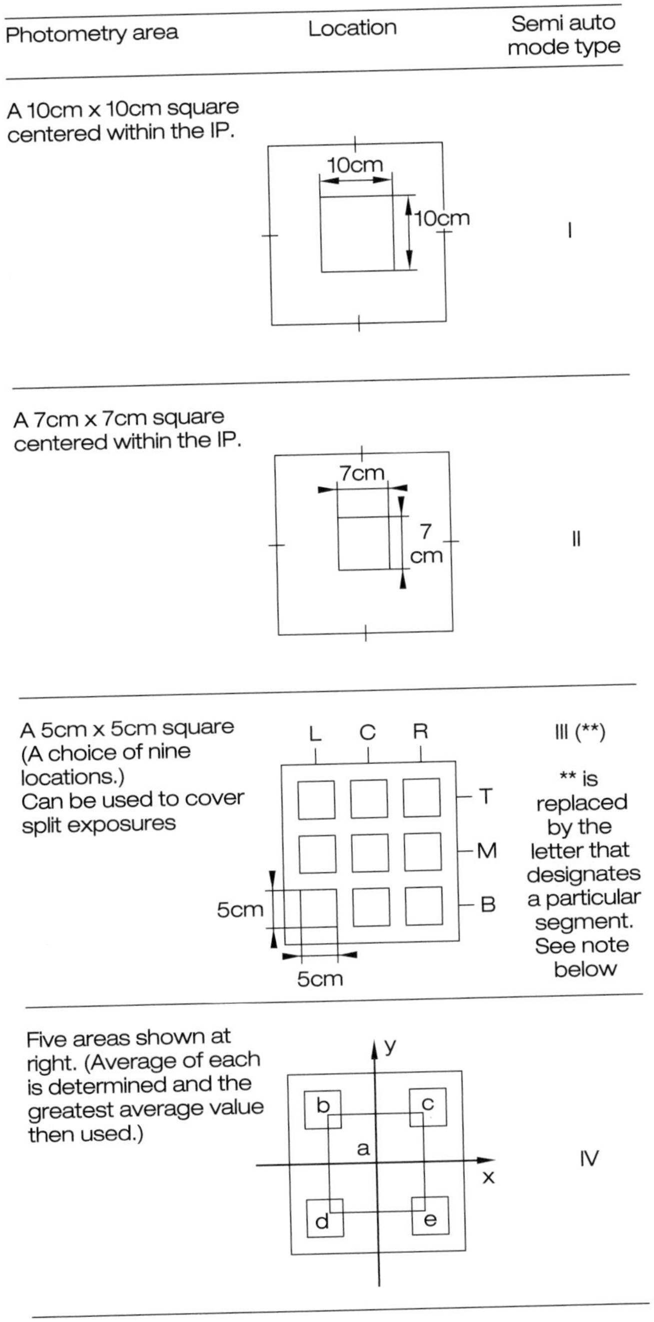

Photometry area
Location
Semi auto mode type
A 10cm x 10cm square centered within the IP.
10cm
10cm
I
A 7cm x 7cm square centered within the IP.
7cm
7 cm
II
A 5cm x 5cm square (A choice of nine locations.) Can be used to cover split exposures
L C R
T
M
B
5cm
5cm
III (**)
** is replaced by the letter that designates a particular segment. See note below
Five areas shown at right. (Average of each is determined and the greatest average value then used.)
y
x
a
b
c
d
e
IV

FIGURE 43–4. An example of different scanning detection patterns available on a Fuji system set for semiautomatic exposure data recognition (EDR) mode. *(Courtesy of Fuji Photo Film Co., Ltd.)*

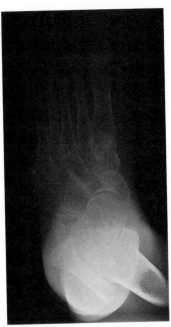

FIGURE 43–5. Nonparallel collimation artifact. Histograms require that collimation edges be parallel to the sides of the imaging plate.

is used by Kodak, and Agfa is using a MUSCIA (multiscale image contrast algorithm) system.

The correct algorithm must be selected prior to processing the imaging plate, otherwise the image will not possess the correct density and contrast. Figure 43–7 is

Max
Count
0
289
Pixel value
2817

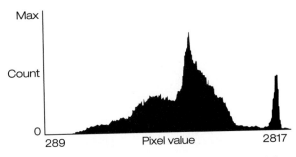

FIGURE 43–6. Histogram of the gray scale generated from a computed radiography image by Laurie Cesar from the Mayo Clinic. The vertical axis represents the number of pixels. The horizontal axis represents the quantity of information (image density). Low density is to the left, high density to the right. *(Reprinted by permission of the American Society of Radiologic Technologists, 1997)*

an example of a typical chest histogram with the various anatomical areas annotated on the histogram. Figure 43–8 illustrates how a computed radiography system can analyze a pediatric chest histogram and then display regions of interest outside the lung. Finally, Figure 43–9 emphasizes the critical importance of adhering to uniform positioning and collimation procedures when using a computed radiography system. The reading system must be given consistent data to analyze if it is to provide consistent diagnostic quality results.

The knee images in Figure 43–10 illustrate the ability of a CR system to adjust the histogram into the visible diagnostic density range. Look carefully at Figures 43–10A&B as compared to C&D and then to E&F. While it may appear that all three CR images (B, D, and F) have appropriate density ranges as compared to the conventional radiography images, a careful inspection will show that CR image 43–10B is extremely grainy and as a result is outside the acceptable range for detail. This is an example of the CR histogram adjusting for density but lacking adequate data to fill in an acceptable level of detail.

A CR system reacts in a similar manner if an inappropriate histogram is selected. For example, if a chest histogram was selected rather than the knee, then the incoming data will not match the histogram and the computer will attempt to manipulate the image to correspond to the histogram algorithm that was selected (Figure 43–11). Once the imaging plate is placed in the

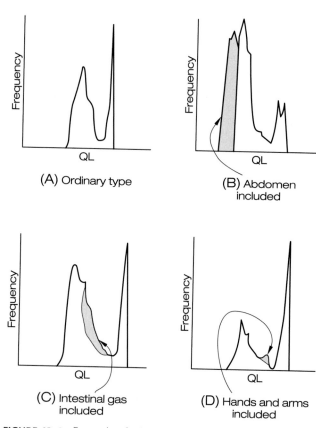

FIGURE 43–8. Example of a histogram that would be produced by a pediatric chest with potential computerized enhancements possible by displaying density ranges typical of other regions of interest outside normal lung densities. *(Courtesy of Fuji Photo Film Co., Ltd.)*

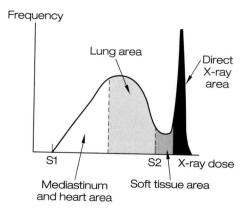

FIGURE 43–7. Example of a histogram that would be produced by a normal chest radiograph. *(Courtesy of Fuji Photo Film Co., Ltd.)*

processor and read, if the algorithm is wrong the plate cannot be processed again and the information is lost.

The raw data has to go through a number of manipulations to achieve the optimum gray scale range to give a useful diagnostic image. A gradation processing function maps the density values in a nonlinear curve as a basis for adjusting density and contrast. These gradation curves serve to match image contrast requirements to specific exam types or to emphasize specific densities, such as lung fields. The curves are manufacturer specific, but can function in much the same way as $D_{log}E$ curves of different film types. Programs within the computer can manipulate the contrast scale, or the slope of the $D_{log}E$ curve. For example, if the slope becomes steeper,

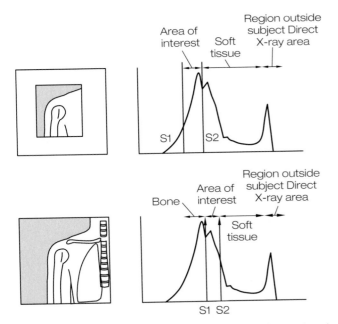

FIGURE 43–9. Example of a histogram that would be produced by two different positioning and collimation methods for a normal shoulder. Observe the radical difference that is necessary for the computed radiography reading system to produce a diagnostic range of densities for each method. This illustrates the critical importance of developing consistent procedures for positioning and collimation when using a CR system. *(Courtesy of Fuji Photo Film Co., Ltd.)*

contrast increases in the image. Most CR systems allow you to view the response ($D_{log}E$) curve on the workstation monitor as the image is manipulated.

Spatial frequency processing is also possible with CR systems. It should be used when it is necessary to increase image sharpness. Edge enhancement is obtained with an unsharp mask technique. In this technique the original image is blurred by a low pass filter, which is subtracted from the original to leave only high spatial frequency signal. This signal is amplified and added back into the exam data to produce an image with higher frequencies or edge enhancement. The process is demonstrated in Figure 43–12. It is important to understand that edge enhancement techniques usually increase noise and as a result may produce lower quality images with higher base fog levels and lower contrast.

Computed Radiography Image Quality

Although the image reader device analyzes the imaging plate exposure and adjusts the sensitivity of the receptors to assure maximum data acquisition, it is still important for the radiographer to understand how to assess image quality. The computed radiography processing system indicates several values that are useful for this purpose. Although different manufacturers use different systems for this information, the basic concept is similar.

Fuji System

The Fuji computed radiography system uses an S number to assist in evaluating exposure. It is inversely proportional to the exposure reaching the imaging plate. For example, an S value of 200 indicates that the imaging plate received about 1 mR (approximately the same exposure necessary to produce a diagnostic density image with a typical 300 RS film-screen combination). A higher S value indicates that the imaging plate (IP) was underexposed, while a lower S value indicates overexposure of the IP. Properly exposed imaging plates should produce S values of 150-250. Figure 43–13 demonstrates a full range of over- and underexposed images.

Kilovoltage for computed radiography will control contrast similar to film radiography. However, some computed radiography manufacturers recommend avoiding the use of more than 80 kVp for non-grid imaging because higher kVp levels produce excessive fog that will decrease contrast significantly more than the same increase with a film-screen imaging receptor.

The Fuji system uses two types of CR plates with different speeds and resolution. The standard plate (ST-V) is used for exams that would typically use a 400 relative speed film-screen speed system and has resolution of around 5.0 lp/mm. The ST-V has a reflective layer between the phosphor layer and the conductive layer. For exams requiring lower speed and increased resolution, the high resolution plate (HR) is used; it is comparable to a 100 film-screen speed system and has a resolution slightly greater than 5 lp/mm.

One advantage to CR is the wide dynamic range response of the imaging plate detector. Rather than the

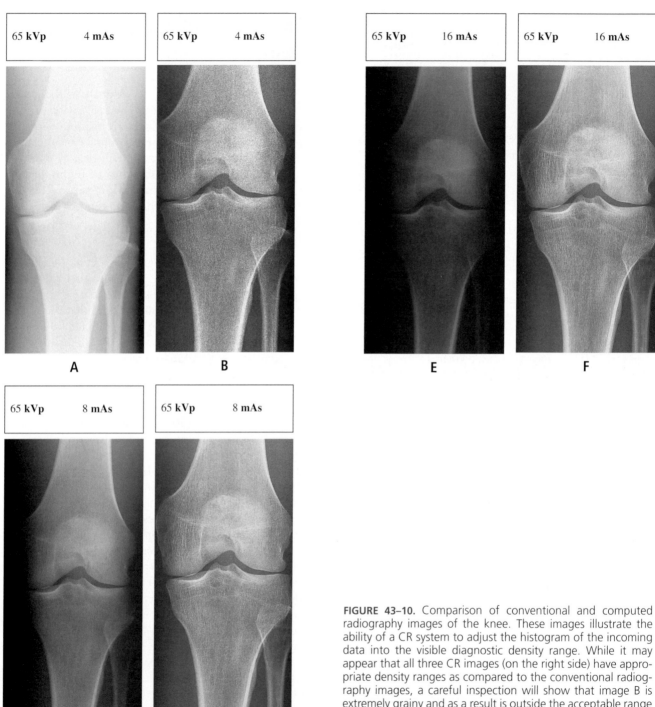

| 65 kVp | 4 mAs | | 65 kVp | 4 mAs |
| 65 kVp | 16 mAs | | 65 kVp | 16 mAs |

A   B   E   F

| 65 kVp | 8 mAs | | 65 kVp | 8 mAs |

C   D

FIGURE 43–10. Comparison of conventional and computed radiography images of the knee. These images illustrate the ability of a CR system to adjust the histogram of the incoming data into the visible diagnostic density range. While it may appear that all three CR images (on the right side) have appropriate density ranges as compared to the conventional radiography images, a careful inspection will show that image B is extremely grainy and as a result is outside the acceptable range for detail. This is an example of the CR histogram adjusting for density but lacking adequate data to fill in an acceptable level of detail.

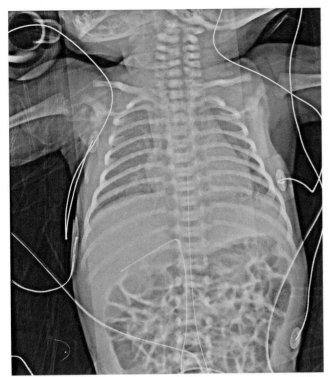

FIGURE 43–11. Histogram error artifact. Selection of an adult histogram used on a pediatric chest.

characteristic curve of film screen systems, the response of an imaging plate to x-ray is linear. This linear response gives the imaging plate increased exposure latitude over film-screen (Figure 43–14). This means that areas that receive very little radiation can be enhanced by the computer instead of all the densities clumping around the toe of the $D_{log}E$ curve as they do when using a film receptor. Conversely, areas receiving greater exposure can be separated and brought down into the visible density range by the computer instead of all clumping around the shoulder of the $D_{log}E$ curve.

An important extension of the density range occurs with CR with areas of much greater exposure because the imaging plate does not have a D_{max}. When film is exposed beyond D_{max}, it actually reverses and begins to get lighter (as with duplicating film). The CR imaging plate continues to record the exposure and the computer can bring these densities down into the visible range. This is why a CR system can compensate for gross overexposure. This is also why the radiographer using CR must realize that **there is great danger in permitting personal professional standards to relax and routinely overexposing all patients with the intention of the CR system adjusting the histogram to correct the exposure.** This practice is unethical, violates ALARA radiation protection guidelines, and is to be avoided at all times.

There are multiple benefits inherent in this increased latitude, such as the ability to image structures of widely different attenuation values such as the chest, on the same image without loss of visibility of structures with widely different densities (such as lung vasculature and the mediastinum). (See Figures 43–7 and 43–8.)

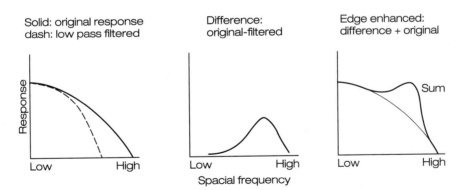

FIGURE 43–12. Spatial frequency edge enhancement technique. The histogram of the image on the left has a dashed line added as a result of a second analysis with a low pass filter added. The center histogram represents only the difference between the two histograms from the figure on the left. The final histogram is a combination of the original data with the data from the center added to produce the enhancement of the edge. *(Reprinted with permission of the American Association of Physicists in Medicine, 1997)*

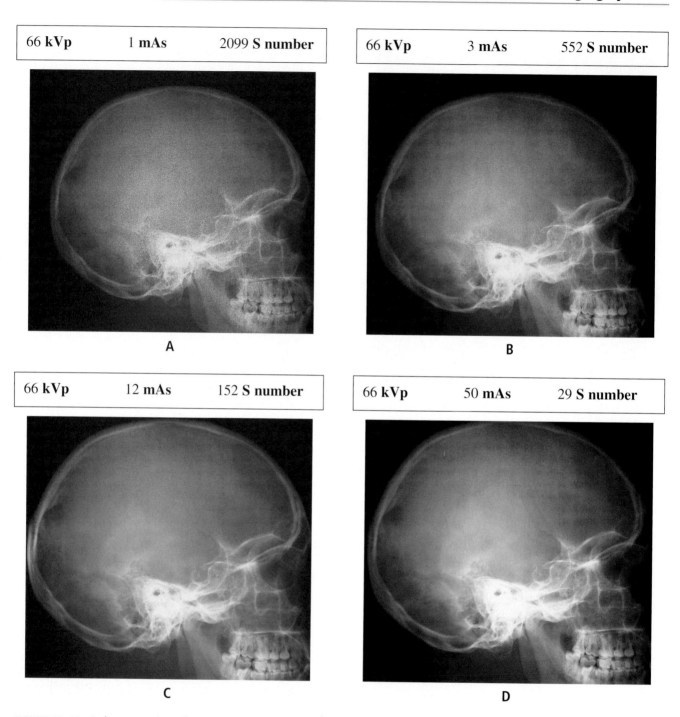

FIGURE 43–13. A demonstration of over- and underexposure with a CR system. While it may appear that all four CR images have appropriate density ranges, a careful inspection will show that with the exception of image C, the Fuji S numbers are outside the optimal range of 150–250. Image A has an S number of 2099, which indicates that it was grossly underexposed, As a result, it exhibits excessive loss of detail and graineness. Image D has an S number of 29, which indicates that patient exposure was probably close to 10 times more than it should have been.

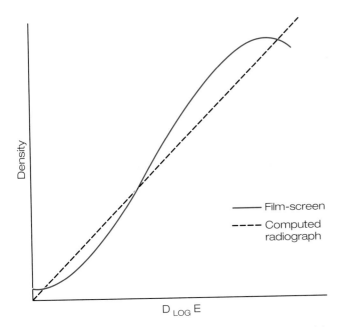

FIGURE 43–14. Comparison of $D_{log}E$ curves of radiographic film and intensifying screens versus a digital computed radiography system. Note that the computed radiography system response is linear and does not have a toe or shoulder as the film-screen curve.

Another benefit is the increased margin for error in over- and underexposure to the receptor. CR can maintain a useful density over a wider latitude than allowable with film-screen. However, even though density can be maintained, the overall image quality may be poor if exposures range too far from optimal. **Images that are underexposed will show quantum mottle, even though the density is acceptable, while overexposed images will tend to suffer from low contrast.**

Table 43–2 provides a summary of the Fuji computed radiography system.

Image Acquisition Elements

CR offers many advantages over traditional film-screen for obtaining diagnostic images; however, as with any system, there are pitfalls that must be recognized. To obtain high quality images with minimal patient dose, a deeper understanding of CR is required. One of the big advantages of CR is the reduction of repeat exposures due to incorrect technique or to image various densities in the same anatomical region without repeat exposures. Two reasons CR has this advantage are the wide dynamic range of the imaging plate and the ability to use windowing and leveling in the image.

The exposure sensitivity of the imaging plate ranges from a minimum of 0.1 mR up to a maximum of 100 mR, a range of approximately 10,000:1. If soft tissue and bone densities are required, one exposure will give the information owing to the ability to change window levels. In order to evaluate the exposure for a CR image, most manufacturers have an exposure indicator that provides information on the average amount of radiation used for an image (see Table 43–3).

Fuji uses a sensitivity, or S, number that is related to the amount of amplification required by the PM tube to adjust the digital image. The S number is inversely related to exposure in mR, so a large S number indicates a low exposure to the imaging plate, while a small S number reflects high mR. For example, an exposure of 1 mR has an S value of 200. Properly exposed images should have an S value around 150–250 for ST-V plates, reflecting appropriate patient dose. Kodak's CR indicator system is called the exposure index, which is directly proportional to the radiation striking the imaging plate. An exposure of 0.1 mR has an exposure index of 1,000 while 1 mR in this system gives an exposure index of 2,000, and 10 mR results in an exposure index of 3,000. Properly exposed images should have an exposure index that ranges from 1,800 to 2,200. The Agfa system is optional and uses a relative exposure value, which compares the exposure level of an image to a database of previous exposures.

The increased latitude of the imaging plate allows for correction of exposure errors, but as the exposure error increases, image quality will decrease. If a substantial overexposure occurs, the resulting image will not offer optimum image quality. Basic principles regarding the production of poor low contrast images when using film-screen do not change with the use of CR. Factors that produce low contrast include high kVp, no grid or inadequate grid efficiency, inadequate beam limitation, and increased part size or tissue thickness (Table 43–4). As with film-screen, kVp selection should be based on

TABLE 43–2. Fuji Computed Radiography System Summary

System Limitations and Guidelines for Use

Corrects exposure errors >2X.

Images with low contrast or high mottle may be produced for expo
sure errors up to 50X.

To achieve optimal quality exposure must be set within a range of 2X.

Cannot compensate for low photon intensity (underexposure).

Cannot compensate for excessive scatter radiation.

The system cannot compensate for:

exposure >2X

insufficient mAs

insufficient kVp

excessive part size

excessive kVp

inadequate grid use

Photostimulable Phosphor Imaging Plates

Standard Plate (ST-V) ~ 300RS (~5.0 lp/mm)

High Resolution Plate (HR) ~100RS (~5.0 lp/mm)

Exposure Data Recognition (EDR) Preprocessing Modes

AUTOmatic

entire image plate is scanned

requires beam and part centered to image plate

requires image margins parallel to image plate

requires image margins equidistant from edges

SEMIautomatic

center of image plate is scanned

requires image at center of image plate

FIXED

eliminates preprocessing

designed for use when anatomy cannot be centered to image plate

density and contrast depend on exposure set by radiographer

Image Labeling

L value

subject contrast (differential light intensities)

changes with kVp, scatter, part size

appropriate range 1.6–1.8

>2.2 = low inherent data contrast

S value

photomultiplier tube sensitivity used for final reading
(exposure index)

Standard Plate (ST-V) appropriate range 150–250

<50 = gross patient overexposure
(may produce residual exposure on next use of image plate)

<100 = substantial patient overexposure

>400 = objectionable mottle

High Resolution Plate (HR) appropriate range 50–100

<10 = gross patient overexposure (may produce residual
exposure on next use of image plate)

<25 = substantial patient overexposure

>100 = objectionable mottle

inversely proportional to image plate exposure
(reciprocal roentgen value)

2 = 100 mR

20 = 10 mR

200 = 1 mR (~400RS)

2,000 = 0.1 mR

20,000 = 0.01 mR

C values

baseline contrast and density shift values in image processing
program

G setting

gradient

R setting

spatial frequency enhancement

desired subject contrast and grid selection. It is recommended that kVp not exceed 80 for all non-grid radiography. Since CR plates have a wide dynamic range they are especially sensitive to fogging, from both scatter and background radiation. The lower K edge of the BaFBr phosphor contributes to the scatter sensitivity of CR when compared to the higher K edge of rare earth inten-sifying screens. Because the imaging plate is so sensitive to background ionizing radiation, **it is recommended that plates be erased daily if not used to eliminate unwanted noise** from these sources.

Grid use in CR occurs more often due to the sensitivity of the imaging plate to scatter. When performing chest radiography, a grid should be used when chest

TABLE 43–3. Exposure Index Numbers Relative to Imaging Plate Exposure

Fuji S Value	2	20	200	2,000	20,000
Kodak Exposure Index		3,000	2,000	1,000	
mR	100	10	1	0.1	0.01

measurements exceed 24 to 26 cm for optimum images. Even when using a grid, if a substantial overexposure (>2×) occurs, enough scatter may be generated to degrade the image. Selecting the proper grid will depend on part size, kVp desired, scatter cleanup desired, and grid frequency (lines per cm or inch). The imaging plate is scanned line by line; **if the scan frequency and the grid frequency are similar and oriented in the same direction a moire effect will be observed.** Recommendations for grid frequency are 85 lines/in (33–34 lines/cm) for a 14 × 17 and 103 (40–44 lines/cm) for a 10 × 12.

Indirect Silicon Flat Panel Imaging Plate Systems

Amorphous silicon cannot directly convert x-rays into an electric charge, but it does work as a light detector (photo-diode) to capture fluorescent light. Because the atomic number of silicon is only 14, it is necessary to have a relatively thick silicon layer to provide adequate sensitivity to the incoming x-ray photons. Amorphous

TABLE 43–4. Factors That Produce Low Contrast and Are Prone to Cause CR Imaging Plate Fogging

high kVp
no grid or inadequate grid efficiency
inadequate beam limitation
increased part size or tissue density

silicon requires a scintillator, such as cesium iodide (CsI)(which is currently used by Philips and General Electric) or a rare earth intensifying screen composed of gadolinium and lanthanium with osysulfides (this system is currently used by Canon). Scintillators emit light isotropically, which can reduce spatial resolution. To minimize light spread, CsI is manufactured as structured crystals in the form of needles or columns 10 to 20 micrometers in diameter. This significantly reduces light spread and channels light toward the amorphous silicon photodiode. The Canon scintillator is designed as a thin screen to minimize light spread. Once the light reaches the amorphous silicon it is converted into an electric signal. Figure 43–15 illustrates the design of an amorphous silicon system.

Charge Coupled Devices (CCD)

Once the image has been converted into an electrical signal, it still needs to be converted into electronic pulses that are correlated to the image matrix for the computer. One method of accomplishing this signal is to place a charged coupled device (CCD) in contact with the scintillator. Companies that are using CCD systems include OEM, Odelft, and Swissray.

Thin Film Transistors (TFTs)

Both the amorphous silicon and amorphous selenium flat plate detectors use thin film transistors (TFT) for electronic readout. The TFT collects the electric charges produced by either the selenium or silicon as an array or matrix of pixel-size detector elements. Each TFT element collects the charge and then, when a gate is activated by the computer, sends a signal. The TFTs are positioned in a matrix that allows the charge pattern to

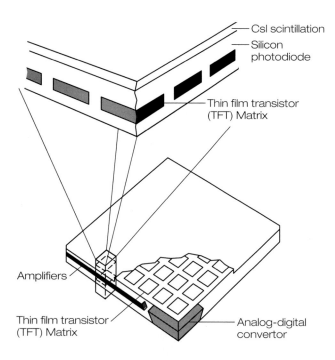

— CsI scintillation
— Silicon photodiode
— Thin film transistor (TFT) Matrix
Amplifiers
Thin film transistor (TFT) Matrix
— Analog-digital convertor

FIGURE 43–15. Indirect amorphous silicon flat panel imaging plate system. When x-ray photons strike the CsI they are converted to light. The columns of CsI reduce the light spread interacting with the amorphous silicon.

be read out on a pixel-by-pixel and column-by-column basis. Philips, General Electric, and Canon are all using TFTs.

Direct Exposure Imaging Systems

Direct conversion systems directly convert incoming x-ray photons to an electronic digital signal. These systems use amorphous selenium and are sometimes referred to as **direct radiography systems.** The term **flat panel** (or **flat field**) **detectors** is also being used to describe both the indirect amorphous silicon and the direct amorphous selenium plates that are being used in some digital radiography systems.

Direct Selenium Flat Panel Imaging Plate Systems

The active layer in the imaging plate is amorphous selenium, which is a semiconductor with excellent x-ray photon detection ability and spatial resolution of >20 lp/mm. Prior to the exposure, a high voltage charge is applied from the top surface of the selenium layer. The ionization caused by the x-ray photons results in the selenium atoms freeing electrons for collection by the electrodes at the bottom of the selenium layer. The charge that is collected is then transmitted through TFTs to the computer for processing. This process is illustrated in Figure 43–16.

DICOM Standard

The Digital Imaging and Communications in Medicine (DICOM) standard is a system of computer software standards that permit a wide range of digital imaging programs to understand one another. The DICOM-3 standard is currently in use and it is responsible for much of the acceptance of digital imaging modalities in recent years. Prior to the widespread use of DICOM-3, many medical imaging systems, especially those made by different manufacturers, were unable to communicate with each other. DICOM-3 permits the interfacing of diverse systems; for example, a diagnostic radiographic digital radiography system, a computed tomography unit, and a digital chest system can all share the same computer network and software filing system without conflict.

Computed Radiography Artifacts

As with all computerized imaging systems, computed radiography has unique artifact patterns as a result of errors in the systems. Some of the more common CR artifacts include:

- Fogging due to imaging plates being much more sensitive than film

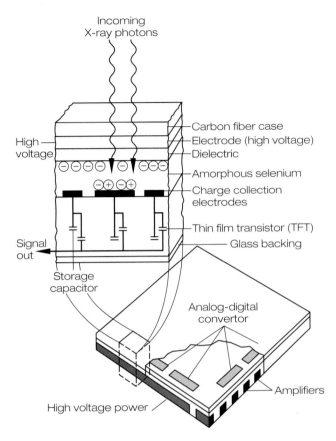

FIGURE 43–16. Direct conversion amorphous selenium flat panel imaging plate. The high voltage charge at the top surface of the selenium layer results in the ionization caused by the x-ray photons to free electrons for collection by the electrodes at the bottom of the selenium layer. The charge that is collected is then transmitted through thin film detectors (TFTs) to the computer for processing.

- Quantum mottle caused by inadequate exposure (usually insufficient mAS)

- Heat blur (Figure 43–17) caused from image receptor being exposed to intense heat

- Histogram error (see Figure 43–11) due to incorrect preprocessing histogram selection - adult histogram used on pediatric chest

- Nonparallel collimation (see Figure 43–5) - histograms require that collimation edges be parallel to the sides of imaging plate

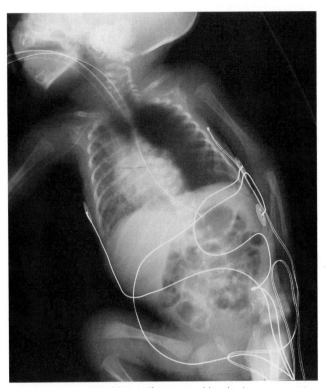

FIGURE 43–17. Heat blur artifact caused by the image receptor being exposed to intense heat.

Summary

Digital radiography replaces traditional film with a reusable detector. Detectors currently used to acquire radiographic images include photostimulable storage phosphor imaging plates (IP), charge coupled devices (CCD), silicon, and selenium. These detectors are classified as either indirect conversion or direct conversion. Silicon and selenium receptors are also known as flat panel detectors.

Indirect conversion systems use a two-part process involving a scintillator (which converts incoming x-ray photons to light) and a photodetector (which converts light into an electronic digital signal). Indirect systems include those that use photostimulable storage phosphor imaging plates (IP), charged coupled devices (CCD), and silicon.

Direct conversion systems directly convert incoming x-ray photons to an electronic digital signal. These systems use selenium and are sometimes referred to as direct radiography (DR) systems.

In order for digital radiography to function, the imaging plate material must have the ability to store and release the image information in a usable form. The imaging plate is more sensitive to scatter both before and after it is sensitized. The latent image will lose about 25 percent of its energy in 8 hours. Pixel size and quantity depend on the size of the phosphor plate being scanned. The smaller the pixels and the larger the matrix the higher the spatial resolution.

When using the Fuji computed radiography systems, it is important to remember that the beam and part need to be centered within each pattern and collimation must be parallel and equidistant from the edges of the imaging plate, and the correct histogram algorithm must be selected prior to processing. The Fuji system uses an S number to assist in evaluating exposure. A higher S value indicates that the imaging plate was underexposed, while a lower S value indicates overexposure.

Kilovoltage for digital radiography will control contrast similar to film radiography, However, some digital radiography manufacturers recommend avoiding the use of more than 80 kVp because higher kVp levels produce excessive fog that will decrease contrast significantly more than the same increase with a film-screen imaging receptor. The primary advantage to digital radiography is the wide dynamic range response of the imaging plate detector. Rather than the characteristic curve of film-screen systems, the response to x-ray is linear, so the imaging plate does not have a D_{max}. When film is exposed beyond D_{max}, it actually reverses and begins to get lighter (as with duplicating film). The digital radiography imaging plate continues to record the exposure and the computer can bring these densities down into the visible range. This is why a digital radiography system can compensate for gross overexposure. This is also why the radiographer using digital radiography must realize that there is great danger in permitting personal professional standards to relax and routinely overexposing all patients with the intention of the digital radiography system adjusting the histogram to correct the exposure. This practice is unethical, violates ALARA radiation protection guidelines, and is to be avoided at all times.

Once the image has been converted into an electrical signal, it still needs to be converted into electronic pulses that are correlated to the image matrix for the computer. One method of accomplishing this signal is to place a charged coupled device (CCD) in contact with the scintillator. Both the amorphous silicon and amorphous selenium flat plate detectors use thin film transistors (TFT) for electronic readout. Each TFT element collects the charge and then, when a gate is activated by the computer, sends a signal.

Digital radiography has unique artifact patterns as a result of errors in the systems. Some of the more common digital radiography artifacts include fogging, quantum mottle, heat blue, histogram error, and nonparallel collimation.

REVIEW QUESTIONS

1. Give an example of the types of image receptors used for both a direct and indirect conversion digital radiography system.

2. Name the image receptors used in one of the flat panel detector systems.

3. Explain the function of two of the layers of a photostimulable phosphor imaging plate.

4. Why are imaging plates more sensitive to radiation than radiographic film?

5. Why do digital radiography cassettes stored for several days after exposure and before processing lose most of their latent image?

6. How is digital radiography spatial resolution controlled?

7. What data are collected during the creation of the histogram from a digital radiography exposure?

8. Why do digital radiography systems have significantly greater latitude than conventional film-screen radiography systems?

9. What elements of computed radiography systems make them prone to violations of ALARA radiation protection concepts?

10. Name as many digital radiography artifacts as you know.

REFERENCE AND RECOMMENDED READING

Bell, J. (1999). A direct image capture system: The future of digital x-ray. *Medical Imaging Technology. 17*(2), 105–109.

Burns, C. (1993). Using computed digital radiography effectively. *Seminars in Radiologic Technology. 1*(1), 24–35.

Bushberg, J., Seibert, J., Leidholdt, E., & Boone, J. (1994). *The essential physics of medical imaging.* Baltimore: Williams & Wilkins.

Cesar, L. (1997). Computed radiography: Its impact on radiographers. *Radiologic Technology. 68*(3), 225–232.

Choatas, H., Dobbins, J., & Ravin, C. (1999) Principles of digital radiography with large-area electronically readable detectors: A review of the basics. *Radiology. 210*(3), 595–599.

Frey, G. & Sprawls, P. (1997) *The Expanding Role of Medical Physicists in Diagnostic Imaging: Proceedings of the 1997 AAPM Summer School.* Madison, WI: Advanced Medical Publishing for American Association of Physicists in Medicine.

Fuji Photo Film Co., Ltd. (1996). *Fujifilm imaging and information: Chapter 2: Information capacity of FCR images.* Tokyo: Fuji Photo Film Co., Ltd., Ref. No. CR-008040C2 (CR-96-9).

Fuji Photo Film Co., Ltd. (1996). *Fujifilm imaging and information: Chapter 3: Auto density control (EDR).* Tokyo: Fuji Photo Film Co., Ltd., Ref. No. CR-008040C3 (CR-96-9).

Fuji Photo Film Co., Ltd. (1996). *Fujifilm imaging and information: Chapter 4: Image processing.* Tokyo: Fuji Photo Film Co., Ltd., Ref. No. CR-008040C4 (CR-96-9).

Fuji Photo Film Co., Ltd. (1996.) *Fujifilm imaging and information: Chapter 5: Special image processing.* Tokyo: Fuji Photo Film Co., Ltd., Ref. No. CR-008040C5 (CR-96-9).

Fuji Photo Film Co., Ltd. (1996). *Fujifilm imaging and information: Appendix 1: Clinical effects of FCR.* Tokyo: Fuji Photo Film Co., Ltd., Ref. No. CR-008040A1 (CR-96-9).

Fuji Photo Film Co., Ltd. (1996). *Fujifilm imaging and information: Appendix 2: Case studies.* Tokyo: Fuji Photo Film Co., Ltd., Ref. No. CR-008040A2 (CR-96-9).

Hamers, S. & Freyschmidt, J., (Eds.) (1998). Digital radiography with an electronic flat-panel detector: First clinical experience in skeletal diagnostics. *MedicaMunda. 42*(3), 2–6.

Hillman, B. & Fajardo, L. (1989). Clinical assessment of phosphor-plate computed radiography: Equipment, strategy, and methods. *Journal of Digital Imaging. 2*(4), 220–227.

Hindel, R. (1983). Digital imaging—the technology of the future. *The Canadian Journal of Medical Radiation Technology. 14*(4), 128.

Lim, A. (1996). *Image quality in film digitizers: Testing and quality assurance. Syllabus: A Course in Physics.* Chicago: Radiological Society of North America, 183–193.

Long, B.W. (1989). Computed radiography: Photostimulable phosphor image plate technology. *Radiologic Technology. 61*(2), 107–112.

Mixdorf, M. & Tortorici, M. (1993). Practical Considerations in Computed Radiography. *Seminars in Radiologic Technology. 1*:1, 16–23.

Murphey, M., Quale, J., Martin, N., Bramble, J., Cook, L. & Dwyer, S. (1992). Computed radiography in musculoskeletal imaging: State of the art. *American Journal of Roentgenology. 158*, 19–27.

Neitzel, U. (1999). *Integrated digital radiography with a flat electronic detector.* www.de.ms.philips.com/sections/rad/digbucky/news/html/neitzel.htm, 7-16-99.

Solomon, S., Jost, R., Glazer, H., Sagel, S., Anderson, D., & Molina, P. (1991). Artifacts in computed radiography. *American Journal of Roentgenology. 157,* 181–185.

Wilson, P. (1984). Digital imaging: An introduction. *Radiography. 50*(590), 449.

Yamazaki, T., Satoh, M., Eguchi, Y., Yamada, K., Endo, Y., & Kaga, Y. (1998). *Image quality of the digital radiography system using the flat panel detector compared with the storage phosphor based computed radiography system.* Radiological Society of North American Scientific Exhibit 0499PH, Chicago, IL.

CHAPTER 44

Computed Tomography

The physicians seem to be quite keen on it.

Allan Cormack upon being informed that he and Godfrey Hounsfield
were to share the 1979 Nobel Prize for Medicine for the invention of computed tomography.

OBJECTIVES

Upon completion of this chapter, the student should be able to:

▶ Relate the invention of computed tomography.

▶ Describe typical gantry components.

▶ Explain the basic features of each generation of CT scanners, especially third and fourth generation units.

▶ Explain why CT tabletops have patient weight limits.

▶ Compare the requirements for a CT x-ray tube with those of a routine diagnostic tube.

▶ Explain the operation of a scintillation crystal and photomultiplier tube CT detector.

▶ Explain the operation of a xenon gas-filled ionization chamber CT detector.

▶ Discuss the importance of detector alignment and calibration.

▶ Discuss the use of a CT computer menu or index.

▶ Describe the major display features possible with advanced software.

▶ Describe the calculation and use of Hounsfield units.

▶ Explain reformatting image reconstruction.

▶ Explain how CT display image density and contrast are controlled.

▶ Describe the factors affecting resolution, including voxel, pixel and matrix size.

▶ Discuss methods of reducing CT image noise and motion.

▶ Illustrate section shape, partial volume effect and scan arc to scanning procedures.

▶ Explain a variety of common CT artifacts.

▶ Discuss radiation protection of the patient and others during CT examinations.

Computed tomography (CT) produces a digital tomographic image from diagnostic x-rays. The basic principle of CT involves digitizing an image received from a slit scan projection of the patient's body and then back-projecting the image through mathematical algorithms.

Although CT scanning is usually performed transversely, digital processing of information can produce sagittal and coronal sections (Figure 44–1). Because the CT x-ray beam is confined to a slit, much scatter radiation is eliminated from the image. The combination of the transverse sectioning procedure with slit scanning produces an image of significantly better quality than that available with other imaging methods. Primarily the image differentiates various types of soft tissues (e.g., gray matter, white matter, blood, tumor, cerebrospinal fluid, etc.). When digital image data manipulation is added, CT provides more diagnostic information than any other ionizing radiation imaging modality.

As with other tomographic modalities, the terms "cut" and "slice" are used in clinical practice. Because these phrases can easily cause distress when overheard by a patient, the radiographer should strive to adhere to the term "section," avoiding "cut" and "slice."

The Invention of Computed Tomography

The invention of computed tomography has been credited to Godfrey N. Hounsfield for his work in 1970–71, although preliminary work was done by Oldendorf in 1961 and Cormack in 1963, and all three based their work on the investigations of the Austrian mathematician J. Radon, who proved in 1917 that an image of a three-dimensional object could be produced from its mathematical projections. Hounsfield was a research engineer with Electro-Musical Instruments Ltd. (EMI), the English firm that gained international renown as the Beatles' music publishers during the 1960s. His original scanner was built on a lathe bed and required nine days to produce a single section image. Although the company sold its CT business, it continues to operate American and British EMI record labels. Hounsfield and Cormack were awarded the 1979 Nobel Prize for Medicine. Hounsfield's invention parallels Röntgen's discovery of x-rays as the two most outstanding contributions to medical imaging.

Early CT units were capable of only axial tomography, and the term computerized axial tomography (CAT) scanning became a popular acronym. Modern CT units are capable of diverse modes much more complex than simple axial scanning. However, the term CAT scanning may endure, as have other antiquated radiologic terms (e.g., flat plate and wet reading). A modern CT unit includes a gantry, table, x-ray tube, detectors, computer, display console and image storage units (Figure 44–2).

Gantry

The gantry is the movable frame of the CT unit. It contains the x-ray tube and detectors and is the most visible part of the unit. The gantry frame maintains the alignment of the tube and detectors and contains the equipment necessary to perform the scanning movements. The gantry includes a 50–85 cm (20"–34") aperture for the patient. Obese patients who exceed the tabletop weight limits must never be forced into the aperture. They may become stuck.

Most gantrys can be angled up to 30° to permit positioning for partial coronal images. This is especially desirable in obtaining transverse scans perpendicular to the vertebral column. Table angulation can sometimes be used in place of gantry angulation. Scanners with the x-ray beam placed near the table side of the aperture permit more comfortable positioning of the patient and may permit coronal or sagittal scanning of some body parts, especially of the head. Both magnetic resonance imaging and CT reconfiguration software may be used in place of positions designed to achieve coronal or sagittal sections.

Positioning lights are usually mounted on the gantry as well. Intense white halogen lights and low-power red laser lights are used for positioning. The body part of interest must be properly centered to the aperture because the extreme edge of the scanning field produces a severely degraded image. There are often three positioning lights for accurate sagittal, coronal and transverse centering.

Scanner Generations

Computed tomography technology advanced very rapidly after Hounsfield's discovery. Scanners are sometimes described by their generation, with the original EMI head scanner considered to be the first. Descriptions of various computed tomography equipment refer to both rays and projections (also called views). A **ray** is a pencil thin beam of radiation that strikes a single detector. A **projection** (or **view**) is composed of a set of rays striking a detector array (a group of detectors). Although there are no distinct lines between the generations, Table 44–1 illustrates the major characteristics of each.

First Generation   First generation CT scanners were single ray systems designed for examination of the head only (Figure 44–3). The head was surrounded by a water bag to eliminate air interfaces. A single x-ray tube and a pair of detectors were aligned on a fixed C-arm. The detectors were sodium iodide scintillation crystals with photomultiplier tubes. A pencil-thin slit field, 3 mm × 26 mm, scanned a 180° arc around the patient's head. Each detector was exposed to a 3 mm × 13 mm field. First generation units used a rotating scan and index system that scanned the head linearly (from one

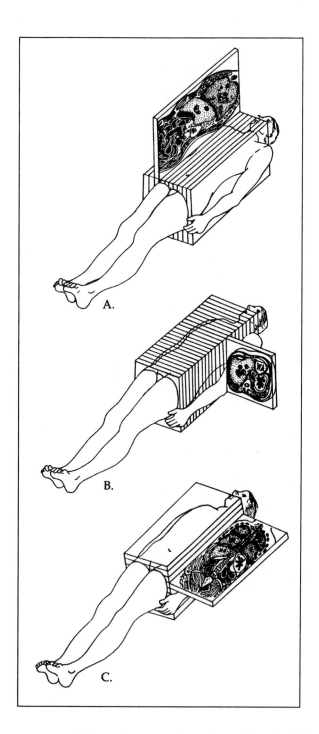

FIGURE 44–1. Computed tomography sections: (A) sagittal, (B) transverse, and (C) coronal.

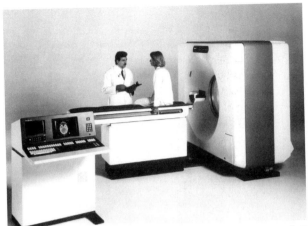

FIGURE 44–2. A computed tomography unit. *(Courtesy of GE Medical Systems)*

TABLE 44–1. Major Characteristics Of CT Unit Generations

First generation	head only linear scan and rotate (180 scans, 1° rotations) paired detectors (160 measurements per scan) 4.5–5 minute scan time single ray pencil beam single detector
Second generation	single projection fan-shaped beam (permitting whole body scanning) up to 30 detectors 10–90 second scan time linear scan and rotate (6 scans, 30° rotations)
Third generation	single projection fan-shaped beam up to 300 detectors 2–10 second scan time 360° rotation of x-ray tube and detectors crude dynamic capabilities
Fourth generation	single projection fan-shaped beam 360° ring of stationary detectors 2–10 second scan time 360° rotation of x-ray tube dynamic capabilities
Helical/Spiral	multiple projection fan-shaped beam 360° ring of stationary detectors 360° rotation of x-ray tube computer controlled table movement through gantry bore continuous scanning throughout entire examination
Other Designs	nutating detector ring multiple anode ring (cardiac system) 50 msec scan time multiple x-ray tube to video (DSR system) 16 msec scan time

side to the other), indexed 1°, repeated the scanning process, indexed another 1°, etc., for the entire 180° (Figure 44–4). This is also called a translate (scan) and rotate (index) system. The x-ray tube was on during scanning and off during indexing. Although the pair of detectors did not decrease the 180° scanning time, they permitted two anatomical sections to be scanned simultaneously, thus reducing the total examination time by half.

The detectors measured the attenuation coefficient of the exit radiation beam at overlapping 1.7 mm intervals 240 times during each scan. The unit required 4.5 minutes to complete a pair of full 180° scans and 5 minutes to reconstruct the images. Each section was derived from 43,200 measurements (180° × 240) and was displayed on an 80 × 80 matrix. Each display pixel represented a voxel of tissue 3 mm × 3 mm × 13 mm although a 1.5 mm pixel display became available. A common examination routine for the head consisted of 10–12 sections, which required 25–35 minutes to obtain.

Second Generation
Second generation CT units used a single projection fan-shaped beam instead of a pencil slit and a linear array of as many as 30 detectors (Figure 44–5). They too are no longer available. The fan-shaped beam and increased number of detectors permitted scanning and rotation with fewer linear movements. For example, a 30 detector unit could complete the 180° linear movement in only six rotations of 30° each.

However, the loss of collimation increased the amount of scatter radiation detected. This is a major disadvantage of all fan beam scanners. A lead mask was added to the detectors to assist in reducing the scatter reaching the detectors. Scan time was reduced to between 10 and 90 seconds, a reasonable respiratory suspension time, thus permitting examination of the whole body.

Third Generation
Third generation CT units used a wider fan-shaped beam and a curved array of 250–750 detectors to achieve a single projection (Figure 44–6). The fan-shaped beam was wide enough to include the entire body in a single exposure and rotated 360° within the gantry, thus eliminating the linear scan and rotate system. A typical third generation scanner might pro-

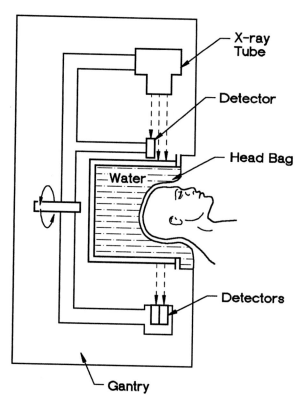

FIGURE 44–3. A first generation CT head scanner.

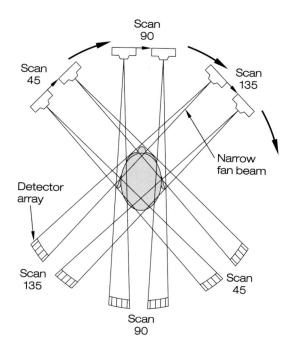

FIGURE 44–4. First generation CT scan and rotate system. Only three scans (the 45th, 90th, and 135th) are shown to simplify the illustration. A single scan and rotate required 180 scans, each 1° apart.

duce 700,000 measurements per section. Various scanning arcs were usually possible, for example 220° or 360°. Scan time was reduced to between 1 and 12 seconds, permitting sequential images to crudely approximate dynamic functions. Third generation units that featured dynamic scanning usually performed at about four scans per minute, which equals the routine scanning time of a fourth generation unit. Because they had only a single detector array, third generation scanners were prone to ring artifacts (Figure 44–21).

Fourth Generation
Fourth generation CT units were developed as a result of a competitive contract awarded to the American Science and Engineering Company (AS&E) by the United States National Institutes of Health (NIH). They use a single projection fan-shaped beam with 600–2,000 stationary detectors arrayed in a 360° ring (Figure 44–7). The ring of detectors eliminates movement of detectors, thereby decreas-

ing calibration requirements. As many as 1,200,000 measurements may be processed per section. A wider range of scan arcs, including arcs over 360°, are usually possible with scan times ranging from 0.5 to 10 seconds.

Some fourth generation scanners are capable of dynamic scanning rates in the range of 15 scans per minute. The limiting factor is the interscan time and the computer processing time, not the actual scanning time. Dynamic scanning is usually achieved by reducing the interscan time to 1–2 seconds and not indexing the gantry. Scanning occurs first in a clockwise direction, then counterclockwise, etc. Another technique, called overscan, may also be available. Overscanning uses a scan of more than 360°. The overscan may be displayed as segmented data from 2, 3 or 4 scans as a single image.

Helical/Spiral Computed Tomography
Helical (spiral) scanners were made possible by advances in slip ring connection technology. Slip rings consist of brushes that fit into grooves to permit the current and voltage to

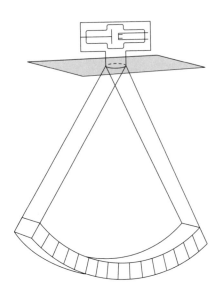

FIGURE 44–5. A fan-shaped beam.

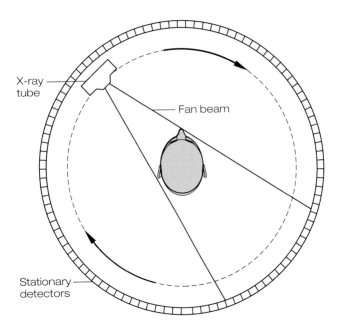

FIGURE 44–7. A fourth generation CT scanner.

the x-ray tube to be supplied while the tube is in continuous rotation around the gantry (Figure 44–8). This permits scanning of the entire body in a helical pattern without stopping the tube. When the patient table is

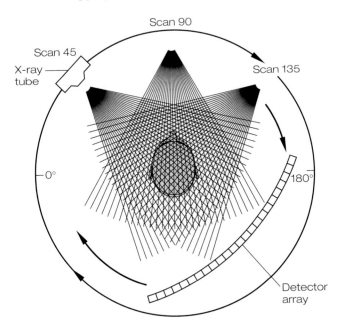

FIGURE 44–6. A third generation CT scanner.

moved slowly during the x-ray exposure while the tube is in continuous rotation, data comprising a continuous helical scan of the patient is acquired. Both low and high voltage slip rings have been developed by different manufacturers.

The term spiral is a misnomer. A spiral is a circular motion with a decreasing or increasing diameter. The actual scanning motion has a set circular diameter, which is a helix. The data is acquired in a helical, not a spiral, motion.

The primary advantage of helical scanning is a much shorter total scan time (30–40 sec. for the entire abdomen). This in turn permits the use of less contrast media. Not only are patients at less risk of contrast media reaction, the throughput of patients is greatly increased. Another advantage is that for many patients the entire examination can be completed in one breath hold, eliminating overlaps and missed areas due to variations in the amount of air in the lungs between scan sections. This also reduces the possibility of motion artifacts.

The primary disadvantage is that a full 360° set of data is not acquired for each section because the patient is continuously advancing through the gantry bore during the exposure. The sectional image is created from

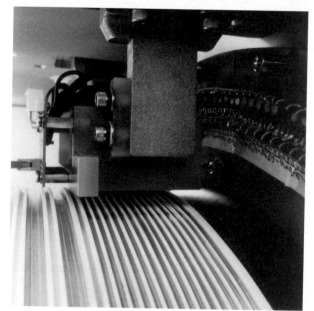

FIGURE 44–8. A helical computed tomography scanner slip ring. The brushes are contained in the large unit at the center of the photograph. They fit into grooves in the ring underneath. As the x-ray tube rotates, the necessary electrical connections are maintained without interruption. *(Courtesy of Picker International, Cleveland, OH)*

Example: If the table is moving at 15 mm/sec. and a section thickness of 10 mm is being acquired, what is the pitch?

Answer: $P = \dfrac{I}{S}$

$$P = \frac{15}{10} = 1.5$$

Example: If a pitch of 0.8 is being used and a section thickness of 8 mm is being acquired, what is the proper table speed?

Answer: $P = \dfrac{I}{S}$ or $I = PS$

$I = 0.8 \times 8$

$I = 6.4$ mm/sec.

Example: If the table is moving at 5 mm/sec. and a pitch of 1.0 is being used, what is the section thickness?

Answer: $P = \dfrac{I}{S}$ or $S = \dfrac{I}{P}$

$$S = \frac{5}{1.0}$$

$S = 5$ mm

computer reconstructions of planar sections that approximate the acquisition of planar reconstruction data. Reconstruction can take up to 3 minutes, during which time the unit cannot be used for other purposes without interrupting the process. Both the advantages and disadvantages are detailed in Table 44–2.

Because the patient table moves during the exposure a method to measure and reproduce this motion must be established. Pitch is the term that is used to define this extension or contraction of the helix. Pitch is simply the ratio of the distance the table moves during one tube rotation to the section thickness. Although 360° is the most common rotation, lesser rotations are possible during quick scan procedure. The formula for pitch is:

$$P = \frac{I}{S}$$

where   P = pitch
         I = table increment in mm/sec.
         S = section thickness in mm

Increasing the pitch value permits a greater field of view (FOV) to be imaged in a shorter time. However, it is important to understand that **pitch values less than 1.0 imply data oversampling. Pitch values greater than 1.0 imply that some data is being missed.** The ability to set the pitch less than 1.0 and produce oversampling of areas of interest is also an advantage of helical scanning. Another major advantage is that image reconstruction can be set for smaller section thicknesses than those that were acquired.

Double Helix Computed Tomography   Double helix computed tomography is the first major advancement in helical CT. It is made possible by using a dual beam from a double focus x-ray tube combined with a dual detector system. It permits scan time or section thickness to be reduced by half. For example, a 30 second scan can be completed in 15 seconds with the same section thickness. The same 30 second scan could also produce 5 mm sections instead of 10 mm sections if increased detail was desired but the scan time could remain constant.

TABLE 44–2. Advantages and Disadvantages Of Helical (Spiral) Computed Tomography

Advantages

Requires less contrast media resulting in decreased patient risk of contrast media reactions.

Eliminates overlap and missed areas due to variations in breathing for some patients and examinations where the entire scan can be completed in one breath hold.

Motion artifacts are reduced.

Faster scan time increases patient throughput.

Pitch settings can be set to oversample sections of interest.

Reconstruction section thickness can be smaller than the acquisition section thickness.

Disadvantages

Full 360° projection data is not acquired for each section.

Sections are reconstructed to represent approximate acquisition of planar data.

Other Designs   Other CT designs have been produced. A **nutating** unit is one in which a 360° ring of detectors wobbles to continually intercept a perpendicular beam from a tube which is also rotating 360°. The term nutating is derived from a similar motion observed in astronomy. This unit is capable of dynamic scanning. Two other designs also exist: the cardiac and the dynamic spatial reconstructor (DSR).

The **cardiac scanner** replaces the x-ray tube with a huge electron gun that directs an electron beam in a circular pattern at a 360° anode ring. The fan beam that is produced is intercepted by a 360° detector array. The patient is placed within the anode ring, somewhat akin to being inside the x-ray tube itself. This unit is a dynamic scanner as it can produce four sections simultaneously within 50 msec. The **dynamic spatial reconstructor** (DSR) was developed at the Mayo Clinic in Rochester, Minnesota. It uses 14 x-ray tubes with fluorescent screens and video cameras and is capable of producing an image in 16 msec.

Table

The CT table may be either flat or curved. It is usually made of carbon graphite fiber to decrease beam attenuation. Because the top must extend beyond the table to move the patient into the gantry aperture, it must be capable of supporting the entire weight of the patient without sagging when fully extended. Tabletops are rated for maximum weight and it is critical that the radiographer make sure that this weight is not exceeded. Extensive damage to the table may result when attempts are made to examine very large patients who exceed the tabletop weight limit. Physicians must be informed if the CT unit cannot move obese patients into the aperture for examination. Examinations of patients over the weight limit may remove the CT unit from clinical use for all patients for a considerable time while the top is replaced. The top is motor-driven to permit the patient to be moved the exact desired distance between sections. Section intervals may be controlled automatically by a program initiated at the control console. The table must also be capable of vertical movement, both for positioning within the aperture and for ease of patient transfer.

X-Ray Tubes

The rapid sequential exposures required to produce CT images produce massive amounts of heat in the x-ray tube. Most CT x-ray tube difficulties have revolved around attempts to solve this problem. The early scanners used a stationary anode with a 2 mm × 16 mm focal spot operating at 120 kVp and 30 mA. This reduced image resolution significantly. However, since first generation images were usually displayed on an 80 × 80 matrix, the x-ray tube was not the problem in this system.

As matrix size increased to 512 × 512, rotating anode tubes with focal spots as small as 0.6 mm × 1.2 mm came into use. Small focal-spot scanners use a pulsed beam to reduce the heat load. Modern pulsed scanner tubes operate at 120 kVp, 1–5 msec pulses, and up to 1,000 mA. Some units permit 80 and 140 kVp to be selected, sometimes in alternate pulses, for dual-energy scanning in which comparisons can be made between images at different kVp values. In addition, 0.5–5.0 million heat unit anodes of layered alloys, cylindrical anodes and liquid-cooled and air-cooled tube housing designs have been developed. A CT tube may produce 30 exposures per examination. Because most CT units are scheduled for 10–20 examinations per day, a tube may accumulate 10,000 exposures in a single month. It is not unusual for a CT tube to fail after several months. Only a few last a full year.

The radiation beam is double collimated, once at the tube exit and again at the detector entrance. This assists in eliminating scatter information. Collimation controls the voxel length. Collimation is variable from 1 mm to 13 mm and is usually controlled by the software program. The dimension of the collimation width determines the voxel length, or section thickness.

Detectors

Detectors must be capable of responding with extreme speed to a signal, without lag, must quickly discard the signal, and prepare for the next. They must also respond consistently and be small in size. They are usually placed with a source-to-image receptor distance of 44" (110 cm).

CT detectors should have high **capture efficiency**, high **absorption efficiency**, and high **conversion efficiency**. These three parameters are called the **detector dose efficiency**.

$$\begin{array}{r} \text{capture efficiency} \\ \text{absorption efficiency} \\ \underline{+ \text{ conversion efficiency}} \\ \text{dose efficiency} \end{array}$$

The capture efficiency is how well the detectors receive photons from the patient. It is controlled primarily by detector size and the distance between detectors. Absorption efficiency is how well the detectors convert incoming x-ray photons. It is determined primarily by the materials used (for example, the scintillation crystal or the gas) as well as the size and thickness of the detector. Conversion efficiency is determined by how well the detector converts the absorbed photon information to a digital signal for the computer.

CT detectors should also have high **stability**, fast **response time**, and a wide **dynamic range**. Stability is controlled by how often the detectors must be recalibrated to meet quality control standards. Response time is the speed with which the detector can react to recognize an incoming photon and recover for the next input. The dynamic range is the ratio of the largest signal that

can be measured to the smallest. Typical modern scanners are capable of dynamic ranges of 1,000,000 to 1.

Scintillation Crystals and Photomultiplier Tubes

Early detectors consisted of a scintillation crystal in contact with a photomultiplier tube (Figure 44–9). This system was used in nuclear medicine for many years prior to the advent of CT. A sodium iodide (NaI) crystal absorbs an x-ray photon and produces light flashes (scintillations) in proportion to the energy of the photon and at the exact location where the photon struck within the crystal. This light (photo) is then amplified (multiplied) by the photomultiplier (PM) tube. The light photon strikes the cathode of the PM tube, where it is converted into electrons. The electrons are then amplified by a series of dynodes as they move through the tube. Each dynode has a higher voltage, thereby increasing the number and voltage of the electrons as they move toward the anode. Upon striking the anode, the electrons are converted into a digital signal which can be processed by the computer.

Although sodium iodide scintillation crystals are nearly 100 percent efficient within the diagnostic x-ray range, they exhibit phosphorescent afterglow, or lag. This makes them useless with the rapid sequential exposures in the later generation scanners. Some units have been produced using calcium fluoride (CaF_2), bismuth

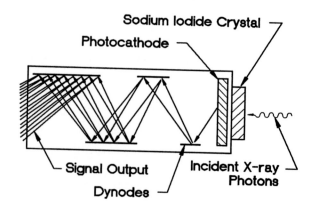

FIGURE 44–9. A scintillation crystal and photomultiplier tube detector.

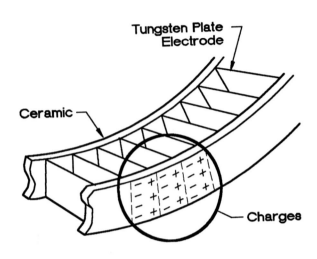

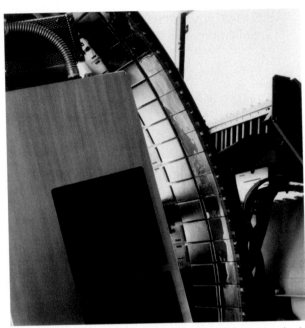

FIGURE 44–10. (A) A xenon gas-filled ionization chamber CT detector. The tungsten plate electrodes are alternately charged with positive and negative voltages. (B) A detector ring in a helical CT unit. *(Photograph courtesy of Picker International, Inc., Cleveland, OH)*

germinate ($Bi_4Ge_3O_{12}$), cesium iodine (CsI), gadolinium ceramics, and cadmium tungstate ($CdWO_4$) scintillation crystals, which, although less efficient (≅ 90 percent), have minimal afterglow. These materials are often bonded directly to the photocathode. A major disadvantage of scintillation-PM detectors is their size and interspace material, which prohibit packing them closer in the detector array. This reduces their total detection efficiency to less than 50 percent.

Xenon Gas-Filled Ionization Chambers

Some CT detectors use xenon gas-filled ionization chambers (Figure 44–10). They operate on the same principle as an ionization chamber. Essentially, they measure ionization in air by attracting to an electrode the ions created by x-ray photons in the air. The electrodes are usually thin tungsten plates spaced 1.5 mm apart. This spacing determines the maximum detector (and therefore display pixel size) resolution. The electrodes are alternately charged with positive and negative voltages. The quantity of ionic charge at the electrode is proportional to the energy of the photons detected between the electrodes. The detected energy comprises a digital signal that is sent to the computer.

Gas detectors range in efficiency from 60 to 90 percent but exhibit no lag. Ion chamber detectors were not used in the original EMI scanner because they were not sensitive enough. This disadvantage was overcome by using a long ion chamber and filling it with krypton or xenon, the heaviest inert gas, at high compression (20–30 atmospheres).

Although gas-ion detector efficiency may be only 60 percent, these detectors can be packed extremely close in the detector array, permitting a detection efficiency of slightly less than 50 percent, which is similar to that of scintillation-PM detectors.

Xenon detectors are highly directional. In other words, they must be set in a fixed position oriented to the x-ray source. This is why fourth generation and helical scanners cannot use xenon detectors.

A comparison of the advantages and disadvantages of solid-state and xenon detectors is presented in Table 44–3.

TABLE 44–3. Advantages and Disadvantages of Solid State and Xenon CT Detectors

Advantages

Solid State

Near 100 percent efficiency

Capable of reception of primary beam from a moving tube

Xenon

Tight packing ability increases total detector efficiency to around 50 percent

Tight packing ability increases resolution

Negligible lag time

Highly directional to receive maximum primary beam

Disadvantages

Solid State

Cannot be packed as tight as xenon detectors so total detector efficiency is around 50 percent

Cannot be packed as tight as xenon detectors so resolution is decreased

Xenon

60–90 percent efficiency

Highly directional prohibits efficient reception of primary beam from a moving tube

Alignment

Tube and detector alignment is critical in CT because of the tight collimation of the tube and the collimator mask at the detector. The slightest misalignment may produce a concentric ring artifact image that completely overrides clinical information.

Rotating anode tubes are aligned with their long axis perpendicular to the scanning plane. This prevents the anode heel effect within the useful beam while eliminating the gyroscopic effect on the rotating anode.

Stability

Detectors must remain in close calibration at all times. Some scanners calibrate detectors one per day while others calibrate them during scanning. One fourth generation scanner calibrates each detector immediately before and after it detects the fan beam. Detectors that

are out of calibration may cause artifacts that destroy image quality.

Computer

The CT computer is designed to control data acquisition, process and display, and storage. The computer itself is usually enclosed in a room that has controlled temperature and humidity. The CT console provides the radiographer with access to the software program that controls data acquisition, processing and display. Remote consoles may also be linked to the system to permit display and storage functions. Control of data storage may be available at the control console, remote consoles or at the storage units themselves.

A systems program is used to start up the CT unit. This program turns on and performs quality assurance checks on numerous components in both the x-ray equipment and computer hardware systems, warms up the x-ray tube, etc. It also permits the radiographer to record various problems that need the attention of the service engineer. One of its main functions is to perform calibration checks on the detectors, although this may be an ongoing process during scanning. A diagnostics program with specific quality assurance tests is used by service engineers to troubleshoot the systems.

The CT console operates from a "menu" or index directory of operations. The radiographer simply uses a keyboard, light pen or other input device to indicate the desired operation. At the beginning of each examination, patient information, such as identification, history, etc., is entered. This information permits retrieval of the images at a later date and will also be displayed adjacent to each image.

Data Acquisition

The data acquisition program controls a variety of operations, including tube and detector collimation (pixel size), matrix size, gantry angle, tabletop entrance into the gantry aperture, section increment movements of the tabletop, x-ray tube voltage and amperage, scan speed (the scanning operation itself) and the direction of detector signals to the digital image processing section of the computer.

Display Console

The processing and display program controls the digital image production process, including the series of mathematical formulas (algorithms) that compile the image and the display parameters, such as window level and width.

The display console is often part of the main console and appears as a separate CRT with controls (Figure 44–11). Also available are separate reporting consoles that permit radiologists to display images and electronically report the results, and independent consoles that contain their own CPU to retrieve and display images from the memory storage units and to receive images from examinations in progress.

Features

Most CT display units permit a wide range of display features to enhance diagnosis. These vary by manufacturer but often include the following.

Scanogram A localization image or **scanogram** is often displayed as the first image of an examination. It is achieved prior to the examination by slit scanning as the tabletop moves the patient through the tightly collimated primary beam. The resolution of the image is affected by the speed of the scan and the exposure output of

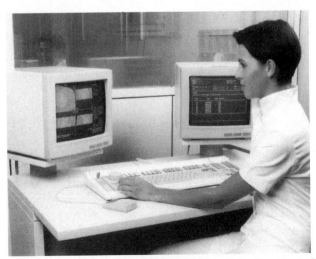

FIGURE 44–11. CT main console with display CRT. *(Courtesy of Siemens Medical Systems, Inc.)*

the tube. The poorer the scan, the less the patient dose. Because these images are used primarily for localization, image quality is seldom important. The radiographer should advocate the highest-speed scan and the lowest exposure output possible. The addition to the slit scan of dotted lines corresponding to the section intervals provides a convenient reference guide when viewing the sectional images. The scanogram can serve as a diagnostic tool in radiation therapy treatment planning by using a cursor to delineate the margins of a tumor on a series of transverse sections. The scanogram can then compile the cursor delineations to provide a coronal and sagittal outline of the tumor. The scanogram is sometimes called by one of a number of trademark names.

Grid Application A grid pattern may be added to any image. Radiographers use the grid to confirm exact centering of the patient; radiologists use the grid pattern to describe precise structural locations.

Cursor A cursor can be used to outline an area of interest. The area can be recorded on film and the Hounsfield unit mean or standard deviation can be displayed for the tissue within the marked area. Hounsfield units (HU) are discussed below. A line can be drawn between any two cursor locations, displaying the area's measurement within the patient. A cursor can also be used by itself to mark an area of interest.

Density Contouring Software is available that permits selection of a single point by a cursor, with the program highlighting all pixels of matching HU. This feature can be used to outline a tumor or other object.

Radiation Therapy Planning Special software is available to facilitate radiation therapy treatment planning through the use of cursors and integration with dosimetric data from a dosimetry computer.

Reverse Display Reverse display is available to reverse the image from left to right and/or reverse the density display so that blacks appear white and whites appear black.

Magnification Although nearly unlimited magnification may be accomplished, distortion usually becomes objectionable beyond 3×.

Suppression Originally designed to suppress the information from surgical clips, this feature permits a problem area, such as a surgical clip, to be outlined and then deleted from the reconstruction data.

Annotation
Text may be added to images for descriptions or anatomical labeling.

Histograms
A histogram is a bar graph which may provide useful diagnostic data in some instances. Software is available to produce these graphs by Hounsfield units and by time versus motion. Volumetric analysis is possible with some histographic data.

Hounsfield Units (HU) (CT Number) A histogram of the Hounsfield units along a line drawn between two cursor points may be useful in some diagnoses.

Time-Motion Histograms of various motions versus time may also be displayed for diagnosis of vascular flow or heart motion. These histograms are of limited value in CT because other modalities, especially ultrasonography and nuclear medicine, produce more accurate information.

Three-Dimensional Imaging
Software and separate image processing units are available that will reconstruct CT data into a three-dimensional image (Figure 44–12) that can be manipulated in a manner similar to a draftsman's CAD/CAM computer graphics system. The image can be rotated, tumbled or tilted to demonstrate structures that would otherwise be hidden. Images can be adjusted to various degrees of translucency and can be divided. For example, an image of the head may have soft tissue density reduced to 25 percent, bone density reduced to 50 percent, and the right half of the image removed to permit viewing of the left side of the sella turcica.

CT Numbers (Hounsfield Units)

The true linear attenuation coefficients of the tissue voxels are not exactly represented by the data received by the CT computer. Therefore a series of tissue density values has evolved for CT measurements. Originally named computed tomography numbers, they were renamed Hounsfield units (HU) after the Nobel Prize was awarded to Godfrey Hounsfield in 1979. These numbers are calculated by comparing the linear attenuation coefficient of each pixel to the linear attenuation coefficient of water, according to the following formula:

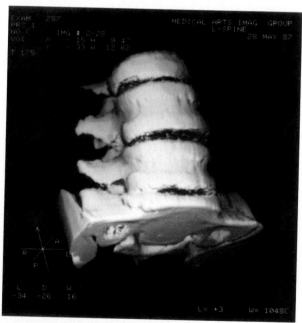

FIGURE 44–12. Three-dimensional CT reconstructions. (A) pelvis and (B) spine. (*Courtesy of GE Medical Systems*)

$$CT\ Number\ =\ 1{,}000\ \frac{\mu_p - \mu_w}{\mu_w}$$

where: μ_p = linear attenuation coefficient of measured pixel, and

μ_w = linear attenuation coefficient of water.

Therefore the HU of water is always 0, average bone +1,000, and air −1,000. Table 44–4 illustrates the HU of other tissues. The CT unit can display the HU of any given volume of tissue. Most units use a cursor to delineate the pixels to be measured and then display the HU on the CRT next to the image. Radiologists may use HUs occasionally to assist in diagnosis even though the original hope of defining HUs for specific pathologies has not been realized. The attenuation data received by CT detectors is accurate ± 0.2 percent; therefore HUs are accurate ±2.

Image Reconstruction

The detectors send information proportional to the attenuation coefficient of the voxel of tissue lying between the detector and the x-ray tube. The CT image is then reconstructed using a mathematical algorithm (Fourier transformation or a combination of convolution and back-projection) of the digitized information received by the computer.

The programs used by CT scanners compensate for numerous intrinsic and extrinsic factors, including the emission spectrum of the beam, and weighting factors for the geometrical aberrations caused by beam divergence and semicircular detector arrangement. Reconstruction often requires up to 30 seconds. However, when an array processor is used, reconstruction time can be decreased to less than one second, which is desirable for dynamic studies.

Reformatting

Reconstruction software is available that permits reformatting the information from a series of sectional images to produce an image of a section not actually

TABLE 44–4. Hounsfield Units (HU) (CT Numbers) Of Various Tissues

Tissue	HU
Bone, petrous	+ 3,000
Bone, average	+ 1,000
Bone, cortical	+ 800
Blood, clotted	+ 55–75
Spleen	+ 50–70
Liver	+ 40–70
Pancreas	+ 40–60
Kidney	+ 40–60
Aorta	+ 35–50
Muscle	+ 35–50
Brain, white matter	+ 36–46
Cerebellum	+ 30
Brain, gray matter	+ 20–40
Blood	+ 13–18
Cerebrospinal fluid	+ 15
Tumors	+ 5–35
Gallbladder	+ 5–30
Water	0
Orbits	− 25
Fat	− 100
Lungs	− 150–400
Air	− 1,000

scanned. For example, the extracted coronal image could be formed by reconstruction of only the appropriate voxels from each of the transverse sections. A typical reformatted CT image is shown in Figure 44–13.

Reformatting may also be used for a magnification technique called **targeting**, which permits an area of interest to be selected for reformatting. The reformatting process reconstructs the image data in a smaller pixel size to permit magnification with less distortion. This technique is used for regions in which extremely fine detail is necessary, such as the inner ear.

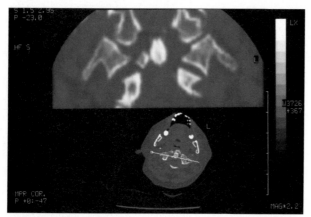

FIGURE 44–13. A reformatted CT image. The upper image is a coronal reconstruction from data acquired during axial transverse scanning of the cervical spine. Note the square bone fragment from the fracture. It is against the left side of the circular dens of C-2 at the center of the image. *(Courtesy of Barbara Imber and St. Rita's Medical Center, Lima, OH)*

TABLE 44–5. Appropriate Computed Tomography Window Widths

Area of Interest	Window Width (HU)
Head	70–200
Spine	350–750
Orbits	350–700
Heart	250–350
Abdomen	250–450
Thorax for lungs	1,200–1,400
Inner ear	2,000–4,000

Image Quality

Computed tomography image quality is primarily controlled by resolution and noise considerations. Density and contrast, as with any digitized image, can be manipulated by the computer. The prime consideration of the radiographer when making decisions regarding how to perform a particular CT examination must involve obtaining the necessary resolution while limiting noise.

Density and Contrast

Display density and contrast differences are varied with window level and width controls. Most CT images can demonstrate contrast differences of as little as 0.4 percent (4 HU), as compared to a minimum of 10 percent for a diagnostic radiograph. Appropriate CT window widths are shown in Table 44–5.

Resolution

The resolution of the CT image depends on pixel, voxel and matrix size. High contrast objects 1.5 times the pixel size or larger can be imaged reliably. For example, a pixel size of 0.5 mm can resolve an object 0.75 mm in size. Low contrast objects may require a larger pixel size to permit the detectors to provide sufficient data to reach a visible difference between the attenuation coefficients. Therefore low contrast objects may actually be seen better with a larger pixel size, although the total resolution is reduced. The current spatial resolution possible is about 0.35 mm, as compared to 0.25 mm and better with diagnostic radiography. However, this resolution is not possible under routine scanning conditions.

Voxel, Pixel and Matrix Size　Discussion of CT imaging detail must consider voxel, pixel and matrix size. It is possible to have pixels and matrix size equal yet the voxel width may have a considerable effect on image quality. Matrix sizes offered on CT units have included 256 × 256, 320 × 320, 360 × 360, and 512 × 512. Because most CT images are processed and displayed with a circular field, the actual number of image pixels is less than if the matrix were square. For example, a 512 × 512 circular field matrix has slightly over 200,000 pixels.

Voxel width may be varied between 8 mm and 13 mm. A common voxel size might be 1 mm × 1 mm × 10 mm with 10 mm representing the voxel width. The 20 percent additional tissue volume of a 13 mm voxel requires 60 percent more radiation exposure to produce an image of comparable quality. Therefore patient dose considerations in CT are similar to those in diagnostic radiography. Improved image quality can only be achieved through increased exposure to the patient.

Interface Artifacts Depending on the mathematical algorithm used, imaging aberrations displayed as density differences may occur when two objects have more than a 60 percent difference in attenuation coefficients. These artifacts are called undershoot and overshoot. Any object of greatly different contrast, such as metallic surgical clips, bullets, an old contrast medium and air, is likely to cause a star pattern artifact. The effect can be somewhat modified by using a larger matrix. However, different reconstruction algorithms that mathematically filter or compensate for the effect have been designed for various body parts. For example, a soft tissue algorithm is useless during examination of the inner ear. A special bone algorithm is required to produce useful information when a number of small bony structures are in close proximity to one another.

Magnification The **display or reconstruction field of view** (FOV) is different from the scan field of view. True CT magnification is achieved by choosing a smaller display field of view. This produces an image with less tissue per voxel, which in turn provides higher resolution and a larger image of a smaller area of interest. Magnification of the matrix field size has no effect on image resolution. When a CT image matrix is magnified it may be possible to perceive individual pixels. This causes the image to appear less sharp. Therefore most radiologists prefer to diagnose from images of a smaller size that are sharp.

Noise

All digital images have noise problems. Noise on a CT image is directly related to the amount of data collected by the detector. It appears as quantum mottle (best seen in an image of a water phantom) and normally comprises 3–5 percent of the image. Most CT image noise is a result of statistical fluctuation in the information recorded by the detector, not a result of computer reconstruction mathematics. **The amount of noise controls the low contrast resolving ability of the CT unit.** A standard CT quality assurance measurement is a daily noise evaluation that is done by imaging a phantom and using a cursor to read the HUs for control areas. Each reading should average at least 100 pixels (10 × 10 matrix).

Motion Motion on a CT image is a function of exposure time, just as in diagnostic radiography. The exposure time in CT is controlled by the quantity of data detected. Because insufficient data results in a poor quality image, motion during a CT scan is displayed as a series of very poor quality images. For example, a rib that moves is recorded in a series of locations due to the movement instead of in a stationary location if respiration had been suspended. Each of the movement images is of poor quality because the detector received too little data to permit reconstruction of a normal quality image. Some CT units are capable of analyzing a motion image, deleting the portion of the data that made up the motion, and then reconstructing a stationary image from the remaining data. Although these images do not contain as much information as originally planned, they do eliminate the motion (Figure 44–14).

Scanning Procedures

Section Interval and Thickness

The section interval is the distance between scan sections. The section thickness is the width of the volume of tissue being examined (the voxel). Section thickness is usually slightly less than voxel width because of the divergence of the beam. Both the section interval and the thickness are affected by the section shape.

Section Shape Although section thickness is equivalent to voxel width, or slightly less, a section does not have parallel sides due to the divergence of the x-ray beam. Figure 44–15 illustrates the section shape problem that either overlaps or excludes tissue between sections. One author has described the total scan volume as more like a stack of frisbees than a stack of coins (Figure 44–16). The scanning procedure must take this geometry into account. Overlapping, which occurs with section intervals equal to voxel width, is desirable. For example, a voxel width of 13 mm should use section intervals of 13 mm. In most procedures it is important that no sections of tissue miss examination. Overlap and exclusions must be considered when designing the section interval sequence for the scanning procedure. Most

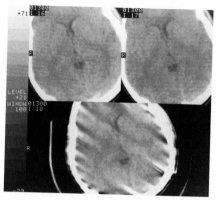

FIGURE 44–14. Computer correction of motion: (A) motion artifacts obscuring information, (B) separate images for each third of the scan time reveal all the motion that occurred during the final third of the scan, and (C) reconstruction using only the first two thirds of the scan time produces a diagnostic quality image.

CT unit programs have standardized scanning procedures for the various examinations, although they can be modified to fit specific circumstances and institutional requirements.

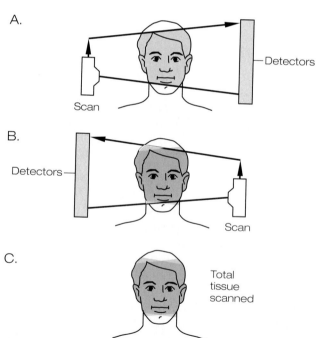

FIGURE 44–15. Section shape due to divergent beam geometry. (A and B) The first scan produces a wedge-shaped volume of scanned tissue. (C) The final scan produces a concave volume of double-scanned tissue with a convex volume of single-scanned tissue at the edges.

Scan Arc

Third and fourth generation scanners permit selection of the scanning arc. Common scan arcs are 220°, 360°, and 400° or 440° overscan on fourth generation units. The scan arc is sometimes called **half scan, full scan or overscan**. Wider scan arcs require more time to reconstruct the image and provide higher resolution.

Exposure Factors

Most CT scanning is performed at 120 kVp. Time is not a factor, as it must be controlled by the scanning program to provide sufficient exposure to the detectors (much as in fluoroscopy and conventional tomography). The CT radiographer usually varies the mA to control the primary beam. However, dual energy scanning units require scanning with different kVp values, usually 80 kVp or 140 kVp.

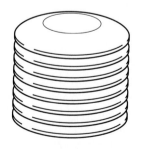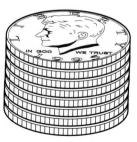

FIGURE 44–16. The total scan volume is more like a stack of frisbees than a stack of coins.

Algorithms

As discussed earlier under image reconstruction techniques, the proper reconstruction algorithm must be used to mathematically filter unwanted artifacts. The CT console often combines the proper algorithm with the scanning procedure. As with digital subtraction radiography, high-pass and low-pass filters and other mathematical manipulations can also be performed to improve image quality.

Scan Field Size

The scan field size, or field of view, is set to accommodate the size of the part under examination. The smaller the scan field size, the better the image resolution and the faster the scan time. Common field sizes are 25 cm for the head and magnification of the spine, 35 cm for small bodies and 48 cm for large bodies.

Artifacts

Motion

Motion is a problem in CT because it produces streak artifacts through the image (Figure 44–17). The algorithm faults when it receives the changes in attenuation that occur at the edges of the moving part. This produces blank pixels, which appear as streaks in these regions.

Metal or Star

The presence of metallic materials in the patient also cause streak artifacts but may also produce star artifacts (Figure 44–18). The metal objects attenuate nearly 100 percent of the primary beam, which produces an incomplete projection. This may produce a star artifact if the reconstruction algorithm has been unable to create a full set of surrounding projections to smooth the edges of the object. Some CT units have software algorithms designed to reduce and partially correct for these artifacts.

Beam Hardening

Beam hardening artifacts are a result of the attenuation of the beam as it passes through the patient. The CT number of a posterior structure may be much different from a similar anterior structure because the beam reaching the posterior structure has already been significantly attenuated. Beam hardening artifacts are often described as broad dark bands or streaks known as cupping artifacts (Figure 44–19). A capping artifact occurs when the

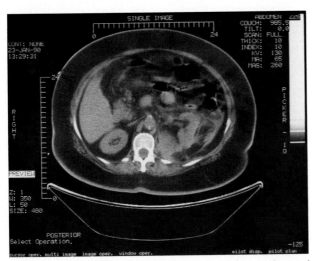

FIGURE 44–17. A typical computed tomography motion artifact. *(Courtesy of Wil Reddinger, Lima Technical College, Lima, OH)*

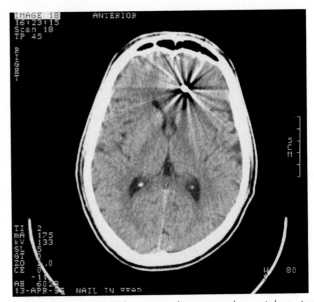

FIGURE 44–18. A typical computed tomography metal or star artifact. *(Courtesy of Wil Reddinger, Lima Technical College, Lima, OH)*

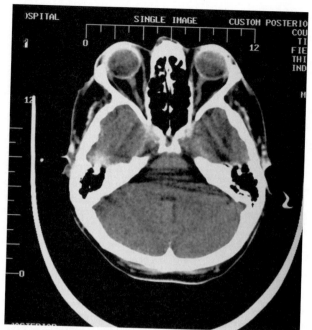

FIGURE 44–19. A typical computed tomography cupping or beam hardening artifact. *(Courtesy of Wil Reddinger, Lima Technical College, Lima, OH)*

algorithm overcompensates for the beam hardening artifact. Cupping artifacts have lower CT numbers than expected while capping artifacts have higher CT numbers than expected. Software algorithms are available to reduce or partially correct for their effect on the image.

Partial Volume Effect

Because the data from an entire section thickness is averaged together to form the image, the exact location of a section may cause small structures or portions of large structures to be hidden when they comprise only a small percentage of the total section. This is a common concern during CT of the vertebral column when a section interval happens to produce a section where an intervertebral disc comprises a small percentage of the total section volume (Figure 44–20). This is called the partial volume effect. It may obscure any object that is smaller than the voxel width (section thickness) when that object is scanned by two sections. Compensation for the partial volume effect may be overcome in some instances by slightly overlapping sections.

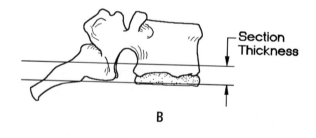

B

A

FIGURE 44–20. (A) A typical computed tomography out of field artifact demonstrating a severe partial volume averaging effect. *(Courtesy of Wil Reddinger, Lima Technical College, Lima, OH).* (B) A graphic illustration of the partial volume effect.

Ring Artifacts

When a single detector goes out of calibration and does not properly record incoming attenuation data the projection (or view) includes a detector error as shown in Figure 44–21A. When this error is multiplied during the scan, an annular or ring artifact, such as that illustrated in Figures 44–21B and C, is produced.

A number of artifacts are unique to computed tomography. The more common include motion, metal, beam hardening, partial volume effect, and ring artifacts.

Radiation Protection

Patient Dose

Patient dose during computed tomography was originally measured according to the concepts of diagnostic radiology. Because the CT scan irradiates tissue via a tightly collimated beam that is moved over the patient, it became necessary to find a new method to measure patient dose during CT examinations. In 1981 the U.S.

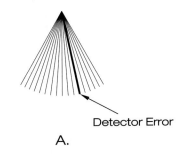

Detector Error

A.

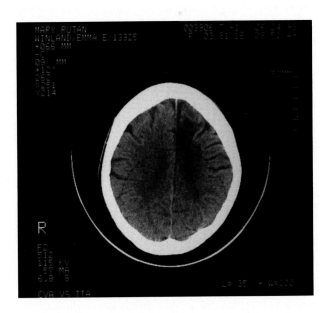

C.

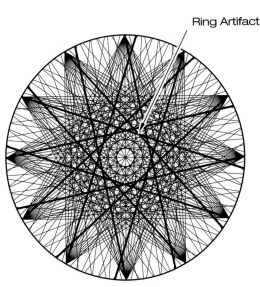

Ring Artifact

B.

FIGURE 44–21. A typical tomography ring artifact. (A) The effect of a defective detector cell on a single projection. (B) The sum effect of the multiple projections that comprise the entire image. (C) An example scan with a ring artifact. *(Courtesy of Wil Reddinger, Lima Technical College, Lima, OH)*

Food and Drug Administration (FDA) Bureau of Radiological Health (BRH), now known as the Center for Devices and Radiological Health (CDRH), developed the computed tomography **dose** index (CTDI) and the multiple scan average dose (MSAD). The CTDI measures the radiation dose to the patient measured within the primary beam of the CT scanner. The MSAD represents the average dose a patient receives during an examination, which would include numerous individual scans (or in the case of a helical scanner, a moving scan). These are actual tissue doses, not the entrance skin exposure that is often used to describe diagnostic radiography examinations.

Example MSAD readings for a head scan vary from 4–8 rads (4–8 cGy). This is very much greater than the typical entrance skin exposure for a single skull radiograph, which may range from 0.105–0.24 rad (0.105–0.24 cGy). Of course, the comparisons are somewhat absurd as the CT examination provides vastly more information than a single radiograph, or even the entire skull series of exposures, which would comprise a full skull examination.

Filtration is used in CT in a manner similar to that in diagnostic radiography, although CT uses much greater amounts of filter. A special "bow tie" filter has been developed for CT that matches the beam divergence and shape of the patient's body in transverse section (Figure 44–22).

Dose to Others

Dose to other persons in the scanning room results primarily from scatter from the patient, as during fluoroscopy. Lead aprons and other appropriate protective equipment should be used by anyone in the scanning room during examinations. A routine scan might produce a scatter dose of 2 to 5 mrads per section at one meter from the patient. Unless absolutely necessary, no one should be present in the scanning room while the unit is in operation. When someone must be present, he or she should remain as far from the patient as possible to take best advantage of the inverse square law. Standard radiation protection procedures should be followed. The most desirable person to stay with a patient is a relative, then a nonradiology staff member. A radiology department member is the last to be considered. Although use of a remotely controlled power injector is preferred, per-

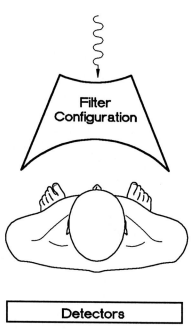

FIGURE 44–22. A CT bow tie filter.

sons who must manually inject a contrast medium during scanning procedures should stand behind a lead shield, as far from the gantry as possible.

Summary

Computed tomography (CT) produces a digital tomographic image from diagnostic x-rays. The basic principle of CT involves digitizing an image received from a slit scan projection of the patient's body and then back-projecting it through mathematical algorithms.

A modern CT unit includes a gantry, table, x-ray tube, detectors, computer, display console and image storage units. The gantry is the movable frame of the CT unit. It contains the x-ray tube and detectors and is the most visible part of the unit. The gantry frame maintains the alignment of the tube and detectors and contains the equipment necessary to perform the scanning movements. CT tables are usually made of carbon graphite fiber to decrease beam attenuation and must support the entire weight of the patient without sagging when fully extended. They are rated for maximum weight. Modern pulsed scanner x-ray tubes operate at 120 kVp, 1–5 msec pulses, and up to 1,000 mA. The most common CT detector is a xenon gas-filled ionization chamber which measures ionization in air by attracting to an electrode the ions created by x-ray photons in the air.

The CT computer is designed to control data acquisition, process and display, and storage. The CT console operates from a "menu" or index directory of operations. The radiographer uses a keyboard, light pen or other input device to indicate the desired operation. The data acquisition program controls a variety of operations, including tube and detector collimation (pixel size), matrix size, gantry angle, tabletop entrance into the gantry aperture, section increment movements of the tabletop, x-ray tube voltage and amperage, scan speed and direction of detector signals to the digital image processing section of the computer. The processing and display program controls the digital image production process. The display console permits a wide range of display features, including the scanogram, grid pattern, cursor, density contouring, radiation therapy planning, reverse display, magnification, suppression, annotation, histograms and three-dimensional imaging. Hounsfield units (HU), or CT numbers, represent the tissue density values for each pixel.

Computed tomography image quality is primarily controlled by resolution and noise considerations. Density and contrast, as with any digitized image, can be manipulated by the computer and are varied with window level and width controls. The resolution of the CT image depends on pixel, voxel and matrix size. Imaging aberrations (artifacts) displayed as density differences may occur when two objects have more than a 60 percent difference in attenuation coefficients. Noise on a CT image is directly related to the amount of data collected by the detector. Motion on a CT image is a function of exposure time, just as in diagnostic radiography.

The section interval is the distance between scan sections. Its determination is effected by the section shape and the partial volume effect. Section thickness is equivalent to voxel width, or slightly less. Because the data from an entire section thickness is averaged together to form the image, the exact location of a section may cause small structures or portions of large structures to be hidden when they comprise only a small percentage of the total section. This is called the partial volume effect.

A number of artifacts are unique to computer tomography. The more common include motion, metal, beam hardening, partial volume effect, and ring artifacts.

Because of the strictly collimated primary beam, most CT examinations have a patient dose much greater than that of the same part in diagnostic radiography examinations. Filtration is used in CT in a manner similar to that in diagnostic radiography. Dose to other persons in the scanning room results primarily from scatter from the patient, as during fluoroscopy. Lead aprons and other appropriate protective equipment should be used by anyone in the scanning room during examinations.

REVIEW QUESTIONS

1. What are the major components of a modern CT unit?

2. What is the gantry?

3. Why are tabletops rated for maximum weight?

4. What is the purpose of the detectors in a CT unit?

5. What operations are controlled by the data acquisition program?

6. What is a scanogram?

7. How are Hounsfield units (HU) (CT numbers) calculated?

8. What controls the density, contrast and resolution of the CT image?

9. Explain the partial volume effect.

10. Explain how a ring artifact is produced.

11. How does patient dose in CT compare to the doses for routine radiography?

REFERENCES AND RECOMMENDED READING

Ambrose, J. & Hounsfield, G. (1973). Computerized transverse axial tomography. *British Journal of Radiology.* 46(148), 1,023–1,047.

Berland, L. L. (1987). *Practical CT technology and techniques.* New York: Raven Press.

Brooker, M. J. (1986). *Computed tomography for radiographers*. Lancaster: MTP Press Limited.

Brooks, R. A. & DiChiro, G. (1977). Slice geometry in computer assisted tomography. *Journal of Computer Assisted Tomography. 1*(2), 191–199.

Brooks, R. A. & DiChiro, G. (1975). Theory of image reconstruction in computed tomography. *Radiology. 117*, 561.

Bushberg, J. T., Seibert, J. A., Leidholdt, E. M., & Boone, J. M. (1994). *The essential physics of medical imaging*. Baltimore: Williams & Wilkins.

Bushong, S. C. (1997). *Radiologic science for technologists: Physics, biology, and protection*. (6th ed.). St. Louis: C. V. Mosby.

Chiu, L. C., Lipcamon, J. D., & Yiu-Chiu, V. S. (1995). *Clinical computed tomography for the technologist*. (2nd ed.). New York: Raven.

Coulam, C. M., Erickson, J. J., Rollo, F. D., & James, A. E. (1981). *The physical basis of medical imaging*. New York: Appleton-Century-Crofts.

Curry, T. S., Dowdey, J. E., & Murry, R. C. (1990). *Christensen's introduction to the physics of diagnostic radiology*. (4th ed.). Philadelphia: Lea and Febiger.

Forster, E. (1985). *Equipment for diagnostic radiography*. Lancaster: MTP Press.

General Electric. (1976). *Introduction to computed tomography*. Milwaukee: General Electric Company, Medical Systems Division, publication 4691.

Harper, C. (1979). CT scanners: The industry behind the science. *Radiologic Technology. 51*(2), 199–202.

Hendee, W. R. (1983). *The physical principles of computed tomography*. Boston: Little, Brown and Co.

Hounsfield, G. N. (1979). Computed tomography: Past, present, and future. *Medical Imaging*. Ed. Kreel, L. & Steiner, R. E. Chicago: Year Book.

Hounsfield, G. N. (1973). Computerized transverse axial scanning (tomography): Part I. Description of system. *British Journal of Radiology. 46*, 1,016–1,022.

Kalender, W.A., Arkadiusz, P. & Christoph, S. (1994). A comparison of conventional and spiral CT: An experimental study on the detection of spherical lesions. *Journal of Computer Assisted Tomography. 18*(2), 167–176.

Knapp, R. H., Vannier, M. W., & Marsh, J. L. (1985). Generation of 3-D images from CT scans: Technological perspective. *Radiologic Technology. 56*(6), 391–398.

Kreel, L. & Steiner, R. E. Ed. (1979). *Medical imaging*. Chicago: Year Book.

Kuni, C. C. (1988). *Introduction to computers and digital processing in medical imaging*. Chicago: Year Book.

Lee, J. K., Sagel, S. S., & Stanley, R. J. (1990). *Computed body tomography*. (2nd ed.). New York: Raven Press.

McCullough, E. C. & Payne, J. T. (1977). X-Ray transmission computed tomography. *Medical Physics. 4*, 85.

Morgan, C. L. (1983). *Basic principles of computed tomography*. Baltimore: University Park Press.

Moss, A. A., Gamsu, G., & Genant, H. K. (1984). *Computed tomography of the body*. Philadelphia: W. B. Saunders.

Parker, J. A. (1990). *Image reconstruction in radiology*. Boca Raton, FL: CRC Press.

Parkinson, L. (1991). Assessment of dose in computerized tomography. *Radiography Today. 57*(650), 23–28.

Ritman, E. L., Kinsey, J. H., Robb, R. A., Harris, L. D., & Gilbert, B. K. (1980). Physical and technical considerations in the design of the DSR: A high temporal resolution volume scanner. *American Journal of Roentgenology. 134*, 369–374.

Romans, L. E. (1995). *Introduction to computed tomography*. Baltimore: Williams & Wilkins.

Seeram, E. (1994). *Computed tomography: Physical principles, clinical applications, and quality control*. Philadelphia: W. B. Saunders.

Seeram, E. (1989). *Computers in diagnostic radiology*. Springfield, IL: C. Thomas Publishers.

Seeram, E. (1983). A course on CT for radiologic technologists: A conceptual framework. *The Canadian Journal of Medical Radiation Technology. 14*(1), 11.

Seeram, E. (1978). Computed tomography: An overview. *Radiologic Technology. 49*(4), 491–496.

Short, A. J. (1981). Reconstructions in computerized transverse axial radiography. *Radiography. 47*(557), 119.

Shrimpton, P. (1994). Patient dose in CT and recommendations for reduction. *Radiography Today. 60*(683), 9–11.

Ter-Pogossian, M. M. (1983). Physical principles and instrumentation. *Computed Body Tomography.* Edited by Lee, J. K. T., Sagel, S. S., & Stanley, R. J. New York: Raven.

Whitmore, R. C., Bushong, S., Archer, B., & Glaze, S. A. (1979). Radiation dose in neurological computed tomography scanning. *Radiologic Technology. 51*(1), 21–26.

Wolbarst, A. B. (1993). *Physics of radiology.* Norwalk, CT: Appleton & Lange.

Yaffe, M., Fenster, A., & Johns, H. E. (1977). Xenon ionization detectors for fan beam computed tomography scanners. *Journal of Computer Assisted Tomography. 1*(2), 419–428.

Yoshizumi, T. T., Suneja, S. K., & Teal, J. S. (1989). Practical CT dosimetry. *Radiologic Technology. 60*(6), 505.

The Case of the Mysterious Mammal

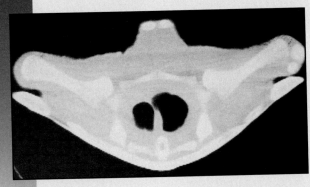

This computed tomography is of an animal found on the roadside near Jolly Beach, South Carolina. Look carefully at the bone structure to determine what it is.

(Courtesy of Stephen I. Schabel, M.D., Medical University of South Carolina)

Answers to the case studies can be found in Appendix E.

CHAPTER 45

Magnetic Resonance Imaging

We are dealing not merely with a new tool but with a new subject, a subject I have called simply nuclear magnetism . . . the history of ordinary magnetism . . . has been rich in difficult and provocative problems, and full of surprises. Nuclear Magnetism . . . is like that too.

Edward M. Purcell from his Nobel Lecture, December 11, 1952.

OBJECTIVES

Upon completion of this chapter, the student should be able to:

▶ Describe the source of the magnetic fields within the body that are used during MRI.

▶ Describe the properties of proton precession as used in MRI.

▶ Define T_1, T_2, p, TR, TE, and TI.

▶ Explain the functions of x, y, and z gradient coils in selecting an image section by the use of the Larmor equation and a gradient magnetic field.

▶ Describe the use of RF pulses in the various MRI pulse sequences.

▶ Analyze the various events during a spin-echo pulse sequence.

▶ Describe the components of an MRI unit, including the stationary magnet, gradient and RF coils, table, and computer consoles.

▶ Explain how MRI image contrast is controlled.

▶ Describe the use of paramagnetic contrast agents.

▶ Discuss methods of reducing MRI image noise.

▶ Discuss safety measures for protection of all persons who approach the MRI unit magnetic field.

*T*he typical magnetic resonance imaging (MRI) unit looks similar to a CT unit. It has a computer, computerized console, gantry, and table. However, because MRI uses magnetism and radio frequencies (RF) to create diagnostic sectional images of the body (Figure 45–1), the internal construction is quite different. The phenomena that permit MRI are based on magnetism and radio frequencies applied according to the principles of nuclear physics and quantum mechanics. For this reason the imaging process was originally called nuclear magnetic resonance (NMR). Also for this reason, it is critical to understand new physical concepts in order to comprehend how MR images are created and viewed.

The Physics of Magnetic Resonance

In 1924 Wolfgang Pauli suggested that some nuclei spin. It was not until 1946 that nuclear magnetic resonance was first reported by Swiss physicist Felix Bloch (1905–1983) at Stanford and American physicist Edward Purcell (1912–) at Harvard. These men shared the 1952 Nobel Prize in physics for their work. In the late 1960s and early 1970s the basis for diagnostic MRI was developed by several researchers. In 1967 Jasper Jackson produced the first MR signals from a live animal, in 1971 Raymond Damadian reported NMR differences between normal tissue and tumors, in 1972 Paul Lauterbur produced the first magnetic resonance image, in 1975 Damadian produced the first live animal MR images, and by 1977 the first diagnostic human images had been obtained.

Nuclear Magnetism

The nucleus of an atom is a tiny but highly charged piece of matter. The spinning nucleus has angular momentum, or **nuclear magnetic moment**. This rotating charge acts as a current loop and produces a magnetic field, thus causing the nucleus to behave as a microscopic spinning bar magnet; it rotates and flips within the atom like a tiny gyroscope on perfect bearings. When nuclei having magnetic moments are placed in a magnetic field, they tend to align with the field, as does any magnet.

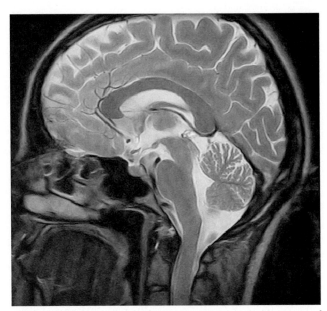

FIGURE 45–1. A sagittal MR image of the head. *(Courtesy of GE Medical Systems)*

In addition to having a charge, a nucleus also has mass. The spinning mass has a moment of inertia as well as a magnetic moment. The moment of inertia resists changes to angular momentum, thus inhibiting the nucleus from aligning in a magnetic field. This inhibiting factor is measured as the ratio of the magnetic moment to the moment of inertia and is called the gyromagnetic (or magnetogyric) **ratio**. It is represented by the Greek letter gamma (γ) and is measured in units of **megahertz per tesla (MHz/T)**. Recall from Chapter 4 that the tesla and the gauss are the units of magnetic flux density. One tesla equals 10,000 gauss. Each isotope has a specific gyromagnetic ratio, which allows it to be differentiated during MR imaging (Table 45–1).

Variations in gyromagnetic ratios and in the length of relaxation time after the application of an RF pulse permit the differentiation of various metabolites. This is the general basis of spectroscopy, which, when coupled with static MR images, may provide additional diagnostic information.

Precession of Nuclei Although the dynamics of rapidly rotating objects are quite complex, several of their properties are easily understood. The most important property is that of a rapidly spinning nucleus when

TABLE 45–1. Magnetic Resonance Properties of Diagnostically Important Nuclei

Nucleus	Gyromagnetic Ratio (MHz/T)
^{1}H	42.6
^{14}H	3.1
^{13}C	10.7
^{19}F	40.0
^{23}Na	11.3
^{31}P	17.2
^{39}K	2.0

it is subjected to a magnetic field; not only will the nucleus's magnetic field align with the external magnetic field, but it will also begin to wobble. This wobbling, like that of a spinning top when it begins to lose momentum, is actually a rotation of the axis of rotation, or **precession** (Figure 45–2). The rotational precession of the nucleus causes the magnetic field itself to precess. Therefore the direction of precession indicated in Figure 45–2 also represents the precession of the rotational magnetic field. MR imaging is accomplished through various measurements of this movement of the nuclear magnetic field.

The nuclear magnetic field is continually changing direction as it rotates around the axis of the external magnetic field's lines of flux. The **rate of precession** is indicated by the Greek letter omega (ω) and is calculated as:

$$\omega = \gamma B_O$$

where:
ω = rate of precession
γ = gyromagnetic ratio
B_O = static magnetic field strength

The rate of precession (ω) is also known as the angular velocity of the nuclear magnetic field.

Larmor Frequencies

The gyromagnetic ratio (γ) is fixed for each element. Therefore the precessional frequency is fixed for a given magnetic field strength. This means that in a static homogeneous magnetic field, all protons in a nucleus of a given type element will rotate with exactly the same frequency. This frequency is called

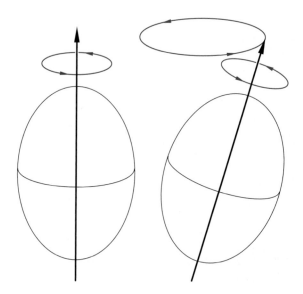

FIGURE 45–2. Precession.

the **Larmor frequency** and is critical to MR imaging. Only those elements with nuclear angular momentum have nuclear magnetic moments and are capable of producing nuclear magnetic resonance signals. The most important of those that do is the proton, which is also the major isotope of hydrogen (^{1}H), because it is abundant in the human body and has a high gyromagnetic ratio (γ). **The precessional frequency is the Larmor frequency. It is the RF that induces magnetic resonance as well as the RF of the emitted nuclear magnetic resonance signal.**

Production of the Nuclear Magnetic Resonance Signal

The laws of quantum mechanics permit protons to align either with the external magnetic field or against it. This creates two populations of proton orientations relative to the main magnetic field: parallel and antiparallel. When an electromagnetic RF field that is alternating, or resonating, at the Larmor frequency is applied in addition to the static field, protons will alternate from parallel to antiparallel. This phenomenon is called **magnetic resonance**. Protons that are antiparallel have excessive energy, which they emit as electromagnetic radiation in the **radio frequency (RF)** range.

Magnetic resonance imaging data is accumulated by measuring detection differences of only one millionth of a percent (0.000001 percent). When a large number of protons are subjected to a magnetic field, the nuclear magnetic moments immediately begin lining up with the field; some line up in the same direction as the magnetic field while others line up in the opposite direction. For every 200,000,000 hydrogen atoms, about two more will align themselves *with* the predominate external magnetic field. In other words, 100,000,001 atoms will align with the field while 99,999,999 will align against it. This means that the body tissue has become almost imperceptibly magnetized.

The Larmor equation predicts the exact RF that will be emitted by a specific element. When the RF is detected with an antenna and a radio receiver that is tuned to the proper frequency, magnetic resonance imaging is possible.

Production of the nuclear magnetic resonance signal requires applying a Larmor frequency RF and then listening to the RF emissions from the protons. Digital imaging reconstruction techniques are then used to create sectional and three-dimensional images.

MRI Parameters

The primary parameters controlling the MRI process include **proton spin density (N(H) or ρ), spin-lattice or longitudinal relaxation time (T_1), spin-spin or transverse relaxation time (T_2), repetition time (TR), echo time (TE), inversion time (TI), and flip angle**. The parameters that are used vary depending on the pulse sequence used.

Proton (spin) density ($ρ$ or N(H)) is the quantity of resonating spins in a tissue. It is expressed as a percentage of the proton density of water and determines the MR signal strength (sometimes called image brightness) (Table 45–2). Various authors refer to it as proton density (N(H) or PD), spin density (SD), or by the Greek letter rho ($ρ$). Proton density weighted images are achieved by using a long repetition time (TR) between pulses. This permits the RF signal from a larger number of protons to be detected, thus creating the image from a greater number, or density, of spinning protons. Proton density images have relatively low contrast due to the slight differences between the percentages of hydrogen present in various tissues (Table 45–2).

Spin-lattice relaxation time (T_1) is the time required for precessing spins to align with the constant external

TABLE 45–2. Effect Of Parameter Variation On MR Image Density (Brightness)

| | | | Effect on MR Signal With: | | |
Image Weighting	TR	TE	$ρ$ Increased	Longer T_1	Longer T_2
Proton Spin Density ($ρ$)	long	short	+	−*	+*
T_1	short	short	+	−	+*
T_2	long	long	+	−*	+

* = some tissues only

magnetic field to 63 percent of the maximum possible strength. It is also known as longitudinal relaxation time and is sometimes called thermal relaxation time.

T_1 is the time required for the sum of the magnetic moments, or M_O, to regain its original orientation following a 90° RF pulse. It varies depending on thermal interactions between resonating protons and other nuclear magnetic fields in the atomic lattice. The value of T_1 increases with the strength of the magnetic field. The term longitudinal was originally applied in reference to the time required for precessing to cease and the proton spin to reorient with the original "longitudinal" magnetic field.

The T_1 of hydrogen is approximately three seconds in water but this time varies considerably for hydrogen in different types of tissues. This phenomenon provides the contrast necessary for the MR image. T_1 relaxation characteristics for various body tissues are shown in Table 45–3. Relaxation times vary with the amount of water available. In fact, dehydrated tissues will demonstrate significantly different relaxation times.

When a magnetic field is applied, almost all the proton spins will have aligned after several T_1 times have passed. Magnetic resonance imaging uses only those spins that have not been cancelled out by a corresponding spin in the opposite direction. Although these protons occur in only one out of 100,000,000 atoms, the vast quantity of atoms in even a small voxel of tissue produce a large number of eligible protons. Only these protons are capable of producing an RF when subjected to a magnetic field at the appropriate Larmor frequency.

The mechanism by which protons emit RF is especially complex because it occurs in three dimensions. However, careful consideration of a few simple illustra-

TABLE 45–3. Example T$_1$ and T$_1$ Relaxation Times In A 0.15 Tesla Field

Relaxation times vary considerably depending on numerous factors, including the specific conditions surrounding the tissue and external magnetic field strength.

Tissue	T$_1$	T$_2$	T$_1$/T$_2$	Proton Density (Percent ρ Water)
Fat	170 ms	80 ms	2.1	9.6
Muscle	580 ms	40 ms	14.5	9.3
Brain, white matter	350 ms	80 ms	4.4	10.6
Brain, gray matter	500 ms	100 ms	5.0	10.6
Blood	720 ms	175 ms	4.1	
Cerebrospinal fluid	1,500 ms	260 ms	5.8	10.8
Water	2,500 ms	2,500 ms	0.0	11.0

T$_1$/T$_2$ is an indication of contrast differences between T$_1$ and T$_2$ weighted images. (Adapted with permission from Elster, Allen D., *Magnetic Resonance Imaging: A Reference Guide and Atlas.* Philadelphia: J. B. Lippincott Company, 1986.)

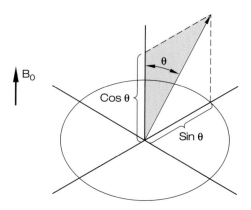

FIGURE 45–3. Gradient echo imaging preserves longitudinal magnetization by utilizing a flip angle of less than 90°.

tions will reveal that once the three-dimensional aspect is understood, the basic principle is not so difficult. The sum of the magnetic moments, or M$_O$, is always in the same direction as B$_O$ (the static magnetic field strength) when the body is within the static external magnetic field. When M$_O$ precesses, it produces a rotating magnetic field which is perpendicular to the original direction of M$_O$ (Figures 45–4A, B). To cause protons to emit an RF, another magnetic field (B$_1$) must be applied for a brief moment. In Figure 45–4B the magnetic field in the x^1–y^1 plane is precessing synchronously with M$_O$ (at the same angular speed). This precessing magnetic field is stationary in its relationship with M$_O$. This relationship is more easily understood by comparing it to riding on a carousel. Although the carousel is spinning (like M$_O$), when one rides on one of the horses the other horses appear to be stationary (x^1–y^1) while objects outside the carousel appear to be spinning around (x–y). If an alternating magnetic field (B$_1$) is applied in the direction of x, it will simply cause M$_O$ to rotate further away from z toward y (Figure 45–4C). In order to apply B$_1$ in the direction of the moving x axis, it is simply pulsed so that it is applied only during the moment that x is aligned with x^1 during every rotation (Figure 45–4C). The con-

cept of T$_1$ as M$_O$ returns to equilibrium after an RF pulse is shown graphically in Figure 45–9. Because x is rotating at the Larmor frequency with M$_O$, **the applied magnetic field must be pulsed at the Larmor frequency**.

The Larmor frequency is very high, usually in the MHz range, for the 0.2–4.0 Tesla fields used in MR imaging. For example, the Larmor frequency for hydrogen in a 1.5 T field is 64 MHz, which is within RF bands of the electromagnetic spectrum (see Figure 2–10). The MHz frequency magnetic field for MRI is produced by a properly tuned radio transmitter coil, very similar to the coil used to receive UHF frequency television signals.

Spin-spin relaxation time (T$_2$) is the time required, after precessing spins have aligned at an angle to the external magnetic field due to an RF pulse, for them to lose 63 percent of their coherence (alignment with each other) due to interactions between the spins. It varies depending on the tissue. It is also known as transverse relaxation time. T$_2$ is always shorter than T$_1$. The symbol T$_2$* is used to indicate T$_2$ due to inhomogeneities in the magnetic field and due to spin-spin relaxation. T$_2$* is always shorter than T$_2$. Of all the parameters described, PD, T$_1$, and T$_2$ are intrinsic. The others are extrinsic or controllable by the operator.

Repetition time (TR) is the time interval between pulse sequences. It is usually between 300 and 3,000 ms but is highly variable, always being the longest of the parameters used to describe the sequence.

Echo time (TE) is the time between a 90° pulse and the echo during a spin-echo pulse sequence. It is usually

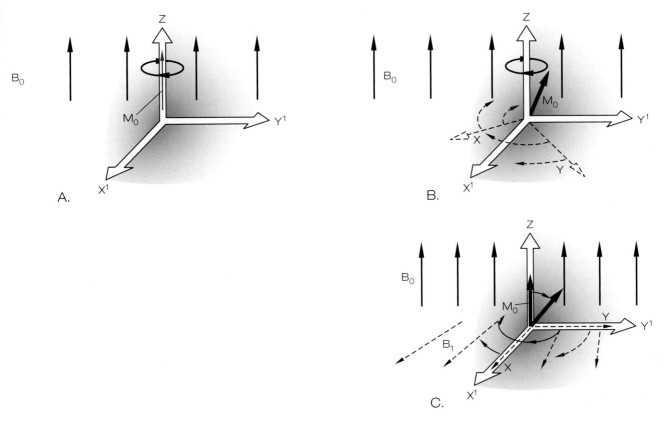

FIGURE 45–4. Proton emission of radio frequencies (RF). (A) B_0 is the direction of the static external magnetic field. M_0 is the direction of the sum of the predominant proton magnetic moments. (B) When M_0 is tipped slightly off the z axis, it immediately begins precessing around the z axis at its Larmor frequency. This causes a perpendicular magnetic field to rotate in the x–y plane, also at the Larmor frequency. (C) If an alternating magnetic field (B_1) is applied in the direction of x, it causes M_0 to rotate further away from z toward y. B_1 is pulsed so it is applied only during the moment x is aligned with x^1 during every rotation. Because x is precessing at the Larmor frequency, the applied magnetic field must also be pulsed at the Larmor frequency.

between 10 and 100 ms but is always the shortest time used for a sequence. When more than one echo is recorded, the TE is designated as TE_1, TE_2, etc.

Inversion time (TI) is the time between a 180° pulse and a 90° inversion pulse in an inversion recovery pulse sequence. It is usually between 200 and 2,000 ms.

Flip angle: in gradient echo imaging, increasing flip angle will increase T_1 weighting (Figure 45–3)

Nuclear Magnetic Resonance Pulses
The distance that M_0 precesses from the z axis is determined by the strength of B_1 and by the duration of the pulse. It is measured by the angle of the precession. For example, a 45° pulse tips the rotational axis of M_0 45° away from the z axis. The most common MRI pulses are 90° and 180°. A 180° pulse aligns M_0 with the –z axis or, in other words, aligns it perfectly in the opposite direction. A 360° pulse would return the rotational axis to its original position and therefore have no effect. During all pulsing only the protons spinning at the Larmor frequency that matches the pulse frequency will respond. The actual response of proton spin to an RF pulse is to change M_0 in a precessing corkscrew motion (Figure 45–5).

A 90° pulse is used to tip the rotational axis of the protons so that they are spinning around the z axis in the x–y plane. Because the protons are functioning as spinning magnets, an electromagnetic force is produced when a coil of wire is positioned within the lines of flux. **The voltage that is detected from this arrangement is the magnetic resonance imaging signal.** The coil is aligned to detect only precession in the x^1–y^1 plane. The frequency of the voltage matches the Larmor frequency of the precessing protons, thus making it possible to detect which element emitted the signal.

Nuclear Magnetic Resonance Decay

The signal that is emitted by the precessing protons decays exponentially. This occurs because the protons' magnetic fields are not exactly the same, even though they are all within the Larmor frequency range. Just as individual atoms of the same element have slight differences, precessional rates also differ slightly. For example, if a hydrogen proton is spinning at its Larmor frequency of 64,000,000 rotations per second and a second proton is spinning at 64,000,001 rotations per second, in 0.5 second the two protons will be exactly opposite one another. When this occurs, their magnetic fields cancel one another. The millions of protons that comprise M_O quickly become out of phase with each other by this process, which is called dephasing. **When a tissue sample has dephased, M_O ceases to exist and the magnetic resonance signal disappears.**

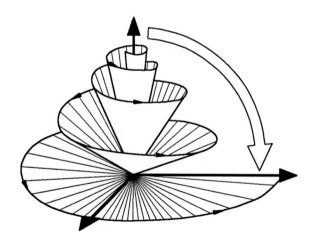

FIGURE 45–5. The precessing corkscrew motion of proton spin to an RF pulse. *(Used by permission from Edelman, R. R., Hesselink, J. R. [1990]. Clinical magnetic resonance imaging. Philadelphia: W. B. Saunders)*

Free induction decay (FID) is the simplest example of this process. It produces the most basic type of MRI signal, as shown in Figure 45–6. Because an FID signal will vary depending on how many protons are spinning in the tissue volume, it is known as a **proton spin density (ρ) image**. Because proton density does not vary much in soft tissue, this imaging technique produces an extremely low contrast image.

Production of the Magnetic Resonance Image

The localization of information for the MR image occurs very differently from computed tomography or any other digital imaging modality, although the final computerized digital image reconstruction algorithms are very similar. Three electromagnetic coils are required to produce magnetic field gradients corresponding to the x, y, or z axis to be imaged. The RF that are detected from these gradient coils, as they are called, can then be analyzed to determine not only the type of atom they came from but also the atom's precise location within the imaging matrix.

Gradient Coils

Data localization in MRI is accomplished through the use of a gradient magnetic field that is superimposed on the static external magnetic field. The gradient coil field system was developed by the American physicist Paul Lauterbur in 1972 at the State University of New York (SUNY) at Stony Brook. Gradient coils can be resistive or superconducting and are located within the bore of the stationary magnet. They superimpose their magnetic fields on the uniform magnetic field produced by the stationary magnet. A gradient field coil produces a magnetic field somewhat like a magnetic penetrometer in that it grows in strength from one end to the other, varying the field strength in proportion to distance.

Since the strength of the magnetic field affects the precessional frequency of the proton spins, the result is different precessional frequencies according to location along the gradient field. This technique permits the MRI computer to determine the location of an RF signal with digital imaging calculations. It also permits the calcula-

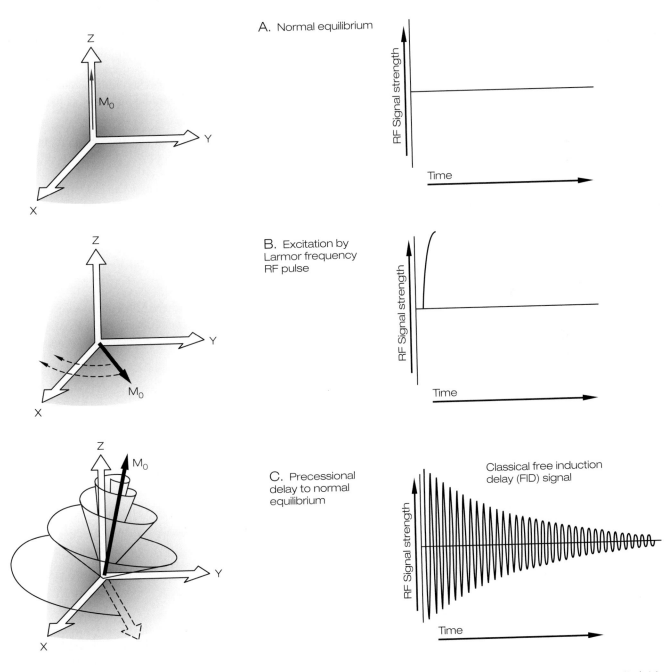

A. Normal equilibrium

B. Excitation by Larmor frequency RF pulse

C. Precessional delay to normal equilibrium

Classical free induction delay (FID) signal

FIGURE 45–6. Classical free induction decay (FID). (A) Normal spin equilibrium. (B) When a Larmor frequency RF pulse is applied, M_0 precesses 90° into the x–y plane, thus producing a maximum strength MR signal. (C) As M_0 emits RF, it loses energy and precesses in a corkscrew back to normal equilibrium while emitting a gradually decaying RF signal.

tion of T_1 and T_2 as a function of distance along the axis of the magnetic field. Changing the x axis permits detection from an opposite direction and the use of many of the digital reconstruction algorithms employed in computed tomography (see Chapters 42 and 43). Other variations between the three gradient coils also permit various oblique sections to be constructed. The basic algorithm in MRI is a two-dimensional Fourier transform (2DFT) method. It is often expanded to a 3DFT to permit faster data acquisition.

Magnetic resonance imaging requires the use of three gradient coils, one each for the x, y, and z axes (Figure 45–12B). Each coil must be linear and uniform to within a few percentage points. **The gradient coils determine the section thickness as well as the resolution and plane of the image.**

The z axis coil is perpendicular to the imaging plane. It is called the slice selection gradient because it determines the exact location of the section and its thickness. A thicker section is produced by increasing the RF bandwidth or by increasing the magnitude (or slope) of the gradient. The z axis coil can be set to produce transverse, coronal, or sagittal sections by varying the orientation of the z axis so it is replaced by the x or y axis.

The y axis coil is called the phase encoding gradient because it selectively precesses the protons to define the x–y coordinates within the section. This phase gradient must be repeated for each x coordinate in the matrix array. For example, a 256×256 matrix requires the phase gradient to be repeated 256 times to collect data for the entire matrix. This is the basic process of a two-dimensional Fourier transform (2DFT) data projection method.

The x axis coil is called the frequency encoding gradient or the readout gradient because it is applied for each value of the y axis coil. Three-dimensional MR imaging uses the z axis coil to cause a large volume of tissue to begin precessing. X and y encoding gradients are then compared and the collected data is reconstructed in three dimensions.

Although these phasing methods are not always applied to the x and y axes in the order described, spatial location is achieved by phase encoding for one axis while frequency encoding for the other. Variations in the use of all three gradient coils permit the acquisition of various oblique sections through the subject.

Magnetic Resonance Imaging Operations Sequence

The production of MR imaging data varies depending on the pulsing sequence used and on the manufacturer. As an example, a spin-echo pulse sequence of operations might include the following steps to produce an MR image:

1. A gradient is applied along the z axis. A 90° pulse is applied at a desired Larmor frequency. The z gradient selects an x–y plane (section selection). The z gradient is turned off. This produces a precessing M_O in the selected plane. The M_O in the other planes are still aligned along the z axis (Figure 45–7A).

2. A gradient is applied along the y axis for a short time. This produces precessing M_O at various rates depending on their location along the y axis gradient. The phasing of the precessing spins now indicates their location in the y–z plane (phase encoding) (Figure 45–7B).

3. A gradient is applied along the z axis again and a 180° pulse is applied with a frequency that will affect only the x–y plane that is being imaged. The z gradient is then turned off.

4. A gradient is applied along the x axis. This causes the precessing M_O to return a spin-echo at differing frequencies that will indicate their positions along the x axis (readout frequency encoding) (Figure 45–7C). The RF receiver is then turned on and the signals received are sent to the MRI computer for digital image reconstruction.

Radio Frequency Pulse Sequences

The primary variable in the data collection procedure during MRI is the sequence of RF pulses that are used to cause the protons to precess. There is a dramatic difference in the information that becomes visible with the various sequences. The operator must select the appropriate pulsing sequence as well as the proper intervals for the specific examination.

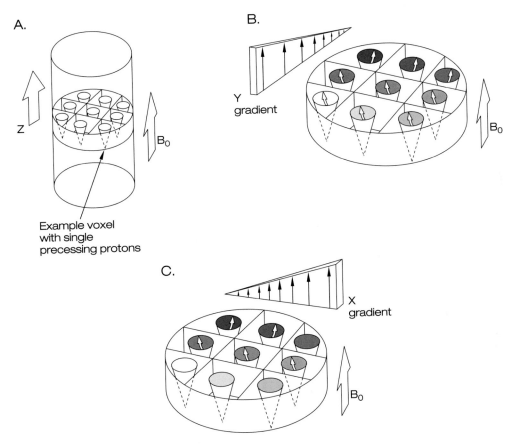

FIGURE 45–7. Spatial location by gradient fields. (A) Application of the z gradient field produces precession within the selected section (the z axis). (B) Application of the y gradient field produces phase encoding along the y axis. Note that there is still no differentiation of spatial location along the x axis. (C) Application of the x gradient field produces frequency encoding along the x axis. Note that each voxel now has a different precession rate, thus permitting spatial location in the x, y, and z axes.

Similar to many computed tomography units, the MRI control console includes programmed selections of sequences for various examinations. However, the knowledgeable MRI technologist can increase the quantity and quality of diagnostic information by understanding which sequences and intervals are best for specific tissues. The sequences are a series of various magnetic fields from the x, y, and z gradients, RF pulses, flip angles applied at various angles, repetition times (TR), inversion times (TI), and echo times (TE).

Partial Saturation

Partial saturation is also referred to as saturation recovery (SR) or repeated free induction decay (repeated FID). The pulse sequence is a series of 90° RF pulses with the signal measured after each (Figure 45–8A). Note that the y gradient is changed for each pulse sequence to record data from a different anatomical section. The TR is set according to the tissue of interest.

If a 90° pulse is repeated before M_O is fully re-established along the z axis, the angle of M_O precession will depend on the first time interval (T_1). Images produced with data collected at this point are known as partial saturation images because they vary with both proton density and the length of T_1. Because different tissues have different T_1 values, contrast can be varied by changing the repetition time (TR). However, when very short recovery times are encountered, the M_O is weak and this produces a very weak RF signal. When long recovery times are encountered, the M_O has time to recover and the T_1 contrast is lost. For this reason partial saturation is not used for most MR imaging. However, short TR T_1 partial saturation sequencing is useful in demonstrating cysts and subdural fluids and has been used for blood flow studies as well.

Spin-Echo

Spin-echo is the most popular pulse sequence because it reduces scan time significantly (Figure 45–8B). It was first described by Carr and Purcell and is therefore also known as the Carr-Purcell (CP) sequence. The basic spin-echo sequence consists of a 90° pulse which initiates a partial saturation sequence. However, it is followed by a 180° pulse (the refocusing pulse) at 50 percent of the TE. The refocusing pulse flips the proton precession and produces a spin-echo RF signal that grows, then fades in intensity. The y gradient is changed for each pulse sequence to record data from a different anatomical section. The TR and TE are set according to the tissue of interest.

The decay or dephasing process is used to advantage in spin-echo imaging by allowing dephasing to continue until it is nearly undetectable. This permits the faster spinning protons to precess further and further out of synch. When the 180° refocusing pulse is used to flip M_O in the opposite direction, the protons that have precessed faster and are the furthest out of synch now begin precessing back into synchrony with those that were slower. At an equal time after the 180° pulse, all the precessions will again be equal. This has the effect of an echo and produces the spin-echo signal. The process operates exactly as if the Indianapolis 500 auto race were begun and allowed to run for one hour. If each car were stopped at the end of the hour, turned around and run for a second hour at exactly the same speed, the race would end with all the cars crossing the finish line together. Although this would be a very boring race, in MRI it provides enough time to measure the differences between the precessional rates.

The T_2 term is used during spin-echo MRI to describe where the data collection occurs after the second time interval when 63 percent of the spins have lost their alignment with each other as they decay back toward equilibrium. The T_2 relaxation characteristics for various body tissues are shown in Table 45–4.

Spin-echo pulses are weighted for T_1 by using short TR and TE (Figure 45–15B). Although a T_1 image is valuable when used in conjunction with a T_2 image, it is not considered useful information by itself. Spin-echo pulses are weighted for T_2 by using long TR and TE (Figure 45–15C).

Gradient Echo

Gradient echo sequences use a single RF pulse of less than 90°. The signal of the echo is produced by using gradient pulses, rather than RF pulses. Because the RF pulse only slightly decreases the longitudinal magnetization, the recovery time is much quicker. This allows for shorter TR and, therefore, more rapid imaging. Image contrast in gradient echo imaging is controlled largely by flip angle. Gradient echo imaging is used in a wide variety of neuro, body, and orthopedic applications.

Inversion Recovery

Inversion recovery is a three pulse sequence. It consists of a 180° pulse followed by a spin-echo sequence (Figure 45–8C). Because of the time required to accumulate data, it is seldom used in current clinical imaging. Note that the y gradient is changed for each pulse sequence to record data from a different anatomical section. The TR and TI are set according to the tissue of interest.

The first pulse is an inverting pulse to invert M_O into the −z axis. TI is an interpulse time delay that permits M_O to begin to recover, becoming less and less negative, then rising along the +z axis. No signal is generated during this process because M_O is not in the x–y plane. However, at a set interval a 90° pulse rotates M_O into the x–y plane, producing precession and an RF signal. The strength of this signal at the time of the 90° pulse will depend on the TI recovery time that was allowed. Because this is different for each tissue, useful MRI data can be collected. Inversion recovery provides good

TABLE 45–4. Example T_1 and T_1 Relaxation Times

Tissue	T_1	T_2
Fat	170 ms	80 ms
Example tumor	580 ms	80 ms
Muscle	580 ms	40 ms

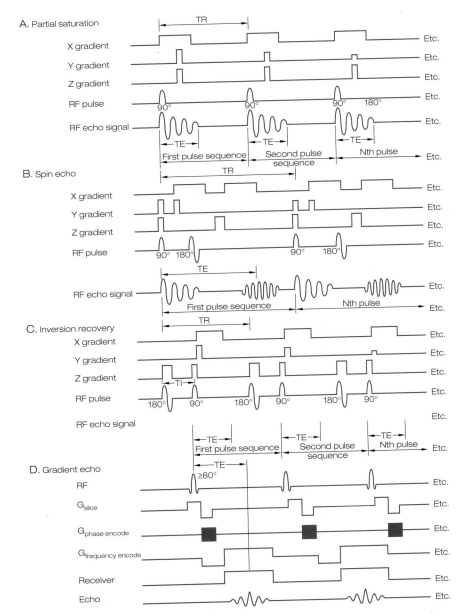

FIGURE 45–8. Magnetic resonance pulse sequences. (A) Partial saturation is a simple series of 90° RF pulses sequenced with short y and z gradient pulses and a long x gradient pulse. The RF signal is classical free induction decay. (B) Spin-echo uses a partial saturation sequence followed by a 180° (refocusing) RF pulse sequenced with an x and z gradient pulse but without a second y gradient pulse. The refocusing pulse flips the proton precession and produces the spin-echo RF signal. The RF signals that are received are a free induction decay followed by the spin-echo that begins faintly, increases to maximum strength , then fades away. TE is measured between the first and the echo RF signals. (C) Inversion recovery uses a 180° RF pulse sequenced with a z gradient pulse prior to a partial saturation sequence. The RF signal is a classical free induction decay that occurs with the 90° pulse. TI is measured between the two RF pulses. Gradient echo imaging uses gradients rather than RF to produce flip angles of less than 90° and low TRs. (D) Gradient echo imaging uses a flip angle other than 90° with a gradient refocusing pulse (rather than a 180° refocusing RF pulse), which takes less time to generate an echo that is sampled at time TE.

anatomical contrast because T_1 values for normal tissues vary considerably. Finally, a 180° pulse is used to create the signal.

Because of the reversal of M_O, the RF signal decreases with a short TI, then flips and increases as TI increases (Figure 45–9). The MR unit is usually programmed to display the reversed (negative) range of M_O so that it is shown to be returning to its original equilibrium. This permits the image to be displayed lighter as the negative signal decreases and then to continue lighter as the positive signal increases. Short TI inversion recovery techniques are sometimes called STIR imaging.

Other Pulse Sequences   Numerous other pulse sequences have been developed to increase the amount of data collected or to decrease the scanning time. These include various gradient refocused echo (GRE) techniques, including steady-state free precession (SSFP), fast low-angle shot (FLASH), fast-imaging steady-state precession (FISP), and gradient-recalled acquisition steady state (GRASS). Short TI inversion recovery (STIR) and fluid attenuated inversion recovery (FLAIR) are variations of the IR pulse sequence. Echo planar imaging (EPI) is a very efficient sequence for many applications and is the sequence used for diffusion and perfusion imaging.

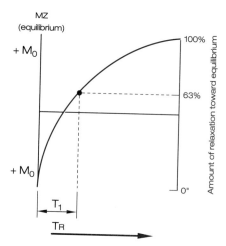

FIGURE 45–9. Relaxation after reversal of M_0 during an inversion recovery pulse. Although the precession is decaying back toward equilibrium, it flips from the −z axis to +z at the solid horizontal line. By definition, T_1 occurs when 63 percent of the return to the maximum field strength (equilibrium) has been attained.

By using the special contrast properties of blood flow during pulse sequences, magnetic resonance angiography (MRA) is rapidly becoming a routine study. Cardiac gating is often used to trigger each pulse sequence from the electrical signals of the heart, thus decreasing phase mismapping produced from heart motion. Methods used in dynamic MR for cardiac and blood flow studies include gradient motion rephasing (GMR), gradient motion nulling (GMN), motion artifact suppression technique (MAST), presaturation (dark blood sequence), and spatial modulation of magnetization (SPAMM).

Special Acquisition (Fast Spin Echo Techniques)

Because many T_1 relaxation times are relatively long, most MRI units begin to acquire data from additional sections while the first section is still proceeding through the pulse sequence. The TR interval between pulses is used to begin the pulse sequencing of other sections.

K-Space   Fast spin echo (FSE) can be achieved by generating two or more echoes within a single repetition of a sequence. This is accomplished by applying multiple 180° pulses (echo train length) following the first echo. This is done within a single-phase encoding gradient at the beginning of the sequence. The incoming data is then filed in multiple lines of **k-space**. The process continues until all lines are full. Although there are some signal-to-noise ratio (S/N) problems the computer must resolve, FSE sequences can reduce scan time by a factor of the ETL without changing the repetition time (TR), resolution matrix, or the number of acquisitions (NEX), thus significantly reducing overall scan time.

Magnetic Resonance Imaging Equipment

The typical MRI unit looks similar to a CT unit (Figure 45–10A, B). However, its internal construction is unique, consisting of a stationary magnet within which are fitted gradient and radio frequency (RF) coils (Figure 45–11). The stationary magnet must be extremely strong; field strengths for clinical imaging range from 0.06–4.0 T. A table for the patient and a large computer

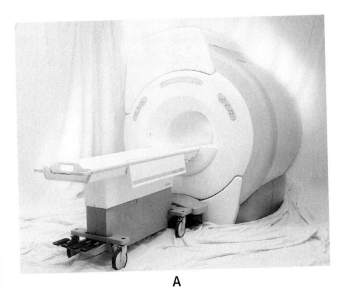

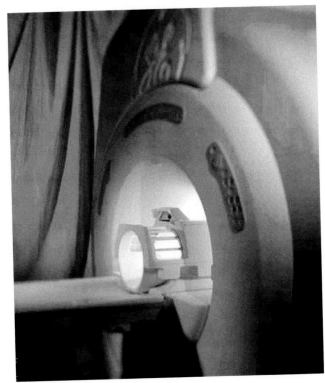

A   B

FIGURE 45–10. (A) A typical MRI unit. (B) Birdcage headcoil. *(Courtesy of GE Medical Systems)*

for image processing, display, and storage complete the MRI system.

Stationary Magnet

Magnetic resonance imaging has been achieved with resistive, permanent, and superconducting magnets. Each has significant differences in potential field strength, stability, uniformity, and cost.

Resistive
Resistive magnets produce a strong field in the range of 0.02–0.4 T from the flow of current in large numbers of turns of wire or conducting ribbons. These magnets are called resistive because of the large amount of resistance produced by this type of wiring configuration. The heat produced by the resistance is so great that resistive magnets are severely limited by their cooling requirements.

Resistive magnets provide good uniformity of magnetic field and are relatively inexpensive. However, their field strength is limited and somewhat unstable, they often exhibit longitudinal fringe field problems, and they consume a large amount of electrical power.

Permanent
Permanent magnets of up to 0.3 T have been produced by inducing a strong magnetic field in ferromagnetic materials during manufacturing. These magnets are extremely heavy and may weigh up to 200,000 pounds (100 tons). Attempts have been made to use rare earth alloys to reduce the total magnet weight.

Permanent magnets are inexpensive to maintain and offer transverse field imaging. They also exhibit minimal fringe field problems. Because the strength of permanent magnets is limited by the number of magnetic domains available in the material, they have been used only for relatively low field strength MRI units. Their weight and temperature sensitivity can be a problem.

Superconductive
Superconductive magnets may produce field strengths of up to 4 T or more. They use

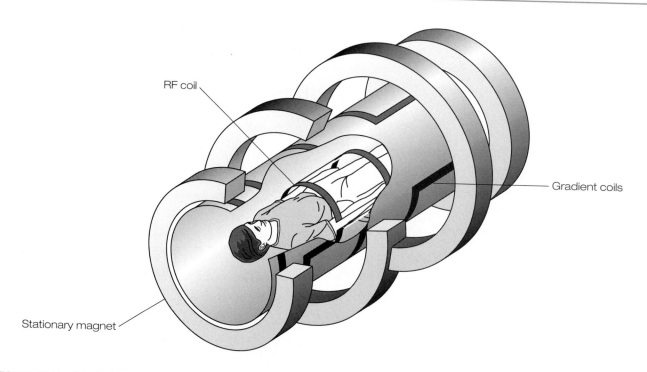

RF coil

Gradient coils

Stationary magnet

FIGURE 45–11. A typical MRI unit, with the relationship of the stationary magnet, gradient coil, and RF coil to the patient illustrated.

liquid cryogens to produce extremely low temperatures that permit some conductors to become superconductive. Much effort is currently being devoted to the development of room temperature superconductors. If these efforts are successful, MRI will become much less expensive and much more important as a diagnostic imaging tool.

Strong magnetic fields require enormous quantities of wire loops. For example, a 1.5 T magnet might require 1,000 loops, each carrying 1,000 A. This amperage in so many loops in the same circuit would produce a large quantity of heat and consume a great deal of power. In fact, a resistive magnet of this strength cannot be produced because of these physical limits. The heat would melt the conducting wire and destroy the circuit.

At temperatures near absolute zero (0° Kelvin) some conductors lose nearly all resistance, thus becoming superconductors. This permits the construction of magnets with the strength necessary to permit MRI at 1 T and higher field strengths. Superconduction has been observed as a basic property of atoms, where electrons have been spinning in tiny electromagnetic fields, apparently since the creation of the universe, without losing rotational energy as heat and slowing down.

Special cooling agents, called **cryogens**, must be used to achieve the extremely low temperatures necessary for superconductive magnets. The electromagnetic coils are placed in an insulated chamber called a **dewar**, or **cryostat**, which contains **liquid helium**. A dewar is constructed much like an insulated Thermos bottle, with the electromagnet inside. Liquid helium has a boiling point of 4° K (–269° C or –452° F) and is used to maintain the coil temperature below 9.5° K (–264° C or –443° F). The liquid helium is then surrounded by another dewar, this one containing **liquid nitrogen**, which has a boiling point of 77° K (–196° C or –320° F). The nitrogen serves as another insulator to help maintain the temperature necessary for the helium to remain liquid. The process of bringing the superconducting magnet to the necessary temperature by using cryogens is called **ramping**.

Superconductive magnets are capable of very high field strengths. They typically produce very stable and uniform fields. However, they are expensive and require expensive site preparation and maintenance. In addition, the high field strengths may cause fringe field problems.

If the temperature of the cryogens rises to the boiling point of helium, both liquids will vaporize into gases. Neither gas can maintain the necessary environment for superconduction and the electromagnetic coil will rapidly overheat. This process is known as **quenching** and is a serious hazard to the electromagnet, the patient, and personnel during superconductive MRI. The rapid vaporization of the gases can replace the oxygen in areas around the MRI unit. Although safety release valves are designed to vent these gases outside the unit, audible oxygen monitors are required to warn personnel in the event of quenching. Although helium and nitrogen are not poisonous, if the gases displace the air in the examination areas asphyxiation becomes a danger and an explosion is also possible. A patient or technologist would lose consciousness quickly and could die within minutes. A mask and nonmagnetic O_2 tank are required to permit the technologist to remove a patient from the unit as rapidly as possible if the alarms sound. The technologist must put on an oxygen mask before attempting to help a patient or anyone else. If the technologist were to lose consciousness there might be no one else to help others.

In addition to these hazards, the heat buildup that occurs in the electromagnet during a quench usually does severe damage to the coil windings and requires extensive repairs or replacement of the entire coil. Quenching is therefore not only dangerous but also prohibitively expensive. Failure to maintain sufficient cryogenic pressures through regular replacement of natural evaporation is the most likely cause of a quench. Therefore, the dependability of the cryogenic supply company to the MRI unit is of critical importance.

Shim Coils

All stationary magnets have irregularities in their fields due to the shape and construction of the magnets themselves, the location of ferromagnetic materials near the MRI unit, and the materials used in the construction of the MRI room. These irregularities are compensated for by adding a series of corrective magnetic coils, called **shim coils**, inside the bore of the main stationary magnet. Shim coils can be resistive or superconducting and are custom fitted for each unit by adjusting the current to each (Figure 45–12A).

Magnetic Field Strength

Magnetic field strength decreases inversely with the cube of the distance. This is much faster than the effect of distance (the inverse square law) that is so important in diagnostic radiography. The inverse cube law is complex but is based on the fact that both magnetic north and south poles are always present. The two poles affect each other with increasing significance as distance increases, the result being that the poles begin to cancel each other. This has the effect of reducing the magnetic field strength exponentially, as compared to the inverse square law.

This rapid fall-off of magnetic field strength makes it difficult to establish and maintain a homogeneous field for imaging. Because distance has such a dramatic effect on field strength, it becomes extremely difficult to perform MRI over a large area, even one the size and thickness of the human body.

The basic principles of magnetism are directly involved in determining magnetic field strength (see Chapter 3). The degree of alignment of induced magnetic domains in a material depends on the strength of the magnetic field that is inducing them and the inverse cube of the distance between them. This is expressed as:

$$M_I = \frac{M_O}{D^3}$$

where: M_I = induced magnetic field
M_O = original magnetic field
D = distance

This is of critical importance in understanding how magnetic attraction occurs. Not only does the attraction increase by the inverse cube with distance, but the number of magnetic domains also increases by the inverse cube. These two factors function mathematically so that their product represents the total attraction. In other words, the actual increase is not the inverse cube of the distance but rather the inverse cube of the distance times the inverse cube of the number of magnetic domains. Therefore, attraction occurs by the inverse sixth power. Moving ten times closer to the magnet actually causes the magnetic field strength attraction to increase by 1,000,000 times.

A free magnet will move to align itself in a magnetic field. For example, the needle of a compass aligns itself on a north-south axis because it experiences the torque

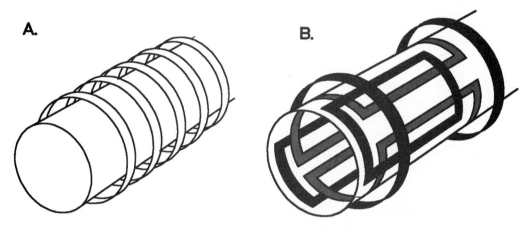

FIGURE 45–12. (A) Shim coils and (B) gradient coils, both surrounding the bore of the stationary magnet.

of the earth's magnetic field. Torque can be a powerful force in a strong magnetic field. For example, this principle of inducing torque is used to activate the motors that move trains and lift elevators. However, torque also acts on the nucleus of an atom and can cause a nucleus to align with a magnetic field. This is a basic principle in MRI.

Gradient Coils

There are three sets of gradient coils, one each for the x, y, and z axes (Figure 45–12B). They can be operated as required to achieve the appropriate pulse sequence and spatial localization within the anatomical section.

Radiofrequency Coils

Radiofrequency (RF) coils may serve as both the transmitter and the receiver of the MRI signal (although some units use separate RF coils for each function). Because it is desirable to position RF coils as close as possible to the body part to be imaged, they are often sized and shaped to fit specific body parts. This type of coil is known as a **surface coil. Head, neck, and extremity** surface coils are commonly used in either **saddle** or **solenoid** shapes (a solenoid head coil is shown in Figure 45–10B). **Solenoid (or birdcage) coils are used in a transverse magnetic field.** A solenoid extremity coil is shown in Figure 45–13A. **Saddle coils are used in a longitudinal**

magnetic field. However, the best images are produced with surface (or local) coils that are placed directly on the patient, as close to the region of interest as possible. Body coils permit resolution to the depth of the entire body section but decreased signal-to-noise ratio (SNR) can be a problem. Surface coils permit thinner sections and increased SNR, but they are limited to a depth of resolution of half their diameter (usually 5–6 cm).

It is important to select the RF coil appropriate to the structure being examined. For example, a birdcage coil (Figure 45–13B) would image the entire head quite well but a small surface coil would produce the best image of the TMJ (Figure 45–13C).

Table

The MRI table is usually slightly curved for patient comfort and to conform to the circular shape of the bore of the magnet. As with CT units, tabletops are rated for maximum weight and it is critical that this weight not be exceeded. Extensive damage to the table may result when attempts are made to examine very large patients who exceed the limit. Most tables are driven by hydraulics to move the patient smoothly into the bore of the magnet.

Computer

Data acquisition sequences are complex in most MRI units. The computer must precisely control the gradient

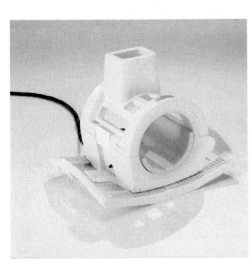

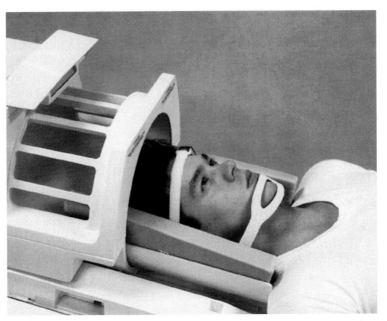

A

B

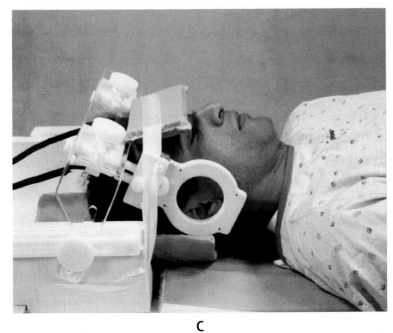

C

FIGURE 45–13. (A) Extremity coil. (B) Head coil. (C) 3-inch general purpose coils positioned very close to the temporomandibular joint in a dual-array offer increased SNR. *(Courtesy of GE Medical Systems)*

and RF coils and their pulsing sequences, as well as collect and process the received RF data. Most data is collected by sampling the received signal during a series of RF windows. All data and images can be stored electronically on magnetic or optical tape or disk. The operator can access the computer through two consoles, one for operating the MRI unit to acquire data, the other for manipulation of images for which data has been collected although some units use a single console.

Operating Console   The MRI unit operator controls the scanning procedure by specifying the radio frequency, RF pulse sequence, pulsing time intervals, matrix size, number of excitations (NEX) or acquisitions, field of view, and section parameters.

The radio frequency is adjusted by tuning the system to the proper Larmor frequency for the tissue to be examined and by tuning the RF coils to receive the desired RF signal that will be emitted from the tissues.

The RF pulse sequences are classified as partial saturation, inversion recovery, spin-echo, or one of the other fast data sequences discussed previously. The MRI computer is programmed to initiate the RF and magnetic field pulses to accomplish the selected sequence. These sequences are usually extremely complex as they commonly use multisection and multiecho techniques to reduce scan time by acquiring data for numerous sections simultaneously. Although the operator does not have to initiate the various pulses, an appropriate sequencing method for the particular examination must be selected.

The most common variable in operating an MRI unit is the time interval (TI, TE, and TR) used to enhance image quality. Appropriate intervals determine how tissue characteristics (such as T_1, T_2, T_2^*, or ρ) are demonstrated on MR images. T_1 and T_2 can vary depending on the tissue of interest, suspected pathology, and clinical experience (Table 45–3). The time interval (TR) directly affects the total scan time.

As in all digital imaging, the matrix size controls the resolution of the image. The matrix size that is selected also has a direct effect on the total scan time, with a larger matrix producing higher resolution but requiring longer scan times. This is often set as the number of phase encoding steps, with 256 or 512 being common selections. Interpolation schemes can also be implemented to enhance apparent resolution.

The quantity of protons precessing and emitting RF determines the proton density (ρ). The longer the TR, the more time is available for RF emission. The larger the tissue sample or the greater the number of precessing protons in the tissue, the greater is the proton spin density. These factors determine the strength of the RF signal and therefore the intensity (brightness) of the image.

The number of signals used to create the image also has a linear effect on the total scan time. Several terms are used to represent this parameter. These include number of excitations (NEX), number of signal averages (NSA), and number of acquisitions. It also determines the strength of the RF signal.

The field of view (FOV) also affects resolution. A larger FOV decreases resolution.

The section, the interval between sections, and the section thickness can all be controlled by the operator.

Display Console   The image reconstruction algorithms used for MRI are similar to those used in CT (see Chapters 42 and 43). However, there are differences because of the increased data that is collected during the MRI pulse sequences. Depending on the pulse sequence and quantity of data collected, this permits oblique sections as well as routine sagittal, coronal, and even 3D reconstructions.

Most display consoles also permit the addition of software **filters**. Smoothing filters average pixel values but decrease resolution. Noise reduction filters eliminate image densities below a selected level. Edge (contour) enhancement filters accentuate the differences between pixels when those differences exceed a selected value. Other filters for special uses may be created with custom algorithms.

MRI display consoles permit density level windows and contrast widths to be set as with any digital image processing technology. However, MRI units collect significantly more data than CT units and they have the ability to perform more complex data analysis as well. MR angiograms can be projected into multiple planes or rotated about an axis. Reformatting of data to display transverse, sagittal, and coronal images, as well as oblique and three-dimensional images, is also possible without additional data collection (Figure 45–14). Region of interest (ROI) controls permit calculations of pixel values, histograms, and highlighting of specific regions. Scanograms for anatomical reference, grid application,

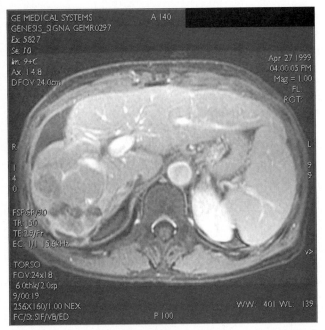

GE MEDICAL SYSTEMS A 140
GENESIS_SIGNA GEMR0297
Ex: 5827
Se: 10
Im: 9+C
Ax 14.8   Apr 27 1999
DFOV 24.0cm   04:00:05 PM
                                           Mag = 1.00
                                                FL
                                                R.O.T.
R   L

I   9
4   9
0

FSPGR/90
TR: 150
TE: 2.9/Fr
EC: 1/1 15.6kHz

TORSO
FOV:24x18
6.0thk/2.0sp
9/00:19
256X160/1.00 NEX   W/W: 401 W/L: 139
FC/St: S/F/VB/ED   P 100

FIGURE 45–14. A coronal projection image from a 3D Time-of-Flight MR angiogram. *(Courtesy of GE Medical Systems)*

reverse display, annotation, and simultaneous image display (collaging) are all possible. Electronic magnification of the field of view (FOV) is often used when filming MRI studies.

Image Quality

Numerous factors directly affect image quality. The primary visual factor is often called brightness, which is actually the density of the MR image. The RF signal strength determines brightness, although other factors affect it.

Field Strength

Higher strength magnetic fields produce a stronger RF signal. There is a dramatic difference between the imaging parameters and the resultant image for the same tissues when examined under different strength magnets. Although the most efficient field strength has not yet been determined, it most likely is between 1 and 3 T.

Section Thickness

Section thickness is determined by the size (or depth) of the tissue voxel. It is the primary factor of image quality because all signals from a single voxel are mathematically combined to give a single image value for the voxel. Therefore the voxel size determines the smallest tissue differences that can be imaged.

The dimension of a voxel is determined by dividing the size of the field of view by the matrix size:

$$d = \frac{F}{M}$$

where: d = voxel dimension
F = field of view
M = matrix size

Example: What is the voxel dimension for a 256×256 matrix showing a field of view of 22 cm?

Answer: $d = \dfrac{F}{M}$

$d = \dfrac{22 \text{ cm}}{256}$

$d = 0.0859 \text{ cm} = 8.59 \text{ mm}$

This formula must be applied in both directions (x and y) as many matrices have different x and y sizes.

Effect of MRI Parameters

The effects of the major MRI parameters, proton spin density (ρ), repetition time (TR), echo time (TE), inversion time (TI), spin-lattice relaxation time (T_1), and spin-spin relaxation time (T_2) are summed in Table 45–2.

The present state of MRI diagnosis demands that each examination include at least one T1 weighted image and at least one T_2 weighted image. This is because proton precession (and therefore the frequency of the RF signal emitted) varies depending on adjacent tissues. As an example, a tumor might have a T_1 and T_2 as shown in Table 45–4. If the tumor were imbedded in fat, a T_1 weighted image would provide the contrast to permit its detection; the tumor would be hidden in a T_2 image because the T_2 relaxation times of the tumor and of fat are identical, making them appear at the same image density. However, if the same tumor were imbedded in muscle, a T_2 weighted image would be required to provide contrast; the tumor would be hidden in a T_1 image because the T_1 of the tumor and of muscle are identical. Chemical saturation techniques can also be employed to minimize signal from certain structures containing fat or water.

Motion

Motion (temporal resolution) is a special problem in MRI because of the extremely long scan times that must be used. Good communication with the patient is the best method of assuring cooperation in reducing motion artifacts. Much has been written about patient claustrophobia due to the small diameter and long length of the bore of most MRI units. However, only about 5 percent of all patients cannot be examined due to claustrophobia. Cardiac gating procedures that use an electrocardiographic wave to trigger scanning pulses have proven effective in reducing motion in thoracic, cardiac, and cervical spine imaging. Some patients can be led through a breath holding technique in which the technologist activates the pulse sequence at expiration to eliminate diaphragmatic motion. This technique is most effective with pulse sequences of 30 seconds or less.

Spatial Resolution

Resolution is the ability to distinguish one structure from another. Spatial resolution is determined by the homogeneity of the static external magnetic field, the steepness of the gradient fields, and the scan time. Its quality is limited by noise, or the signal-to-noise ratio; when this ratio becomes low, image quality begins to decrease. Current MRI units are capable of resolving objects as small as 0.1 mm.

Signal-to-Noise Ratio

Noise, or extraneous visual information, is measured as the signal-to-noise ratio (S/N). It is determined by the voxel size and detection volume, the quantity of precessing protons, the pulse sequence, and the field strength. It is undesirable because it reduces the visibility of low contrast structures. **The S/N is enhanced by reducing TE and using optimal TR.** It can also be enhanced by **averaging** a series of RF signals and by the use of a **stronger magnetic field**.

RF coils are sensitive enough that they can detect the tiny electrical currents produced by normal Brownian motion of body electrolytes. Because the quantity of Brownian motion increases with body temperature, it is referred to as **thermal noise**.

Scan Time

As with all digital imaging methods, scan time depends on the quantity of data that must be processed by the computer. In MRI it depends on the pulse sequences, the number of phase encoding steps, and the number of excitations. For example, a 256×256 matrix with a TR of 2 seconds for 2 excitations requires a 17-minute scan time. For three-dimensional MRI, the scan time is usually much greater. Multisection and multiecho pulse sequences are the prime methods of reducing scan time.

Image Contrast

Contrast resolution is dependent upon image contrast, which in turn is determined by the tissue characteristics (T_1 and T_2) and the pulse sequence variables (especially TR and TE). By using knowledge of these parameters, a technologist can produce images to maximize the contrast between tissues. In spin-echo sequences, this relates to the appropriately named T_1 weighted, T_2 weighted, and proton density weighted images. As MRI continues to develop, new techniques are constantly being researched to improve contrast as well as spatial resolution. It is the responsibility of the MR technologist to apply the proper sequences and algorithms to maximize the visualization of both anatomy and pathology.

Image contrast can be controlled to a great extent by the manipulation of the sequence of radio frequency pulses, ρ, TI, TR, and TE. Maximum contrast is obtained when the RF signal strength is at its greatest difference between two tissues. For example, in Figure 45–15A, the T_1 relaxation curves become further apart as time increases. Therefore, the contrast increases with increasing time.

A **T_1 weighted image** is usually produced with a short TR (300–800 ms) to maximize T_1 and a short TE to minimize T_2 (Figure 45–15B). A **T_2 weighted image** is usually produced with a **long TR** (2–3 sec) to minimize T_1 and a **long TE** to maximize T_2 (Figure 45–15C). However, there are some situations in which image density actually reverses (Figure 45–15C). In these instances a short TE produces greater T_1 contrast while a long TE produces greater T_2 contrast. When TE is set at the crossover point, no contrast is produced. This is most common in proton density images produced by a moderate length TR. The subject contrast of a T_1 image varies with the magnetic field strength, while T_2 values remain essentially constant.

Whereas CT uses Hounsfield units, there are no standardized units for tissue measurements in MRI because subject contrast depends on the differences between the signals received from the tissues. There are so many different pulse and frequency sequences and algorithms in use that no unit system is yet feasible.

Most pathologies increase both T_1 and T_2. This produces a black, negative contrast image on a T_1 weighted image and a white, positive contrast image on a T_2 weighted image. This contrast disappears when images are not weighted toward either T_1 or T_2. Consequently, efforts should be made to produce weighted images when pathological conditions are to be demonstrated.

The effects of the most common parameter weighting, proton spin density (ρ), T_1, and T_2, on image density (brightness) are shown in Table 45–2.

Chemical Shift Artifact

The chemical shift is the slight difference between the resonating frequencies of similar protons. The differences are so slight that they are expressed in parts per million (ppm). For example, hydrogen in fat resonates at a slightly higher frequency than hydrogen in water (about 3 ppm). This produces a bright band next to a dark band on the MR image at water-fat interfaces and is considered an imaging artifact, although some studies have indicated that proper manipulation of the RF spectrum data can produce useful information from chemical shift. Chemical shift artifacts can be reduced or eliminated by increasing the strength of the gradient fields, although this may also increase the visible noise in the image.

Paramagnetic Contrast Agents

Magnetic resonance imaging contrast agents are primarily **paramagnetic agents designed to enhance the T_1 and T_2 relaxation times of adjacent hydrogen nuclei**. Some agents are classified as T_1 active or T_2 active. They produce complex effects that vary depending on the RF pulsing sequence. For example, T_1 shortening increases the RF signal intensity but T_2 shortening decreases it. In many instances paramagnetic contrast agents permit the visualization of lesions with shorter TR, thus decreasing scan time.

Paramagnetic contrast agents have been developed for oral, intravenous, and inhalation administration, and although this is an active research area in MRI, at the present time the IV agents have predominated. Gadolinium^{+3} (Gd^{+3}), which has seven unpaired electrons, has the strongest relaxation rate properties and has proven effective in demonstrating various types of lesions. However, alone it is extremely toxic and is administered in a chelate with DTPA (diethylenetriaminepentaacetic acid) (Gd-DTPA) to ensure detoxification. IV administration is common, especially for neuroimaging and MR angiography.

Safety and Biological Hazards

As yet, there is no known biological risk from the magnetic field of an MRI unit. However, magnetic resonance imaging units require special consideration of the environment in which they are installed because of possible interactions between their extremely strong magnetic fields with ferromagnetic materials and electromagnetic devices. Included among devices that are affected by MRI units are cathode ray tubes, gamma cameras, cardiac pacemakers, and radio broadcasting and receiving equipment. Other equipment affected by magnetic fields includes computers (including the MRI computer itself), x-ray tubes, image intensification systems, computed tomography units, ultrasound units, electron microscopes, credit cards, analog watches, and any other devices that operate on electromagnetic principles. Safe operating distances for these devices depend on the strength of the MRI magnet and may range up to 500 feet for a 1.5 T magnet.

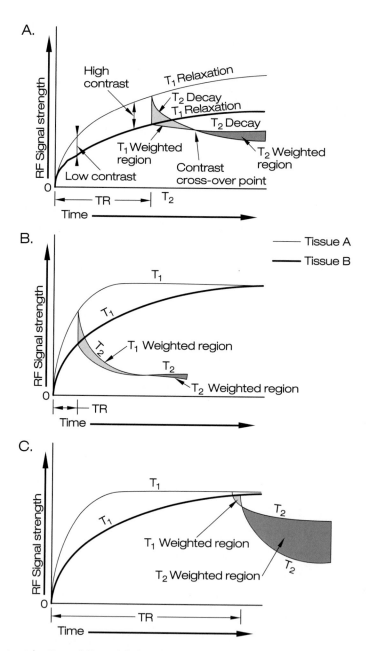

FIGURE 45–15. Obtaining contrast by T_1 and T_2 weighting during spin-echo imaging. The T_1 curves demonstrate recovery back toward equilibrium after the first pulse. The T_2 curves demonstrate decay from the refocusing pulse back toward equilibrium. (A) Relatively equal T_1 and T_2 weighting with a medium TR. Note the contrast crossover point. A short TE after the TR would produce a T_1 weighted image. A long TE after the TR would produce a T_2 weighted image. (B) T_1 weighting occurs with a short TR. The shorter the TE after the TR, the greater the signal difference (contrast) between the tissues. (C) T_2 weighting occurs with a long TR. The longer the TE before the TR, the greater the signal difference (contrast) between the tissues. *(Adopted by permission from Friedman, B. R., Chaves-Munoz, G., & Merritt, C. R. B. [1989].* Principles of MRI. *New York: McGraw-Hill, Inc.)*

The MRI unit itself can be seriously affected by moving ferromagnetic devices, such as elevators and automobiles, and by strong electromagnetic devices, such as power transformers and radio broadcasting antennas. Although ferromagnetic sheets can be used to shield the MRI unit and the main resonance frequency can be adjusted slightly to avoid ranges conflicting with other equipment, these measures can compromise the imaging ability of the unit.

Safety Factors

Because magnetic fields change so dramatically with distance, it is easy for someone who is not knowledgeable about them to be misled on safety considerations. Accidents around MRI units occur when ferromagnetic materials such as oxygen tanks, IV poles, mop buckets, scissors, and personal items such as earrings and belt buckles enter the field. These items can become lethal projectiles. Magnetic media, such as computer and audio disks, and magnetized information strips on credit cards may be erased.

Other electronic devices, such as cardiac pacemakers and pocket pagers, and physiologic monitors, such as electrocardiographic monitors, may be damaged or turned off and will not work properly in a strong magnetic field. It is also possible that metal objects that have been surgically implanted, such as replacement hips, aneurysm clips and surgical staples, or foreign objects, such as buckshot or metallic debri in the eye, may be torqued during MRI examinations with catastrophic consequences. For example, torquing an aneurysm clip could open an artery and cause a fatal hemorrhage. Careful histories and, in some cases, fluoroscopic screening, are safety precautions that must be taken before MRI. Patients with histories of surgical implants or with employment histories in metal working must be interviewed with special care. The objects considered to contraindicate MRI examination are listed in Table 45–5.

A few steps closer to an MRI unit will increase the magnetic field attraction by the inverse cube law. A distance of as little as one inch can make the difference between being able to hold onto an object and having it fly at incredible speed directly to the bore of the MRI unit. Remembering that an industrial electromagnet is capable of lifting an automobile or railroad car may help in understanding the power of an extremely strong magnetic field.

TABLE 45–5. Objects That Contraindicate MRI Examination

Pacemakers
Ferromagnetic cranial aneurysm clips
Shrapnel or other metallic objects in vital locations
Cochlear implants

Within 10–20 feet of the magnet, wheelchairs and carts may begin to roll toward the MRI unit and within 5–10 feet, hairpins and pens may become projectiles. A cart may begin to roll from 20 feet away, but as it approaches the bore of the magnet the field may become strong enough to cause an oxygen tank or other object on the cart to become a projectile. It is important to emphasize to others that the magnetic field is operating at all times. Many persons assume that, as with most electromagnetic devices, the magnetic field is on only when the unit is in operation. The doors to the MRI scanning room should not only be locked, but padlocked during hours the unit is closed. This procedure prevents entry by persons with master passkeys during these hours.

Because of the cryogenically established superconductive conditions, superconductor magnets maintain their fields at all times and are therefore hazardous at all times. The extremely strong field must be treated with respect. The attractive force on an object as large as an oxygen tank makes it possible to fatally injure a patient or technologist if he or she is caught between the object and the MRI unit.

Biological Factors

The term used to describe the absorption of RF radiation is the **specific absorption rate (SAR)**. The SAR is indicated in units of watts per kilogram (W/kg). The United States Environmental Protection Agency (EPA) has concluded that adverse human health effects are associated with whole-body average SARs of 1–4 W/kg or greater. A primary concern is increased effects due to heating in geriatric and dehydrated patients. Consequently many agencies are considering RF radiation as a noncarcinogen but with uncertainty factors used in deriving exposure limits. The current FDA safe levels for exposure to RF during MR procedures are:

The exposure to RF energy below the level of concern is an SAR of 0.4 W/kg or less averaged over the body; 8.0 W/kg or less spatial peak in any 1 g of tissue, and 3.2 W/kg or less averaged over the head, OR

The exposure to RF energy that is insufficient to produce a core temperature increase of 1°C and localized heating to no greater than 38°C in the head, 39°C in the trunk, and 40°C in the extremities, except for patients with impaired system blood flow and/or perspiration (i.e., those with compromised thermoregulatory systems).

These conclusions are consistent with the recommendations of other agencies such as the United States National Council on Radiation Protection and Measurements (NCRP), International Radiation Protection Association (IRPA), the United States Food and Drug Administration (FDA), and the American National Standards Institute (ANSI). Although there have not been any published reports of harmful effects due to the use of MRI, the issue is under intense study and much additional information is expected in the years to come. In the United States, the FDA requires prominent posting of triangular warning signs at the 5 G (0.0005 T) line. There are two signs, one indicating a strong magnetic field, the other with markings and wording prohibiting pacemakers or loose metal objects.

Static magnetic fields appear to augment the T wave amplitude of the heart. This may occur when conductive fluids, such as blood, pass through the static magnetic field, thus generating low potentials that may affect the biopotentials of the heart. No arrhythmias or other heart rate alterations have yet been produced in laboratory animals or observed in patients undergoing MRI.

Intense gradient magnetic fields have been shown to induce electrical currents in body tissues such as nerve, muscle, skeletal, and heart. Light flashes due to physiological stimulation of the retina have also been observed. However, these field strengths are far above that used in MRI.

Radio frequency magnetic fields are known to produce thermal effects. Potential biological damage would depend on the ability of the specific biological system to metabolically absorb and distribute heat. Some effects, including ocular cataractogenesis due to thermal heating of the eye, have been recorded, although again at field levels well above those used in MRI.

Because of the lack of definitive data on the biological effects of MRI, pregnant women are seldom examined. However, when necessary, MRI studies are considered less hazardous to the fetus than computed tomography studies.

Summary

Magnetic resonance imaging (MRI) uses magnetism and radio frequencies (RF) to create diagnostic sectional images of the body. The nucleus is spinning, thus creating a nuclear magnetic moment. This rotating charge acts as a current loop and produces a magnetic field. When a rotating nucleus is subjected to a magnetic field, it will begin to precess. MR imaging is accomplished through various measurements of this movement of the nuclear magnetic field.

The frequency of precession is called the Larmor frequency and is critical to MR imaging. Production of the nuclear magnetic resonance signal requires applying a Larmor frequency RF and then listening to the RF emissions from the protons. Digital imaging reconstruction techniques are then used to create sectional and three-dimensional images.

The primary parameters controlling the MRI process include proton spin density (PD, NEX or NSA, or ρ), repetition time (TR), echo time (TE), inversion time (TI), spin-lattice or longitudinal relaxation time (T_1), and spin-spin or transverse relaxation time (T_2). The parameters that are used vary depending on the pulse sequence used.

The localization of information for the MR image requires three electromagnetic coils to produce magnetic field gradients corresponding to the x, y, and z axes to be imaged. The RF that are detected from these gradient coils can then be analyzed to determine not only the type of atom they came from but also the atom's precise location within the imaging matrix.

The primary variable in the data collection procedure during MRI is the sequence of RF pulses that are used to cause the protons to precess. Partial saturation, spin-echo, inversion recovery, and gradient-echo are the major sequences, although most MRI is done with spin-echo pulse sequences. There are many modifications of spin-echo sequences, including multisection and multi-echo sequences.

A typical MRI unit consists of a stationary magnet within which are fitted gradient and radio frequency (RF) coils. The stationary magnet must be extremely strong; current field strengths range from 0.06–3.0 T. A table for the patient and a large computer for image processing, display, and storage complete the system.

The primary image quality factor is often called brightness, which is actually the density of the MR image. The RF signal strength determines brightness, although it is also affected by field strength, section thickness, the MRI parameters (ρ, TI, TE, TR, T_1, T_2), motion, spatial resolution, S/N, and scan time. Image contrast is controlled by manipulating the MRI parameters to produce T_1 and T_2 weighted images. Chemical shift artifacts may occur at fat-water interfaces although chemical shift imaging may provide useful diagnostic information in the future. Paramagnetic contrast agents are used to enhance image contrast. As yet, there is no known biological risk from the magnetic field of an MRI unit. However, magnetic resonance imaging units require special restrictions to their access because of possible interactions between their extremely strong magnetic fields and ferromagnetic materials and electromagnetic devices. Accidents around MRI units occur when ferromagnetic materials such as oxygen tanks, IV poles, mop buckets, scissors, and personal items such as earrings and belt buckles enter the field. These items can become lethal projectiles.

The Food and Drug Administration suggests limiting whole or partial body exposure to 2.0 T for static magnetic fields, 3.0 T/sec for gradient fields, and a specific absorption rate (SAR) of 0.4 W/kg for RF fields.

REVIEW QUESTIONS

1. What is the source of the magnetic fields within the body that are used during MRI?

2. What is precession?

3. What is TI? TR? TE? T_1? T_2?

4. How do the gradient coils select an image section?

5. What is accomplished by an RF pulse during a pulse sequence?

6. What occurs at each step during a spin-echo pulse sequence?

7. How is MR image contrast increased? decreased?

8. How can MR image noise be reduced by improving the S/N?

9. Describe appropriate safety measures for protection of all persons who approach the MRI unit magnetic field.

REFERENCES AND RECOMMENDED READING

Andrew, E. R. (1982). Nuclear magnetic resonance imaging. *Scientific Basis of Medical Imaging*. Edited by Wells, P. N. T. Edinburgh: Churchill Livingstone.

Atkinson, D. J. (1990). Pulse sequence design. *Clinical Magnetic Resonance Imaging*. Edited by Edelman, R. R. & Hesselink, J. R. Philadelphia: W. B. Saunders.

Axel, L. (1988). Chemical shift imaging. *Magnetic Resonance Imaging*. Edited by Stark, D. D. & Bradley, W. G. St. Louis: C. V. Mosby.

Ayton, V. T., Smith, M. A., & Bingham, J. B. (1989). Practical consideration for patient investigation using a high field magnetic resonance system. *Radiography Today*. 55(620), 12.

Barrafate, D. (1985). MRI: A technologist's perspective. The *Canadian Journal of Medical Radiation Technology*. 16(3), 73.

Barrafate, D. & Henkelman, M. (1985). MRI and surgical clips. *The Canadian Journal of Medical Radiation Technology*. 16(3), 101.

Bloch, F. (1964). The principle of nuclear induction. *Nobel Lectures in Physics: 1942–1962*. New York: Elsevier Publishing Company.

Bloch, F. (1946). Nuclear induction. *Physics Review*. 70, 460–474.

Bloch, F., Hansen, W. W., & Packard, M. E. (1946). Nuclear induction. *Physics Review*. 69, 127.

Bushberg, J. T., Seibert, J. A., Leidholdt, E. M., & Boone, J. M. (1994). *The essential physics of medical imaging*. Baltimore: Williams & Wilkins.

Bushong, S. C. (1997). *Radiologic science for technologists: Physics, biology, and protection.* (6th ed.). St. Louis: C. V. Mosby.

Bushong, S. C. (1988). *Magnetic resonance imaging: Physical and biological principles.* (5th ed.). St. Louis: C. V. Mosby.

Curry, T. S., Dowdey, J. E., & Murry, R. C. (1990). *Christensen's introduction to the physics of diagnostic radiology.* (4th ed.). Philadelphia: Lea and Febiger.

Damadian, R. (1971). Tumor detection by nuclear magnetic resonance. *Science. 171,* 1151–1153.

Damadian, R., Goldsmith, M., & Minkoff, L. (1977). NMR in cancer XVI: FONAR image of the live human body. *Physiological Chemistry and Physics. 9,* 97–100.

Damadian, R., Zaner, K., Hor, D., DiMaio, T., Minkoff, L., & Goldsmith, M. (1973). Nuclear magnetic resonance as a new tool in cancer research: Human tumors by NMR. *Annals of the New York Academy of Science. 222,* 1,048–1,076.

Damadian, R. *(NMR) in medicine.* Berlin: Springer-Verlag.

Davis, P. (1981). Potential hazards in NMR imaging: Heating effects of changing magnetic fields and RF fields on small metallic implants. *American Journal of Roentgenology. 137,* 857–860.

Edelman, R. R. & Hesselink, J. R. (1990). *Clinical magnetic resonance imaging.* Philadelphia: W. B. Saunders.

Elster, A. D. (1986). *Magnetic resonance imaging: A reference guide and atlas.* Philadelphia: J. B. Lippincott.

Fitzsimmons, J. R. & Mick, R. C. (1985). Image quality and magnetic field strength in NMR imaging. *Applied Radiology. 14*(2), 52.

Fodor, J. & Mallot, J. (1984). MRI: A new imaging modality. *Radiologic Technology. 56*(1), 17.

Forster, E. (1985). *Equipment for diagnostic radiography.* Lancaster: MTP Press.

Friedman, B. R., Jones, J. P., Chaves-Munoz, G., Salmon, A. P., & Merritt, C. R. B. (1989). *Principles of MRI.* New York: McGraw-Hill.

Grey, M. L. & Coffey, C. W. (1987). Methods for evaluating image quality in magnetic resonance imaging. *Radiologic Technology. 58*(4), 339.

Heiken, J. P. & Brown, J. J. (Eds.). (1991). *Manual of clinical magnetic resonance imaging.* (2nd ed.). New York: Raven.

Hendee, W. R. & Ritenour, R. (1993). *Medical imaging physics.* (3rd ed.). St. Louis: C. V. Mosby.

Hinshaw, W. S., Bottomley, P. A., & Holland, G. N. (1977). Radiographic thin-section image of the human wrist by nuclear magnetic resonance. *Nature. 270*(22/29), 722–723.

Kaut, C. (1992). *MRI workbook for technologists.* New York: Raven.

Lauterbur, P. C. (1973). Image formation by induced local interactions: Examples employing nuclear magnetic resonance. *Nature. 242,* 190–191.

Lipcamon, J. D., Chiu, L. C., Phillips, J. J., & Pottany, P. M. (1988). MRI of the upper abdomen using motion artifact suppression technique. *Radiologic Technology. 59*(5), 415.

Lufkin, R. B. (1990). *The MRI manual.* St. Louis: C. V. Mosby.

Morgan, C. J. & Hendee, W. R. (1984). *Introduction to magnetic resonance imaging.* Denver: Multi-Media Publishing.

Nelson, T. R., Ritenour, E. R., Davis, K., & Pretorius, D. H. (1985). MRI: The basic physical and clinical concepts Part 1. *Radiologic Technology. 56*(6), 410.

Nelson, T. R, Ritenour, E. R., Davis, K., & Pretorius, D. H. (1985). MRI: The basic physical and clinical concepts Part 2. *Radiologic Technology. 57*(1), 26.

Nelson, T. R., Ritenour, E. R., Davis, K., Pretorius, D. H., & Hendrick, R. E. (1985). MRI: The basic physical and clinical concepts Part 3. *Radiologic Technology. 57*(2), 142.

Olendorf, W. & Olendorf, W., Jr. (1991). *MRI primer.* New York: Raven.

Philips Medical Systems. (1984). *Principles of MR imaging.* The Netherlands: Philips Medical Systems Publication 1984–11.

Purcell, E. (1964). Research in nuclear magnetism. *Nobel Lectures in Physics: 1942–1962.* New York: Elsevier.

Purcell, E. M., Torrey, H. C., & Pound, R. V. (1946). Resonance absorption by nuclear magnetic moments in a solid. *Physics Review. 69,* 37–83.

Rollo, F. D. & Patton, J. A. (1981). Nuclear magnetic resonance imaging. Radiographic films and screen-film systems. *The Physical Basis of Medical Imaging.* Editors: Coulam, C. M., Erickson, J. J., Rollo, F. D., & James, A. E. New York: Appleton-Century-Crofts.

Russel, R., Dallas-Hultema, C., & Cohen, M. D. (1986). MRI techniques in children. *Radiologic Technology. 57*(5), 428.

Schellock, F. G. & Kanal, E. (1994). *Magnetic resonance bio-effects, safety, and patient management.* New York: Raven.

Seeram, E. (1985). *X-ray imaging equipment: An introduction.* Springfield: Charles C. Thomas.

Sigal, R. (1988). *Magnetic resonance imaging: Basis for interpretation.* Berlin: Springer-Verlag.

Smith, H. & Ranallo, F. N. (1989). *A non-mathematical approach to basic MRI.* Madison, WI: Medical Physics Publishing.

Sobol, W. T. (1994). Artifacts in magnetic resonance imaging. *Applied Radiology. 23*(8), 11–16.

Stark, D. D. & Bradley, W. (Eds.). (1988). *Magnetic resonance imaging.* St. Louis: C. V. Mosby.

Westbrook, C. (1994). *Handbook of MRI technique.* Oxford: Blackwell Scientific.

Westbrook, C. & Kaut, C. (1993). *MRI in practice.* Oxford: Blackwell Scientific.

Wolbarst, A. B. (1993). *Physics of radiology.* Norwalk, CT: Appleton & Lange.

Wolfe, G. & Popp, C. (1984). *NMR: A primer for medical imaging.* Thorofare, NJ: Slack Book Division.

Woodward, P. & Freimarck, R. D. (1995). *MRI for technologists.* New York: McGraw-Hill.

Young, S. W. (1984). *Nuclear magnetic resonance imaging: Basic principles.* New York: Raven.

On a New Kind of Rays*

by W. C. Röntgen

(1) A discharge from a large induction coil is passed through a Hittorf's vacuum tube, or through a well-exhausted Crookes' or Lenard's tube. The tube is surrounded by a fairly close-fitting shield of black paper; it is then possible to see, in a completely darkened room, that paper covered on one side with barium platinocyanide lights up with brilliant fluorescence when brought into the neighbourhood of the tube, whether the painted side or the other be turned towards the tube. The fluorescence is still visible at two metres distance. It is easy to show that the origin of the fluorescence lies within the vacuum tube.

(2) It is seen, therefore, that some agent is capable of penetrating black cardboard which is quite opaque to ultra-violet light, sunlight, or arc-light. It is therefore of interest to investigate how far other bodies can be penetrated by the same agent. It is readily shown that all bodies possess this same transparency, but in very varying degrees. For example, paper is very transparent; the fluorescent screen will light up when placed behind a book of a thousand pages; printer's ink offers no marked resistance. Similarly the fluorescence shows behind two packs of cards; a single card does not visibly diminish the brilliancy of the light. So, again, a single thickness of tinfoil hardly casts a shadow on the screen; several have to be superposed to produce a marked effect. Thick blocks of wood are still transparent. Boards of pine two or three centimetres thick absorb only very little. A piece of sheet aluminium, 15 mm. thick, still allowed the x-rays (as I will call the rays, for the sake of brevity) to pass, but greatly reduced the fluorescence. Glass plates of similar

thickness behave similarly; lead glass is, however, much more opaque than glass free from lead. Ebonite several centimetres thick is transparent. If the hand be held before the fluorescent screen, the shadow shows the bones darkly, with only faint outlines of the surrounding tissues.

Water and several other fluids are very transparent. Hydrogen is not markedly more permeable than air. Plates of copper, silver, lead, gold, and platinum also allow the rays to pass, but only when the metal is thin. Platinum .2 mm. thick allows some rays to pass; silver and copper are more transparent. Lead 1.5 mm. thick is practically opaque. If a square rod of wood 20 mm. in the side be painted on one face with white lead, it casts little shadow when it is so turned that the painted face is parallel to the x-rays, but a strong shadow if the rays have to pass through the painted side. The salts of the metals, either solid or in solution, behave generally as the metals themselves.

(3) The preceding experiments lead to the conclusion that the density of the bodies is the property whose variation mainly affects their permeability. At least no other property seems so marked in this connection. But that the density alone does not determine the transparency is shown by an experiment wherein plates of similar thickness of Iceland spar, glass, aluminium, and quartz were employed as screens. Then the Iceland spar showed itself much less transparent than the other bodies, though of approximately the same density. I have not remarked any strong fluorescence of Iceland spar compared with glass (see below, No. 4).

(4) Increasing thickness increases the hindrance offered to the rays by all bodies. A picture has been impressed on a photographic plate of a number of superposed layers of tinfoil, like steps, presenting thus a regu-

* This article was reprinted from Nature, No. 1369, Vol. 53, January 23, 1896. By W. C. Röntgen. Translated by Arthur Stanton from the *Sitsungsberichte der Würsburger Physik-medic. Gesellschaft,* 1895.

larly increasing thickness. This is to be submitted to photometric processes when a suitable instrument is available.

(5) Pieces of platinum, lead, zinc, and aluminium foil were so arranged as to produce the same weakening of the effect. The annexed table shows the relative thickness and density of the equivalent sheets of metal.

	Thickness	Relative thickness	Density
Platinum	.018 mm.	1	21.5
Lead	.050 "	3	11.3
Zinc	.100 "	6	7.1
Aluminium	3.500 "	200	2.6

From these values it is clear that in no case can we obtain the transparency of a body from the product of its density and thickness. The transparency increases much more rapidly than the product decreases.

(6) The fluorescence of barium platinocyanide is not the only noticeable action of the x-rays. It is to be observed that other bodies exhibit fluorescence, e.g. calcium sulphide, uranium glass, Iceland spar, rock-salt, &c.

Of special interest in this connection is the fact that photographic dry plates are sensitive to the x-rays. It is thus possible to exhibit the phenomena so as to exclude the danger of error. I have thus confirmed many observations originally made by eye observation with the fluorescent screen. Here the power of the x-rays to pass through wood or cardboard becomes useful. The photographic plate can be exposed to the action without removal of the shutter of the dark slide or other protecting case, so that the experiment need not be conducted in darkness. Manifestly, unexposed plates must not be left in their box near the vacuum tube.

It seems now questionable whether the impression on the plate is a direct effect of the x-rays, or a secondary result induced by the fluorescence of the material of the plate. Films can receive the impression as well as ordinary dry plates.

I have not been able to show experimentally that the x-rays give rise to any calorific effects. These, however, may be assumed, for the phenomena of fluorescence show that the x-rays are capable of transformation. It is also certain that all the x-rays falling on a body do not leave it as such.

The retina of the eye is quite insensitive to these rays: the eye placed close to the apparatus sees nothing. It is clear from the experiments that this is not due to want of permeability on the part of the structures of the eye.

(7) After my experiments on the transparency of increasing thicknesses of different media, I proceeded to investigate whether the x-rays could be deflected by a prism. Investigations with water and carbon bisulphide on mica prisms of 30° showed no deviation either on the photographic or the fluorescent plate. For comparison, light rays were allowed to fall on the prism as the apparatus was set up for the experiment. They were deviated 10 mm. and 20 mm. respectively in the case of the two prisms.

With prisms of ebonite and aluminium, I have obtained images on the photographic plate, which point to a possible deviation. It is, however, uncertain, and at most would point to a refractive index 1.05. No deviation can be observed by means of the fluorescent screen. Investigations with the heavier metals have not as yet led to any result, because of their small transparency and the consequent enfeebling of the transmitted rays.

On account of the importance of the question it is desirable to try in other ways whether the x-rays are susceptible of refraction. Finely powdered bodies allow in thick layers but little of the incident light to pass through, in consequence of refraction and reflection. In the case of the x-rays, however, such layers of powder are for equal masses of substance equally transparent with the coherent solid itself. Hence we cannot conclude any regular reflection or refraction of the x-rays. The research was conducted by the aid of finely-powdered rock-salt, fine electrolytic silver powder, and zinc dust already many times employed in chemical work. In all these cases the result, whether by the fluorescent screen or the photographic method, indicated no difference in transparency between the powder and the coherent solid.

It is, hence, obvious that lenses cannot be looked upon as capable of concentrating the x-rays; in effect, both an ebonite and a glass lens of large size prove to be without action. The shadow photograph of a round rod is darker in the middle than at the edge; the image of a cylinder filled with a body more transparent than its walls exhibits the middle brighter than the edge.

(8) The preceding experiments, and others which I pass over, point to the rays being incapable of regular

reflection. It is, however, well to detail an observation which at first sight seemed to lead to an opposite conclusion.

I exposed a plate, protected by a black paper sheath, to the x-rays, so that the glass side lay next to the vacuum tube. The sensitive film was partly covered with star-shaped pieces of platinum, lead, zinc, and aluminium. On the developed negative the star-shaped impression showed dark under platinum, lead, and more markedly, under zinc; the aluminium gave no image. It seems, therefore, that these three metals can reflect the x-rays; as, however, another explanation is possible, I repeated the experiment with this only difference, that a film of thin aluminium foil was interposed between the sensitive film and the metal stars. Such an aluminium plate is opaque to ultra-violet rays, but transparent to x-rays. In the result the images appeared as before, this pointing still to the existence of reflection at metal surfaces.

If one considers this observation in connection with others, namely, on the transparency of powders, and on the state of the surface not being effective in altering the passage of the x-rays through a body, it leads to the probable conclusion that regular reflection does not exist, but that bodies behave to the x-rays as turbid media to light.

Since I have obtained no evidence of refraction at the surface of different media, it seems probable that the x-rays move with the same velocity in all bodies, and in a medium which penetrates everything, and in which the molecules of bodies are embedded. The molecules obstruct the x-rays, the more effectively as the density of the body concerned is greater.

(9) It seemed possible that the geometrical arrangement of the molecules might affect the action of a body upon the x-rays, so that, for example, Iceland spar might exhibit different phenomena according to the relation of the surface of the plate to the axis of the crystal. Experiments with quartz and Iceland spar on this point lead to a negative result.

(10) It is known that Lenard, in his investigations on kathode rays, has shown that they belong to the ether, and can pass through all bodies. Concerning the x-rays the same may be said.

In his latest work, Lenard has investigated the absorption coefficients of various bodies for the kathode rays, including air at atmospheric pressure, which gives 4.10, 3.40, 3.10 for 1 cm., according to the degree of exhaustion of the gas in discharge tube. To judge from the nature of the discharge, I have worked at about the same pressure, but occasionally at greater or smaller pressures. I find, using a Weber's photometer, that the intensity of the fluorescent light varies nearly as the inverse square of the distance between screen and discharge tube. This result is obtained from three very consistent sets of observations at distances of 100 and 200 mm. Hence air absorbs the x-rays much less than the kathode rays. This result is in complete agreement with the previously described result, that the fluorescence of the screen can be still observed at 2 metres from the vacuum tube. In general, other bodies behave like air; they are more transparent for the x-rays than for the kathode rays.

(11) A further distinction, and a noteworthy one, results from the action of a magnet. I have not succeeded in observing any deviation of the x-rays even in very strong magnetic fields.

The deviation of kathode rays by the magnet is one of their peculiar characteristics; it has been observed by Hertz and Lenard, that several kinds of kathode rays exist, which differ by their power of exciting phosphorescence, their susceptibility of absorption, and their deviation by the magnet; but a notable deviation has been observed in all cases which have yet been investigated, and I think that such deviation affords a characteristic not to be set aside lightly.

(12) As the result of many researches, it appears that the place of most brilliant phosphorescence of the walls of the discharge-tube is the chief seat whence the x-rays originate and spread in all directions; that is, the x-rays proceed from the front where the kathode rays strike the glass. If one deviates the kathode rays within the tube by means of a magnet, it is seen that the x-rays proceed from a new point, *i.e.* again from the end of the kathode rays.

Also for this reason the x-rays, which are not deflected by a magnet, cannot be regarded as kathode rays which have passed through the glass, for that passage cannot, according to Lenard, be the cause of the different deflection of the rays. Hence I conclude that the x-rays are not identical with the kathode rays, but are produced from the kathode rays at the glass surface of the tube.

(13) The rays are generated not only in glass. I have obtained them in an apparatus closed by an aluminium plate 2 mm. thick. I purpose later to investigate the behaviour of other substances.

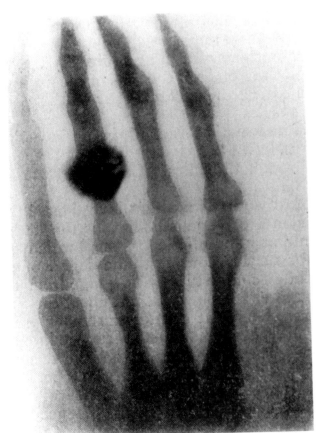

FIGURE A–1. Photograph of the bones in the fingers of a living human hand. The third finger has a ring upon it.

(14) The justification of the term "rays," applied to the phenomena, lies partly in the regular shadow pictures produced by the interposition of a more or less permeable body between the source and a photographic plate or fluorescent screen.

I have observed and photographed many such shadow pictures. Thus, I have an outline of part of a door covered with lead paint; the image was produced by placing the discharge-tube on one side of the door, and the sensitive plate on the other. I have also a shadow of the bones of the hand (Figure A–1), of a wire wound upon a bobbin, of a set of weights in a box, of a compass card and needle completely enclosed in a metal case (Figure A–2), of a piece of metal where the x-rays show the want of homogeneity, and of other things.

For the rectilinear propagation of the rays, I have a pin-hole photograph of the discharge apparatus covered with black paper. It is faint but unmistakable.

(15) I have sought for interference effects of the x-rays, but possibly, in consequence of their small intensity, without result.

(16) Researches to investigate whether electrostatic forces act on the x-rays are begun but not yet concluded.

(17) If one asks, what then are these x-rays; since they are not kathode rays, one might suppose, from their power of exciting fluorescence and chemical action, them to be due to ultra-violet light. In opposition to this view a weighty set of considerations presents itself. If x-rays be indeed ultra-violet light, then that light must possess the following properties.

(a) It is not refracted in passing from air into water, carbon bisulphide, aluminium, rock-salt, glass or zinc.

(b) It is incapable of regular reflection at the surfaces of the above bodies.

(c) It cannot be polarised by any ordinary polarising media.

(d) The absorption by various bodies must depend chiefly on their density.

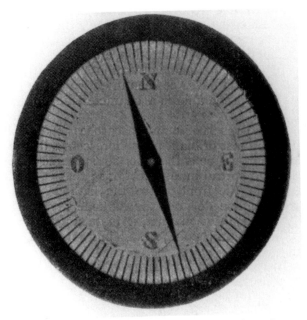

FIGURE A–2. Photograph of a compass card and needle completely enclosed in a metal case.

That is to say, these ultra-violet rays must behave quite differently from the visible, infrared, and hitherto known ultra-violet rays.

These things appear so unlikely that I have sought for another hypothesis.

A kind of relationship between the new rays and light rays appears to exist; at least the formation of shadows, fluorescence, and the production of chemical action point in this direction. Now it has been known for a long time, that besides the transverse vibrations which account for the phenomena of light, it is possible that longitudinal vibrations should exist in the ether, and, according to the view of some physicists, must exist. It is granted that their existence has not yet been made clear, and their properties are not experimentally demonstrated. Should not the new rays be ascribed to longitudinal waves in the ether?

I must confess that I have in the course of this research made myself more and more familiar with this thought, and venture to put the opinion forward, while I am quite conscious that the hypothesis advanced still requires a more solid foundation.

Agfa's Troubleshooting the Radiographic System: Symptoms and Possible Causes*

Low Density

A. Underexposure

1. Wrong Exposure Factors
   a. Too low kilovoltage
   b. Too low milliamperage
   c. Too short exposure
   d. Too great focal-film distance
2. Meters out of calibration
3. Timer out of calibration
4. Inaccurate setting of meters or timer
5. Drop in incoming line voltage
   a. Elevators, welders, furnaces, blowers, etc. on same circuit
   b. Insufficient size of power line or transformers
6. Photocell timer out of adjustment
7. Incorrect centering of patient to photocell
8. Central ray of X-ray tube not directed on film
   a. X-ray tube rotated in casing
9. Distance out of grid radius
10. Bucky timer inaccurate
11. One or more valve tubes burned out (Full wave rectifying machines)

B. Underdevelopment

1. Improper development
   a. Time too short
   b. Temperature too low (Hydroquinone inactive below 55° F, or 13° C)

*Reprinted with permission from Agfa Matrix Division of Agfa Corporation, 100 Challenger Road, Ridgefield Park, NJ 07660.

   c. Combination of both
   d. Inaccurate thermometer
2. Exhausted developer
   a. Chemical activity used up
   b. Activity destroyed by contamination
3. Diluted developer
   a. Water overflowed from wash tank
   b. Insufficient chemical mixed originally due to tank actually larger than rating
   c. Improper additions
4. Incorrectly mixed developer
   a. Exact capacity of tank unknown
   b. Mixing ingredients in wrong sequence
   c. Omission of ingredients
   d. Unbalanced formula composition

High Density

A. Overexposure

1. Wrong exposure factors
   a. Too high kilovoltage
   b. Too high milliamperage
   c. Too long exposure
   d. Too short focal-film distance
2. Meters out of calibration
3. Timer out of calibration
4. Inaccurate setting of meters or timer
5. Surge in incoming line voltage
6. Photocell timer out of adjustment
7. Incorrect centering of patient to photocell

B. Improper development

1. Time too long
2. Temperature too high
3. Combination of both
4. Inaccurate thermometer
5. Insufficient dilution of concentrated developer
6. Omission of bromide when mixing

C. Fog—see section on "FOG"

1. Light struck
2. Radiation
3. Chemical
4. Film deterioration

Low Contrast

A. Overpenetration from too high kilovoltage

1. Overmeasurement of part to be examined
2. Incorrect estimate of material or tissue density
3. Meters out of calibration
4. Meters inaccurately set
5. Surge in incoming line voltage
6. Undermeasurement of focal-film distance

B. Scattered radiation

1. Failure to use Bucky diaphragm
2. Failure to use stationary grid
3. Failure to use cutout diaphragm
4. Failure to use suitable cones
5. Failure to use lead backing cassette

C. Too short exposure

1. Timer out of calibration
2. Timer inaccurately set
3. Overload relay kicked out

D. Improper development

High Contrast

A. Underpenetration from too low kilovoltage

1. Undermeasurement of part to be examined
2. In parts of varying thickness, setting of kilovoltage for thinner sections
3. Meters out of calibration
4. Meters inaccurately set
5. Drop in incoming line voltage
   a. Elevators, welders, furnaces, etc. on same line
   b. Insufficient size of power line or transformer
6. Overmeasurement of focal-film distance

B. Too long exposure

1. Timer out of calibration
2. Timer inaccurately set

C. Improper development

Fog

A. Unsafe light

1. Light leaks into processing room
   a. Leaks through doors, windows, etc.
   b. Poorly designed labyrinth entrance
      1. Bright light at outer entrance
      2. Reflection from white uniforms of persons passing through
   c. Sparking of motors
      1. Ventilating fans
      2. Dryer fans
      3. Mixers-barium
      4. Light leaks in film carrying box
2. Safelights
   a. Bulb too bright
   b. Improper filter
      1. Not dense enough
      2. Cracked
      3. Bleached
      4. Shrunken

3. Luminous clock and watch faces
4. Lighting matches in darkroom
5. Where film is carried from machine to darkroom in containers, container may leak light

B. Radiation

1. Insufficient protection
   a. During delivery or transportation in laboratory or shop
   b. Film storage bin
   c. Loaded cassette racks—steel back should face toward source of radiation
   d. Not enough protection for loading darkroom
2. Improper storage
   a. Radium
   b. Isotopes
   c. X-ray machines

C. Chemical

1. Prolonged development (See item B under "HIGH DENSITY")
2. Developer contaminated
   a. Foreign matter of any kind (Metals, etc.)
3. Contaminated chemicals

D. Deterioration of film

1. Age (Use oldest film first)
2. Storage conditions
   a. Too high temperatures
      1. Hot room
      2. Cool room but near radiator or hot pipe
   b. Too high humidity
      1. Damp room
      2. Moist air
      3. Ammonia or other fumes present in darkroom or other work area
3. Delivery conditions
   a. Moisture precipitation when cold box of film is opened in hot, humid room
   b. Fresh boxes should be stored overnight at room temperature before opening

E. Excessive pressure on emulsions of unprocessed film

1. During storage
2. During manipulation in darkroom

F. Loaded cassettes stored near heat, sunlight or radiation

Stains on Radiographs

A. Yellow

1. Exhausted, oxidized developer
   a. Old
   b. Covers left off
   c. Scum on developer surface
      1. Oil from pipelines
      2. Impure water used when mixing
      3. Dust
2. Prolonged development
3. Insufficient rinsing
4. Exhausted fixing bath

B. Dichroic

1. Old, exhausted developer
   a. Colloidal metallic silver
2. Nearly exhausted fixer
3. Developer containing small amounts of fixer or scum
4. Films partially fixed in weak fixer, exposed to light and refixed
5. Prolonged intermediate rinse in contaminated rinse water

Green tinted

1. Insufficient fixing or washing

Deposits on Radiographs

A. Metallic

1. Oxidized products from developer
2. Silver salts reacting with hydrogen sulfide in air to form silver sulfide
3. Silver loaded fixer

B. White or crystalline

1. Milky fixer
   a. Hardener portion added too fast while mixing
   b. Hardener portion added when too hot
   c. Excessive acidity
   d. Developer splashed into fixer
   e. Insufficient rinsing
2. Prolonged washing

C. Grit

1. Dirty water
2. Dirt in dryer

Marks on Emulsion Surfaces

A. Runs

1. Insufficient fixing
   a. Weakened fixer
   b. Unbalanced formula
   c. Exhausted ingredients
   d. Low acid content
      1. Deficient when fresh
      2. Diluted from rinse water
      3. Neutralized by developer because of insufficient or no rinsing
2. Drying temperature too high
3. Contact with hot viewing box

B. Blisters

1. Formation of gas bubbles in gelatin
   a. Carbonate of developer reacting with acid of fixer
   b. Unbalanced processing temperatures
      1. Combination of hot fixer and cool developer
      2. Combination of cool fixer and hot developer
   c. Excessive acidity of fixer
   d. No agitation of film when first placed in fixer

C. Reticulation

1. Non-uniform processing temperatures
   a. Developer (Hot)
   b. Fixer (Cool)
   c. Wash
2. Weakened fixer with little hardening action

D. Frilling

1. Weakened fixer with little hardening action
2. Hot processing solutions
   a. Developer
   b. Fixer
   c. Wash

E. Drying marks from uneven drying of gelatin

1. Excessive drying temperatures
2. Extremely low humidity
3. Puddies (Buckshot marks)
   a. Drops of water striking semi-dried emulsion surface
4. Streaks
   a. Drops of water running down semi-dried emulsion surface
      1. Water splashes
      2. Drying air flow too rapid
      3. Insufficient or uneven squeeze last roller pair waterrack

F. White spots

1. Screens pitted
2. Grit or dust present on film or screens
3. Chemical dust settling on film or screens (Particles of certain chemical dusts will also cause black spots)

G. Artifacts

1. Crescents — rough handling
2. Smudge marks — fingerprints or finger abrasions
3. Bands in marginal areas usually due to screen mounting medium

Slow Drying

A. Waterlogged films

1. Insufficient hardening in fixer
   a. Too short fixing period
   b. Weakened fixer from splashing
   c. Exhausted fixer
   d. Insufficient acidity (carry over dev. fixer)
2. Wash water too warm

B. Incoming air too humid

C. Incoming air too cold

D. Air velocity too low

Streaks on Radiographs

A. Insufficient agitation while processing

B. Fog

C. Chemically active deposits (Dried chemicals)

D. Pressure fog

E. Scratches

1. Careless handling
2. Grit present in air, cassettes, or on illuminator

F. Exposure to white light before complete fixing

G. Uneven drying due to high temperature and low humidity

Lack of Detail or Fuzziness

A. Motion (Tube, film, subject)

1. Inadequate immobilization
2. Too long exposure
3. Vibration of floor
4. Slipping of subject on mount
5. Stepping on and off operator's platform during exposure where control and tube are mounted on common mobile base
6. Failure to arrest tube vibration after positioning before making exposure

B. Poor contact of intensifying screens

C. Improper distance relationship

1. Object film distance too great
2. Target film distance too short

D. Improper focal spot

1. Too large
2. Damaged (Cracked or pitted)

Static

A. Low humidity

B. Insulation

1. Use of rubber gloves, shoes, finger cots, etc.
2. Insulated flooring

C. Improper handling in:

1. Removal from box
2. Removal from interleaving paper
3. Loading cassette
4. Unloading cassette
5. Loading hanger
6. Films stacked before processing

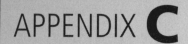

Du Pont Bit System

WHAT THE BIT SYSTEM DOES

The Bit System helps to change techniques, create new exposure and processing conditions, estimate patient skin exposure, and understand the factors affecting radiographic quality. It supplements practical experience by helping you make changes quickly and accurately.

HOW IT WORKS

Bit values are relative exposure units common to all radiographic variables and assigned according to the effect of the variable on film density. They serve the same trading purpose as money. Values are arranged in tables so that reading up the column increases film exposure and density and vice versa. A + 1.0 Bit increase doubles exposure and a –1.0 Bit decrease halves exposure (see Table "T").

The Bit System has these versatile features. You can:

- make changes with the speed and mathematical accuracy of simple addition and subtraction.
- use either centimeter or inch distances; Fahrenheit or Centigrade temperatures.
- be compatible with existing technique change methods. Table T lists equivalent % and mAs factor changes.
- incorporate new radiographic variables as their control becomes desirable.
- put the Bit System into a computer as we have done in the Micro Quality Manager® computerized quality control system.

Bit tables are accurate under average conditions of use. However, normal generator variations in beam quality, milliampere seconds and other variables introduce errors into the Bit System as well as all other technique conversion systems. Usually an exposure or processing variation of .2 Bits (15%) is not recognized in a radiograph because of the latitude of the system. A .4 Bit (32%) variation is obvious and may require a repeat exposure.

OPTIMIZING TECHNIQUES

Technique charts frequently need to be changed due to individual preference, new equipment, film, screens, processing conditions, etc. Some of the typical changes that can be made with the Bit System and their benefits follow:

- Convert to Rare Earth film-screen systems to optimize image quality/skin exposure.
- Raise kVp and shorten time to stop motion.
- Change from no grid to grid and raise kVp to increase exposure latitude.
- Use faster screens and shorter time to reduce skin exposure.
- Increase illuminator brightness and mAs to increase radiographic contrast.
- Increase distance and kVp to reduce penumbra unsharpness.
- Increase screen speed and reduce focal spot size to reduce penumbra unsharpness.
- Lower developer temperature and increase mAs to reduce quantum mottle.

WAYS TO USE THE BIT SYSTEM

1. Change Techniques by Measuring on the Tables

All radiographic variables are spaced on this card so that a distance change on one table will have the same effect on exposure as the same distance on another table.

Example: **Increase kVp from 64 to 85 and Decrease Time from 2/5 sec. to Reduce Contrast**

1. Place edge of a piece of paper beside kVp Table H.
2. Mark the paper edge at 64 and 85 kVp in this case.
3. To indicate a kVp increase, place an up arrow between the marks on the paper.
4. Move paper edge to "time" Table K and place the mark beside the original 2/5 sec. and extending in the down direction.
5. Read new exposure time (1/10 sec.) at the other mark.

2. Change The Techniques with Slide Rule Supplement

The Slide Rule Supplement contains time, mAs and kVp tables in inverted form. When one of these scales is placed beside one on the fold out card with known **original** factors side-by-side, other combinations providing the same radiographic density can be read direct. Use as in the following example:

Example: **Change from Original Technique of 64 kVp and 2/5 sec. to 85 kVp and New Time to Reduce Contrast.**

1. Place kVp scale of supplement beside time scale (Table K) of this folder.
2. Move scales vertically until original technique, 64 kVp and 2/5 sec., are beside each other.
3. Read new time, 1/10 sec., beside new kVp—85 kVp.
4. Read any other combinations desired.

3. Change Techniques by Totaling Bits

As with phototiming, it should not make any difference to the film what combination of technical factors within reason are selected to make an exposure as long as a certain total number of exposure units (Bits) are provided.

Assuming you want the same film density as the original, total the Bits of the **original** factors to be changed and subtract the Bit Value of the **new** factor to be used. The remainder will be the Bit Value of the other new factor.

Example: **kVp Increase and Time Decrease to Reduce Contrast**

Original kVp	:	64	=	6.4 Bits
Original sec	:	2.5	=	+11.0
Original Total	:			17.4
New kVp	:	85	=	±8.4
Unknown sec	:			9.0 Bits or 1/10 sec.

4. Create New Techniques Using Bit Totals Provided

This extension of the totaling method discussed on the opposite page is used when techniques are non-existent. A technique is selected to exactly meet the Guide Bit Total provided. Two applications of this principle follow:

- Correct exposure exists when kVp Bits +mAs Bits + Film-Screen Bits + Grid Bits + F-F Distance Bits + Anatomical Thickness Bits = Guide Bit Total.

    Guide Total may be obtained by totaling Bits on all important variables used to expose excellent radiographs. These Totals are then used when new techniques are needed.

BIT SYSTEM SLIDE RULE TABLES

% Increase (+)
% Decrease (−)

+3100%	
+2720%	
+2360%	
+2040%	
+1760%	
+1500%	
+1310%	
+1130%	
+ 970%	
+ 812%	
+ 700%	
+ 592%	
+ 503%	
+ 425%	
+ 357%	
+ 300%	
+ 247%	
+ 200%	
+ 163%	
+ 130%	
+ 100%	
+ 74%	
+ 51%	
+ 32%	
+ 15%	
0	
− 13%	
− 24%	
− 34%	
− 42%	
− 50%	
− 56%	
− 62%	
− 67%	
− 71%	
− 75%	
− 78%	
− 81%	
− 83%	
− 86%	
− 87%	
− 89%	
− 91%	
− 92%	
− 93%	
− 94%	
− 95%	
− 95.5%	
− 96%	
− 96.5%	
− 97%	

To Use
1. Select one factor above and another factor to be changed from the folding bit card
2. Lay **original** techniques side by side.
3. Read any new techniques.

kVp	mAs
25−	.63 −
26−	.72 −
27−	.83 −
28−	.94 −
29−	1.08 −
30−	1.25 −
31−	1.45 −
33−	1.66 −
34−	1.80 −
35−	2.16 −
37−	2.50 −
38−	2.90 −
39−	3.33 −
41−	3.75 −
42−	4.4 −
43−	5.0 −
44−	5.7 −
45−	6.6 −
46−	7.5 −
47−	8.7 −
49−	10 −
50−	11.2 −
51−	13 −
53−	15 −
54−	17.5 −
55−	20 −
56−	23 −
58−	26 −
60−	30 −
62−	35 −
64−	40 −
66−	45 −
68−	52 −
70−	60 −
72−	70 −
74−	80 −
76−	92 −
78−	105 −
80−	120 −
82−	140 −
85−	160 −
88−	182 −
91−	210 −
94−	240 −
98−	280 −
102−	320 −
106−	365 −
110−	420 −
115−	485 −
120−	550 −
125−	640 −
130−	−
135−	−
141−	−
147−	−
153−	−

Seconds

−1/1000	=	.0010
−1/860	=	.0012
−1/780	=	.0013
−1/666	=	.0015
−1/560	=	.0017
−1/500	=	.0020
−1/430	=	.0023
−1/360	=	.0026
−1/333	=	.0030
−1/280	=	.0035
−1/250	=	.0040
−1/215	=	.0046
−1/180	=	.0053
−1/160	=	.0063
−1/140	=	.0072
−1/120	=	.0083
−1/105	=	.0095
−1/90	=	.0110
−1/80	=	.0125
−1/72	=	.0143
−1/60	=	.0166
−1/50	=	.019
		.022
−1/40	=	.025
		.029
−1/30	=	.033
−1/24	=	.038
		.044
−1/20	=	.050
		.057
−1/15	=	.066
−1/12	=	.075
		.087
−1/10	=	.100
		.115
−2/15	=	.132
−3/20	=	.151
		.175
−1/5	=	.200
−1/4	=	.230
		.265
		.300
−3/10	=	.350
−2/5	=	.400
		.455
−1/2	=	.525
−3/5	=	.600
		.700
−3/4	=	.800
		.920
−1	=	1.05
−1·1/5	=	1.20
		1.40
−1·1/2	=	1.60
		1.83
−2	=	2.10
−2·1/2	=	2.50
		2.80
−3	=	3.20
		3.70
−4	=	4.20
−5	=	5.00
−6	=	5.50
		6.32

TABLE E
Generator Output*
80 kVp & 20 inches Distance

	mr/mAs	=	Bits
	60	=	4.4
	52	=	4.2
	45	=	4.0
	40	=	3.8
	35	=	3.6
Av. 3 phase	30	=	3.4
	26	=	3.2
	23	=	3.0
	20	=	2.8
	17.5	=	2.6
Av. 1 phase	15	=	2.4
	13	=	2.2
	11.2	=	2.0
	10	=	1.8

*mr measured in air at 80 kVp
20" distance and normal filtration

TABLE F
FOCAL-FILM DISTANCE

Inches	=	Bits	=	Centimeters
6.7	=	12.0	=	17
7.3	=	11.8	=	18.5
7.7	=	11.6	=	19.5
8.3	=	11.4	=	21
9.0	=	11.2	=	22.5
9.5	=	11.0	=	24
10.0	=	10.8	=	25.5
10.6	=	10.6	=	27
11.4	=	10.4	=	29
12.2	=	10.2	=	31
13	=	10.0	=	33
14	=	9.8	=	35
15	=	9.6	=	38
16	=	9.4	=	40
17	=	9.2	=	43
18	=	9.0	=	46
19	=	8.8	=	48
21	=	8.6	=	53
22	=	8.4	=	56
24	=	8.2	=	61
25	=	8.0	=	64
27	=	7.8	=	69
29	=	7.6	=	74
31	=	7.4	=	79
33	=	7.2	=	84
36	=	7.0	=	91
39	=	6.8	=	99
41	=	6.6	=	104
44	=	6.4	=	112
48	=	6.2	=	122
51	=	6.0	=	130
55	=	5.8	=	140
58	=	5.6	=	147
63	=	5.4	=	160
67	=	5.2	=	170
72	=	5.0	=	183
77	=	4.8	=	196
83	=	4.6	=	211
88	=	4.4	=	224
95	=	4.2	=	241
102	=	4.0	=	259
109	=	3.8	=	277
116	=	3.6	=	295
125	=	3.4	=	318
136	=	3.2	=	345
144	=	3.0	=	366
154	=	2.8	=	391
165	=	2.6	=	419
176	=	2.4	=	447
180	=	2.2	=	457
203	=	2.0	=	516
218	=	1.8	=	554

TABLE G
ANATOMICAL THICKNESS

Centimeters	=	Bits
1	=	10.8
2	=	10.6
3	=	10.4
4	=	10.2
5	=	10.0
6	=	9.8
7	=	9.6
8	=	9.4
9	=	9.2
10	=	9.0
11	=	8.8
12	=	8.6
13	=	8.4
14	=	8.2
15	=	8.0
16	=	7.8
17	=	7.6
18	=	7.4
19	=	7.2
20	=	7.0
21	=	6.8
22	=	6.6
23	=	6.4
24	=	6.2
25	=	6.0
26	=	5.8
27	=	5.6
28	=	5.4
29	=	5.2
30	=	5.0
31	=	4.8
32	=	4.6
33	=	4.4
34	=	4.2
35	=	4.0
36	=	3.8
37	=	3.6
38	=	3.4
39	=	3.2
40	=	3.0
41	=	2.8
42	=	2.6
43	=	2.4
44	=	2.2

TABLE H

kVp	=	Bits
153	=	11.4
147	=	11.2
141	=	11.0
135	=	10.8
130	=	10.6
125	=	10.4
120	=	10.2
115	=	10.0
110	=	9.8
106	=	9.6
102	=	9.4
98	=	9.2
94	=	9.0
91	=	8.8
88	=	8.6
85	=	8.4
82	=	8.2
80	=	8.0
78	=	7.8
76	=	7.6
74	=	7.4
72	=	7.2
70	=	7.0
68	=	6.8
66	=	6.6
64	=	6.4
62	=	6.2
60	=	6.0
58	=	5.8
56	=	5.6
55	=	5.4
54	=	5.2
53	=	5.0
51	=	4.8
50	=	4.6
49	=	4.4
47	=	4.2
46	=	4.0
45	=	3.8
44	=	3.6
43	=	3.4
42	=	3.2
41	=	3.0
39	=	2.8
38	=	2.6
37	=	2.4
35	=	2.2
34	=	2.0
33	=	1.8
31	=	1.6
30	=	1.4
29	=	1.2
28	=	1.0
27	=	.8
26	=	.6
25	=	.4

TABLE I

mAs	=	Bits
640	=	22.0
550	=	21.8
485	=	21.6
420	=	21.4
365	=	21.2
320	=	21.0
280	=	20.8
240	=	20.6
210	=	20.4
182	=	20.2
160	=	20.0
140	=	19.8
120	=	19.6
105	=	19.4
92	=	19.2
80	=	19.0
70	=	18.8
60	=	18.6
52	=	18.4
45	=	18.2
40	=	18.0
35	=	17.8
30	=	17.6
26	=	17.4
23	=	17.2
20	=	17.0
17.5	=	16.8
15	=	16.6
13	=	16.4
11.2	=	16.2
10	=	16.0
8.7	=	15.8
7.5	=	15.6
5.7	=	15.2
5.0	=	15.0
4.4	=	14.8
3.75	=	14.6
3.33	=	14.4
2.90	=	14.2
2.50	=	14.0
2.16	=	13.8
1.80	=	13.6
1.66	=	13.4
1.45	=	13.2
1.25	=	13.0
1.08	=	12.8
.94	=	12.6
.83	=	12.4
.72	=	12.2
.63	=	12.0

TABLE J

mA	=	Bits
2100	=	11.4
1840	=	11.2
1600	=	11.0
1400	=	10.8
1200	=	10.6
1060	=	10.4
900	=	10.2
800	=	10.0
700	=	9.8
600	=	9.6
530	=	9.4
450	=	9.2
400	=	9.0
350	=	8.8
300	=	8.6
260	=	8.4
225	=	8.2
200	=	8.0
175	=	7.8
150	=	7.6
130	=	7.4
112	=	7.2
100	=	7.0
87	=	6.8
75	=	6.6
65	=	6.4
56	=	6.2
50	=	6.0
43	=	5.8
38	=	5.6
33	=	5.4
28	=	5.2
25	=	5.0
22	=	4.8
19	=	4.6
16	=	4.4
14	=	4.2
12	=	4.0
11	=	3.8
9.5	=	3.6
8.3	=	3.4
7.2	=	3.2
6.3	=	3.0
5.4	=	2.8
4.7	=	2.6
4.1	=	2.4
3.6	=	2.2
3.2	=	2.0
2.7	=	1.8
2.35	=	1.6
2.05	=	1.4
1.80	=	1.2
1.55	=	1.0
1.35	=	.8
1.17	=	.6
1.02	=	.4

TABLE K

Fraction Seconds	Bits	Decimal Seconds
6	15.0	6.32
	14.8	5.50
5	14.6	5.00
	14.4	4.20
4	14.2	3.70
	14.0	3.20
3	13.8	2.80
2-1/2	13.6	2.50
	13.4	2.10
2	13.2	1.83
	13.0	1.60
1-1/2	12.8	1.40
1-1/5	12.6	1.20
	12.4	1.05
1	12.2	.920
	12.0	.800
3/4	11.8	.700
3/5	11.6	.600
	11.4	.525
1/2	11.2	.455
2/5	11.0	.400
	10.8	.350
3/10	10.6	.300
	10.4	.265
1/4	10.2	.230
1/5	10.0	.200
	9.8	.175
3/20	9.6	.151
2/15	9.4	.132
	9.2	.115
1/10	9.0	.100
	8.8	.087
1/12	8.6	.075
	8.4	.066
1/15	8.2	.057
1/20	8.0	.050
	7.8	.044
1/24	7.6	.038
1/30	7.4	.033
	7.2	.029
1/40	7.0	.025
	6.8	.022
1/50	6.6	.019
1/60	6.4	.0166
1/72	6.2	.0143
1/80	6.0	.0125
1/90	5.8	.0110
1/105	5.6	.0095
1/120	5.4	.0083
1/140	5.2	.0072
1/160	5.0	.0063
1/180	4.8	.0053
1/215	4.6	.0046
1/250	4.4	.0040
1/280	4.2	.0035
1/333	4.0	.0030
1/360	3.8	.0026
1/430	3.6	.0023
1/500	3.4	.0020
1/560	3.2	.0017
1/666	3.0	.0015
1/780	2.8	.0013
1/860	2.6	.0012
1/1000	2.4	.0010

TABLE L
TECHNIQUE CHANGES REQUIRED FOR PATHOLOGY

RESPIRATION SYSTEMS

Increase kVp	Bits
Atelectasis	+.4
Bronchiectasis	+.4
Carcinoma (advanced)	+.4
Edema	+.4
Empyema	+.6
Hydropneumothorax	+.6
Pleural Effusion	+.6
Pneumoconiosis	+.5
Pneumonia	+.5
Thoracoplasty	+.6
Tuberculosis (calcific-miliary)	+.4

Decrease kVp	Bits
Emaciation	−.5
Emphysema	−.6

OTHER SYSTEMS

Increase kVp	Bits
Acromegaly	+.4
Ascites	+.6
Arthritis (Rheumatoid)	+.4
Cirrhosis of Liver	+.4
Charcot Joint	+.4
Edema	+.4
Hydrocephalus (without air)	+.4
Metastasis (Secondary to prostatic carcinoma)	+.4
Osteochondroma	+.4
Osteoma	+.4
Osteomyelitis (healed)	+.4
Osteopetrosis	+.4
Paget's Disease	+.4

Decrease kVp	Bits
Arthritis (degenerative)	−.5

Atrophy	−.5
Bowel Obstruction	−.5
Cystic Diseases	−.5
Emaciation	−.5
Gout	−.5
Hydrocephalus (with air study)	−.5
Hyperparathyroidism	−.5
Leprosy	−.5
Multiple Myeloma	−.5
Necrosis	−.5
Osteomyelitis (active)	−.5
Pneumoperitoneum	−.5
Sarcoma	−.5
Syphilis (advanced)	−.5

(mAs may be changed instead of kVp.)

TABLE N

Collimation	mAs Bits
8" × 10" or larger	0
5" × 7"	+.3
Cylinder Collapsed	+.5
Cylinder Extended	+.7

TABLE S
GRID TRANSMISSION (80 kVp)

Ratio	% Trans	Bits
None	100	10.0
	87	9.8
6 in. Air Gap	76	9.6
	66	9.4
	58	9.2
4:1 60L	50	9.0
	44	8.8
	38	8.6
5:1 80L, 6:1 103L	33	8.4
8:1 103L	29	8.2
8:1 80L, 10:1 103L	25	8.0
10:1 80L	22	7.8
12:1 103L	20	7.6
5:1 Cross Hatched	17	7.4
16:1 80L	14	7.2
8:1 Cross Hatched	13	7.0

PERCENTAGE

TABLE T

Bit Change	% Increase (+) % Decrease (−)	Dosage or mAs Factor*	Relative mAs or Arithmetic Speed
+5.0	+3100%	32.00×	3200
+4.8	+2720%	28.20×	2820
+4.6	+2360%	24.60×	2460
+4.4	+2040%	21.40×	2140
+4.2	+1760%	18.60×	1860
+4.0	+1500%	16.00×	1600
+3.8	+1310%	14.10×	1410
+3.6	+1130%	12.30×	1230
+3.4	+ 970%	10.70×	1070
+3.2	+ 812%	9.12×	912
+3.0	+ 700%	8.00×	800
+2.8	+ 592%	6.92×	692
+2.6	+ 503%	6.03×	603
+2.4	+ 425%	5.25×	525
+2.2	+ 357%	4.57×	457
+2.0	+ 300%	4.00×	400
+1.8	+ 247%	3.47×	347
+1.6	+ 200%	3.00×	300
+1.4	+ 163%	2.63×	263
+1.2	+ 130%	2.30×	230
+1.0	+ 100%	2.00×	200
+ .8	+ 74%	1.74×	174
+ .6	+ 51%	1.51×	151
+ .4	+ 32%	1.32×	132
+ .2	+ 15%	1.15×	115
0	0	1.00×	100
− .2	− 13%	.87×	87
− .4	− 24%	.76×	76
− .6	− 34%	.66×	66
− .8	− 42%	.58×	58
−1.0	− 50%	.50×	50
−1.2	− 56%	.44×	44
−1.4	− 62%	.38×	38
−1.6	− 67%	.33×	33
−1.8	− 71%	.29×	29
−2.0	− 75%	.25×	25
−2.2	− 78%	.22×	22
−2.4	− 81%	.19×	19
−2.6	− 83%	.17×	17
−2.8	− 86%	.14×	14
−3.0	− 87%	.13×	13
−3.2	− 89%	.11×	11
−3.4	− 91%	.09×	9
−3.6	− 92%	.08×	8
−3.8	− 93%	.07×	7
−4.0	− 94%	.06×	6
−4.2	− 95%	.05×	5
−4.4	− 95.5	.045	4.5
−4.6	− 96%	.04×	4
−4.8	− 96.5	.035	3.5
−5.0	− 97%	.03×	3

* New mAs = Old mAs × mAs Factor
Reprinted with permission from:

E. I. DU PONT DE NEMOURS & CO. (INC.)
MEDICAL PRODUCTS DEPARTMENT
CUSTOMER TECHNOLOGY CENTER
WILMINGTON, DELAWARE 19898
PHONE 1-800-527-2601

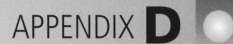

Basic Exposure Table: Siemens Point System

Siemens Exposure Points and Parameter Steps

Exposure Points	Exposure Factor	mAs Steps	kV Steps
−10	0.10000	0.100	—
−9	0.1259	0.125	—
−8	0.1585	0.16	—
−7	0.1995	0.20	—
−6	0.2512	0.25	—
−5	0.3162	0.32	—
−4	0.3981	0.40	—
−3	0.5012	0.50	—
−2	0.6310	0.64	—
−1	0.7943	0.80	—
0	1.0000	1.00	40
1	1.259	1.25	41
2	1.585	1.6	42
3	1.995	2.0	44
4	2.512	2.5	46
5	3.162	3.2	48
6	3.981	4.0	50
7	5.012	5.0	52
8	6.310	6.3	55
9	7.943	8.0	57
10	10.000	10.0	60
11	12.59	12.5	63
12	15.85	16	66
13	19.95	20	70
14	25.12	25	73
15	31.62	32	77
16	39.81	40	81
17	50.12	50	85
18	63.10	63	90

Siemens Exposure Points and Parameter Steps   (continued)

Exposure Points	Exposure Factor	mAs Steps	kV Steps
19	79.43	80	96
20	100.00	100	102
21	125.9	125	109
22	158.5	160	117
23	199.5	200	125
24	251.2	250	133
25	316.2	320	141
26	398.1	400	150
27	501.2	500	—
28	631.0	630	—
29	794.3	800	—
30	1,000.0	1000	—

Guideline values for free setting

The exposure guideline values given apply for optimum development conditions and when a 12 pulse generator or a DC voltage generator is used. If there is a deviation from the given exposure parameters, the required change of the exposure parameters must be made according to the correction and conversion table.

*   *For units with undertable tube: 70 cm*
For units with overtable tube: 115 cm

**   *Cassette on tabletop*

Object		Thickness (cm)	SID (cm)	Screen (Typ)	Grid (Pb 12/40)	Points	kV	mAs
Skull								
Skull survey	p.a./a.p.	19				30	70	50
Face bones	lat.	16	115	Special/TU	with	26	66	25
Skull	lat.	16				27	66	32
Skull	axial	22				35	85	63
Petrous bone	sag.	17	115	Special/TU	with	33	73	80
Petrous bone, Stenvers	view	17				32	70	80
Nasal								
Sinuses	p.a.	22	115	Special/TU	with	32	70	80
Orifice of optic nerve after Rhese		17	115	Special/TU	with	29	66	50
Mandible	lat.	11	105**	Titan D	without	20	57	12,5
Chest								
Ribs 1–7	p.a./a.p.	20				28	66	40
Ribs 8–12	p.a./a.p.	22	115	Titan D	with	34	70	125
Sternum	p.a.	21				31	63	100

Object		Thickness	SID	Screen	Grid	Points	kV	mAs
Sternum	lat.	30				32	66	100
Clavicle	p.a./a.p.	14	115	Titan D	with	25	60	32
Scapula	a.p.	17				28	63	50
Scapula	a.p.	14	115	Titan D		31	63	100
Lung	p.a./a.p.	21	185	Ruby	with	33	125	8
Lung	p.a./a.p.	21	185	Ruby		33	150	4
Lung (in bed)	p.a./a.p.	21	115		without	18	60	6,3
Lung, heart	lat.	30	150	Titan D	with	29	125	4
Lung, heart	lat.	30	185		with	32	150	3,5
Lung, heart	lat.	30	115	Titan D	without	21	77	4
Oesophagus	obl.	28	70/115*	Titan HS	with	24/28	90	4/10
Abdomen								
Kidney, gallbladder	lat.	27				35	81	80
Kidney, gallbladder	a.p.	19	115	Special/TU	with	29	66	50
Urinary bladder	a.p.	19				29	66	50
Urinary bladder	axial	21	115	Special/TU		33	70	100
Gravid uterus	lat.	28	115	Titan HS	with	36	125	20
Content study of stomach	p.a.	22	70/115*	Special/TU		28/32	102	6,3/16
Bulbus	p.a.							
Gastrointestinal tract, survey sup.		22	70/115*	Special/TU	with	28/32	102	6,3/16
Stomach, relief	p.a.							
Spinal column								
Cervical vertebrae, 1–3	oral	13						
Cervical vertebrae, 4–7	a.p.	13	150	Titan D	with	33	70	100
Cervical vertebrae, 1–7	lat.	12						
Cervical vertebrae, 1–7	obl.	13	150	Titan D		33	70	100
Thoracic vertebrae	a.p.	21	115	∓Graduated	with	35	73	125
Thoracic vertebrae	lat.	30	115	±Graduated		35	81	80
Lumbar vertebrae, 1–4	a.p.	19		Special/TU		31	77	40
Lumbar vertebrae, 1–4	lat.	27	115	∓Graduated	with	39	90	125
Lumbar vertebrae, 1–4	obl.	22		Special/TU		33	81	50
Lumbar vertebrae, 5	a.p.	22	115	Titan/TU	with	38	77	63
Lumbar vertebrae, 5	lat.	33				38	90	100
Pelvis								
Pelvis, hip	a.p.	20				30	73	40
Sacrum, coccyx	a.p.	19	115	Special/TU	with	31	73	50
Sacrum, coccyx	lat.	33				37	90	80
Upper extremities								
Shoulder joint	a.p.	11	115		with	26	63	32
Shoulder joint	axial	11	105**	Titan D	without	20	60	10
Upper arm	a.p./lat.	8	105**		without	16	55	6,3
Elbow	a.p.	6				14		4
Elbow	lat.	8	105**	Titan D	without	15	55	5
Forearm	a.p.	6				14		4
Forearm	lat.	7				15	55	5
Wrist	p.a.	4	105**	Titan D	without	9	46	3,2
Wrist	lat.	6				12	52	3,2

Object		Thickness	SID	Screen	Grid	Points	kV	mAs
Hand	p.a.	3				7	42	3,2
Hand	lat./obl.	6	105**	Titan D	without	10	48	3,2
Finger		2				4	40	2,5
Lower extremities								
Neck of femur	axial	22	105*		without	29	70	40
Femur	sup.	13	115	Titan D	with	30	70	50
Femur	inf.	12	115		with	27	60	50
Knee joint	a.p.	12	115		with	24	60	25
Knee joint	lat.	10	115	Titan D	with	23	60	20
Knee joint fissure		12	105**		without	17	57	6,3
Patella	axial	7				16		6,3
Tibia	a.p.	11	105**	Titan D	without	16	55	6,3
Tibia	lat.	9				15		5
Ankle	a.p.	9				17	55	8
Ankle	lat.	7	105**	Titan D	without	15	50	8
Oscalsis	lat.	7				14	50	6,3
Oscalsis	axial	10				18	55	10
Metatarsus	d.pl./p.a.	5	105**	Titan D	without	13	50	5
Metatarsus	obl.	6				12	50	4
Foot	lat.	7	105**	Titan D	without	13	50	5
Toes		3				8	44	3,2

Correction Values

In exposure points† for deviations from the starting conditions

SID	cm	65	75	85	95	105	115	130	145	160	185	210	235	260	290	325	360	400
	Points	−5	−4	−3	−2	−1	0	+1	+2	+3	+4	+5	+6	+7	+8	+9	+10	+11

Screen‡	Type	Titan HS/2 HS		Titan U/2 U/Tit.-Grad./Special		Titan D/2 D		Sapphire/Sapph.-Grad.		Ruby		Ruby Super
	Points (50−90 kV) (90−150 kV)	−7 −8		−3 −4		0 −1		0 0		+3 +3		+6 +6

Generator	Type	DC voltage	12-pulse	Multipulse	Six-pulse	Two-pulse
	Points in kV	0	0	0...+1	+1	+3

Grid	Type	without	Pb 8/40	Pb 10/40	Pb 12/40
	Points	−6	−2	−1	0

Object	State	Thin	Thick	Close collimation	Plaster half-shell	Plaster, dry	Plaster, wet
	Points	−3...−1	+1...+3...	+2	...+3	...+5	...+7

Tomography	Pattern	—	◯	◯	◎ 16°	◎
	Points	+2	+3	+3	+3	+4

† An exposure point difference of three causes doubling or halving of the dose. An exposure point difference of one causes a blackening change of $\Delta_s \approx 0.25$ on the X-ray film.
‡ Guideline Values for the dose requirement of Siemens intensifier screens for the same blackening.

Correction Values (continued)

Zonography	Pattern	—	O
	Points	+1	+1

Screen	Titan HS/2 HS violet	Special Titan U/2 U Graduated green	Sapphire Titan D/2 D Graduated blue	Ruby orange	Ruby Super yellow
dose requirement	$\frac{1}{3}$	$\frac{1}{2}$	1	2	4

Conversion Table

From Exposure points * into mAs or kVp value

kV	Points	mAs		kV	Points	mAs		kV	Points	mAs
—	−10	0,1		46	4	2,5		90	18	63
—	− 9	0,125		48	5	3,5		96	19	80
—	− 8	0,16		50	6	4		102	20	100
—	− 7	0,2		52	7	5		109	21	125
—	− 6	0,25		55	8	6,3		117	22	160
—	− 5	0,32		57	9	8		125	23	200
—	− 4	0,4		60	10	10		133	24	250
—	− 3	0,5		63	11	12,5		141	25	320
—	− 2	0,63		66	12	16		150	26	400
—	− 1	0,8		70	13	20		—	27	500
40	0	1		73	14	25		—	28	630
41	1	1,25		77	15	32		—	29	800
42	2	1,6		81	16	40		—	30	1000
44	3	2		85	17	50				

Reprinted courtesy of Siemens Medical Systems, Inc.

Answers To Case Studies

The Case of the Mysterious Mammals

Chapter 1, p. 19

Bats

The Case of the Unidentified Flying Object in the Skull

Chapter 5, p. 109

This patient was shot in the left temporal region by an arrow. The shaft was broken off prior to the time the radiograph was taken.

The Case of the Double Row of Capsules

Chapter 9, p. 171

This is a pack of fire crackers from Taiwan.

The Case of Lumpy

Chapter 15, p. 247

Theodore Bear

The Case of the Injured Animal

Chapter 16, p. 253

This is a rodent, a muskrat. The cause of death was a severed thoracic vertebral column, the result of being caught in a trap in the Ohio woods.

The Case of the White Snakes

Chapter 17, p. 264

The radiographer failed to observe that the high-voltage cables were within the primary beam field. Observe the sheath of grounding net inside the upper cable.

The Case of the Colon in the Spider's Web

Chapter 20, p. 313

This patient was unable to hold the barium within the colon and the sheet has become barium soaked. The wrinkled sheet is dense enough to make a distinct image under the patient.

The Case of the Line in the Stomach

Chapter 22, p. 341

The stomach is half filled with liquid barium. The line is an air-fluid level between the air and barium.

The Case of the Missing Lower Pelvis

Chapter 23, p. 355

This patient is quite obese and the large volume of soft tissue that has fallen down over the pelvis is demonstrated with an appropriate density. However, these technical factors produce much too much density for the pelvis. A second radiograph to demonstrate the pelvis, shown here, fails to demonstrate the abdomen. A case of "You can't have your cake and eat it too."

The Case of the Animal with the Large Calcified Tumor-like Mass

Chapter 25, p. 381

A chicken's egg about to be laid

The Case of the Last Dinner

Chapter 32, p. 474

There are no skeletal remains of the snake's last dinner on this image, but it's good practice to always examine your radiographs with careful attention to detail; the last dinner could have been demonstrated if it had been eaten more recently.

The Case of the Very Dense Object

Chapter 34, p. 501

The object is a bullet that was absorbed by the patient, a Chicago policeman, many years previous. Because it did not cause any discomfort, it was never removed. Notice the fragments lodged in the soft tissue down the right side of the thoracic vertebral column.

The Case of the Dripping Film

Chapter 36, p. 517

The horizontal lines are pi lines, so called because they are spaced apart by pi times the diameter of the first film processing roller. They are caused when developer precipitates onto the top rollers at the level of the chemistry when left in the tank overnight. When the first film is processed, the precipitate is deposited on the film emul-

sion each time the roller turns. The drip marks are most likely from developer solution that was splattered onto the film while it was being held vertically before processing.

The Case of Do You Know Your Whole Grains?

Chapter 38, p. 551

Wheat

The Case of the Ghostly Plants

Chapter 39, p. 564

A peony

The Case of the Deep Sea Rodeo

Chapter 42, p. 631

A seahorse

The Case of The Mysterious Mammal

Chapter 44, p. 673

Loggerhead turtle *(Caretta, caretta)*

Epigraph Sources and Credits

Chapter 1 "Helping with the Math Homework" reprinted with permission of Louisiana State University Press from *In All This Rain* by John Stone. Copyright 1980 by John Stone.

Chapters 2, 3, 7, 8, 9, 34, and 36 from Otto Glasser, *Dr. W. C. Röntgen*, 2nd edition, 1972. Courtesy of Charles C. Thomas, Publisher, Springfield, Illinois.

Chapters 4 and 28 from *The Magic Mountain (Der Zauberberg)* by Thomas Mann, originally published by S. Fischer Verlag, Berlin, 1924; translated from the German by H. T. Lowe-Porter, New York: Alfred A. Knopf, 1965.

Chapter 5 by permission from "One More Time," copyright, Patricia Goedicke.

Chapters 6, 13, and 26 from W. D. Coolidge, "Experiences with the Roentgen-Ray tube," *American Journal of Roentgenology, 54*: 6, 1945.

Chapter 10 by permission, copyright Celia Gilbert, "X-Ray" from *Queen of Darkness*, Viking Press, New York, NY, 1977.

Chapters 11, 25, 29, and 33 from E. C. Jerman, "An analysis of the end-result: The radiograph," *Radiology, 6*: 59–62, 1926.

Chapter 12 from A. H. Compton in the preface to the first edition of *X-Rays and Electrons*, reprinted in *X-Rays in Theory and Experiment*, by A. H. Compton and H. K. Allison, 2nd edition, New York: Van Nostrand and Company, 1935.

Chapter 14 by Lawrence K. Russell, *Life*, March 12, 1896.

Chapter 15 lyrics from the song "X-Ray Vision" from the Capitol-EMI album *Mystery Ticket*, by Moon Martin, Pete Sinfield, and Terry Taylor, copyright 1982, Paper Music, Ltd.

Chapter 16 from William Carlos Williams, *The Autobiography of William Carlos Williams*, copyright 1951, William Carlos Williams. Reprinted by permission of New Directions Publishing Corporation.

Chapter 17 lyrics from the song "I'm Looking Through You" from the Capitol-EMI Records, Inc. album, *Rubber Soul*, by John Lennon and Paul McCartney, Northern Songs, Ltd., copyright 1965, EMI Records, Inc.

Chapter 18 from Hollis E. Potter, "The Bucky diaphragm principle applied to roentgenography," *The American Journal of Roentgenology, 7*: 292–295, 1920.

Chapter 19 quoted from the Jerman Memorial Lecture given by Arthur W. Fuchs during the 1950 Annual Meeting of the American Society of X-Ray Technicians in Cincinnati, Ohio.

Chapter 20 reprinted by permission of Margaret Atwood, from *Selected Poems I*, published by Houghton Mifflin, U.S.A and *Selected Poems 1966–1984*, published by McClelland and Stewart, Canada, copyright 1968.

Chapter 21 reprinted by permission of the estate of Howard Moss from "In The X-Ray Room" from *New Selected Poems*, Antheneum Press, copyright MacMillan Publishing Company, 1985.

Chapter 22 as quoted in *From Immigrant to Inventor*, the autobiography of M. Pupin, in *Trail of the Invisible Light* by Otto Glasser as published by Charles C. Thomas, Publisher, Springfield, Illinois, 1965.

Chapter 23 as quoted from *Pall Mall Gazette*, March, 1986 by Arthur W. Fuchs in "Radiography of 1896," Image 9: 4–17, 1960.

Chapter 24 from Gerhart S. Schwarz, *Unit-Step Radiography*, 1961. Courtesy of Charles C. Thomas, Publisher, Springfield, Illinois.

Chapter 27 quoted from Merrill C. Sosman

Chapter 30 William B. Hendee and Raymond P. Rossi in *Quality Assurance for Radiographic X-Ray Units and Associated Equipment*, Rockville, MD: U.S. Department of Health, Education, and Welfare, Public Health Service, Food and Drug Administration, Bureau of Radiological Health, HEW Publication FDA 79–8094, 1979.

Chapter 31 from Arthur W. Fuchs in the Preface to *Principles of Radiographic Exposure and Processing*, 1st edition, 1949. Charles C. Thomas, Publisher, Springfield, Illinois.

Chapter 32 quoted from the Jerman Memorial Lecture given by John B. Cahoon, Jr. during the 1961 Annual Meeting of the American Society of X-Ray Technicians.

Chapter 35 from the text of the chapter.

Chapter 37 from William Shakespeare, *Hamlet*, III, iv, 18.

Chapter 38 Arthur W. Fuchs, "Edison and Roentgenology," *The American Journal of Roentgenology and Radium Therapy, 57*: 2, 145–156, 1947.

Chapter 39 from French patent 536464, June 3, 1921 by Andre-Edmund-Marie-Bocage, entitled Method of, and apparatus for, radiography on a moving plate, as quoted by J. T. Littleton in *Tomography: Physical Principles and Clinical Applications*. Section 17: Golden's Diagnostic Radiology Series. Baltimore, MD: Williams & Wilkins, 1976.

Chapter 40 attributed to Hippocrates.

Chapter 41 from Margaret Hoing (The First Lady of Radiologic Technology) in *A History of the American Society of X-Ray Technicians*, Chicago: American Society of Radiologic Technologists, 1952.

Chapter 42 by permission from Christopher C. Kuni, *Introduction to Computers and Digital Processing in Medical Imaging*, Chicago, Mosby-Year Book, Inc., 1988.

Chapter 43 quoted from Allan Cormack, upon being informed that he and Godfrey Hounsfield were to share the 1979 Nobel Prize for Medicine for the invention of computed tomography.

Chapter 44 from Edward M. Purcell, "Research in nuclear magnetism," *Nobel Lectures: Physics 1942–1962*, Amsterdam: Elsevier Publishing Company, 210–231, 1964.

INDEX